Additional Features

- **Chapter Outlines** provide an overview of each chapter.
- **"A Step Further"** topics, which expand on the material covered in the textbook.
- **Flashcards** for each chapter offer a convenient way to learn and review the many new terms introduced in the textbook.

Media Links

Using your smartphone or computer, type in the easy Web links that appear throughout the textbook to instantly access animations, videos, activities, and visual summaries on the Companion Website.

To see the video
Narcoleptic Dachshund,
go to
3e.mindsmachine.com/av10.6

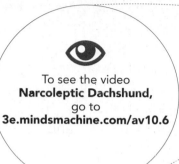
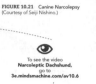
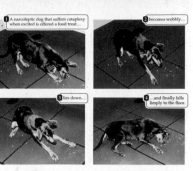

312   CHAPTER 10

FIGURE 10.21   Canine Narcolepsy
(Courtesy of Seiji Nishino.)

To see the video
Narcoleptic Dachshund,
go to
3e.mindsmachine.com/av10.6

① A narcoleptic dog that suffers cataplexy when excited is offered a food treat…
② becomes wobbly…
③ lies down…
④ …and finally falls limply to the floor.

Several strains of dogs exhibit narcolepsy (Aldrich, 1993), complete with sudden collapse and very rapid sleep onset (**FIGURE 10.21**). Just like humans who suffer from narcolepsy, these dogs often show REM signs immediately upon falling asleep. Abrupt collapse in these dogs is suppressed by the same drugs (discussed shortly) that are used to treat human cataplexy.

Finding the mutant gene responsible for narcoleptic dogs revealed a hypothalamic system that is responsible for narcolepsy in people too. This was the gene for a neuropeptide called *orexin* (also known as *hypocretin*; see Chapter 9) (L. Lin et al., 1999). Mice with the *orexin* gene knocked out also display narcolepsy (Chemelli et al., 1999). Genetically normal rats can be made narcoleptic if injected with a toxin that destroys neurons possessing orexin receptors (Gerashchenko et al., 2001). The narcoleptic dogs start losing orexin neurons at about the age when symptoms of narcolepsy appear (Siegel, Nienhuis et al., 1999).

Similarly, humans with narcolepsy have lost about 90% of their orexin neurons (**FIGURE 10.22**) (Thannickal et al., 2000). This degeneration of orexin neurons seems to cause inappropriate activation of the cataplexy pathway that normally happens only during REM sleep. So, orexin normally keeps sleep at bay and prevents the transition from wakefulness directly into REM sleep.

The neurons that produce orexin are found almost exclusively in the hypothalamus. Where do these neurons send their axons to release the orexin? Not so coincidentally, the axons go to each of the three brain centers that we mentioned before: basal forebrain, reticular formation, and locus coeruleus (Sutcliffe and de Lecea, 2002). The orexin neurons also project axons to the hypothalamic tuberomammillary nucleus—the same structure that is inhibited by the basal forebrain to induce SWS. So, it looks as if the hypothalamus contains an orexin-based "switching station" (see Figure 10.19) that switches the brain between states, from wakefulness to non-REM sleep to REM sleep (Saper et al., 2010). This system normally triggers paralysis only during REM, so loss of the system in narcolepsy leads to paralysis while awake (cataplexy).

The traditional treatment for narcolepsy was the use of amphetamines in the daytime. The drug GHB (gamma-hydroxybutyrate, trade name Xyrem) helps some narcoleptics (although there are concerns about potential abuse of this drug [Tuller, 2002]). A newer drug, modafinil (Provigil), is sometimes effective for preventing narcoleptic attacks and has been proposed as an "alertness drug" for people with attention deficit hyperactivity disorder. There is also debate about whether modafinil should be

orexin   Also called *hypocretin*. A neuropeptide produced in the hypothalamus that is involved in switching between sleep states, in narcolepsy, and in the control of appetite.

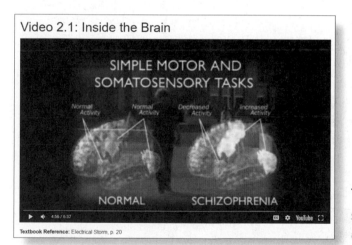

Video 2.1: Inside the Brain

SIMPLE MOTOR AND SOMATOSENSORY TASKS

Normal Activity   Normal Activity   Decreased Activity   Increased Activity

NORMAL   SCHIZOPHRENIA

4:56 / 6:37   YouTube

Textbook Reference: Electrical Storm, p. 20

Videos present real-world examples of some of the key concepts and conditions discussed in the textbook.

BIOLOGICAL PSYCHOLOGY NewsLink
3e.mindsmachine.com/news

This invaluable online resource helps you make connections between the science of biological psychology and your daily life, and keeps you apprised of the latest developments in the field. The site is updated 3–4 times a week and contains thousands of news stories organized both by keyword and by textbook chapter.

BioPsychology NewsLink

Search Article Summaries

Most Recent Links

Links By Chapter:

1. An Introduction to Brain and Behavior
2. Cells and Structures: The Anatomy of the Nervous System
3. Neurophysiology: The Generation, Transmission, and Integration of Neural Signals
4. The Chemistry of Behavior: Neurotransmitters and Neuropharmacology
5. The Sensorimotor System
6. Hearing, Balance, Taste, and Smell
7. Vision: From Eye to Brain
8. Hormones and Sex
9. Homeostasis: Active Regulation of the Internal Environment
10. Biological Rhythms and Sleep
11. Emotions, Aggression, and Stress
12. Psychopathology: The

Chapter 5. The Sensorimotor System

Follow us on Facebook and Twitter, or subscribe to our mailing list, to receive news updates. Learn more.

Links 1 - 20 of 2883

Why this rare childhood brain cancer is so difficult to fight

Marcy Cuttler - CBC News Janaya Chekowski-McKenzie was born with the odds against her. On the day she arrived in 2009, she was non-responsive, and she spent a month in hospital with a lung infection. At three months, she had a seizure. Janaya needed hormone replacements to grow and doctors determined she had underdeveloped optic nerves. In spite of these early difficulties, the Beaumont, Alta., youngster has grown up to be a sassy, funny, bright girl with a lion's mane of curly-brown hair. When Janaya started complaining of worsening headaches last January, her mother, Amanda Chekowski, thought it was yet another medical hurdle to overcome. Instead, doctors told her Janaya had a rare, incurable form of brain cancer called diffuse intrinsic pontine glioma, or DIPG. Hearing the news, Chekowski and her family were stunned. They had to figure out how to explain this to an eight-year-old in terms she would understand. Initially, they made a bit of a joke of it. Janaya was told that "we found a booger in your brain that's not supposed to be there and we're going to try to shrink it," said Chekowski. The truth is very different. DIPG is a cancer that targets kids, and thus far, none have survived. But doctors around the world are trying to change that. ©2018 CBC/Radio-Canada.

Keyword: Movement Disorders
Link ID: 25416 - Posted: 09.05.2018

Preventing Muscle Loss Among the Elderly

By Jane E. Brody "Use it or lose it." I'm sure you're familiar with this advice. And I hope you've been following it, as I certainly thought I was. I usually do two physical activities a day, alternating among walking, cycling and swimming. I do floor exercises for my back daily, walk up and down many stairs and tackle myriad physical tasks in and around my home. My young friends at the Y say I'm in great shape, and I suppose I am compared to most 77-year-old women in America today. But I've noticed in recent years that I'm not as strong as I used to be. Loads I once carried rather easily are now difficult, and some are impossible. Thanks to an admonition from a savvy physical therapist, Marilyn Moffat, a professor at New York University, I now know why. I, like many people past 50, have a condition called sarcopenia — a decline in skeletal muscle with age. It begins as early as age 40 and, without intervention, gets increasingly worse, with as much as half of muscle mass lost by age 70. (If you're wondering, it's replaced by fat and fibrous tissue, making muscles resemble a well-marbled steak.) "Sarcopenia can be considered for muscle what osteoporosis is to bone," Dr. John E. Morley, geriatrician at Saint Louis University School of Medicine, wrote in the journal Family Practice. He pointed out that up to 13 percent of people in their 60s and as many as half of those in their 80s have sarcopenia. As Dr. Jeremy D. Walston, geriatrician at Johns Hopkins University School of Medicine, put it, "Sarcopenia is one of the most important causes of functional decline and loss of independence in older adults." Yet few practicing physicians alert their older patients to this condition and tell them how to slow or reverse what is otherwise an inevitable decline that can seriously impair their physical and emotional well-being and ability to carry out the tasks of daily life. Sarcopenia is also associated with a number of chronic diseases, increasingly worse insulin resistance, fatigue, falls and, alas, death. © 2018 The New York Times Company

Keyword: Muscles; Development of the Brain
Link ID: 25415 - Posted: 09.05.2018

COMPANION WEBSITE Resources (3e.mindsmachine.com)

The Mind's Machine Companion Website includes animations, videos, and activities for each chapter (listed below) as well as an interactive version of each chapter's visual summary. All three media categories are referenced throughout the book with the "eye" icon and direct Web addresses, on the textbook pages listed below. They are also referenced in each chapter's summary.

Animations & Videos

1.1 Nature and Nurture, p. 3

1.2 Brain Explorer, p. 4

2.1 Inside the Brain, p. 23

2.2 Brain Explorer, p. 24

2.3 Brain Development, p. 41

2.4 Visualizing the Living Human Brain, p. 48

3.1 Electrical Stimulation of the Brain, p. 55

3.2 Brain Explorer, p. 56

3.3 The Resting Membrane Potential, p. 59

3.4 The Action Potential, p. 61

3.5 Action Potential Propagation, p. 63

3.6 Spatial Summation, p. 68

3.7 Synaptic Transmission, p. 70

4.1 Synaptic Transmission, p. 83

4.2 Brain Explorer, p. 84

4.3 Neurotransmitter Pathways, p. 89

4.4 Agonists and Antagonists, p. 93

5.1 Sensory Systems, p. 119

5.2 Brain Explorer, p. 120

5.3 Somatosensory Receptive Fields, p. 124

5.4 The Stretch Reflex Circuit, p. 142

6.1 Inside the Ear, p. 153

6.2 Brain Explorer, p. 154

6.3 Sound Transduction, p. 158

6.4 Mapping Auditory Frequencies, p. 161

6.5 The Vestibular System, p. 170

6.6 The Human Olfactory System, p. 176

7.1 Object Recognition, p. 183

7.2 Brain Explorer, p. 184

7.3 Visual Pathways in the Human Brain, p. 192

7.4 Receptive Fields in the Retina, p. 196

7.5 Spatial Frequencies, p. 200

8.1 Gender, p. 217

8.2 Brain Explorer, p. 218

8.3 Chemical Communication Systems, p. 220

8.4 Mechanisms of Hormone Action, p. 222

8.5 The Hypothalamus and Endocrine Function, p. 228

8.6 Organizational Effects of Testosterone, p. 249

9.1 Regaining the Weight, p. 263

9.2 Brain Explorer, p. 264

9.3 Negative Feedback, p. 265

9.4 Thermoregulation in Humans, p. 266

9.5 Anorexia, p. 283

10.1 Narcolepsy, p. 289

10.2 Brain Explorer, p. 290

10.3 Biological Rhythms, p. 291

10.4 A Molecular Clock, p. 295

10.5 Animal Sleep Activity, p. 310

10.6 Narcoleptic Dachshund, p. 312

10.7 REM Behavior Disorder, p. 314

11.1 The Case of S.M., p. 319

11.2 Brain Explorer, p. 320

11.3 Stress, p. 342

12.1 Lobotomy, p. 347

12.2 Brain Explorer, p. 348

12.3 Tardive Dyskinesia, p. 357

13.1 Memory, p. 379

13.2 Brain Explorer, p. 380

13.3 AMPA and NMDA Receptors, p. 399

13.4 Morris Water Maze, p. 401

13.5 Stages of Neuronal Development, p. 404

13.6 Migration of a Neuron along a Radial Glial Cell, p. 406

14.1 Attention and Perception, p. 419

14.2 Brain Explorer, p. 420

14.3 Inattentional Blindness, p. 421

14.4 From Input to Output, p. 425

14.5 Reconstructing Brain Activity, p. 440

15.1 Global Aphasia, p. 451

15.2 Brain Explorer, p. 452

15.3 Split-Brain Research, p. 453

15.4 Face Blindness, p. 458

A.1 Gel Electrophoresis, p. A-2

Activities

2.1 Major Components and Classification of Neurons, p. 27

2.2 The Cranial Nerves, p. 34

2.3 Gross Anatomy of the Spinal Cord, p. 35

2.4 Concept Matching: Sympathetic vs. Parasympathetic, p. 36

2.5 Gross Anatomy of the Human Brain: Lateral View, p. 39

2.6 The Developing Brain, p. 41

2.7 The Basal Ganglia, p. 43

2.8 The Limbic System, p. 43

2.9 Gross Anatomy of the Human Brain: Midsaggital View, p. 44

2.10 Gross Anatomy of the Human Brain: Basal View, p. 44

2.11 The Cerebral Ventricles, p. 46

3.1 Distribution of Ions, p. 57

4.1 Families of Transmitters, p. 91

5.1 Receptors in Skin, p. 122

5.2 Ascending Pain Pathways in the CNS, p. 133

5.3 Subcortical Systems Involved in Movement, p. 148

6.1 Organ of Corti, p. 159

6.2 Taste Buds and Taste Receptor Cells, p. 173

7.1 The Structure of the Eye, p. 184

8.1 Major Endocrine Glands, p. 218

9.1 An Appetite Controller in the Hypothalamus, p. 279

10.1 Stages of Sleep, p. 298

10.2 Sleep Mechanisms, p. 310

11.1 Conditioned Fear Response, p. 331

11.2 The Stress Response and Consequences of Prolonged Stress, p. 342

12.1 Concept Matching: Psychopathology, p. 375

13.1 The "Tower of Hanoi" Problem, p. 386

13.2 Learning and Memory, p. 388

13.3 Development of the Nervous System, p. 403

14.1 Subcortical Sites Implicated in Visual Attention, p. 433

14.2 Cortical Regions Implicated in the Top-Level Control of Attention, p. 434

15.1 Speech and Language Areas, p. 461

15.2 The Connectionist Model of Aphasia, p. 464

15.3 Song Control Nuclei of the Songbird Brain, p. 475

The Mind's Machine

Foundations of Brain and Behavior

THIRD EDITION

The Mind's Machine

FOUNDATIONS OF BRAIN AND BEHAVIOR

THIRD EDITION

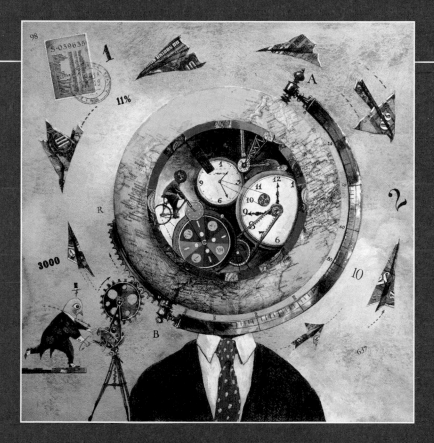

Neil V. Watson • S. Marc Breedlove
Simon Fraser University   *Michigan State University*

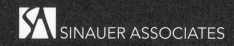

SINAUER ASSOCIATES

NEW YORK   OXFORD
OXFORD UNIVERSITY PRESS

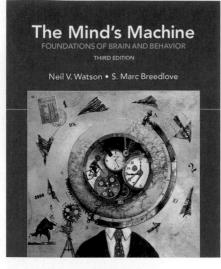

About the Cover and Chapter Opener Images

Bruno Mallart is one of the most talented European artists, his work having appeared in some of the world's premier publications: The New York Times, The Wall Street Journal, and the New Scientist, to name a few. A freelance illustrator since 1986, Mallart first worked for several children's book publishers and advertising agencies, using a classical realistic watercolor and ink style. Some years later he began working in a more imaginative way, inventing a mix of drawing, painting, and collage. His work speaks of a surrealistic and absurd world and engages the viewer's imagination and sense of fun. Despite the recurring use of the brain in his art, Mallart's background is not scientific—though his parents were both neurobiologists. He uses the brain as a symbol for abstract concepts such as intelligence, thinking, feeling, ideas, and knowledge. Attracted to all that is mechanical, Mallart's art frequently includes machine parts such as gears and wheels that imply movement and rhythm. These features together, in their abstract representation, beautifully illustrate the topics discussed in *The Mind's Machine*, Third Edition. To see more of Bruno Mallart's art, please go to his website: www.brunomallart.com.

Eye icon © AlexAlmighty/Shutterstock.com.

The Mind's Machine: Foundations of Brain and Behavior, Third Edition

Oxford University Press is a department of the University of Oxford. It furthers the University's objective of excellence in research, scholarship, and education by publishing worldwide. Oxford is a registered trade mark of Oxford University Press in the UK and certain other countries.

Published in the United States of America by Oxford University Press
198 Madison Avenue, New York, NY 10016, United States of America

Address editorial correspondence to:
Sinauer Associates
23 Plumtree Road
Sunderland, MA 01375 USA

Address orders, sales, license, permissions, and translation inquiries to:
Oxford University Press USA
2001 Evans Road
Cary, NC 27513 USA
Orders: 1-800-445-9714

Library of Congress Cataloging-in-Publication Data
    Names: Watson, Neil V. (Neil Verne), 1962- author. | Breedlove, S. Marc, author.
    Title: The mind's machine : foundations of brain and behavior / Neil V. Watson (Simon Fraser University), S. Marc Breedlove (Michigan State University).
    Description: Third edition. | Sunderland, Massachusetts : Sinauer Associates, Inc., [2019] | Includes bibliographical references and index.
    Identifiers: LCCN 2018032509 | ISBN 9781605357300 (paperback)
    Subjects: LCSH: Brain--Textbooks. | Brain--Physiology--Textbooks. | Human behavior--Physiological aspects--Textbooks. | Psychobiology--Textbooks. | Neurophysiology--Textbooks. | Neuropsychology--Textbooks. | LCGFT: Textbooks.
    Classification: LCC QP376 .W26 2019 | DDC 612.8/2--dc23
    LC record available at https://lccn.loc.gov/2018032509

9 8 7 6 5 4 3 2
Printed in the United States of America

Brief Contents

1 ■ An Introduction to Brain and Behavior   2

2 ■ Cells and Structures   The Anatomy of the Nervous System   22

3 ■ Neurophysiology   The Generation, Transmission, and Integration of Neural Signals   54

4 ■ The Chemistry of Behavior   Neurotransmitters and Neuropharmacology   82

5 ■ The Sensorimotor System   118

6 ■ Hearing, Balance, Taste, and Smell   152

7 ■ Vision   From Eye to Brain   182

8 ■ Hormones and Sex   216

9 ■ Homeostasis   Active Regulation of the Internal Environment   262

10 ■ Biological Rhythms and Sleep   288

11 ■ Emotions, Aggression, and Stress   318

12 ■ Psychopathology   The Biology of Behavioral Disorders   346

13 ■ Memory, Learning, and Development   378

14 ■ Attention and Higher Cognition   418

15 ■ Language and Lateralization   450

Table of Contents

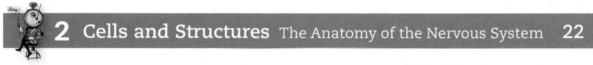

1 An Introduction to Brain and Behavior   2

PART I   The Birth of a Science of Brain and Behavior   4

Behavioral Neuroscience Spans Past, Present, and Future   4

An understanding of the brain's role in behavior has developed over centuries   4

The future of behavioral neuroscience is in interdisciplinary discovery and knowledge translation   9

PART II   Research Design   13

Careful Design of Studies Is Essential for Progress in Behavioral Neuroscience   13

Three types of study designs probe brain-behavior relationships   13

Research objectives reflect specific theoretical orientations   15

Animal research is an essential part of life sciences research, including behavioral neuroscience   15

BOX 1.1 We Are All Alike, and We Are All Different   16

Behavioral neuroscientists use several levels of analysis   17

Looking Forward: A Glimpse inside the Mind's Machine   18

■ **Visual Summary   21**

2 Cells and Structures   The Anatomy of the Nervous System   22

PART I   The Cellular Components of the Nervous System   24

The Nervous System Contains Several Types of Cells   24

The neuron has four principal divisions   24

Information is transmitted through synapses   28

BOX 2.1 Visualizing the Cellular Structure of the Brain   29

The axon integrates and then transmits information   30

Glial cells protect and assist neurons   31

PART II   The Large Scale Structure of the Nervous System   32

The Nervous System Extends throughout the Body   33

The peripheral nervous system has two divisions   33

The central nervous system consists of the brain and spinal cord   36

BOX 2.2 Three Customary Orientations for Viewing the Brain and Body   38

PART III   The Functional Organization of the Nervous System   42

The Brain Is Described in Terms of Both Structure and Function   42

The cerebral cortex performs complex cognitive processing   42

Important nuclei are hidden beneath the cerebral cortex   43

The midbrain has sensory and motor components   43

The brainstem controls vital body functions   44

Networks of connections between brain regions determine behavior   45

Specialized Support Systems Protect and Nourish the Brain   45

The brain floats within layers of membranes   45

The brain relies on two fluids for survival   45

SIGNS & SYMPTOMS Stroke   47

Brain-Imaging Techniques Reveal the Structure and Function of the Human Brain   48

CT uses X-rays to reveal brain structure   48

MRI maps density to deduce brain structure with high detail   48

Functional MRI uses local changes in metabolism to identify active brain regions   48

PET tracks radioactive substances to produce images of brain activity   49

RESEARCHERS AT WORK   Subtractive analysis isolates specific brain activity   50

Magnetism can be used to study the brain   51

■ Visual Summary   52

3 Neurophysiology The Generation, Transmission, and Integration of Neural Signals   54

PART I   Electric Neurons   56

Electrical Signals Are the Vocabulary of the Nervous System   56

A threshold amount of depolarization triggers an action potential   59

Ionic mechanisms underlie the action potential   61

Action potentials are actively propagated along the axon   63

BOX 3.1   How Is an Axon Like a Toilet?   65

SIGNS & SYMPTOMS   Multiple Sclerosis   66

Synapses cause local changes in the postsynaptic membrane potential   66

Spatial summation and temporal summation integrate synaptic inputs   68

PART II   Synaptic Transmission   70

Synaptic Transmission Requires a Sequence of Events   70

Action potentials cause the release of transmitter molecules into the synaptic cleft   71

Receptor molecules recognize transmitters   72

The action of synaptic transmitters is stopped rapidly   73

Neural circuits underlie reflexes   73

PART III   Gross Potentials   75

EEGs Measure Gross Electrical Activity of the Human Brain   75

Electrical storms in the brain can cause seizures   76

RESEARCHERS AT WORK   Surgical probing of the brain revealed a map of the body   78

■ Visual Summary   80

4 The Chemistry of Behavior Neurotransmitters and Neuropharmacology   82

PART I   Chemical Neurotransmission   84

Synaptic Transmission Involves a Complex Electrochemical Process   85

Many Neurotransmitters Have Been Identified   86

RESEARCHERS AT WORK   The first transmitter to be discovered was acetylcholine   87

Neurotransmitter Systems Form a Complex Array in the Brain   88

Four amine neurotransmitters modulate brain activity   89

Many peptides function as neurotransmitters   91

Some neurotransmitters are gases   92

PART II   Drug Actions in the Brain   92

Drugs Fit Like Keys into Molecular Locks   93

The effects of a drug depend on its dose   94

Drugs are administered and eliminated in many different ways   94

Repeated treatments may reduce the effectiveness of drugs   96

Drugs Affect Each Stage of Neural Conduction and Synaptic Transmission   96

Some drugs alter presynaptic processes   97

Some drugs alter postsynaptic processes   98

PART III   Psychopharmacology: Effects of Drugs on Behavior   100

Some Neuroactive Drugs Ease the Symptoms of Psychiatric Illness   100

Antipsychotics relieve symptoms of schizophrenia   100

Antidepressants reduce chronic mood problems   101

Anxiolytics combat anxiety   101

Opiates have powerful painkilling effects   101

Some Neuroactive Drugs Are Used to Alter Conscious Experience   103

Cannabinoids have many effects   103

Stimulants increase neural activity   104

Alcohol acts as both a stimulant and a depressant   106

Hallucinogens alter sensory perceptions   107

Substance Abuse and Addiction Are Global Social Problems   109

Competing models of substance abuse have been proposed   111

SIGNS & SYMPTOMS   **Medical Interventions for Substance Abuse   113**

■ **Visual Summary   115**

5 The Sensorimotor System   118

PART I   Sensory Processing and the Somatosensory System   120

Sensory Systems Detect Various Forms of Energy   120

Receptor Cells Convert Sensory Signals into Electrical Activity   122

Sensory Information Processing Is Selective and Analytical   123

Sensory events are encoded as streams of action potentials   124

Sensory neurons respond to stimuli falling in their receptive fields   125

Receptors may show adaptation to unchanging stimuli   125

Sometimes we need receptors to be quiet   126

Successive Levels of the CNS Process Sensory Information   126

Sensory cortex is highly organized   128

Sensory brain regions influence one another and change over time   129

PART II   Pain: The Body's Emergency Signaling System   130

Human Pain Varies in Several Dimensions   130

A Discrete Pain Pathway Projects from Body to Brain   130

Peripheral receptors get the initial message   130

SIGNS & SYMPTOMS   **A Professional Eater Meets His Match   132**

Special neural pathways carry pain information to the brain   132

Pain Control Can Be Difficult   134

Analgesic drugs are highly effective   134

Electrical stimulation can sometimes relieve pain   135

Placebos effectively control pain in some people, but not all   135

Activation of endogenous opioids relieves pain   135

PART III   Movement and the Motor System   136

Behavior Requires Movements That Are Precisely Programmed and Monitored   137

A Complex Neural System Controls Muscles to Create Behavior   138

Muscles and the skeleton work together to move the body   138

Sensory feedback from muscles, tendons, and joints regulates movement   140

The spinal cord mediates "automatic" responses and receives inputs from the brain   142

Motor cortex plans and executes movements—and more   144

RESEARCHERS AT WORK   **Mirror neurons in premotor cortex track movements in others   146**

Extrapyramidal systems regulate and fine-tune motor commands   148

Damage to extrapyramidal systems impairs movement   148

■ **Visual Summary   150**

6 Hearing, Balance, Taste, and Smell 152

PART I   Hearing and Balance   154

Pressure Waves in the Air Are Perceived as Sound   154

  BOX 6.1 The Basics of Sound   155

  The external ear captures, focuses, and filters sound   156

  The middle ear concentrates sound energies   156

  The cochlea converts vibrational energy into neural activity   156

  RESEARCHERS AT WORK Georg von Békésy and the cochlear wave   158

  The hair cells transduce movements of the basilar membrane into electrical signals   159

Auditory Signals Run from Cochlea to Cortex   160

Our Sense of Pitch Relies on Two Signals from the Cochlea   162

Brainstem Systems Compare the Ears to Localize Sounds   163

The Auditory Cortex Processes Complex Sound   164

Hearing Loss Is a Widespread Problem   165

SIGNS & SYMPTOMS Restoring Auditory Stimulation in Deafness   168

The Inner Ear Provides Our Sense of Balance   169

Some Forms of Vestibular Excitation Produce Motion Sickness   170

PART II   The Chemical Senses: Taste and Smell   171

Chemicals in Our Food Are Perceived as Five Basic Tastes   171

  Tastes excite specialized receptor cells on the tongue   172

  The five basic tastes are signaled by specific sensors on taste cells   172

  Taste information is transmitted to several parts of the brain   174

Chemicals in the Air Elicit Odor Sensations   175

  The sense of smell starts with receptor neurons in the nose   175

  Olfactory information projects from the olfactory bulbs to several brain regions   177

  Many vertebrates possess a vomeronasal system   178

■ **Visual Summary   180**

7 Vision From Eye to Brain 182

PART I   Vision Pathways   184

The Visual System Extends from the Eye to the Brain   184

  Visual processing begins in the retina   185

  Photoreceptors respond to light by releasing less neurotransmitter   186

  Different mechanisms enable the eyes to work over a wide range of light intensities   188

  Acuity is best in foveal vision   189

  Neural signals travel from the retina to several brain regions   191

  The retina projects to the brain in a topographic fashion   193

PART II   Visual Analysis   194

Neurons at Different Levels of the Visual System Have Very Different Receptive Fields   194

  Neurons in the retina and the LGN have concentric receptive fields   195

RESEARCHERS AT WORK Neurons in the visual cortex have varied receptive fields   198

  Spatial-frequency analysis is unintuitive but efficient   199

  Neurons in the visual cortex beyond area V1 have complex receptive fields and help identify forms   201

  Visual perception of motion is analyzed by a special system that includes cortical area V5   202

PART III   Color Vision   203

Color Vision Depends on Special Channels from the Retinal Cones through Cortical Area V4   203

  Color perception requires receptor cells that differ in their sensitivities to different wavelengths   204

  BOX 7.1 Most Mammalian Species Have Some Color Vision   207

  Some retinal ganglion cells and LGN cells show spectral opponency   208

Some visual cortical cells and regions appear to be specialized for color perception   209

SIGNS & SYMPTOMS   Correcting "Color Blindness"?   210

PART IV   What versus Where   211

The Many Cortical Visual Areas Are Organized into Two Major Streams   211

Visual Neuroscience Can Be Applied to Alleviate Some Visual Deficiencies   212

Impairment of vision often can be prevented or reduced   213

Increased exercise can restore function to a previously deprived or neglected eye   213

■ **Visual Summary**   214

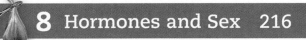

8 Hormones and Sex   216

PART I   The Endocrine System   218

Hormones Act in a Great Variety of Ways throughout the Body   218

RESEARCHERS AT WORK   Our Current understanding of hormones developed in stages   219

Hormones are one of several types of chemical communication   220

Hormones can be classified by chemical structure   220

Hormones Act on a Wide Variety of Cellular Mechanisms   221

Hormones initiate actions by binding to receptor molecules   221

Hormones can have different effects on different target organs   222

BOX 8.1 Techniques of Behavioral Endocrinology   223

Each Endocrine Gland Secretes Specific Hormones   225

The posterior pituitary releases two hormones directly into the bloodstream   226

Posterior pituitary hormones can affect social behavior   226

Feedback control mechanisms regulate the secretion of hormones   227

Hypothalamic releasing hormones govern the anterior pituitary   228

Two anterior pituitary tropic hormones act on the gonads   230

The gonads produce steroid hormones, regulating reproduction   230

Hormonal and neural systems interact to produce integrated responses   232

PART II   Reproductive Behavior   234

Reproductive Behavior Can Be Divided into Four Stages   234

Copulation brings gametes together   236

Gonadal steroids activate sexual behavior   236

RESEARCHERS AT WORK   Individual differences in mating behavior   237

The Neural Circuitry of the Brain Regulates Reproductive Behavior   238

Estrogen and progesterone act on a lordosis circuit that spans from brain to muscle   238

Androgens act on a neural system for male reproductive behavior   238

Maternal behaviors are governed by several sex-related hormones   240

The Hallmark of Human Sexual Behavior Is Diversity   241

Hormones play only a permissive role in human sexual behavior   243

PART III   Sexual Differentiation and Orientation   244

Genetic and Hormonal Mechanisms Guide the Development of Masculine and Feminine Structures   244

Sex chromosomes direct sexual differentiation of the gonads   244

Gonadal hormones direct sexual differentiation of the body   244

Changes in sexual differentiation processes result in predictable changes in development   245

Dysfunctional androgen receptors can block masculinization of the body   246

Some people seem to change sex at puberty   247

SIGNS & SYMPTOMS Defining an
Athlete's Sex   248

How should we define sex—by genes, gonads,
genitals?   248

RESEARCHERS AT WORK Gonadal hormones
direct sexual differentiation of behavior and
the brain   249

Early testicular secretions result in masculine behavior
in adulthood   250

Several regions of the nervous system display
prominent sexual dimorphism   251

Social influences also affect sexual differentiation
of the nervous system   254

Do Fetal Hormones Masculinize Human Behaviors
in Adulthood?   255

What determines a person's sexual orientation?   256

■ Visual Summary   259

9 Homeostasis Active Regulation of the Internal Environment   262

PART I   Principles of Homeostasis   264

Homeostatic Systems Share Several Key
Features   264

Negative feedback allows precise control   264

Redundancy ensures critical needs are met   265

Animals use behavioral compensation to adjust to
environmental changes   266

PART II   Fluid Regulation   267

Water Moves between Two Major Body
Compartments   267

Two Internal Cues Trigger Thirst   269

Osmotic thirst occurs when the extracellular fluid
becomes too salty   269

Hypovolemic thirst is triggered by a loss of fluid
volume   270

We don't stop drinking just because the throat and
mouth are wet   271

PART III   Food and Energy Regulation   272

Nutrient Regulation Helps Prepare for Future
Needs   272

Insulin is essential for obtaining, storing, and using
food energy   275

The Hypothalamus Coordinates Multiple Systems
That Control Hunger   276

RESEARCHERS AT WORK Lesion studies
showed that the hypothalamus is crucial for
appetite   276

Hormones from the body drive a hypothalamic
appetite controller   277

Other systems also play a role in hunger
and satiety   280

Obesity Is Difficult to Treat   281

Eating Disorders Can Be Life-Threatening   283

SIGNS & SYMPTOMS Friends with
Benefits   284

■ Visual Summary   286

10 Biological Rhythms and Sleep   288

PART I   Biological Rhythms   290

Many Animals Show Daily Rhythms in
Activity   290

Circadian rhythms are generated by an endogenous
clock   290

The Hypothalamus Houses a Circadian Clock   292

RESEARCHERS AT WORK Transplants prove that
the SCN produces a circadian rhythm   293

In mammals, light information from the eyes reaches
the SCN directly   293

Circadian rhythms have been genetically dissected
in flies and mice   295

PART II   Sleep   297

Human Sleep Exhibits Different Stages   297

We do our most vivid dreaming during REM sleep   300

Different species provide clues about the evolution
of sleep   301

Our Sleep Patterns Change across the
Life Span   301

Mammals sleep more during infancy than in adulthood   301

Most people sleep appreciably less as they age   302

Manipulating Sleep Reveals an Underlying Structure   303

Sleep deprivation impairs cognitive functioning but does not cause insanity   303

SIGNS & SYMPTOMS   Total Sleep Deprivation Can Be Fatal   304

Sleep recovery may take time   304

What Are the Biological Functions of Sleep?   305

Sleep conserves energy   306

Sleep enforces niche adaptation   306

Sleep restores the body and brain   306

Sleep may aid memory consolidation   307

Some humans sleep remarkably little, yet function normally   307

At Least Four Interacting Neural Systems Underlie Sleep   308

RESEARCHERS AT WORK   The forebrain generates slow wave sleep   308

The reticular formation wakes up the forebrain   309

The pons triggers REM sleep   309

PART III   Sleep Disorders   311

Sleep Disorders Can Be Serious, Even Life-Threatening   311

A hypothalamic sleep center was revealed by the study of narcolepsy   311

Some minor dysfunctions are associated with sleep   313

Some people appear to be acting out their nightmares   313

Insomniacs have trouble falling asleep or staying asleep   314

Although many drugs affect sleep, there is no perfect sleeping pill   315

Everyone should practice good sleep hygiene   315

■ **Visual Summary   317**

11   Emotions, Aggression, and Stress   318

PART I   Emotional Processing   320

Broad Theories of Emotion Emphasize Bodily Responses   320

Do emotions cause bodily changes, or vice versa?   321

BOX 11.1   Lie Detector?   322

RESEARCHERS AT WORK   Stanley Schachter proposed a cognitive interpretation of stimuli and visceral states   323

Is There a Core Set of Emotions?   324

Facial expressions have complex functions in communication   326

Facial expressions are mediated by muscles, cranial nerves, and CNS pathways   327

Do Distinct Brain Circuits Mediate Different Emotions?   328

Electrical stimulation of the brain can produce emotional effects   328

Brain lesions also affect emotions   329

The amygdala is crucial for emotional learning   330

Different emotions activate different regions of the human brain   332

PART II   Aggression   334

Neural Circuitry, Hormones, and Synaptic Transmitters Mediate Violence and Aggression   334

Androgens seem to increase aggression   334

Brain circuits mediate aggression   336

The biopsychology of human violence is a topic of controversy   336

PART III   Stress and Health   337

Stress Activates Many Bodily Responses   337

The stress response progresses in stages   338

There are individual differences in the stress response   339

Stress and emotions affect our health   341

Why does chronic stress suppress the immune system?   341

SIGNS & SYMPTOMS   Long-Term Consequences of Childhood Bullying   343

11 ■ **Visual Summary   344**

12 Psychopathology The Biology of Behavioral Disorders 346

PART I   Schizophrenia 348

The Toll of Psychiatric Disorders Is Huge 348

Schizophrenia Is a Major Neurobiological Challenge in Psychiatry 349

Schizophrenia is characterized by an unusual array of symptoms 349

Schizophrenia has a heritable component 349

RESEARCHERS AT WORK Stress increases the risk of schizophrenia 352

An integrative model of schizophrenia emphasizes the interaction of factors 353

The brains of some people with schizophrenia show structural and functional changes 353

Antipsychotic medications revolutionized the treatment of schizophrenia 356

BOX 12.1 Long-Term Effects of Antipsychotic Drugs 357

PART II   Mood Disorders 361

Depression Is the Most Prevalent Disorder of Mood 361

Inheritance is an important determinant of depression 361

The brain changes with depression 362

A wide variety of treatments are available for depression 362

SIGNS & SYMPTOMS Mixed Feelings about SSRIs 364

Why do more females than males suffer from depression? 365

Sleep characteristics change in affective disorders 366

Scientists are still searching for animal models of depression 366

In Bipolar Disorder, Mood Cycles between Extremes 367

RESEARCHERS AT WORK The entirely accidental discovery of lithium therapy 368

PART III   Anxiety Disorders 369

There Are Several Types of Anxiety Disorders 369

Drug treatments provide clues to the mechanisms of anxiety 369

In Post-Traumatic Stress Disorder, Horrible Memories Won't Go Away 370

In Obsessive-Compulsive Disorder, Thoughts and Acts Keep Repeating 372

BOX 12.2 Tics, Twitches, and Snorts: The Unusual Character of Tourette's Syndrome 374

12 ■ Visual Summary 375

13 Memory, Learning, and Development 378

PART I   Types of Learning and Memory 380

There Are Several Kinds of Learning and Memory 380

For Patient H.M., the present vanished into oblivion 380

RESEARCHERS AT WORK Which brain structures are important for declarative memory? 383

Damage to the medial diencephalon can also cause amnesia 384

Brain damage can destroy autobiographical memories while sparing general memories 385

Different Forms of Nondeclarative Memory Involve Different Brain Regions 386

Different types of nondeclarative memory serve varying functions 386

Animal research confirms the various brain regions involved in different attributes of memory 387

Brain regions involved in learning and memory: A summary 388

Successive Processes Capture, Store, and Retrieve Information in the Brain 388

BOX 13.1 Emotions and Memory 390

Long-term memory has vast capacity but is subject to distortion 390

PART II   Neural Mechanisms of Memory   392

Memory Storage Requires Physical Changes in the Brain   392

Plastic changes at synapses can be physiological or structural   392

Varied experiences and learning cause the brain to change and grow   392

Invertebrate nervous systems show synaptic plasticity   394

Classical conditioning relies on circuits in the mammalian cerebellum   396

Synaptic Plasticity Can Be Measured in Simple Hippocampal Circuits   398

NMDA receptors and AMPA receptors collaborate in LTP   399

Is LTP a mechanism of memory formation?   401

PART III   Development of the Brain   402

Growth and Development of the Brain Are Orderly Processes   402

Development of the Nervous System Can Be Divided into Six Distinct Stages   404

Cell proliferation produces cells that become neurons or glia   404

In the adult brain, newly born neurons aid learning   406

The death of many neurons is a normal part of development   407

An explosion of synapse formation is followed by synapse rearrangement   407

Genes Interact with Experience to Guide Brain Development   410

Genotype is fixed at birth, but phenotype changes throughout life   411

Experience regulates gene expression in the developing and mature brain   411

The Brain Continues to Change as We Grow Older   413

Memory impairment correlates with hippocampal shrinkage during aging   413

Alzheimer's disease is associated with a decline in cerebral metabolism   414

SIGNS & SYMPTOMS Imaging Alzheimer's Plaques   415

13 ■ Visual Summary   416

14 Attention and Higher Cognition   418

PART I   Effects of Attention on Behavior   420

Attention Focuses Cognitive Processing on Specific Objects   420

There are limits on attention   420

Attention Is Deployed in Several Different Ways   422

RESEARCHERS AT WORK We can choose which stimuli we will attend to   423

Some stimuli grab our attention   424

BOX 14.1 Reaction-Time Responses, from Input to Output   425

We use visual search to make sense of a cluttered world   426

PART II   Neural Mechanisms of Attention   428

Attention Alters the Functioning of the Brain   428

Distinctive patterns of brain electrical activity mark shifts of attention   429

Attention affects the activity of neurons   431

A Network of Brain Sites Creates and Directs Attention   433

Two subcortical systems guide shifts of attention   433

Several cortical areas are crucial for generating and directing attention   433

Brain disorders can cause specific impairments of attention   435

SIGNS & SYMPTOMS Difficulty with Sustained Attention Can Sometimes Be Relieved with Stimulants   436

PART III   Consciousness, Thought, and Executive Function   437

Consciousness Is a Mysterious Product of the Brain   438

Which brain regions are active when we are conscious?   438

Some aspects of consciousness are easier to study than others   440

BOX 14.2 Building a Better Mind Reader   442

The frontal lobes are a crucial part of the executive system that guides our thoughts, feelings, and choices 444

Frontal lobe injury in humans leads to emotional, motor, and cognitive changes 444

BOX 14.3 Neuroeconomics Identifies Brain Regions Active during Decision Making 446

14 ■ Visual Summary 447

15 Language and Lateralization 450

PART I Cerebral Lateralization 452

The Left and Right Hemispheres of the Brain Are Different 452

Disconnection of the cerebral hemispheres reveals their individual specializations 452

The two hemispheres process information differently in most people 454

The left and right hemispheres differ in their auditory specializations 455

Handedness is associated with cerebral lateralization 456

Right-Hemisphere Damage Impairs Specific Types of Cognition 457

In prosopagnosia, faces are unrecognizable 458

BOX 15.1 The Wada Test 459

Left Hemisphere Damage Can Cause Aphasia 460

Damage to a left anterior speech zone causes nonfluent (or Broca's) aphasia 460

Damage to a left posterior speech zone causes fluent (or Wernicke's) aphasia 462

Widespread left-hemisphere damage can obliterate language capabilities 462

Disconnection of language regions may result in specific verbal problems 464

BOX 15.2 Studying Connectivity in the Living Brain 465

Brain mapping helps us understand the organization of language in the brain 466

RESEARCHERS AT WORK Noninvasive stimulation mapping reveals details of the brain's language areas 467

Functional neuroimaging technologies let us visualize activity in the brain's language zones during speech 468

PART II Verbal Behavior: Speech and Reading 470

Human Languages Share Basic Features 471

Language Has Both Inborn and Learned Components 472

Nonhuman primates engage in elaborate vocal behavior 473

Many different species engage in vocal communication 475

Reading Skills Are Difficult to Acquire and Are Frequently Impaired 476

Brain damage may cause specific impairments in reading 476

Some people struggle throughout their lives to read 477

PART III Recovery from Brain Damage 478

Stabilization and Reorganization Are Crucial for Recovery of Function 478

BOX 15.3 Contact Sports Can Be Costly 479

Rehabilitation and Retraining Can Help Recovery from Brain and Spinal Cord Injury 480

SIGNS & SYMPTOMS The Amazing Resilience of a Child's Brain 481

15 ■ Visual Summary 483

Appendix
Molecular Biology Basic Concepts and Important Techniques   A–1

Genes Carry Information That Encodes Proteins   A–1

Genetic information is stored in molecules of DNA   A–1

DNA is transcribed to produce messenger RNA   A–2

RNA molecules direct the formation of protein molecules   A–2

Molecular Biologists Have Craftily Enslaved Microorganisms and Enzymes   A–3

Southern blots identify particular genes   A–4

Northern blots identify particular mRNA transcripts   A–6

In situ hybridization localizes mRNA transcripts within specific cells   A–6

Western blots identify particular proteins   A–7

Antibodies can also tell us which cells possess a particular protein   A–7

Glossary   G–1

References   R–1

Author Index   AI–1

Subject Index   SI–I

Preface

Who has not pondered their own consciousness, marveled at their many sensory experiences, or wondered how a small and lumpy organ can process so much information? Neuroscience boils down to the mind studying its own machine, so it's an intrinsically fascinating topic that seems to fill every media channel nowadays. But another reason neuroscience is in the news so frequently is simply that it has become one of the most active branches of science. The pace of discoveries about brain and behavior has increased at an exponential rate over the last few decades, and continues to accelerate.

Every new edition of one of our books requires substantial updating because so much is happening all the time. (It's exciting, but wow, do we read a lot of reports and articles!) In fact, by far the hardest part of our job as authors lies in deciding which discoveries to include and which to (reluctantly) leave out: As the Red Queen remarked to Alice in Wonderland, "it takes all the running you can do, to keep in the same place." Our neuroscience news website (3e.mindsmachine.com/news) boasts a collection of more than 25,000 news stories, drawn from the mainstream media, that relate to the topics covered in the book. You can follow updates on the website, via email, or Facebook (www.facebook.com/BehavioralNeuroscience).

While we are sampling from this almost boundless scientific smorgasbord, we have to watch our weight. Our goal for *The Mind's Machine*, Third Edition is to introduce you to the basics of behavioral neuroscience in a way that focuses on the foundational topics in the field—with a generous sprinkling of the newest and most fascinating discoveries—and leaves you with an appetite for more. Whether you are beginning a program of study centered on the brain and behavior, or are just adding some breadth to your education, you will find that behavioral neuroscience now permeates all aspects of modern psychology, along with related life sciences like physiology, biology, and the health sciences. But that's not all. The tools and techniques of behavioral neuroscience are also creating new ways of looking at questions in many nontraditional areas, such as economics, the performing arts, anthropology, sociology, computer science, and engineering. Researchers are beginning to probe mental processes that seemed impenetrable only a decade or two ago: the neural bases of decision making, love and attachment, memory and learning, consciousness, and much of what we call the mind. A few examples of

formerly mysterious questions that are being answered with cutting-edge research include:

- Do prenatal events influence the development of a person's gender identity and sexual orientation?
- Does the brain make new neurons throughout life, in numbers large enough to make a functional difference?
- Can we improve memory performance with some drugs, and use other drugs to erase unwanted, traumatic memories?
- What happens in the brain as we develop trust in another person?
- How can we share so many genes with chimpanzees and other primates, and yet be so different from them?
- Can recent discoveries about the brain's appetite controller help us to curb the obesity epidemic?
- How can the microorganisms inhabiting the gut alter our brains and, ultimately, our behavior?

To understand the research behind these sorts of questions, it's necessary to become familiar with the physiology of behavior and experience. Our aim in *The Mind's Machine*, Third Edition is to provide a foundation that places these and other important problems in a unified scientific context, delivered in clear, inclusive, and gender-neutral language.

We've found that students enrolled in our courses have diverse academic backgrounds and personal interests. In this book, we've tried to avoid making too many assumptions about our readers, and have focused on providing both behavioral and biological perspectives on major topics. If you've had some high-school level biology you should have no trouble with most of the material in the book.

For those readers who have more experience in science—or who want more detail—we have peppered the chapters with embedded links to more advanced material located on our website. These links, called *A Step Further*, are just one of several novel features we have included to aid your learning. Throughout the book you will find web links that will connect you to animated versions of many figures, video clips, and more.

Each chapter also features at least one segment called *Researchers at Work*, which illustrates the nuts and bolts of experimentation through real-world examples, and a segment called *Signs & Symptoms* that relates a real-world clinical issue relevant to the chapter topic. And to help you gauge your progress, each chapter is divided into several major topics each bracketed by features called *The Road Ahead*, specifying your learning objectives for the material that follows, and *How's It Going?*, providing self-test conceptual questions. Every chapter also ends with a Visual Summary, an innovative combination of the main points and figures from the chapter, which you can also view in an interactive format on the companion website. We encourage you to explore the website for the book (3e.mindsmachine.com), which contains a free comprehensive set of study questions. This website is a powerful companion to the textbook that enhances the learning experience with a variety of multimedia resources.

The chapter lineup in this edition of *The Mind's Machine* encompasses several major themes. In the opening chapters, we trace the origins of behavioral neuroscience and introduce you to the structure of the brain, both as seen by the naked eye and as revealed by the microscope. We discuss how the cells of the brain use electrical signals to process information, and how they transmit that information to other cells within larger circuits. Along the way we'll look at the ways in which drugs affect nerve cells in order to change behavior, as well as some of the remarkable technology that lets us study the activity of the conscious brain as it perceives and thinks.

In the middle part of the book we look at the neural systems that underlie fundamental capabilities like feeling, moving, seeing, smelling, and hearing. We'll also consider biological and behavioral aspects of "mission-critical" functions such as feeding, sleeping, and sexual behavior. And we'll look at how the endocrine system acts as an interface between the brain and the rest of the body, as well as the reverse—ways in which the environment and behavior alter hormones and thus alter brain activity.

In the latter part of the book we turn to some of the high-level emotional and cognitive processes that color our lives and define us as individuals. We'll survey the systems that allow us to learn and remember information and skills, and the brain systems dedicated to language and spatial cognition. Research on processes of attention has made great progress in recent years, and we'll also consider consciousness and decision-making from a neuroscientific perspective. Finally, we'll review some of the consequences of brain dysfunction, ranging from psychopathology to behavioral manifestations of brain damage, and some of the innovative strategies being developed to counter these problems.

As you make your way through the book, you'll learn that one of the outstanding features of the brain is its ability to remodel. Every new experience, every piece of information that you learn, every skill that you master, causes changes in the brain that can alter your future behavior. The changes may involve physical alterations in the connections between cells, or in the chemicals they use to communicate, or even the addition of whole new cells and circuits. It's a property that we neuroscientists refer to as "plasticity." And it's something that we aim to exploit—if we've done our job properly, *The Mind's Machine*, Third Edition should cause lots of changes in your brain. We hope you enjoy the process.

Neil V. Watson   S. Marc Breedlove

We welcome feedback on any aspect of
The Mind's Machine, Third Edition
Simply drop us a line at themindsmachine@gmail.com.

Acknowledgments

This book bears the strong imprint of our late colleagues and coauthors Arnold L. Leiman (1932–2000) and Mark R. Rosenzweig (1922–2009). Arnie and Mark prepared the earliest editions of our more advanced text, *Behavioral Neuroscience*, and many illustrations and concepts in *this* book originated in their minds' machines.

In writing this book we benefited from the help of many highly skilled people. These include members of the staff of Sinauer Associates: Syd Carroll, Editor; Alison Hornbeck and Kathaleen Emerson, Production Editors; Christopher Small, Production Manager; Joan Gemme, Production Specialist; Jason Dirks, Manager, Media Editorial; and Zan Carter, Production Editor for Media and Supplements. Copy Editor Lou Doucette skillfully edited the text, and Photo Researchers Mark Siddall and David McIntyre sourced many of the photographs. Mike Demaray, Craig Durant, and colleagues at Dragonfly Media Group transformed our rough sketches and wish list into the handsome and dynamic art program of this text.

Our greatest source of inspiration (and critical feedback) has undoubtedly been the thousands of students to whom we have had the privilege of introducing the mysteries and delights of behavioral neuroscience, over the course of the last couple of decades. We have benefited from wisdom generously contributed by a legion of academic colleagues, whose advice and critical reviews have enormously improved our books. In particular we are grateful to: John Agnew, Duane Albrecht, Anne E. Powell Anderson, Michael Antle, Benoit Bacon, Scott Baron, Mark S. Blumberg, William Boggan, Eliot A. Brenowitz, Chris Brill, Peter C. Brunjes, Rebecca D. Burwell, Aryn Bush, Evangelia Chrysikou, Catherine P. Cramer, Heidi Day, Betty Deckard, Brian Derrick, Karen De Valois, Russell De Valois, Tiffany Donaldson, Rena Durr, Steven I. Dworkin, Thomas Fischer, Julia Fisher, Loretta M. Flanagan-Cato, Francis W. Flynn, Lauren Fowler, Michael Foy, Joyce A. Furfaro, Kara Gabriel, John D. E. Gabrieli, Jack Gallant, Eric W. Gobel, Kimberley P. Good, Diane C. Gooding, Janet M. Gray, Gary Greenberg, James Gross, Ervin Hafter, Mary E. Harrington, Ron Harris, Christian Hart, Chris Hayashi, Wendy Heller, Mark Hollins, Dave Holtzman, Rick Howe, Karin Hu, Richard Ivry, Lucia Jacobs, Karen Jennings, Janice Juraska, Erin Keen-Rhinehart, Dacher Keltner, Raymond E. Kesner, Mike Kisley, Keith R. Kluender, Leah A. Krubitzer, Joseph E. LeDoux, Diane Lee, Robert Lennartz, Michael A. Leon, Simon LeVay, Jeannie Loeb, Stephen G. Lomber, Jeffrey Love, Donna Maney, Stephen A. Maren, Joe L. Martinez, Jr., John J. McDonald, Robert J. McDonald, James L. McGaugh, Robert L. Meisel, Ralph E. Mistlberger, Jeffrey S. Mogil, Daniel Montoya, Randy J. Nelson, Chris Newland, Miguel Nicolelis, Michelle Niculescu, Antonio A. Nunez, Lee Osterhout, Kathleen Page, John Pellitteri, Linda Perrotti, James Pfaus, Eleni Pinnow, Helene S. Porte, Joseph Porter, George V. Rebec, Thomas Ritz, Scott R. Robinson, David A. Rosenbaum, Lawrence Ryan, Stephen Sammut, Martin F. Sarter, Jeffrey D. Schall, Stan Schein, Frederick Seil, Dale R. Sengelaub, Victor Shamas, Matthew Shapiro, Arthur Shimamura, Rachel Shoup, Rae Silver, Cheryl L. Sisk, Laura Smale, Robert L. Spencer, Jeffrey Stowell, Steve St. John, Patrick Steffen, Steven K. Sutton, Bruce Svare, Harald K. Taukulis, Jessica Thompson, Sandra Trafalis, Lucy J. Troup, Meg Upchurch, Franco J. Vaccarino, David R. Vago, Cyma Van Petten, Charles J. Vierck, Beth Wee, Carmen Westerberg, Robert Wickesberg, Christoph Wiedenmayer, Walter Wilczynski, S. Mark Williams, Richard D. Wright, Mark C. Zrull, and Irving Zucker.

A dedicated group of proofreaders pored over the text under severe time constraints; thanks to Will Vickerman, Evan Caldbick, and Maria Watson for catching errors we repeatedly missed. The following external reviewers read and critiqued chapters of the Second Edition of *The Mind's Machine*; their contributions and corrections really helped us to hone this, the Third Edition. Any errors that remain are thus entirely our fault.

Brian R. Adams, *Norco College*

David L. Allen, *University of Colorado, Boulder*

Dionisio A. Amodeo, *California State University San Bernardino*

A. Michael Anch, *Saint Louis University*

Francis R. Bambico, *Memorial University of Newfoundland*

Alo C. Basu, *College of the Holy Cross*

Jeffrey S. Bedwell, *University of Central Florida*

Beth Bowin, *Northeastern State University*

Sunny K. Boyd, *University of Notre Dame*

Susanne Brummelte, *Wayne State University*

Joshua M. Carlson, *Northern Michigan University*

Vanessa Cerda, *University of Texas at San Antonio*

Suzanne Clerkin, *Purchase College, State University of New York*

Kenneth J. Colodner, *Mount Holyoke College*

Jennifer A. Cummings, *University of Michigan*

Gregory L. Dam, *Indiana University East*

Derek Daniels, *University at Buffalo, State University of New York*

Katherine M. Daniels, *University of Southern Indiana*

Rachel A. Diana, *Virginia Polytechnic Institute and State University*

Gary L. Dunbar, *Central Michigan University*

Lena Ficco, *Fitchburg State University*

Lauren A. Fowler, *Weber State University*

Philip A. Gable, *The University of Alabama*

Christopher Goode, *Georgia State University*

Ian A. Harrington, *Augustana College*

Laura M. Harrison, *Tulane University*

Steven J. Hayduk, *Southern Wesleyan University*

Brian J. Hock, *Austin Peay State University*

Tephillah Jeyaraj-Powell, *University of Central Oklahoma*

Jessica M. Karanian, *Wesleyan University*

Christopher M. Lowry, *Brigham Young University – Idaho*

Melissa Masicampo, *Wake Forest University*

Paul Merritt, *Georgetown University*

Julia E. Meyers-Manor, *Ripon College*

Antonio A. Nunez, *Michigan State University*

John D. Pierce, Jr., *Thomas Jefferson University*

Joseph H. Porter, *Virginia Commonwealth University*

Jennifer K. Roth, *Carlow University*

Andrea J. Sell, *California Lutheran University*

Kezia C. Shirkey, *North Park University*

Ken Sobel, *University of Central Arkansas*

D. J. Spear, *South Dakota State University*

Scott F. Stoltenberg, *University of Nebraska*

Earl Thomas, *Bryn Mawr College*

Jennifer L. Thomson, *Messiah College*

Oscar V. Torres, *San Diego Mesa College*

Brian Trainor, *University of California, Davis*

Thomas E. Van Cantfort, *Fayetteville State University*

Carmen Westerberg, *Texas State University*

Eric P. Wiertelak, *Macalester College*

Christina L. Williams, *Duke University*

Adrienne Williamson, *Kennesaw State University*

Guangying Wu, *The George Washington University*

Melana Yanos, *Seattle Central College*

Heather J. Yu, *Stonehill College*

Finally, we would like to thank all our colleagues whose ideas and discoveries make behavioral neuroscience so much fun.

Media and Supplements
to accompany
The Mind's Machine: Foundations of Brain and Behavior, Third Edition

For the Student

Companion Website (3e.mindsmachine.com)

The Mind's Machine, Third Edition Companion Website contains a wide range of study and review resources to help students master the material presented in the textbook and to help engage them in the subject with fascinating examples. Tightly integrated with the text, with content corresponding to every major heading in the book, this online resource greatly enhances the learning experience. Key resources are linked throughout the textbook via direct Web addresses, making access easy from any smartphone, tablet, or computer. The Companion Website includes:

- *Chapter outlines* provide an overview of each chapter.
- *Animations* and *Videos* help illustrate dynamic processes and show examples of interesting phenomena.
- *Activities* include exercises that help the student learn and understand complex concepts and anatomical (and other) terms.
- *"A Step Further,"* additional coverage of selected topics
- Online, interactive versions of the *Visual Summaries*
- *Flashcards* help the student master the hundreds of new terms introduced in the textbook.

Dashboard (www.oup.com/us/dashboard)

Dashboard delivers a wealth of automatically graded quizzes and study resources for *The Mind's Machine*, along with an interactive eBook, all in an intuitive, web-based learning environment. See below for details.

Biological Psychology NewsLink (3e.mindsmachine.com/news)

This invaluable online resource helps students make connections between the science of biological psychology and their daily lives, and keeps them apprised of the latest developments in the field. The site includes links to thousands of news stories, all organized both by keyword and by textbook chapter. The site is updated 3–4 times per week.

For the Instructor

Ancillary Resource Center (oup-arc.com)

The Ancillary Resource Center provides instructors using *The Mind's Machine* with a wealth of resources for use in course planning, lecture development, and assessment. Content includes:

- *Textbook Figures and Tables*: All the figures and tables from the textbook are provided as JPEGs, all optimized for use in presentation software (such as PowerPoint).
- *PowerPoint Resources*: Two ready-to-use presentations are provided for each chapter:
  - A *Lecture* presentation that includes text covering the entire chapter, with selected figures
  - A *Figures* presentation that includes all the figures and tables from the chapter, with titles on each slide, and complete captions in the Notes field
- *Videos*: A collection of video segments that illustrate interesting concepts and phenomena
- *Instructor's Manual*: The Instructor's Manual provides instructors with a variety of resources to aid in planning their course and developing their lectures. For each chapter, the manual includes:
  - *Chapter overview*
  - *Chapter outline*
  - Detailed *key concepts*
  - *References for lecture development*, including books, journal articles, and online resources
  - Detailed media references for *animations and videos*
  - *Key terms*
- *Test Bank*: The Test Bank consists of a broad range of questions covering all the key facts and concepts in each chapter. Each chapter includes multiple choice, matching, short answer, and essay questions. Also included are all the Dashboard quizzes (multiple choice and essay). All questions are keyed to Bloom's Taxonomy, aligned to Learning Objectives, and referenced to specific textbook sections.

- *Computerized Test Bank*: The entire test bank is provided in Blackboard's Diploma software. Diploma makes it easy to assemble quizzes and exams from any combination of publisher-provided questions and instructor-created questions. In addition, quizzes and exams can be exported to many different course management systems, such as Blackboard and Moodle. Includes the Dashboard quiz questions.

Dashboard (www.oup.com/us/dashboard)

Dashboard by Oxford University Press delivers a wealth of study resources and automatically graded quizzes for *The Mind's Machine* in an intuitive, web-based learning environment. A built-in color-coded gradebook allows instructors to track student progress. Dashboard includes:

- *Interactive eBook*: A complete eBook is integrated into Dashboard and includes in-text links to media resources.
- *All Student Companion Website Resources*: Chapter outlines, animations and videos, activities, A Step Further, visual summaries, and flashcards
- *Study Questions*: A set of self-review questions designed to give students the opportunity to test their understanding of each chapter's material

- *Online Quizzes*: Questions for each chapter in two formats:
  - Multiple choice tests student comprehension of the material covered in each chapter
  - Essays challenge students to synthesize and apply what they have learned
- The complete *Glossary* provides definitions for all textbook bolded terms.

To learn more about any of these resources, or to get access, please contact your local OUP representative.

Value Options

eBook

The Mind's Machine is available as an eBook, in several different formats, including RedShelf, VitalSource, and Chegg. All major mobile devices are supported

Looseleaf Textbook

(ISBN 978-1-60535-835-2)

The Mind's Machine is also available in a three-hole punched, looseleaf format. Students can take just the sections they need to class and can easily integrate instructor material with the text.

The Mind's Machine
Foundations of Brain and Behavior

THIRD EDITION

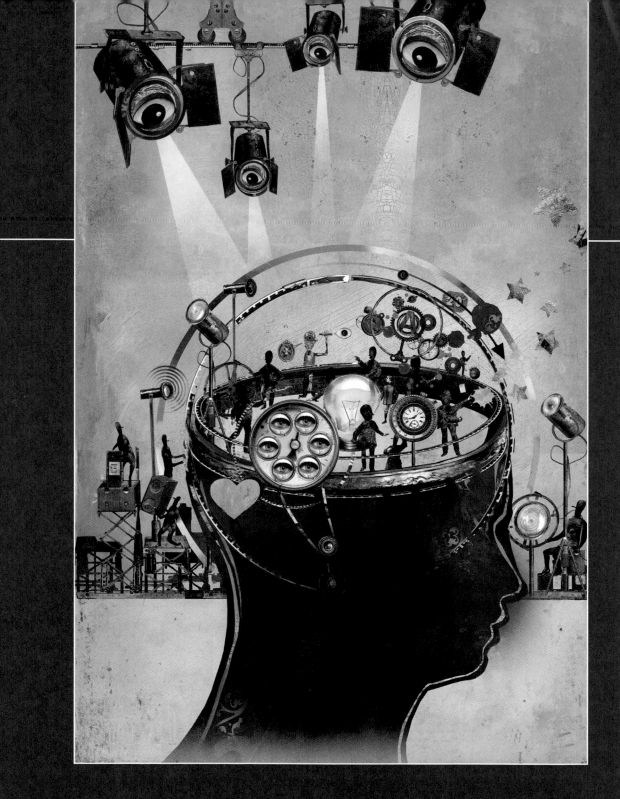

1

An Introduction
to Brain and Behavior

Nature and Nurture: Building the Mind's Machine

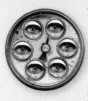

We humans have a long history of using contemporary technology as a metaphor for the mysterious workings of the brain, so today it is commonplace to see the brain described as a computer, complete with "hardware" and "software." Perhaps tomorrow's neuroscientists will describe the brain in terms of holograms, quantum devices, or a technology that has yet to be imagined. But while modern research aims to describe the complicated machine within each of our heads, we also want to know how the operation of the brain produces the *mind*—the perceptions, emotions, thoughts, self-awareness, and other cognitive processes that inform our behavior.

During the twentieth century, a lot of ink was spilled over the "nature-nurture" controversy, with scholars arguing passionately about the extent to which mental characteristics and abilities are the result of learning experiences versus "innate, hardwired" genetic programs. The two perspectives have often been presented as mutually incompatible alternatives, but thanks to more-powerful techniques, we have come to realize that there is nothing controversial about nature versus nurture: they are two sides of the same coin. Consider the case of rat pups who have inattentive mothers. As adults, the formerly neglected pups show elevated stress hormone responses to stressors that have little effect on rats that were not neglected as pups (T. Y. Zhang and Meaney, 2010). How does this lasting reactivity develop—through experience or as a result of inborn biological factors? Both, it turns out. As we'll see later in this chapter, and throughout the book, the mind and its machine are shaped by a precise combination of genes and experience, inextricably tied together.

There are now more than 7.5 billion of us, and while we can debate whether to fear or celebrate that number, there is no doubt that each of those billions of human brains will at times contemplate its own existence and meaning. How does the operation of a three-pound organ generate our sense of self, express our unique personalities, record information, and guide our actions? Evolution has shaped our bodies and brains so that we closely resemble one another, yet our brains remain malleable throughout life, continually remolded by our environments, experiences, and interactions with other people. So, through a remarkable intersection of genetic heritage and environmental influences, 7.5 billion unique individuals have been formed, and we literally change each other's minds on a daily basis.

To see the video
Nature and Nurture,
go to
3e.mindsmachine.com/av1.1

What is this? ──────

In each chapter of the book, you will find two or three of these small features, entitled **THE ROAD AHEAD**. They are intended to provide you with a road map for the reading you are about to do, giving you a sense of where the following section is going and what we hope you will get from it (i.e., your learning objectives).

To view the
Brain Explorer,
go to
3e.mindsmachine.com/av1.2

neuroscience   The scientific study of the nervous system.

behavioral neuroscience   Also called *biological psychology, brain and behavior,* and *physiological psychology*. The study of the biological bases of psychological processes and behavior.

PART I
The Birth of a Science of Brain and Behavior

THE ROAD AHEAD

We open the book with a look at the origins of scientific inquiry into the role of the brain in the guidance of behavior. To do this, we consider the relationships between different branches of brain science, and some of the important developments in the field's history. Reading this section should prepare you to:

1. Define *behavioral neuroscience*, identify its synonyms, describe the scope of the field, and situate it relative to other branches of brain science.
2. Trace the history of our understanding of the role of the brain, as articulated by scholars across the millennia.
3. Name and briefly describe some of the most influential concepts, emerging topics, and future goals for brain research.

Behavioral Neuroscience Spans Past, Present, and Future

The general field of **neuroscience**—the scientific study of the nervous system—is divided into many subdisciplines because the topic is so vast. The first scholars to study the relationships between brain and behavior called themselves philosophers, because it was philosophy that established the scientific method as our best tool for finding new knowledge. Philosophers had long been concerned with the sources of human behavior, so **behavioral neuroscience**, the field that relates behavior to bodily processes, naturally evolved from those beginnings. The names *biological psychology, brain and behavior,* and *physiological psychology* are all synonyms for *behavioral neuroscience*, but whichever name is used, the main goal of this field is to understand the brain structures and functions that respond to experiences and generate behavior.

Researchers with dramatically varied backgrounds—psychologists, biologists, physiologists, engineers, neurologists, psychiatrists, and many others—together make up the field of behavioral neuroscience. It is a field that spans both academia and industry, with focus that ranges from pure research on basic processes to entirely applied work directly translating findings into goods and services (Hitt, 2007). The diverse branches of science that overlap with behavioral neuroscience are mapped in **FIGURE 1.1**.

An early textbook famously opened with the observation that, as a science, "psychology has a long past but only a short history" (Ebbinghaus, 1908). That's certainly an apt description of behavioral neuroscience. The modern era of behavioral neuroscience—characterized by objective experimentation and use of the scientific method to test hypotheses—has a formal history of only 100 years or so. But curiosity about the genesis of behavior reaches much further into the past, shaped by religious ideas, folk knowledge, and ancient observations about the biology of humans and nonhuman animals.

An understanding of the brain's role in behavior has developed over centuries

The elaborate preparation of tombs and careful mummification of important people in ancient Egypt (especially about 1500–1000 BCE) reflected the belief that the dead would enter an afterlife that entailed both struggle and—for the adequately equipped individual—great reward. So, in addition to embalming the body with special salts and oils, the usual practice was to preserve four important organs in alabaster jars in the tomb: liver, lungs, stomach, and intestines. The heart, being especially esteemed, was preserved in its place within the body. The brain, however, was picked out though the nostrils and thrown away; apparently, it was considered to be of little value in the afterlife.

There is little or no mention of the brain in the Quran, and it is likewise never mentioned in either the Old Testament or New Testament of the Bible, but the heart

FIGURE 1.1 How Behavioral Neuroscience Relates to Other Fields

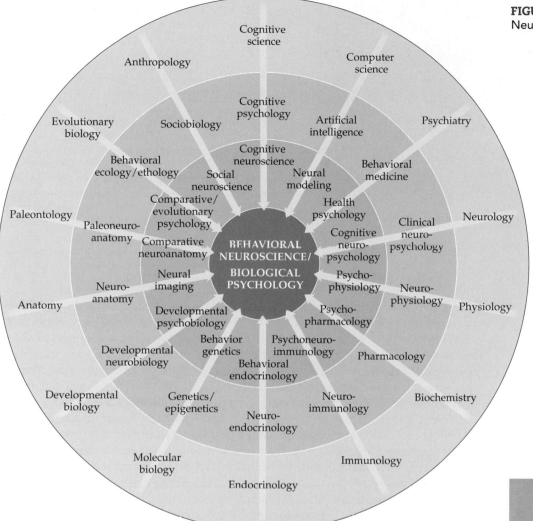

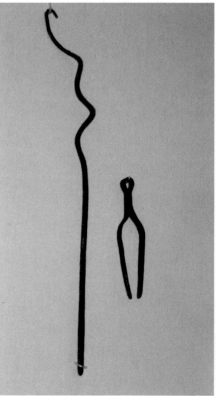

is mentioned hundreds of times, along with several references each to the liver, the stomach, and the bowels as the seats of passion, courage, and pity, respectively. Aristotle (about 350 BCE), the most prominent scientist of ancient Greece, likewise considered mental capacities to be properties of the heart. When we call people kindhearted, openhearted, fainthearted, hardhearted, or heartless, and when we speak of learning by heart, we are using language echoing this ancient notion. Aristotle thought the brain was little more than a cooling system for hot blood from the heart. But Aristotle's near contemporary, the great Greek physician Hippocrates (about 400 BCE), already suspected that Aristotle's view was—ahem—wrongheaded, and he instead ascribed emotion, perception, and thought to the functioning of the brain.

By the second century CE, this brain-centered view of mental processes had become more accepted, appearing in the writings of the Greco-Roman physician Galen

Brain Extraction Kit   It seems the ancient Egyptians had little regard for the brain. During the mummification process, embalmers used specialized tools, like these examples in the British Museum, to first break up the small bones behind the nose and then extract the brain through the opening. Unlike other major organs, the brain was discarded, and the cranium was stuffed with linen or straw. (Photograph by Neil Watson.)

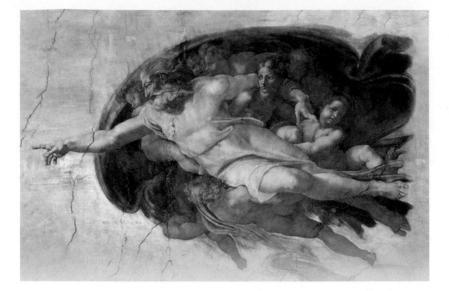

A Brain on the Ceiling of the Sistine Chapel?
Between 1508 and 1512, Michelangelo painted the Sistine Chapel in the Vatican. In one panel of Michelangelo's masterpiece, God is depicted reaching out to bestow the gift of life upon humanity, through Adam. But neuroscientists have noted that the oddly shaped drapery behind God, and the arrangement of his attendants, closely resembles the human brain (Meshberger, 1990); compare it with the midsagittal view in Figure 2.16A. A keen student of anatomy, Michelangelo probably knew perfectly well what a dissected human brain looks like. So, was Michelangelo having some fun, making a subtle commentary about the origins of human behavior? We probably will never know, but modern research tools are helping us to understand how our distinctive human qualities—language, reason, emotion, and the rest—are products of the brain. (© Scala/Art Resource, NY.)

(the "Father of Medicine"). Galen's experiences in treating head injuries of gladiators led him to propose that behavior results from the movement of "animal spirits" from the brain through nerves to the body, but his understanding of the relevant anatomy was poor. Not until much later were techniques developed for making highly detailed anatomical studies of the fine structure of the brain.

Skillfully applying newly developed innovations in drawing technique, Renaissance painter and scientist Leonardo da Vinci (1452–1519) produced exquisite neuroanatomical illustrations of nerves and brain structures (**FIGURE 1.2**). Religious dogma dominated Renaissance science—just ask Galileo—with the result that scientific writing from that era often presents the brain as a mysterious and intricate gift from God. But perhaps some thinkers of the day secretly held a more secular view of neuroscience; for example, it has been observed that certain depictions of God on the ceiling of the Sistine Chapel, painted by Michelangelo (1475–1564) (see above), bear a striking resemblance to the human brain (Meshberger, 1990; Suk and Tamargo, 2010). It is believed that Michelangelo was conducting dissections of cadavers at about the time that the painting was created.

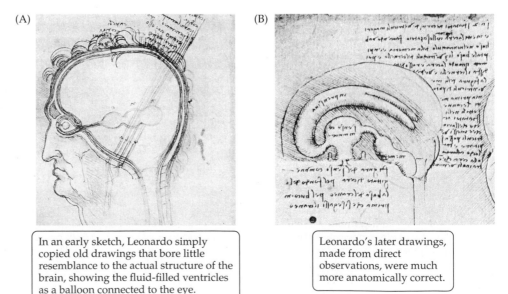

(A) In an early sketch, Leonardo simply copied old drawings that bore little resemblance to the actual structure of the brain, showing the fluid-filled ventricles as a balloon connected to the eye.

(B) Leonardo's later drawings, made from direct observations, were much more anatomically correct.

FIGURE 1.2 Leonardo da Vinci's Changing View of the Brain (Reproduced with gracious permission of Her Majesty Queen Elizabeth II, copyright reserved.)

In any event, weighing religious notions of the soul against increasingly mechanistic views of the brain became a major preoccupation for later scholars. Among his many contributions to math and science, René Descartes (1596–1650) tried to explain how the control of behavior might resemble the workings of a machine, proposing the concept of spinal reflexes and a neural pathway for them (**FIGURE 1.3**). But Descartes also argued (perhaps in order to deflect criticism) that free will and moral choice could not arise from a mere machine. So Descartes asserted that humans, at least, had a nonmaterial soul as well as a material body and that the soul governed behavior through a point of contact (possibly the pineal gland) in the brain. This notion of **dualism** spread widely and left other thinkers with the task of trying to explain how a nonmaterial soul could exert influence over a material body and brain. Today, almost all neuroscientists have discarded dualism in favor of the much simpler view that the workings of the mind can be understood as purely physical processes taking place in the material brain.

Thanks in large part to systematic studies of the relation between various disorders and damage to regions of the human brain that were conducted by the English physician Thomas Willis (1621–1675), the notion that the brain coordinates and controls behavior eventually became widely accepted (Zimmer, 2004). A pseudoscientific fad of the early 1800s called **phrenology** (**FIGURE 1.4A**) capitalized on the emerging idea that specific behaviors, feelings, and personality traits were controlled by corresponding specific regions of the brain. Although phrenology was plainly wrong in several fundamental ways—for example, phrenologists believed they could "read" a person's character by feeling the bumps on that person's head—the field helped establish the concept of **localization of function**, which asserts that different brain regions specialize in specific behaviors.

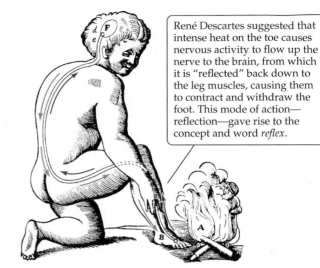

René Descartes suggested that intense heat on the toe causes nervous activity to flow up the nerve to the brain, from which it is "reflected" back down to the leg muscles, causing them to contract and withdraw the foot. This mode of action—reflection—gave rise to the concept and word *reflex*.

FIGURE 1.3 An Early Account of Reflexes (Bettman/Corbis.)

dualism The notion, promoted by René Descartes, that the mind has an immaterial aspect that is distinct from the material body and brain.

phrenology The belief that bumps on the skull reflect enlargements of brain regions responsible for certain behavioral faculties.

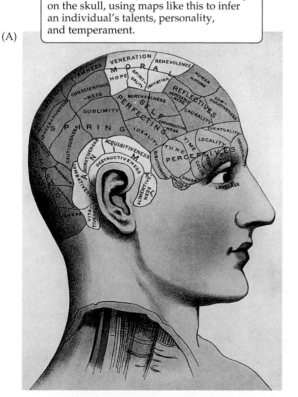

In the nineteenth century phrenologists associated arbitrary "faculties" with bumps on the skull, using maps like this to infer an individual's talents, personality, and temperament.

(A)

FIGURE 1.4 Mapping Behavior: Then and Now (Part A © The Print Collector/Alamy; Part B after M. J. Nichols and W. T. Newsome, 1999. *Nature* 402: C35.)

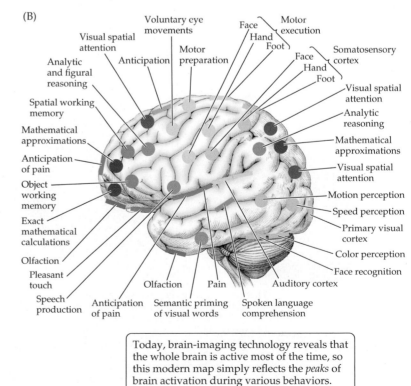

(B)

Today, brain-imaging technology reveals that the whole brain is active most of the time, so this modern map simply reflects the *peaks* of brain activation during various behaviors.

localization of function The concept that different brain regions specialize in specific behaviors.

Later researchers found that damage to specific regions of the brain causes predictable impairments in people; for example, Paul Broca (1824–1880) noted that damage to a particular region of the left side of the brain reliably causes problems with speech production (see Chapter 15). Neuroscientists today accept that the localization of function within the brain is more or less true. Although the whole brain is active most of the time, when we are performing particular tasks, certain brain regions become even more activated, and different tasks activate different brain regions. So modern functional maps of the human brain track the locations where these peaks of activation occur (**FIGURE 1.4B**). A parallel concern that harks back to the phrenologists has been the importance of brain size to intellectual function. After a couple of centuries of study, the evidence indicates that while the overall size of your brain matters, it matters a lot less than you might expect (**FIGURE 1.5**).

In 1890, William James's book *Principles of Psychology* signaled the beginnings of a modern approach to behavioral neuroscience. In James's work, psychological ideas such as consciousness and other aspects of human experience came to be seen as properties of the nervous system. A true behavioral neuroscience began to emerge from this approach. By the beginning of the twentieth century, researchers were applying newly developed tools to study mental processes that had previously seemed unknowable. Rapid progress was made in developing techniques for measuring learning and memory in humans and animals, and Russian physiologist Ivan P. Pavlov (1849–1936) made his landmark discoveries of classical conditioning in animals—Nobel Prize–winning work that influences scientists to this day.

This rapid progress prompted a parallel interest in understanding the neural basis of learning, marked by one of the first true behavioral neuroscience research programs: the "search for the engram" by Karl Lashley (1890–1958). Although he would not accomplish his goal of linking a specific brain region to the formation of a specific long-term memory (an "engram"), Lashley gave us the idea (now well established) that memory is not localized to only one region of the brain. Behavioral neuroscience also bears the strong imprint of Canadian psychologist Donald O. Hebb (1904–1985), a student of Lashley (Brown and Milner, 2003). Hebb showed that cognitive processing

FIGURE 1.5 Does Size Matter? (Part A from the Bettmann Archive; B courtesy of Nancy Andreasen.)

(A)

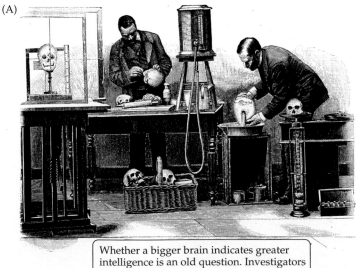

Whether a bigger brain indicates greater intelligence is an old question. Investigators in the nineteenth century measured the volumes of skulls of various groups and estimated intelligence on the basis of people's occupations, teachers' guesstimates, and other doubtful criteria.

(B)

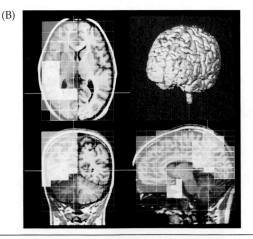

IQ tests improved the objectivity of intelligence measurement. When carefully controlled, MRI studies like this one do find a correlation between brain size and IQ scores (Andreasen et al., 1993), and IQ seems to correlate better with the volume of the front of the brain than the back (Colom et al., 2009). So it seems that bigger is better, but the correlations are of only modest size, meaning that other factors must also contribute to IQ scores (Stanovich, 2009).

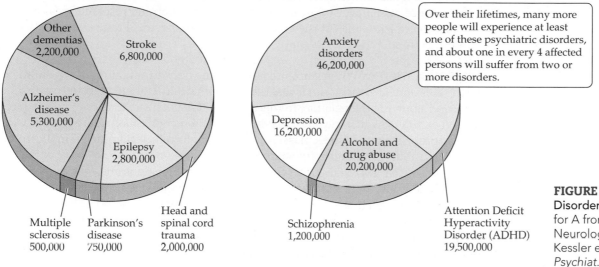

(A) Lifetime incidence of neurological disorders

Other dementias 2,200,000
Stroke 6,800,000
Alzheimer's disease 5,300,000
Epilepsy 2,800,000
Multiple sclerosis 500,000
Parkinson's disease 750,000
Head and spinal cord trauma 2,000,000

(B) Incidence of diagnosed psychiatric illnesses in any one year

Anxiety disorders 46,200,000
Depression 16,200,000
Alcohol and drug abuse 20,200,000
Schizophrenia 1,200,000
Attention Deficit Hyperactivity Disorder (ADHD) 19,500,000

> Over their lifetimes, many more people will experience at least one of these psychiatric disorders, and about one in every 4 affected persons will suffer from two or more disorders.

FIGURE 1.6 The Toll of Brain Disorders in the USA (Data for A from D. Hirtz et al., 2007. *Neurology* 68: 326; B from R. C. Kessler et al., 2005. *Arch. Gen. Psychiat.* 62: 593.)

could be accomplished by networks of active neurons, molded by repeated activation patterns into functional circuits. His hypothesis about how neurons strengthen their connections as a consequence of experiences led to the idea of the Hebbian synapse, a type of plastic (changeable) connection between neurons that remains a hot topic in neuroscience, as discussed in Chapter 13.

The future of behavioral neuroscience is in interdisciplinary discovery and knowledge translation

New discoveries from behavioral neuroscience labs are leading to greater understanding of brain disorders and, with time, will result in the development of effective treatments. This is an urgent problem of much greater scale than many people realize: even excluding addiction and developmental disorders, one in five U.S. residents lived with a mental illness in 2016 (SAMHSA, 2017), and for some disorders, such as depression, the prevalence appears to be on the rise (Hidaka, 2012). Neurological and psychiatric disorders vary tremendously both in their severity—from illnesses that can be managed with suitable treatments, to devastating conditions that completely disable—and in their incidence (**FIGURE 1.6**). The economic toll of so much illness is staggering: the cost for treatment of dementia (severely disordered thinking) alone exceeds the costs of treating cancer and heart disease combined.

As the quest to understand and relieve these diseases gathers speed, some of the historical distinction between clinical and laboratory approaches has begun to fade away. For example, when clinicians encounter a pair of twins, one of whom has schizophrenia while the other seems healthy, the discovery of structural differences in their brains (**FIGURE 1.7**) immediately raises questions for laboratory scientists: Did the structural differences arise before the symptoms of schizophrenia, or the other way around? Were the brain differences present at birth, or did they arise during puberty? Does medication that reduces symptoms affect brain structure? (We'll consider schizophrenia again in Chapter 12.)

The twenty-first century has brought an explosion of new research areas and perspectives to behavioral neuroscience. In addition to

FIGURE 1.7 Identical Twins but Nonidentical Brains and Behavior (Images courtesy of E. Fuller Torrey.)

(A)
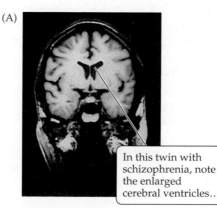

> In this twin with schizophrenia, note the enlarged cerebral ventricles...

(B)
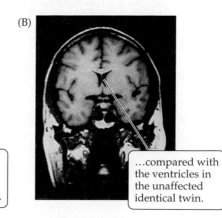

> ...compared with the ventricles in the unaffected identical twin.

the rapid progress that is occurring in the more established topic areas of behavioral neuroscience, which we survey in this book, some emerging research areas are attracting intense interest. In the paragraphs that follow, we'll take a brief look at a handful of these.

NEUROPLASTICITY   When you think about it, the only explanation for our ability to learn skills and form memories is that the brain physically changes in some way to encode and store that information. In this book we'll see many examples of how behavior and experiences alter the physical brain—a phenomenon called **neuroplasticity** (or just *plasticity*; from the Greek plassein, "to mold or form")—but much remains to be discovered about mechanisms of neuroplasticity.

We know that experiences can alter the size of brain regions and interconnections between neurons, and cellular changes have been discovered that could be mechanisms for storing memories; scientists are actively testing that idea. We also know that certain experiences and physiological states can modify the rate at which new neurons are born in the adult brain, but again, the functional significance of this **adult neurogenesis** (see Chapter 13) remains to be determined. Perhaps nothing distinguishes behavioral neuroscience from other neurosciences more clearly than a fascination with neuroplasticity and the role of experience.

SOCIAL NEUROSCIENCE   Because of neuroplasticity, even simple interactions with other people can remodel our brains. Indeed, the whole point of coming to a lecture hall is to have the instructor use words and figures to alter your brain so that you can retrieve that information in the future (in other words, they are teaching you something). Most aspects of our social behavior are learned—from the language we speak to the clothes we wear and the kinds of foods we eat, as well as our identity in belonging to larger groups (clubs, teams, schools, nationalities, and so on).

Social neuroscience is an emerging discipline that uses the tools of neuroscience to discover how biological and social factors continually interact and affect each other as behavior unfolds. For example, the amount of testosterone in a male's circulation affects his dominance behavior and aggression, expressed in social settings ranging from friendly games to overt physical aggression (see Chapter 11). But the outcome of those contests can cause changes in relative testosterone levels—winners show more testosterone, and losers have less—so testosterone concentration in the blood at any particular moment is determined (in part) by the male's recent history of dominant/submissive social experience. The modified testosterone level, in turn, helps determine the male's dominance and aggression in the future. So it goes.

EVOLUTIONARY PSYCHOLOGY   Zoologists have long viewed animal behaviors as adaptations that evolved to solve specific ecological pressures, such as the need to find food and avoid predators. More recently, speculations about how natural selection might have shaped our own behavior, including specific cognitive abilities, have given rise to a lively and controversial field called **evolutionary psychology** (Barkow et al., 1992; Buss, 2013). For example, it has been argued (G. F. Miller, 2000) that sexual selection was crucial for evolution of the human brain. If early ancestors of modern humans came to favor mates who sang, made jokes, or produced artistic works, an "arms race" might have ensued as the ever more discriminating brains of one sex demanded ever more impressive performances from the brains of the other sex. Did humor, song, and art originate from the drive to be sexy? And does sexual selection account for the large size of the human brain?

Although evolutionary psychology excels at generating intriguing hypothetical accounts of the evolution of behaviors, the challenge for the future is to come up with ways to test and potentially disprove these hypotheses.

neuroplasticity   Also called *neural plasticity*. The ability of the nervous system to change in response to experience or the environment.

adult neurogenesis   The creation of new neurons in the brain of an adult.

social neuroscience   A field of study that uses the tools of neuroscience to discover both the biological bases of social behavior and the effects of social circumstances on brain activity.

evolutionary psychology   A field of study devoted to asking how natural selection has shaped behavior in humans and other animals.

EPIGENETICS   Nearly all of the cells in your body have a complete copy of your genome (i.e., a copy of all your genes), but each cell uses only a small subset of those genes at any one time. **Epigenetics** is a young field focusing on factors that have a lasting effect on patterns of **gene expression**—the turning on or off of specific genes—without changing the structure of the genes themselves. In some cases, the acquired alteration in gene expression is passed down through generations, from parent to child, despite the absence of genetic modifications.

At the beginning of the chapter, we briefly discussed rats that will show heightened stress reactivity throughout their lives if neglected by their mothers while they are pups, and we asked whether this phenomenon was more attributable to "nature" or to "nurture." The answer is: neither. Or perhaps both. It is an epigenetic phenomenon, in which the maternal neglect causes lasting inactivation of a gene—a process called *methylation* (see Chapter 13)—that causes the pup to be hyperresponsive to stress for the rest of its life. So, early experience produces a permanent change in the way in which genes are expressed in the brain of the neglected rat, thus altering its behavior in adulthood—nurture and nature.

This same gene is also more likely to be methylated in the postmortem brains of humans who have committed suicide, but only if the victim was subjected to childhood abuse (McGowan et al., 2009). So, methylation of the gene in abused children may make them more susceptible to stress as adults and put them at risk for suicide—a powerful demonstration of epigenetic influences on behavior. Epigenetic modifications are increasingly understood to have a major role in the development of individual differences in mental health disorders such as depression and stress pathology (Gray et al., 2017; Manoli and Tollkuhn, 2018). (For additional examples of social influences on the structure of the brain, see **A STEP FURTHER 1.1**, on the website.)

NEUROECONOMICS   A growing number of neuroscience labs focus on the neural bases of decision making. Involving perspectives ranging from philosophy to social psychology to experimental psychology, neuroscience, and economics, **neuroeconomics** aims to identify brain regions that are especially active when decisions are being made: while playing games, managing resources, making strategic choices, and so on. Naturally, this research has some shorter-term benefits relating to product marketing—what makes us want to buy something—but researchers mostly hope that, over the longer term, we will develop a more complete understanding of both the massive brain networks that are active while we choose among various alternatives and decide what to do next, and the ways in which we perceive and express our free will (as well as if, indeed, we actually *have* free will!).

Early indications are that we possess brain mechanisms dedicated to neuroeconomic evaluations, assessing the relative value of each choice available and then sifting through the evaluated choices in order to make a conscious decision (Kable and Glimcher, 2009; Ojala et al., 2018), along with mechanisms to inhibit impulsive decision making (Muhlert and Lawrence, 2015; Heilbronner and Hayden, 2016). There is good reason to expect exciting new discoveries about how these neural systems interact with other cognitive systems to produce our conscious feeling of self.

THE TRULY FINAL FRONTIER: CONSCIOUSNESS   Ultimately, many of the traditional and emerging topics in behavioral neuroscience converge on the problem of **consciousness**: the personal, private awareness of our emotions, intentions, thoughts, and movements and of the sensations that impinge upon us. How is it possible that you are aware of the words on this page, the room you're occupying, the goals you have in life? Scientists have laid some of the groundwork for conceptualizing consciousness as a property of the brain and for establishing it as an area of scientific inquiry (Zeman, 2002), but the devil is in the details. Later in the book we will consider

epigenetics   The study of factors that affect gene expression without making any changes in the nucleotide sequence of the genes themselves.

gene expression   The turning on or off of specific genes.

neuroeconomics   The study of brain mechanisms at work during economic decision making.

consciousness   The state of awareness of one's own existence, thoughts, emotions, and experiences.

FIGURE 1.8 The Human Brain Project (After M. M. Waldrop, 2012. *Nature* 482: 456.)

The goal of massive projects in both the USA and Europe is to have a digital re-creation of the neurons and connections found in a human brain. As this projection from the European project (bluebrain.epfl.ch) shows, this would require an "exascale" computer capable of a mind-bending quintillion (one billion billion) operations per second, and a truly staggering amount of computer memory.

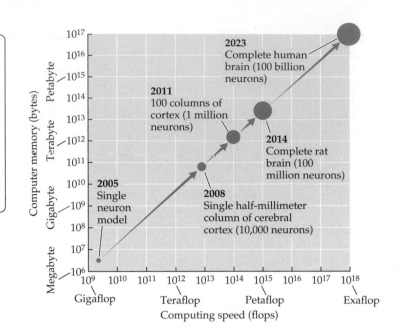

"How Beautifully Blue the Sky"
We would all agree that this sky is the color we call "blue." But in Chapter 14 we'll ask whether everyone who sees that sky has the same experience of the color. (© iStock.com/Roman Sigaev.)

experiments that demonstrate properties of consciousness, including the role of arousal systems of the brain, and evidence that synchronized activity within large cortical networks gives rise to conscious introspection (Raichle, 2015). And some of these experiments lead us to interesting—possibly disturbing—conclusions that our consciousness may track the operation of our brains much less accurately than we perceive (as discussed in Chapter 14).

However it is brought about, any satisfying account of consciousness should be able to explain, for example, why a certain pattern of activity in your brain causes you to experience the sensation of blue when looking at the sky. And a really good theory should tell us how we could cause you to experience the sky as yellow, just by changing your brain activity for you (not, of course, by simply fitting you with colored goggles, but rather through a change in the deeper conscious experience of the world around you). However, we are nowhere near understanding consciousness this clearly. We generally have no idea what the actual inner experience of a human or animal is—only what an individual's behavior tells us about it. So even if you tell me that the sky is blue to you, I can't tell whether blue feels the same in your mind as it does in mine. Until we can get a more complete grasp of these complex issues of brain and behavior, we are in no position to know whether complicated machines like computers are, or might one day be, conscious. Several large research projects are currently engaged in the Herculean task of mapping the neural networks within an entire human brain (Waldrop, 2012), which will require computer systems with almost unimaginable processing power and memory (**FIGURE 1.8**).

What is this?

Sprinkled throughout every chapter, sections entitled **HOW'S IT GOING?** provide conceptual questions that will help you check your learning and ensure you are meeting the objectives set out in **THE ROAD AHEAD**.

HOW'S IT GOING ❓

1. Define *behavioral neuroscience*. Name some fields that are closely allied to behavioral neuroscience.
2. What do we mean when we say that behavioral neuroscience has a long past but only a short history? Review the prehistory of behavioral neuroscience and the gradual process of elimination that linked the brain and behavior.
3. Discuss the concept of localization of function.
4. Comment on the prevalence of psychiatric and neurological disorders in contemporary society, and discuss their economic and emotional impact.
5. Where is behavioral neuroscience headed? Discuss some of the probable hot topics for future behavioral neuroscientists.

PART II
Research Design

THE ROAD AHEAD

In the second part of the chapter, we discuss the factors that neuroscientists consider in designing research: both the formal layout of experiments and the theoretical considerations on which research questions are based. Studying this section should prepare you to:

1. Describe and distinguish between correlational studies and experimental studies—in which either the body is altered and behavior is measured, or behavior is manipulated and bodily changes are measured—and explain how scientists rely on all three types of studies to develop research programs.

2. Discuss the major theoretical perspectives that inform research in behavioral neuroscience.

3. Discuss important issues that modern behavioral neuroscience must contend with, such as the use of animals in research, and the replication crisis in behavioral research.

4. Explain the different levels of analysis that may be focused on by behavioral neuroscientists, and identify how they may relate to one another.

Careful Design of Studies Is Essential for Progress in Behavioral Neuroscience

Because it is both fantastically complex (**FIGURE 1.9**) and somewhat inaccessible, the brain poses special challenges when it comes to formulating research questions and designing experiments to answer those questions. For example, it is difficult to physically manipulate the structure and activity of the brain with pinpoint accuracy, so technological advances have been responsible for the modern explosion in neuroscience research. And because we can't ethically manipulate the brains of human research participants (other than through transient and noninvasive means), we often must rely on alternatives such as purely observational research, in which behavioral means are used to alter brain activity, or research in which we study neural function in lab animals in order to gain insights about our own nervous systems. The complexity of behavior, and the organ by which it is produced, have also been factors in an emerging crisis in behavioral neuroscience: difficulty in replicating numerous influential earlier findings (De Boeck and Jeon, 2018). The development of new research procedures to avoid dead ends and unreproducible or unimportant findings is thus driving a rapid evolution of scientific methodology across the behavioral sciences.

Three types of study designs probe brain-behavior relationships

Behavioral neuroscientists use three general types of studies for research on the biological bases of behavior. In an experiment employing **somatic intervention** (**FIGURE 1.10A**), we alter a structure or function of the brain or body to see how this alteration changes behavior. In this sort of experiment, the physical alteration is an **independent variable** (a general term used to describe the manipulated aspect of any experiment), and the behavioral effect is the **dependent variable** (a general term used to describe the measured consequence of an experimental manipulation). Some examples of somatic intervention experiments include (1) administering a hormone

somatic intervention   An approach to finding relations between body variables and behavioral variables that involves manipulating body structure or function and looking for resultant changes in behavior.

independent variable   The factor that is manipulated by an experimenter.

dependent variable   The factor that an experimenter measures to monitor a change in response to changes in an independent variable.

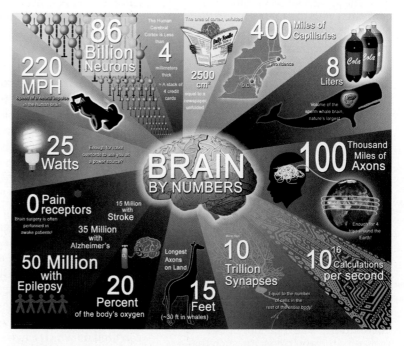

FIGURE 1.9   Your Brain, by the Numbers (© Dwayne Godwin 2011.)

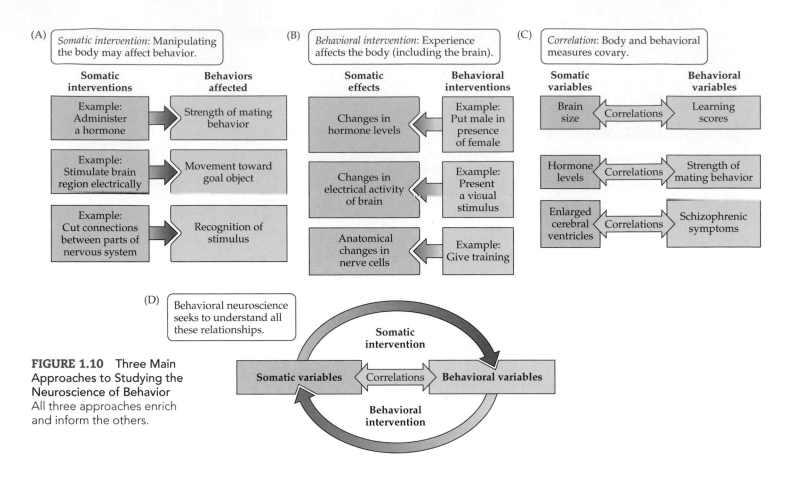

(A) *Somatic intervention*: Manipulating the body may affect behavior.

Somatic interventions	Behaviors affected
Example: Administer a hormone	→ Strength of mating behavior
Example: Stimulate brain region electrically	→ Movement toward goal object
Example: Cut connections between parts of nervous system	→ Recognition of stimulus

(B) *Behavioral intervention*: Experience affects the body (including the brain).

Somatic effects	Behavioral interventions
Changes in hormone levels	← Example: Put male in presence of female
Changes in electrical activity of brain	← Example: Present a visual stimulus
Anatomical changes in nerve cells	← Example: Give training

(C) *Correlation*: Body and behavioral measures covary.

Somatic variables		Behavioral variables
Brain size	←Correlations→	Learning scores
Hormone levels	←Correlations→	Strength of mating behavior
Enlarged cerebral ventricles	←Correlations→	Schizophrenic symptoms

(D) Behavioral neuroscience seeks to understand all these relationships.

Somatic intervention

Somatic variables ←Correlations→ Behavioral variables

Behavioral intervention

FIGURE 1.10 Three Main Approaches to Studying the Neuroscience of Behavior All three approaches enrich and inform the others.

control group In research, a group of individuals that are identical to those in an experimental (or test) group in every way except that they do not receive the experimental treatment or manipulation. The experimental group is then compared with the control group to assess the effect of the treatment.

within-participants experiment An experiment in which the same set of individuals is compared before and after an experimental manipulation. The experimental group thus serves as its own control group.

between-participants experiment An experiment in which an experimental group of individuals is compared with a control group of individuals that have been treated identically in every way except that they haven't received the experimental manipulation.

behavioral intervention An approach to finding relations between body variables and behavioral variables that involves intervening in the behavior of an organism and looking for resultant changes in body structure or function.

correlation The tendency of two measures to vary in concert, such that a change in one measure is matched by a change in the other.

to some animals, but not others, and comparing the later sexual behavior of both groups; (2) electrically stimulating a specific brain region and measuring alterations in movement; and (3) destroying a specific region in the brain and observing subsequent changes in sleep patterns. In each case, the behavioral measurements follow the bodily intervention; furthermore, in each case the behavioral measurements are compared with those of a **control group**. In a **within-participants experiment**, the control group is simply the same individuals, tested before the somatic intervention occurs. In a **between-participants experiment**, the experimental group of individuals is compared with a different group of individuals who are treated identically in every way except that they don't receive the somatic intervention.

The approach opposite to somatic intervention is **behavioral intervention** (**FIGURE 1.10B**). In this approach the scientist alters or controls the behavior of an organism and looks for resulting changes in body structure or function. Here, behavior is the independent variable, and change in the body is the dependent variable. A few examples include (1) allowing adults of each sex to interact and then measuring subsequent changes in sex hormones, (2) having a person perform a cognitive task while in a brain scanner and then measuring changes in activity in specific regions of the brain, and (3) training an animal to fear a previously neutral stimulus and then observing electrical changes in the brain that may encode the newly learned association. As with somatic intervention, these experimental approaches may employ either within-group or between-groups designs.

The third type of study is **correlation** (**FIGURE 1.10C**), which measures how closely changes in one variable are associated with changes in another variable. Two examples of correlational studies include (1) observing the extent to which memory ability is associated with the size of a certain brain structure and (2) noting that increases in a certain hormone are accompanied by increases in aggressive behavior. Note that while this type of study tells us if the measured variables are associated in some way, it can't tell us which causes the other. We can't tell, for example, whether the hormones cause the aggression or aggression increases the hormones. But even though it can't establish **causality**, correlational research can help researchers identify which things are linked, directly or indirectly, and thus it helps us to develop hypotheses that can be tested experimentally using behavioral and somatic interventions.

Combining these three approaches yields the circle diagram of **FIGURE 1.10D**, showing how the three types of studies complement each other. It also underscores that the effects of brain and behavior are reciprocal: each affects the other in an ongoing cycle. We will see examples of these reciprocal relationships throughout the book.

Research objectives reflect specific theoretical orientations

In designing their research programs, behavioral neuroscientists seek answers to well-defined, specific questions that build on the discoveries of scientists who have gone before. In developing the questions that they wish to study, researchers draw on multiple different research perspectives. Here are some of the major ones:

1. *Systematic description of behavior* Until we describe what we want to study, we cannot accomplish much. Depending on our goals, we may describe behavior in terms of detailed acts or processes, or in terms of results or functions. To be useful for scientific study, a description must be precise, using accurately defined terms and units.

2. *The evolution of brain and behavior* Charles Darwin's theory of evolution through natural selection is central to all modern biology and psychology. Behavioral neuroscientists employ evolutionary theory in two ways: by evaluating *similarities* among species due to shared ancestry, and by looking for species-specific *differences* in behavior and biology that have evolved as adaptations to different environments. We will discuss many examples of both perspectives in this book.

3. *Life span development of the brain and behavior* **Ontogeny** is the process by which an individual changes in the course of its lifetime—that is, grows up and grows old. Observing the way a particular behavior changes during ontogeny may give us clues to its functions and mechanisms. For example, we know that learning and memory abilities in monkeys increase over the first years of life. Therefore, we can speculate that prolonged maturation of brain circuits is required for complex learning tasks.

4. *The biological mechanisms of behavior* To understand the underlying mechanisms of behavior, we must regard the organism (with all due respect) as a "machine," made up of billions of nerve cells, or **neurons**. In a sense, the mechanistic questions are the "how" questions of behavioral neuroscience, in contrast to the "why" questions that derive from the evolutionary and developmental perspectives. So in the case of learning and memory, for example, we might try to understand how a sequence of electrical and biochemical processes allows us to store information in our brains, and how a different process retrieves it.

5. *Applications of behavioral neuroscience discoveries* The practical application of fundamental discoveries in behavioral neuroscience can improve our lives, and as in so many other branches of science, basic and applied research inform each other in a reciprocal manner. We'll see numerous examples of this reciprocity in the book, ranging from genome-based treatment of brain diseases to technological approaches for understanding brain mechanisms of learning, memory, and consciousness.

Animal research is an essential part of life sciences research, including behavioral neuroscience

Because we will draw on animal research throughout this book, we should comment on some of the ethical issues of experimentation on animals. Human beings' involvement and concern with other species predates recorded history; early humans had to study animal behavior and physiology in order to escape some species and hunt others. To study the biological bases of behavior inevitably requires research on animals of other species, as well as on human beings. Psychology students usually underestimate the contributions of animal research to psychology because the most widely used

causality The relation of cause and effect, such that we can conclude that an experimental manipulation has specifically caused an observed result.

ontogeny The process by which an individual changes in the course of its lifetime—that is, grows up and grows old.

neuron Also called *nerve cell*. The basic unit of the nervous system.

BOX 1.1
We Are All Alike, and We Are All Different

Each person has some characteristics shared by…

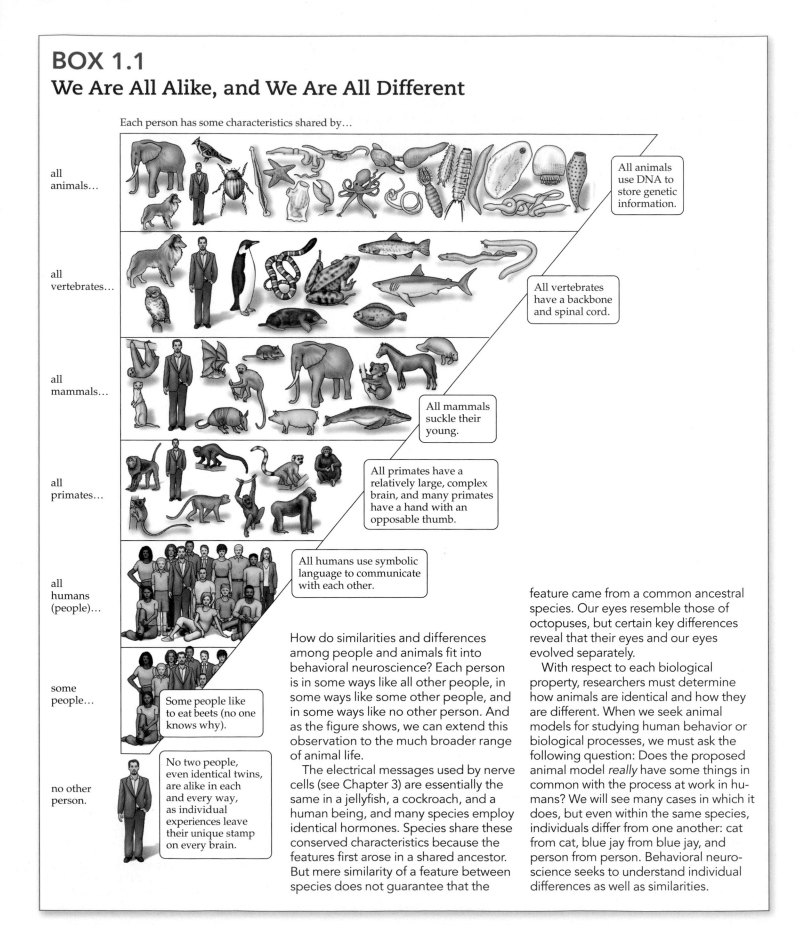

all animals…

All animals use DNA to store genetic information.

all vertebrates…

All vertebrates have a backbone and spinal cord.

all mammals…

All mammals suckle their young.

all primates…

All primates have a relatively large, complex brain, and many primates have a hand with an opposable thumb.

all humans (people)…

All humans use symbolic language to communicate with each other.

some people…

Some people like to eat beets (no one knows why).

no other person.

No two people, even identical twins, are alike in each and every way, as individual experiences leave their unique stamp on every brain.

How do similarities and differences among people and animals fit into behavioral neuroscience? Each person is in some ways like all other people, in some ways like some other people, and in some ways like no other person. And as the figure shows, we can extend this observation to the much broader range of animal life.

The electrical messages used by nerve cells (see Chapter 3) are essentially the same in a jellyfish, a cockroach, and a human being, and many species employ identical hormones. Species share these conserved characteristics because the features first arose in a shared ancestor. But mere similarity of a feature between species does not guarantee that the feature came from a common ancestral species. Our eyes resemble those of octopuses, but certain key differences reveal that their eyes and our eyes evolved separately.

With respect to each biological property, researchers must determine how animals are identical and how they are different. When we seek animal models for studying human behavior or biological processes, we must ask the following question: Does the proposed animal model *really* have some things in common with the process at work in humans? We will see many cases in which it does, but even within the same species, individuals differ from one another: cat from cat, blue jay from blue jay, and person from person. Behavioral neuroscience seeks to understand individual differences as well as similarities.

introductory psychology textbooks often present major findings from animal research as if they were obtained with human participants (Domjan and Purdy, 1995).

A vocal minority of people believe that research with animals, even if it does lead to lasting benefits, is unethical. Others, like Peter Singer in his influential book *Animal Liberation* (1975), argue that animal research is acceptable only when it produces immediate and measurable benefits. The potential cost in taking this perspective lies in the fact that we have no way of predicting which experiments will lead to a breakthrough. The whole point of studying the unknown is that it is unknown; there is a long history of chance observation, based on the steady accumulation of basic knowledge, leading to unexpected benefits.

There's no denying that animal research can cause stress and discomfort, and researchers have a strong ethical obligation to hold pain and stress to the absolute minimum levels possible. Animal research has itself provided us with the drugs and techniques that make most research painless for lab animals, while also leading to improved veterinary care for our animal companions (Sunstein and Nussbaum, 2004), and researchers are ethically bound to continually refine lab practices with animal well-being a primary concern. Researchers are also bound by animal protection legislation and are subject to continual administrative oversight that ensures adherence to nationally mandated animal care policies that emphasize the use of as few animals as possible without jeopardizing research integrity, as well as the use of the simplest species that can answer the questions under study. Selecting the correct animal to study requires a careful evaluation of similarities and differences between species (**BOX 1.1**).

As human beings with the full range of emotions and empathetic feelings toward animals, we all wish there were an alternative to the use of animals in research. But if we want to understand how the nervous system works, we have to actually study it, in detail. The life sciences would slow to a crawl without the basic knowledge that we derive from studying animals.

Behavioral neuroscientists use several levels of analysis

A final consideration that researchers must weigh in designing experiments is the level of complexity at which to work. Even the most complex behavior could, *in theory*, be understood at the level of cellular activity or even lower, at the level of biochemistry and molecular interactions. This idea, that we can understand complex systems by dissecting their simpler constituent parts, is known as **reductionism**. But we wouldn't get very far if we set out to explain, say, the use of grammar in terms of chemical reactions; the behavior is so complex that an explanation at the molecular level would involve a vast amount of data. So instead, the reductionist approach aims to identify **levels of analysis** that are *just simple enough* that they allow us to make rapid progress on the more complex phenomena under study. Finding explanations for behavior often requires several levels of biological analysis, ranging from social interactions, to brain systems, to circuits and single nerve cells and their even simpler, molecular constituents.

Naturally, different problems are carried to different levels of analysis, and fruitful work is often being done simultaneously by different workers at several levels. For example, in their research on visual perception, some cognitive psychologists carefully analyze behavior. They try to determine how the eyes move while looking at a visual pattern, or how the contrast among parts of the pattern determines its visibility. Meanwhile, other behavioral neuroscientists study the differences in visual abilities among species and try to determine the adaptive significance of these differences. For example, how is the presence (or absence) of color vision related to the lifestyle of a species? At the same time, other investigators trace out brain structures and networks involved in different visual tasks. Still other scientists try to understand the electrical and chemical events that occur in the brain during vision (**FIGURE 1.11**).

reductionism   The scientific strategy of breaking a system down into increasingly smaller parts in order to understand it.

level of analysis   The scope of an experimental approach. A scientist may try to understand behavior by monitoring molecules, nerve cells, brain regions, or social environments or using some combination of these levels of analysis.

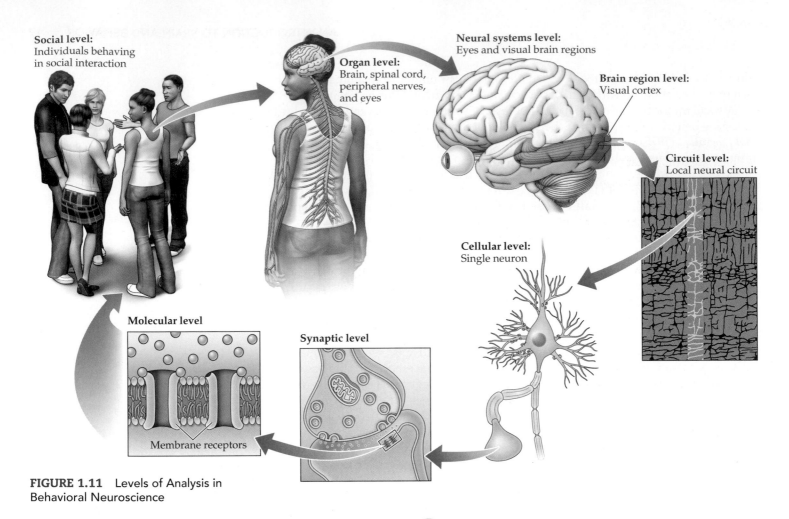

Social level:
Individuals behaving
in social interaction

Organ level:
Brain, spinal cord,
peripheral nerves,
and eyes

Neural systems level:
Eyes and visual brain regions

Brain region level:
Visual cortex

Circuit level:
Local neural circuit

Cellular level:
Single neuron

Molecular level

Membrane receptors

Synaptic level

FIGURE 1.11 Levels of Analysis in
Behavioral Neuroscience

HOW'S IT GOING ?

1. What are the three general forms of research studies in behavioral neuroscience?
   What is the issue of "causality"? How do the three research perspectives inform
   and shape one another?

2. Define *independent variable*, *dependent variable*, *control group*, *within-
   participants experiment*, and *between-participants experiment*.

3. Describe the five major theoretical perspectives employed by modern behavioral neuroscientists that we discussed in the chapter: behavioral description,
   evolution, development, biological mechanisms, and applications.

4. Consider both sides of the debate over animal research, weighing the pros and
   cons of the "for" and "against" positions. How do you think animal use should
   be regulated?

5. What is the general principle behind reductionism? How does this influence the
   level of analysis at which a researcher works? For that matter, what is meant by
   "level of analysis"?

Looking Forward: A Glimpse inside the Mind's Machine

Our mission in this book is to acquaint you with the broad topic of behavioral neuroscience, from historical underpinnings to cutting-edge investigations of the most
complex aspects of our intellect. Along the way, we are going to touch on hundreds of
the most interesting questions in modern neuroscience; here are just a few examples:

- How does the nervous system capture, process, and represent information about
  the environment? For example, sometimes brain damage causes a person to lose
  the ability to identify other people's faces; what does that tell us about how the
  brain works during face recognition?

- What brain sites and activities underlie feelings and emotional expression? Are particular parts of the brain active in romantic love, for example?
- Why are different brain regions active during different language tasks?
- Some people suffer damage to the brain and afterward seem alarmingly unconcerned about dangerous situations and unable to judge the emotions of other people. What parts of the brain are damaged to cause such changes?
- How does the brain manage to change during learning, and how are memories retrieved?
- How does sexual orientation develop? How can gender be defined?

The relationship between the brain and behavior is very mysterious because it is difficult to understand how a physical device, the brain, could be responsible for our subjective experiences of fear, love, and awe. Perhaps it is the "everyday miracle" aspect of the topic that has generated so much folk wisdom—and unfounded mythology—about the brain (Pasquinelli, 2012). For example, the oft-repeated claim that we normally use only 10% of the brain is commonplace—a survey of teachers found that nearly half of them agreed with this cockamamie notion (Howard-Jones, 2014). In fact, brain scans show that the entire brain is active most of the time while we go about normal daily activities. There are lots of other examples of commonplace beliefs about the brain (Macdonald et al., 2017). We've compiled a few of these in **TABLE 1.1**. Some

TABLE 1.1 ■ Neuromythology: Facts or Fables?

Some human nerve cells are more than 3 feet long.	True
Nerve impulses travel at the speed of light.	False
Our bodies make chemicals that are similar in structure to heroin and cannabis.	True
Testosterone is made only by males, and estrogen is made only by females.	False
The adult brain can never grow new nerve cells.	False
Some people are incapable of feeling pain.	True
We have five senses.	False
Different parts of the tongue are specialized to recognize certain tastes.	False
Each side of the brain controls the muscles on the opposite side of the body.	True
There are no anatomical differences between men's and women's brains.	False
Some people are "born gay."	Uncertain
During sleep the brain is relatively inactive.	Not always
Our brain shuts down when we are sleeping.	False
Sleepwalkers are acting out dreams.	False
In some animals, half the brain can be asleep while the other half is awake.	True
All cultural groups recognize the same facial expressions for various emotions.	Uncertain
Scientists are not entirely sure why antidepressant drugs work the way they do.	True
Brain damage can impair your ability to form new memories.	True
Each memory is stored in its own brain cells.	False (probably)
Our memory contains accurate accounts of past experiences.	False (most of the time)
A stimulating environment can change the structure of an animal's brain.	True
We can take in a whole visual scene in just a single glance.	False
My brain decides what I will do next, before my conscious self is aware of the decision.	Uncertain
People are "right-brained" or "left-brained."	False
A child can have half of the brain removed and still develop normal intelligence.	True
Students have different "learning styles" and so should be taught differently.	False
Listening to Mozart and other classical music will make babies smarter.	False
People with dyslexia see letters backward.	False
Physical exercise can improve brain function.	True
Children are less attentive after drinking sugary beverages.	False

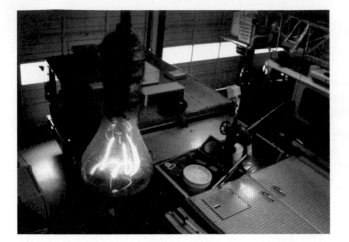

A Bright Idea The symbolic lightbulb coming on over someone's head, representing a sudden insight or idea, is an especially apt metaphor for the functioning of the brain, given the lightbulb's rapid action and ability to penetrate the gloom (both literal and metaphorical). This particular lightbulb, in a fire station in Livermore, California, is the world's longest-burning bulb (you can check in on it, live, at www.centennialbulb.org/cam. htm). It has been continually lit for more than 1 million hours (about 115 years)—since the dawn of the scientific discipline of behavioral neuroscience. (© Caters News/ Zuma Press.)

of them are unfounded; others are true but may sound improbable. No doubt you can think of others.

Of course, it wasn't that long ago that the idea of making light from electricity seemed far-fetched. With each passing year, technological developments and the progress of thousands of neuroscientists in labs around the world provide a clearer view of what is happening when a lightbulb goes on in the mind and someone has a clever idea. Our hope for this book is that it will turn on a few lightbulbs for you too.

Recommended Reading

Decety, J., and Cacioppo, J. T. (2011). *The Oxford Handbook of Social Neuroscience.* New York, NY: Oxford University Press.

Doidge, N. (2007). *The Brain That Changes Itself.* New York, NY: Penguin.

Finger, S. (2001). *Origins of Neuroscience.* New York, NY: Oxford University Press.

Kaku, M. (2015). *The Future of the Mind: The Scientific Quest to Understand, Enhance, and Empower the Mind.* New York, NY: Random House.

Koch, C. (2012). *Consciousness: Confessions of a Romantic Reductionist.* Cambridge, MA: MIT Press.

Wickens, A. P. (2014). *A History of the Brain: From Stone Age Surgery to Modern Neuroscience.* New York, NY: Psychology Press.

You should be able to relate each summary to the adjacent illustration, including structures and processes. If you go to the website for our text (**3e.mindsmachine.com**), you can follow links to figures, animations, and activities that will help you consolidate the material.

1 **Behavioral neuroscience** is a branch of **neuroscience** that focuses on the biological bases of behavior. It is closely related to many other neuroscience disciplines. Review **Figure 1.1**, **Animation 1.2**

2 Although humans have wondered about the control of behavior for thousands of years, only comparatively recently has a mechanistic view of the brain taken hold. Review **Figure 1.3**

3 The concept of **localization of function**, which originated in **phrenology**—despite obvious flaws with the phrenologists' methodology—was an important milestone for behavioral neuroscience. Localization of cognitive functions remains a major focus of behavioral neuroscience. With modern imaging technology and a more carefully validated understanding of cognitive abilities, a detailed view of the organization of the brain is emerging. Today we know that the part of the brain that shows a peak of activity varies in a predictable way depending on what task we're doing. Review **Figure 1.4**

4 The prevalence of neurological and psychiatric disorders exacts a very high emotional and economic toll. Review **Figure 1.6**

5 Although genes can have a major impact on brain function, it is clear that experience physically alters the brain and that genetically identical people will not necessarily suffer from the same brain disorders. Review **Figure 1.7**

6 Behavioral neuroscientists balance three general research perspectives—**correlation**, **somatic intervention**, and **behavioral intervention**—in designing their research. Review **Figure 1.10**

7 Research in behavioral neuroscience is conducted at levels of analysis ranging from molecular events to the functioning of the entire brain and complex social situations. Review **Figure 1.11**

Go to **3e.mindsmachine.com** for study questions, quizzes, flashcards, and other resources.

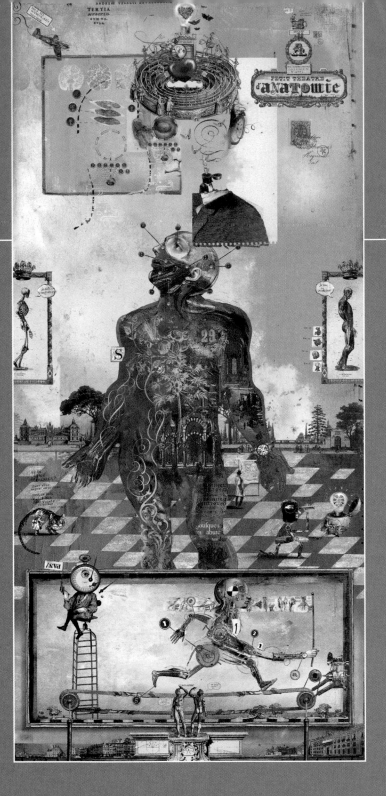

2

Cells and Structures
The Anatomy of the
Nervous System

Electrical Storm

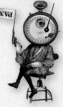

Sam had been complaining about feeling a bit odd all day; he thought perhaps he was coming down with a bug. But when he collapsed unconscious to the floor of the lunchroom at work and began twitching and jerking, it was clear that he had a much bigger problem than the flu. Sam was having a *seizure*, a type of uncontrollable convulsion that he'd never had before. By the time Sam arrived at the hospital, the seizure had stopped, and although he was confused and slow to respond to commands, he didn't seem to be in distress. But when Sam smiled at Dr. Cheng, the attending neurologist, and offered to shake her hand, Dr. Cheng ordered immediate brain scans: Sam could offer only half a smile, because only the left side of his face was working, and he was unable to grip Dr. Cheng's hand at all.

How can an understanding of the pathways between brain and body provide clues about Sam's problem? We now know quite a bit about the neural organization of basic functions, but the control of complex cognition remains a tantalizing mystery. However, the advent of sophisticated brain-imaging technology has invigorated the search for answers to fundamental questions about brain organization: Does each brain region control a specific behavior, or is the pattern of connections within the brain more important? Do some regions of the brain act as general purpose information processors? Is everybody's brain organized in the same way?

Almost everything about us—our thoughts, feelings, and behavior, however serious or silly—is the product of a knobbly three-pound organ that, despite its unremarkable appearance, is the most complicated object in the known universe. In this chapter we'll have a look at the structure of the brain from several different perspectives: the brain's cellular composition, its major anatomical divisions, and its appearance in computerized brain imaging. In later chapters we will build on this information as we learn how cells within the brain communicate through electrical (see Chapter 3) and chemical (see Chapter 4) signals.

To see the video
Inside the Brain,
go to
3e.mindsmachine.com/av2.1

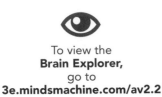

To view the
Brain Explorer,
go to
3e.mindsmachine.com/av2.2

PART I
The Cellular Components of the Nervous System

THE ROAD AHEAD

The first part of the chapter is concerned with the cells of the nervous system. By the end of the section, you should be able to:

1. Name and describe the general function of the four main parts of a neuron.
2. Classify neurons according to both structure and function.
3. Outline the basic structure of a synapse and the steps in neurotransmission.
4. Describe the four principal types of glial cells.

The Nervous System Contains Several Types of Cells

All of your organs and muscles are in communication with the nervous system, which, like all other living tissue, is made up of highly specialized cells. The most important of these are the **neurons** (or *nerve cells*), arranged into the neural circuits that underlie all forms of behavior, from simple reflexes to complex cognition. Each neuron receives inputs from many other cells, integrates those inputs, and then distributes the processed information to other neurons. Your brain contains 80–90 billion of these tiny cellular computers (Herculano-Houzel, 2012), working together to process vast amounts of information with apparent ease. An even larger number of **glial cells** (sometimes called just *glia*) are found in the human brain, mostly providing a variety of support functions but also participating in information processing. Because neurons are larger and produce readily measured electrical signals, we know much more about them than about glial cells.

An important early controversy in neuroscience concerned the functional independence of individual neurons: Was each neuron a discrete component? Or were the cells of the nervous system fused together into larger functional units, like continuous circuits? Through painstaking study of the fine details of individual neurons, the celebrated Spanish anatomist Santiago Ramón y Cajal (1852–1934) was able to show that although neurons come very close together, they are not quite *continuous* with one another. Ramón y Cajal and his contemporaries showed that (1) the neurons and other cells of the brain are structurally, metabolically, and functionally independent; and (2) information is transmitted from neuron to neuron across tiny gaps, later named **synapses**—a notion that came to be known as the *neuron doctrine*.

It's impossible to measure exactly how many synapses there are in the brain, but scientists think there may be as many as 10^{15} (a *quadrillion*) synapses. That's a number too huge for most of us to comprehend: if you gathered a quadrillion grains of sand, each a millimeter in diameter, they would fill a cube that is longer than an American football field on each side—well over a million cubic yards, or 750,000 cubic meters (in more familiar units that's about 260 million gallons of sand, or 750 million liters)! These vast networks of connections are responsible for all of our achievements.

The neuron has four principal divisions

Like most human cells, a neuron contains genes encoded in DNA inside a cell nucleus, as well as a wide assortment of organelles. As in other cells of the body, some organelles (the mitochondria) produce energy, while others (the ribosomes) translate genetic instructions from the nucleus into the specialized proteins needed for the operation of the neuron (consult the Appendix if you need a refresher on cell biology). As we will see, neurons vary widely in size, shape, and function, but almost all neurons also share a set of unique, highly specialized features for

neuron   Also called *nerve cell*. The basic unit of the nervous system, each composed of receptive extensions called dendrites, an integrating cell body, a conducting axon, and a transmitting axon terminal.

glial cells   Also called *glia*. Nonneuronal brain cells that provide structural, nutritional, and other types of support to the brain.

synapse   The cellular location at which information is transmitted from a neuron to another cell.

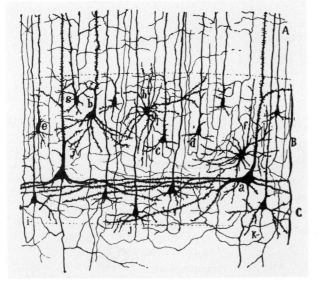

Nineteenth-Century Drawings of Neurons   Santiago Ramón y Cajal perfected methods for visualizing the detailed structure of individual neurons (labeled by Ramón y Cajal with lowercase letters). Ramón y Cajal and his collaborators proposed that neurons are discrete cells that communicate via tiny contacts, which were later named synapses.

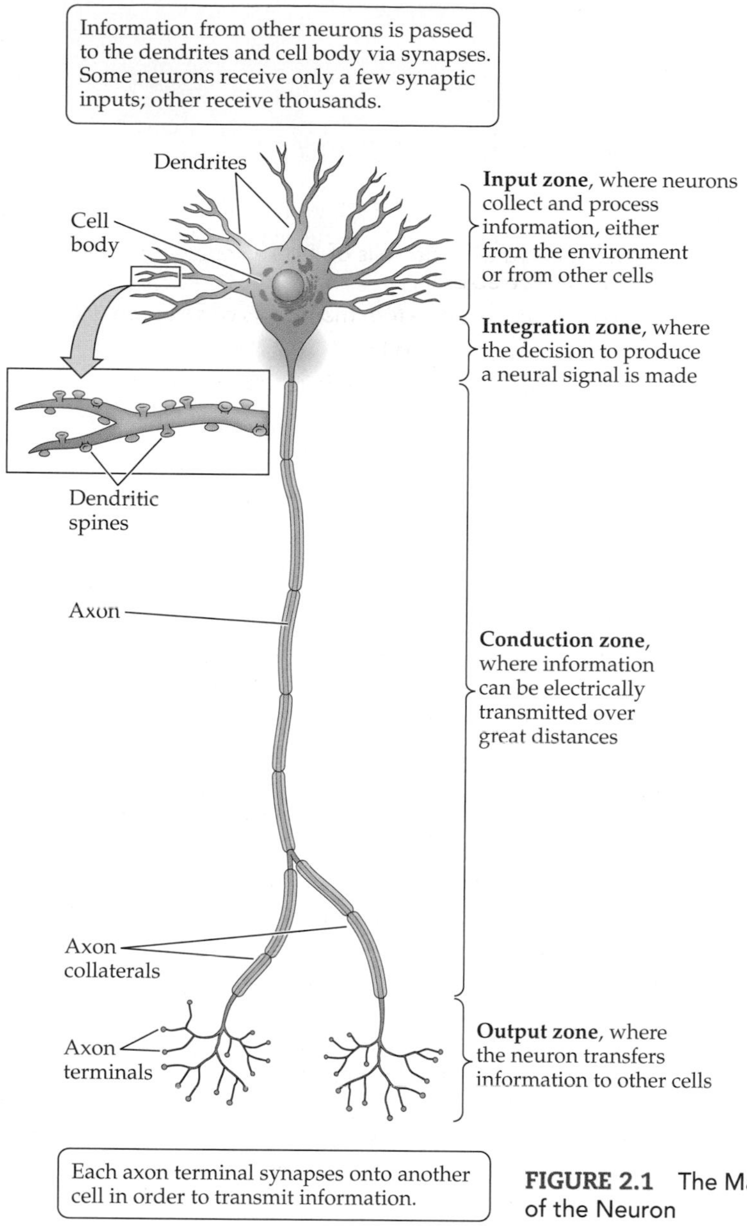

Information from other neurons is passed to the dendrites and cell body via synapses. Some neurons receive only a few synaptic inputs; other receive thousands.

Dendrites

Cell body

Dendritic spines

Axon

Axon collaterals

Axon terminals

Input zone, where neurons collect and process information, either from the environment or from other cells

Integration zone, where the decision to produce a neural signal is made

Conduction zone, where information can be electrically transmitted over great distances

Output zone, where the neuron transfers information to other cells

Each axon terminal synapses onto another cell in order to transmit information.

FIGURE 2.1 The Major Parts of the Neuron

collecting inputs from multiple sources, processing and combining this information, and distributing the results of this processing to other cells. These information-processing features, illustrated in **FIGURE 2.1**, can be viewed as belonging to four functional zones:

1. **Input zone** At cellular extensions called **dendrites** (from the Greek *dendron*, "tree"), neurons receive information via synapses from other neurons. Some neurons have dendrites that are elaborately branched, providing room for many synapses. Dendrites may be covered in *dendritic spines*, small projections from the surface of the dendrite that add additional space for synapses.

2. **Integration zone** In addition to receiving additional synaptic inputs, the neuron's **cell body** (or *soma*, plural *somata*) integrates (combines) the information that has been received to determine whether or not to send a signal of its own.

3. **Conduction zone** A single extension, the **axon** (or *nerve fiber*), carries the neuron's own electrical signals away from the cell body. Toward its end, the axon may split into multiple branches called **axon collaterals**.

4. **Output zone** Specialized swellings at the ends of the axon, called **axon terminals** (or *synaptic boutons*), transmit the neuron's signals across synapses to other cells.

input zone The part of a neuron that receives information from other neurons or from specialized sensory structures.

dendrite An extension of the cell body that receives information from other neurons.

integration zone The part of a neuron that initiates neural electrical activity.

cell body Also called *soma*. The region of a neuron that is defined by the presence of the cell nucleus.

conduction zone The part of a neuron—typically the axon—over which the action potential is actively propagated.

axon Also called *nerve fiber*. A single extension from the nerve cell that carries action potentials from the cell body toward the axon terminals.

axon collateral A branch of an axon.

output zone The part of a neuron at which the cell sends information to another cell.

axon terminal Also called *synaptic bouton*. The end of an axon or axon collateral, which forms a synapse onto a neuron or other target cell and thus serves as the output zone.

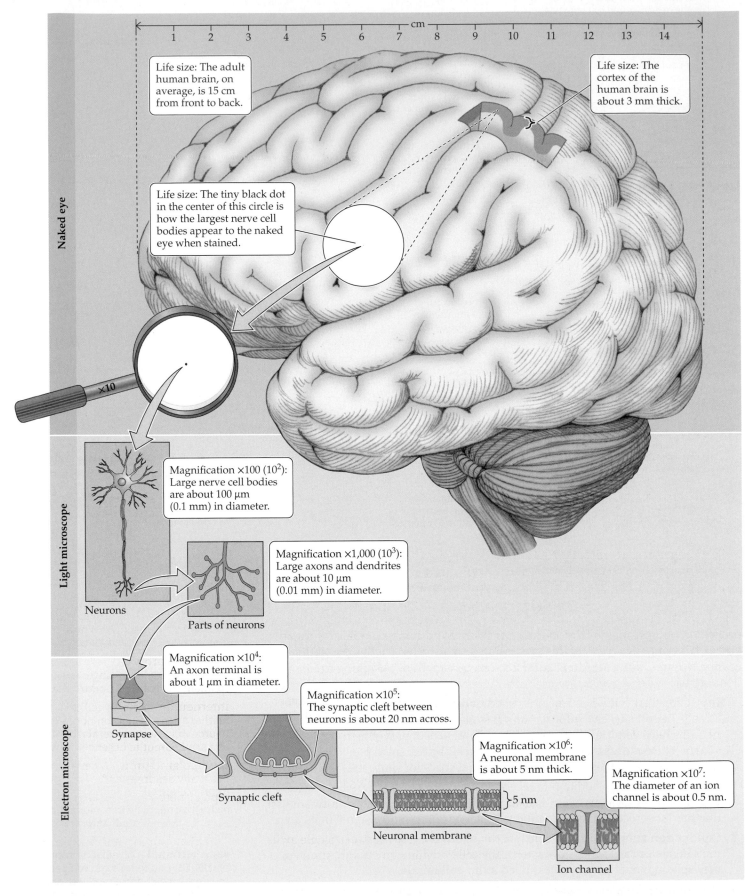

cm

Life size: The adult human brain, on average, is 15 cm from front to back.

Life size: The cortex of the human brain is about 3 mm thick.

Life size: The tiny black dot in the center of this circle is how the largest nerve cell bodies appear to the naked eye when stained.

×10

Naked eye

Light microscope

Magnification ×100 (10^2): Large nerve cell bodies are about 100 μm (0.1 mm) in diameter.

Neurons

Magnification ×1,000 (10^3): Large axons and dendrites are about 10 μm (0.01 mm) in diameter.

Parts of neurons

Electron microscope

Magnification ×10^4: An axon terminal is about 1 μm in diameter.

Synapse

Magnification ×10^5: The synaptic cleft between neurons is about 20 nm across.

Synaptic cleft

Magnification ×10^6: A neuronal membrane is about 5 nm thick.

5 nm

Neuronal membrane

Magnification ×10^7: The diameter of an ion channel is about 0.5 nm.

Ion channel

FIGURE 2.2   Sizes of Some Neural Structures and the Units of Measure and Magnification Used in Studying Them

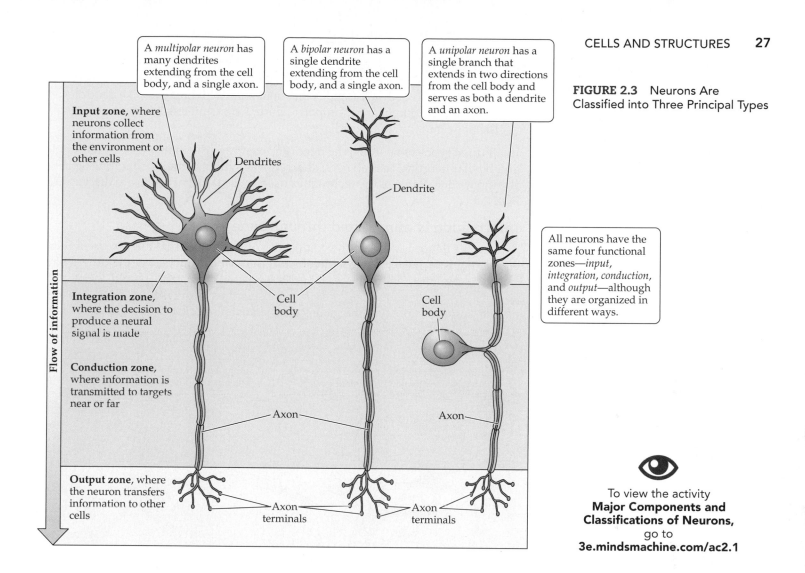

A *multipolar neuron* has many dendrites extending from the cell body, and a single axon.

A *bipolar neuron* has a single dendrite extending from the cell body, and a single axon.

A *unipolar neuron* has a single branch that extends in two directions from the cell body and serves as both a dendrite and an axon.

FIGURE 2.3 Neurons Are Classified into Three Principal Types

Input zone, where neurons collect information from the environment or other cells

Dendrites

Dendrite

All neurons have the same four functional zones—*input, integration, conduction,* and *output*—although they are organized in different ways.

Integration zone, where the decision to produce a neural signal is made

Cell body

Cell body

Flow of information

Conduction zone, where information is transmitted to targets near or far

Axon

Axon

Output zone, where the neuron transfers information to other cells

Axon terminals

Axon terminals

To view the activity **Major Components and Classifications of Neurons,** go to **3e.mindsmachine.com/ac2.1**

There are hundreds of different forms of neurons, specialized to perform different kinds of processing. For example, **motor neurons** (also called *motoneurons*) are large and have long axons reaching out to synapse on muscles, causing muscular contractions. As their name implies, **sensory neurons** are specialized to gather sensory information, and they take many different shapes depending on whether they detect light or sound or touch and so on. Most of the neurons in the brain are **interneurons**, which analyze information gathered from one set of neurons and communicate with others. The axons of interneurons may measure only a few micrometers (μm; a micrometer is a millionth of a meter), while motor neurons and sensory neurons may have axons a meter or more in length, conveying information to and from the most distant parts of the body. In general, larger neurons tend to have more-complex inputs and outputs, cover greater distances, and/or convey information more rapidly than smaller neurons. The relative sizes of neural structures that we will be discussing throughout the book are illustrated in **FIGURE 2.2**.

In addition to size, neuroscientists classify neurons into three general categories of shape, each specialized for a particular kind of information processing (**FIGURE 2.3**):

1. **Multipolar neurons** have many dendrites and a single axon. They are the most common type of neuron.

2. **Bipolar neurons** have a single dendrite at one end of the cell and a single axon at the other end. Bipolar neurons are especially common in sensory systems, such as vision.

3. **Unipolar neurons** (also called *monopolar neurons*) have a single extension (or process), usually thought of as an axon, that branches in two directions after

motor neuron Also called *motoneuron.* A neuron that transmits neural messages to muscles (or glands).

sensory neuron A nerve cell that is directly affected by changes in the environment, such as light, odor, or touch.

interneuron A nerve cell that is neither a sensory neuron nor a motor neuron; interneurons receive input from and send output to other neurons.

multipolar neuron A nerve cell that has many dendrites and a single axon.

bipolar neuron A nerve cell that has a single dendrite at one end and a single axon at the other end.

unipolar neuron Also called *monopolar neuron.* A nerve cell with a single branch that leaves the cell body and then extends in two directions; one end is the input zone, and the other end is the output zone.

leaving the cell body. One end is the input zone with branches like dendrites; the other, the output zone. Unipolar neurons transmit touch information from the body into the spinal cord.

In all three types of neurons, the dendrites comprise the input zone. In multipolar and bipolar neurons, the cell body also receives synaptic inputs, so it is also part of the input zone. Some of the techniques used to visualize neurons are discussed in **BOX 2.1**.

Information is transmitted through synapses

A neuron's dendrites reflect the complexity of the inputs that are received. Some simple neurons have just a couple of short dendritic branches, while others have huge and complex dendritic trees (or *arbors*) covered in many thousands of synaptic contacts from other neurons. At each synapse, information is transmitted from an axon terminal of a **presynaptic** neuron to the **postsynaptic** neuron (**FIGURE 2.4A**).

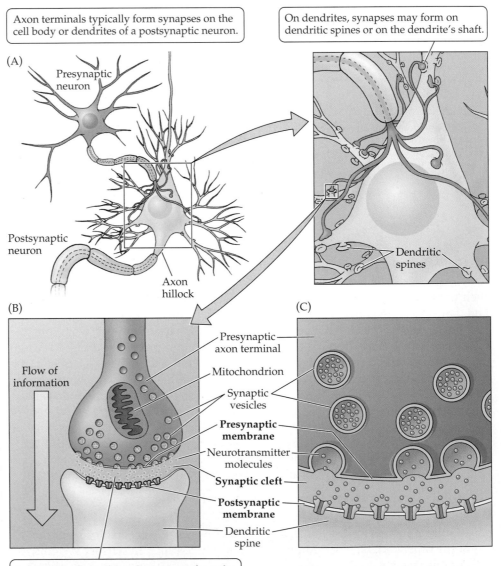

Axon terminals typically form synapses on the cell body or dendrites of a postsynaptic neuron.

On dendrites, synapses may form on dendritic spines or on the dendrite's shaft.

(A)

Presynaptic neuron

Postsynaptic neuron

Axon hillock

Dendritic spines

(B)

Flow of information

(C)

Presynaptic axon terminal

Mitochondrion

Synaptic vesicles

Presynaptic membrane

Neurotransmitter molecules

Synaptic cleft

Postsynaptic membrane

Dendritic spine

Information flows through a synapse from the presynaptic membrane across a gap called the *synaptic cleft* to the postsynaptic membrane.

presynaptic Located on the "transmitting" side of a synapse.

postsynaptic Referring to the region of a synapse that receives and responds to neurotransmitter.

FIGURE 2.4 Synapses

BOX 2.1
Visualizing the Cellular Structure of the Brain

Histology—the scientific study of the composition of tissue—underwent a revolution beginning in the mid-1800s, when derivatives of fabric dyes were found to vividly stain cells in ways that allowed visualization of previously hidden microscopic structure. In the nervous system, it became possible to selectively stain different parts of neurons and glia, such as cell membranes, the cell body, or the sheaths surrounding axons. Nowadays, scientists use specialized staining procedures to study the numbers, shapes, distribution, and interconnections of neurons within targeted regions of the brain.

Counting Cells in Brain Regions

Nissl stains outline all of the cell bodies in a tissue section, allowing us to measure the size and density of cell bodies in particular regions (**FIGURE A**). Many types of Nissl stains and other traditional general-purpose cell stains are available.

Examining the Forms of Individual Neurons

Mysteriously, and in contrast to Nissl stains, **Golgi stains** label only a small minority of neurons in a sample, but the affected cells are stained very deeply and completely, revealing fine details of cell structure such as the branches of dendrites and axons (**FIGURE B**). Golgi-stained neurons stand out in sharp contrast to their unstained neighbors, so Golgi staining is useful for identifying the types and precise shapes of neurons in a region. There are a number of variants on this strategy, such as filling cells with fluorescent molecules.

Mapping the Expression of Cellular Products

Often, neuroscientists would like to know the distribution of neurons that exhibit a specific property, such as sensitivity to a hormone or drug, production of particular proteins, or possession of a particular activated gene. Numerous clever techniques have been developed to trick such neurons into revealing themselves. In **autoradiography**, for example, animals are treated with radioactive versions of experimental drugs, and then thin slices of the brain are placed alongside photographic film. Radioactivity emitted by the labeled compound in the tissue "exposes" the emulsion—as light does striking film—so the brain essentially takes a picture of itself, highlighting the specific brain regions where the drug has become selectively concentrated. An alternative way to visualize cells that have an attribute in common—termed **immunohistochemistry (IHC)**—involves creating antibodies against a protein of interest (we can create antibodies to almost any protein). Equipped with colorful labels, these antibodies can selectively seek out and attach themselves to their target proteins within neurons in a brain slice, revealing the distribution of only those neurons that make the target protein. In the example in **FIGURE C**, antibodies have labeled only those cells containing a protein expressed by *c-fos*, which is an immediate early gene (IEG) that is expressed in cells that have been recently active. Localizing IEG proteins allows researchers to identify brain regions that were active during particular behaviors performed by an animal shortly before it was euthanized. A related procedure called **in situ hybridization** goes a step further and, using radioactively labeled lengths of nucleic acid (RNA or DNA, see the Appendix), labels only those neurons in which a gene of interest has been turned on.

Tracing Interconnections between Neurons

Many research questions are more concerned with the pattern of connections between neurons than with their cellular structure (**FIGURE D**). But tracing the interconnections between regions is a technical challenge, because axons are profuse and tiny, follow intricate routes, and are difficult to disentangle from one another. To accomplish this

(A) Nissl stain

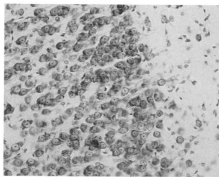

(B) Golgi stain

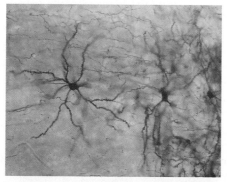

(C) Expression of *c-fos* in activated cells

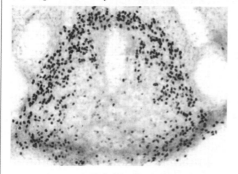

(D) Tract tracing

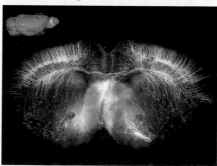

(*Continued*)

goal, scientists have developed many sorts of **tract tracers**, substances that are taken up by neurons and transported over the routes of their axons. In *anterograde labeling* the tract tracer is injected near the dendrites and cell bodies of a region of interest, where it is taken up and transported to the tips of the axons, thus revealing the targets of the neurons under study.

Conversely, in *retrograde labeling*, when a different kind of tract tracer is injected into a region of interest, it is exclusively taken up by axon terminals and then transported back to their originating cell bodies, thus revealing the sources of innervation of the region. Some tract tracers can even jump across synapses and work their way through the length of the neural pathway, leaving

visible molecules of label all along the way. (Figure A courtesy of Dr. Cynthia L. Jordan, Michigan State University; B courtesy of Dr. Timothy DeVoogd; C from N. Sunn et al., 2002. *P. Natl. Acad. Sci. U.S.A.* 99: 3. © National Academy of Sciences, U.S.A; D from J. Yuan et al., 2015. *Front. Neuroanat.* 9: 70, courtesy of Dr. Qingming Luo.)

A synapse typically consists of the following elements (**FIGURE 2.4B**):

1. The specialized **presynaptic membrane** of the axon terminal of the presynaptic (i.e., transmitting) neuron
2. The **synaptic cleft**, a gap of about 20–40 nanometers (nm; billionths of a meter) that separates the presynaptic and postsynaptic neurons
3. The specialized **postsynaptic membrane** on the dendrite or cell body of the postsynaptic (i.e., receiving) neuron

Presynaptic axon terminals contain many tiny hollow spheres called **synaptic vesicles**. Each synaptic vesicle contains molecules of **neurotransmitter**, the special chemical with which a presynaptic neuron communicates with postsynaptic cells. This communication starts when synaptic vesicles fuse to the presynaptic membrane and then rupture, releasing their contents into the synaptic cleft (see Figure 2.4B). After crossing the cleft, the released neurotransmitter molecules interact with matching **neurotransmitter receptors** that stud the postsynaptic membrane. The receptors capture and react to molecules of the neurotransmitter, altering the level of excitation of the postsynaptic neuron. This action affects the likelihood that the postsynaptic neuron will in turn release its own neurotransmitter from its axon terminals. Molecules of neurotransmitter generally do not enter the postsynaptic neuron; they simply bind to the receptors momentarily to induce a response, and then disengage.

The configuration of synapses on a neuron's dendrites and cell body is constantly changing—synapses come and go, dendrites change their shapes, dendritic spines wax and wane—in response to new patterns of synaptic activity and the formation of new neural circuits. We use the general term **neuroplasticity** to refer to this capacity for continual remodeling of the connections between neurons. We will take a much more detailed look at neurotransmission in Chapters 3 and 4.

The axon integrates and then transmits information

Most neurons feature a distinctive cone-shaped enlargement on the cell body called an **axon hillock** ("little hill"), from which the neuron's axon projects. The axon hillock has unique properties that allow it to gather and integrate the information arriving from the synapses on the dendrites and cell body. As we will discuss in more detail later, this process of integration determines when the neuron will produce neural signals of its own. The neuron's output information, encoded in a stream of electrical impulses, then races down the axon toward the targets that the neuron is said to **innervate**.

The axon is a hollow tube, and various important substances, such as enzymes and structural proteins, are conveyed inside the axon from the cell body, where they are produced, to the axon terminals, where they are used. This **axonal transport** works in both directions: *anterograde transport* moves materials toward the axon terminals,

presynaptic membrane   The specialized membrane on the axon terminal of a nerve cell that transmits information by releasing neurotransmitter.

synaptic cleft   The space between the presynaptic and postsynaptic neurons at a synapse.

postsynaptic membrane   The specialized membrane on the surface of a neuron that receives information by responding to neurotransmitter from a presynaptic neuron.

synaptic vesicle   A small, spherical structure that contains molecules of neurotransmitter.

neurotransmitter   Also called *synaptic transmitter*, *chemical transmitter*, or simply *transmitter*. The chemical released from the presynaptic axon terminal that serves as the basis of communication between neurons.

neurotransmitter receptor   Also called simply *receptor*. A specialized protein, that selectively senses and reacts to molecules of a corresponding neurotransmitter or hormone.

neuroplasticity   Also called *neural plasticity*. The ability of the nervous system to change in response to experience or the environment.

axon hillock   The cone-shaped area on the cell body from which the axon originates.

innervate   To provide neural input to.

axonal transport   The transportation of materials from the neuronal cell body toward the axon terminals, and from the axon terminals back toward the cell body.

and *retrograde transport* moves used materials back to the cell body for recycling. Thus the axon has two quite different functions: the rapid transmission of electrical signals along the outer membrane, and the much slower transportation of substances within the axon, to and from the axon terminals.

Glial cells protect and assist neurons

Early neuroscientists had little regard for glial cells, viewing them as a mere filler holding the neurons together (in Greek *glia* means "glue"). But we now know that glial cells are much more important than that. Glial cells directly affect neuronal processes by providing neurons with raw materials, chemical signals, and specialized structural components.

There are as many or more glial cells as there are neurons in the nervous system (Herculano-Houzel, 2014), but in contrast to the hundreds of types of neurons that have been identified, there are just four kinds of glial cells (**FIGURE 2.5**). Two of the four types of glia—**oligodendrocytes** and **Schwann cells**—wrap around successive segments of axons to insulate them with a fatty substance called **myelin**. These myelin sheaths give an axon the appearance of a string of elongated slender beads. Between adjacent beads, small uninsulated patches of axonal membrane, called **nodes of Ranvier**, remain exposed (**FIGURE 2.5A**). Within the brain and spinal cord, myelination is provided by the oligodendrocytes, each cell typically supplying myelin beads to several nearby axons (also illustrated in Figure 2.5A). In the rest of the body, it is Schwann cells that do the ensheathing, with each Schwann cell wrapping itself around a segment of one axon to provide a single bead of myelin. But whether it is provided by oligodendrocytes or by Schwann cells, myelination has the same result: a large increase

oligodendrocyte A type of glial cell that forms myelin in the central nervous system.

Schwann cell A type of glial cell that forms myelin in the peripheral nervous system.

myelin The fatty insulation around an axon, formed by glial cells. This sheath boosts the speed at which nerve impulses are conducted.

node of Ranvier A gap between successive segments of the myelin sheath where the axon membrane is exposed.

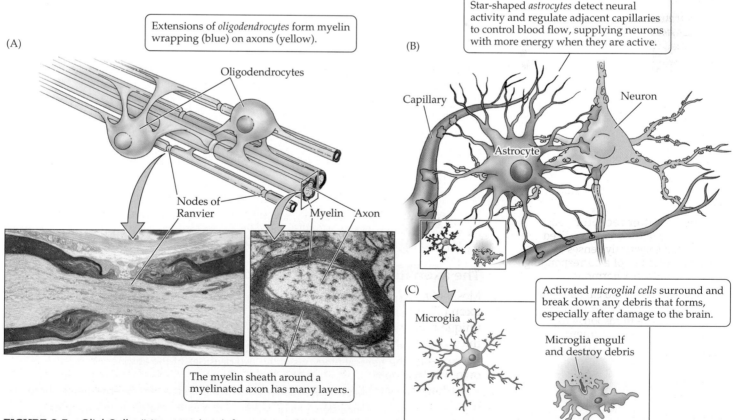

(A)

Extensions of *oligodendrocytes* form myelin wrapping (blue) on axons (yellow).

Oligodendrocytes

Nodes of Ranvier

Myelin Axon

The myelin sheath around a myelinated axon has many layers.

(B)

Star-shaped *astrocytes* detect neural activity and regulate adjacent capillaries to control blood flow, supplying neurons with more energy when they are active.

Capillary

Neuron

Astrocyte

(C)

Microglia

Activated *microglial cells* surround and break down any debris that forms, especially after damage to the brain.

Microglia engulf and destroy debris

FIGURE 2.5 **Glial Cells** (Micrograph A *left* courtesy of Mark Ellisman and the Natl. Ctr. Microsc. Imag. Res.; *right* © ISM/CTμ-UCBL/Medical Images.)

astrocyte A star-shaped glial cell with numerous processes (extensions) that run in all directions.

microglial cells Also called *microglia*. Extremely small motile glial cells that remove cellular debris from injured or dead cells.

edema A general term referring to swelling of any body tissue, including the brain.

gross neuroanatomy Anatomical features of the nervous system that are apparent to the naked eye.

central nervous system (CNS) The portion of the nervous system that includes the brain and the spinal cord.

in the speed with which electrical signals pass down the axon, jumping from one node of Ranvier to the next. (In Chapter 3 we discuss the diverse abnormalities that arise when the myelin insulation is compromised in the disease multiple sclerosis [MS].)

The other two types of glial cells—astrocytes and microglial cells—perform more diverse functions in the brain. **Astrocytes** (from the Greek *astron*, "star") weave around and between neurons with tentacle-like extensions (**FIGURE 2.5B**), helping to define the structure of the brain. Some astrocytes stretch between neurons and fine blood vessels, controlling local blood flow to increase the amount of blood reaching more-active brain regions (Schummers et al., 2008). Astrocytes help to form the tough outer membranes that swaddle the brain, and they also secrete chemical signals that affect synaptic transmission and the formation of synapses (R. D. Fields and Stevens-Graham, 2002; Perea et al., 2009). In contrast, **microglial cells** (or *microglia*) are tiny and mobile (**FIGURE 2.5C**). Their primary job appears to be to contain and clean up sites of injury (Davalos et al., 2005), but research is revealing unexpected additional roles for microglia, such as participation in pain perception and neuronal remodeling (S. Beggs et al., 2012; Chung et al., 2013) and in neurological disease.

Although glial cells perform many beneficial functions, they can also cause problems. For one thing, because they continue to divide in adulthood (unlike neurons), glial cells can give rise to deadly brain tumors. In addition, some glial cells, especially astrocytes, respond to brain injury by swelling. **Edema**—the swelling of tissue—damages neurons and is responsible for many symptoms of brain injuries. Glial cells are also suspected of actively contributing to the synaptic and cognitive impairments seen in various neurodegenerative diseases such as Alzheimer's disease (Chung et al., 2015; Liddelow et al., 2017).

Supported and influenced by glial cells, and sharing information through synapses, neurons form the vast ensembles of information-processing circuits that give the brain its visible form. Powerful anatomical and genetic initiatives, such as the Allen Institute brain mapping project (www.brain-map.org), are now creating detailed maps of the cellular compositions of the major divisions of the brain. These major divisions are our next topic.

─ **HOW'S IT GOING** ❓ ────────────────

1. What are the four "zones" common to all neurons, and what are their functions?
2. Compare and contrast axonal signal transmission and axonal transport.
3. Describe the three main components of the synapse. What are some of the specialized structures found on each side of the synapse?
4. What are the names and general functions of the four types of glial cells?
5. What special properties does myelin have?

PART II
The Large Scale Structure of the Nervous System

━━ **THE ROAD AHEAD** ━━━━━━━━━━━━━━

The second part of the chapter surveys the major components of the nervous system. By the end of the section, you should be able to:

1. Explain what a nerve is, and distinguish between somatic and autonomic nerves.
2. Identify the cranial and spinal nerves by name and function.
3. Describe the general functions of the two divisions of the autonomic nervous system.
4. Name the main anatomical structures that make up the two cerebral hemispheres.
5. Explain the difference between gray matter and white matter, with examples.
6. Describe the fetal development of the brain.

The Nervous System Extends throughout the Body

Large collections of cell bodies and axons form the tissues that define the **gross neuroanatomy** of the nervous system—the neural structures that are visible to the unaided eye (in this context *gross* means "large," not "yucky"). The gross view of the entire human nervous system presented in **FIGURE 2.6** reveals the basic division between the **central nervous system** (**CNS**; consisting of the brain and spinal cord) and the **peripheral nervous system** (everything else). The anatomical organization of these systems is our next topic.

The peripheral nervous system has two divisions

The peripheral nervous system consists of **nerves**—collections of axons bundled together—that extend throughout the body. Some nerves, called **motor nerves**, transmit information from the spinal cord and brain to muscles and glands; others, called **sensory nerves**, convey information from the body to the CNS. The various nerves of the body are divided into two distinct systems:

1. The **somatic nervous system**, which consists of nerves that interconnect the brain and the major muscles and sensory systems of the body
2. The **autonomic nervous system**, which consists of nerves that connect primarily to the viscera (internal organs)

peripheral nervous system The portion of the nervous system that includes all the nerves and neurons outside the brain and spinal cord.

nerve A collection of axons bundled together outside the central nervous system.

motor nerve A nerve that transmits information from the central nervous system to the muscles and glands.

sensory nerve A nerve that conveys information from the body to the central nervous system.

somatic nervous system A part of the peripheral nervous system that supplies neural connections mostly to the skeletal muscles and sensory systems of the body. It consists of cranial nerves and spinal nerves.

autonomic nervous system A part of the peripheral nervous system that provides the main neural connections to the internal organs.

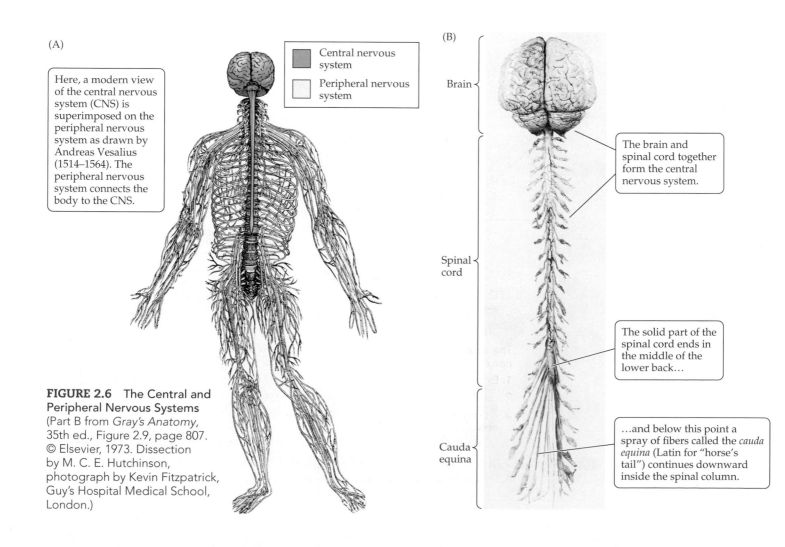

(A)

Here, a modern view of the central nervous system (CNS) is superimposed on the peripheral nervous system as drawn by Andreas Vesalius (1514–1564). The peripheral nervous system connects the body to the CNS.

■ Central nervous system
□ Peripheral nervous system

(B)

Brain

The brain and spinal cord together form the central nervous system.

Spinal cord

The solid part of the spinal cord ends in the middle of the lower back…

Cauda equina

…and below this point a spray of fibers called the *cauda equina* (Latin for "horse's tail") continues downward inside the spinal column.

FIGURE 2.6 The Central and Peripheral Nervous Systems (Part B from *Gray's Anatomy*, 35th ed., Figure 2.9, page 807. © Elsevier, 1973. Dissection by M. C. E. Hutchinson, photograph by Kevin Fitzpatrick, Guy's Hospital Medical School, London.)

cranial nerve A nerve that is connected directly to the brain.

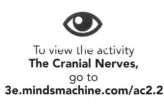

To view the activity
The Cranial Nerves,
go to
3e.mindsmachine.com/ac2.2

THE SOMATIC NERVOUS SYSTEM Taking its name from the Latin word for "body"—*soma*—the somatic nervous system is the main pathway through which the brain controls movement and receives sensory information from the body and from the sensory organs of the head. The nerves that make up the somatic nervous system form two anatomical groups: the cranial nerves and the spinal nerves.

We each have 12 pairs (left and right) of **cranial nerves** that arise from the brain and innervate the head, neck, and visceral organs directly, without ever joining the spinal cord. As you can see in **FIGURE 2.7**, some of these nerves are exclusively sensory: the olfactory (I) nerves transmit information about smell, the optic (II) nerves carry visual information from the eyes, and the vestibulocochlear (VIII) nerves convey auditory and balance information. Five pairs of cranial nerves are exclusively motor pathways from the brain: the oculomotor (III), trochlear (IV), and abducens (VI) nerves innervate muscles to move the eyes; the spinal accessory (XI) nerves control neck muscles; and the hypoglossal (XII) nerves control the tongue. The remaining cranial

FIGURE 2.7 The Cranial Nerves

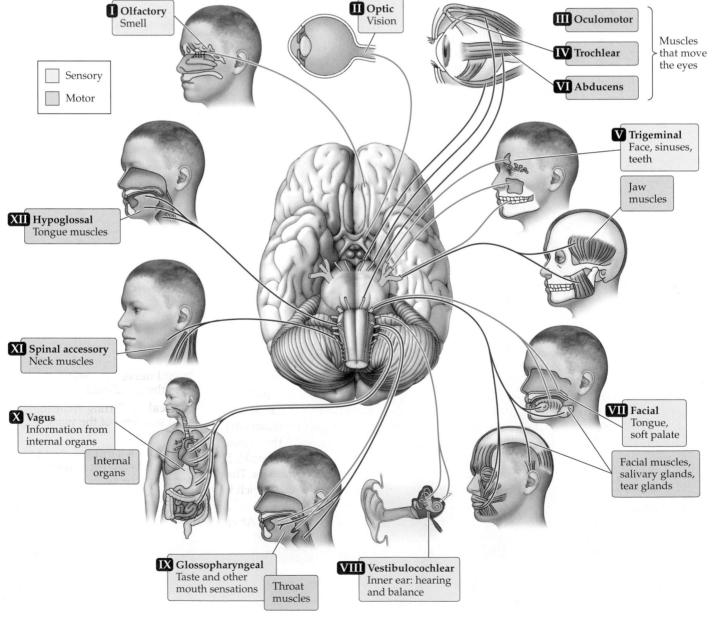

FIGURE 2.8   The Spinal Cord and Spinal Nerves

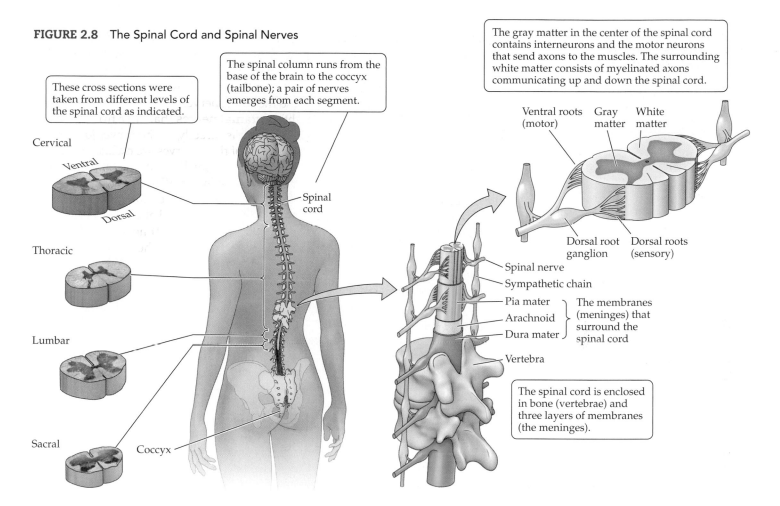

These cross sections were taken from different levels of the spinal cord as indicated.

The spinal column runs from the base of the brain to the coccyx (tailbone); a pair of nerves emerges from each segment.

The gray matter in the center of the spinal cord contains interneurons and the motor neurons that send axons to the muscles. The surrounding white matter consists of myelinated axons communicating up and down the spinal cord.

Cervical

Ventral

Dorsal

Thoracic

Lumbar

Sacral

Coccyx

Spinal cord

Ventral roots (motor)   Gray matter   White matter

Dorsal root ganglion   Dorsal roots (sensory)

Spinal nerve
Sympathetic chain
Pia mater
Arachnoid   } The membranes (meninges) that surround the spinal cord
Dura mater

Vertebra

The spinal cord is enclosed in bone (vertebrae) and three layers of membranes (the meninges).

nerves have both sensory and motor functions. The trigeminal (V) nerves, for example, transmit facial sensation through some axons but control the chewing muscles through other axons. The facial (VII) nerves control facial muscles and receive some taste sensation, and the glossopharyngeal (IX) nerves receive additional taste sensations and sensations from the throat and also control the muscles there. The vagus (X) nerve extends far from the head, running to the heart, liver, and intestines. Its long, convoluted route is the reason for its name, which is Latin for "wandering."

An additional 31 pairs of **spinal nerves**—again, one member of each pair serves each side of the body—are connected to the spinal cord through regularly spaced openings along both sides of the backbone (**FIGURE 2.8**). Each spinal nerve is made up of a group of motor fibers, projecting from the ventral (front) part of the spinal cord to the organs and muscles, and a group of sensory fibers that enter the dorsal (rear) part of the spinal cord. Spinal nerves are named according to the segments of the spinal cord to which they are connected. There are 8 **cervical** (neck), 12 **thoracic** (trunk), 5 **lumbar** (lower back), 5 **sacral** (pelvic), and 1 **coccygeal** (bottom) spinal segments. The name of each spinal nerve reflects the position of the spinal cord segment to which it is connected; for example, the nerve connected to the 12th thoracic segment is called *T12*, the nerve connected to the 7th cervical segment is called *C7*, and so on. After leaving the spinal cord, axons from the spinal nerves spread out in the body and may join with axons from different spinal nerves to form the various peripheral nerves.

THE AUTONOMIC NERVOUS SYSTEM   Although it is "autonomous" in the sense that we have little conscious, voluntary control over its actions, the autonomic nervous

To view the activity
Gross Anatomy of the Spinal Cord,
go to
3e.mindsmachine.com/ac2.3

spinal nerve   A nerve that emerges from the spinal cord.

cervical   Referring to the topmost eight segments of the spinal cord, in the neck region.

thoracic   Referring to the 12 spinal segments below the cervical (neck) portion of the spinal cord, in the torso.

lumbar   Referring to the five spinal segments in the upper part of the lower back.

sacral   Referring to the five spinal segments in the lower part of the lower back.

coccygeal   Referring to the lowest spinal vertebra (the coccyx, or "tailbone").

sympathetic nervous system
The part of the autonomic nervous system that generally prepares the body for action.

parasympathetic nervous system
The part of the autonomic nervous system that generally prepares the body to relax and recuperate.

cerebral hemisphere   One of the two halves—right or left—of the forebrain.

cerebral cortex   Also called simply *cortex*. The outer covering of the cerebral hemispheres, which consists largely of nerve cell bodies and their branches.

gyrus   A ridged or raised portion of a convoluted brain surface.

sulcus   A crevice or valley of a convoluted brain surface.

To view the activity
**Concept Matching:
Sympathetic vs. Parasympathetic,**
go to
3e.mindsmachine.com/ac2.4

system is the brain's main system for controlling the organs of the body. The activity of our organs is determined by a balance between the two major divisions of the autonomic nervous system—called the *sympathetic* and *parasympathetic nervous systems*—that act more or less in opposition to each other (**FIGURE 2.9**).

Axons of the **sympathetic nervous system** exit from the middle parts of the spinal cord, travel a short distance, and then innervate the sympathetic ganglia (small clusters of neurons found outside the CNS), which run in two chains along the spinal column, one on each side (see Figure 2.9 *left*). Axons from the sympathetic ganglia then course throughout the body, innervating all the major organ systems. In general, sympathetic innervation prepares the body for immediate action: blood pressure increases, the pupils of the eyes widen, the heart quickens, and so on. This set of reactions is sometimes called the *fight-or-flight response*.

In contrast to the effects of sympathetic activity, the **parasympathetic nervous system** generally helps the body to relax, recuperate, and prepare for future action—sometimes called the *rest-and-digest response*. Anatomically, nerves of the parasympathetic system originate in the brainstem (above the sympathetic nerves) and in the sacral spinal cord (below the sympathetic nerves), which explains the name: the Greek *para* means "around" (see Figure 2.9 *right*). Compared with sympathetic nerves, parasympathetic nerves travel a longer distance before terminating in parasympathetic ganglia, which are usually located close to the organs they serve.

The sympathetic and parasympathetic systems have very different effects on individual organs because the organs receive different neurotransmitters from the two opposing systems (*norepinephrine* from sympathetic nerves and *acetylcholine* from parasympathetic nerves; see Chapter 3). The balance between the two systems determines the state of the internal organs at any given moment. So, for example, when parasympathetic activity predominates, heart rate slows, blood pressure drops, and digestive processes are activated. As the brain causes the balance of autonomic activity to become predominantly sympathetic, opposite effects are seen: increased heart rate and blood pressure, inhibited digestion, and so on. This tension between parasympathetic and sympathetic activity ensures that the individual is appropriately prepared for current circumstances.

The central nervous system consists of the brain and spinal cord

The spinal cord funnels sensory information from the body up to the brain and conveys the brain's motor commands out to the body. The spinal cord also contains circuits that perform local processing and control simple units of behavior, such as reflexes. We will discuss other aspects of the spinal cord in later chapters, but for now let's focus on the anatomy of the executive portion of the CNS: the brain.

THE OUTER SURFACE OF THE BRAIN   On average, the human brain weighs only 1,400 grams (about 3 pounds), accounting for just 2% of the average body weight. Put your two fists together and you get a sense of the size of the two **cerebral hemispheres**—smaller than most people expect. But what the brain lacks in size and weight it makes up for in intricacy. Anatomists use standard terminology to help identify structures, locations, and directions in the brain, as described in **BOX 2.2**. (It's a bit of a chore, but learning the anatomical lingo now will make later discussions of brain organization much easier to follow.)

One obvious feature of the brain is its lumpy, convoluted surface—the result of elaborate folding of a thick sheet of tissue, mostly the dendrites, cell bodies, and axonal projections of neurons, called the **cerebral cortex** (or sometimes just *cortex*). The resultant ridges of tissue, called **gyri** (singular *gyrus*), are separated from each other by crevices called **sulci** (singular *sulcus*). Folding up the tissue in this way greatly increases the amount of cortex that can be crammed into the confines of the skull, and about two-thirds of the cerebral cortex is hidden in the depths of these folds. The pattern of folding is not random; in fact, it is similar enough between brains that we can name the various gyri and sulci and group them together into *lobes*.

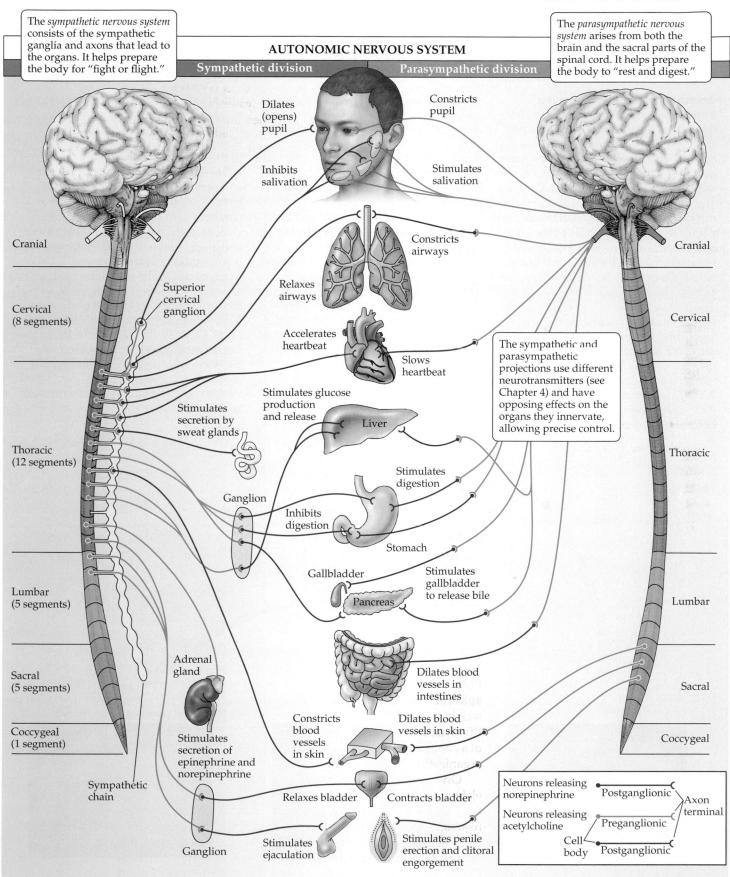

The *sympathetic nervous system* consists of the sympathetic ganglia and axons that lead to the organs. It helps prepare the body for "fight or flight."

The *parasympathetic nervous system* arises from both the brain and the sacral parts of the spinal cord. It helps prepare the body to "rest and digest."

AUTONOMIC NERVOUS SYSTEM

Sympathetic division   Parasympathetic division

Dilates (opens) pupil

Constricts pupil

Inhibits salivation

Stimulates salivation

Cranial

Cervical (8 segments)

Superior cervical ganglion

Constricts airways

Relaxes airways

Accelerates heartbeat

Slows heartbeat

Stimulates glucose production and release

Stimulates secretion by sweat glands

Liver

Thoracic (12 segments)

Ganglion

Inhibits digestion

Stimulates digestion

Stimulates gallbladder to release bile

Gallbladder

Stomach

Pancreas

Lumbar (5 segments)

Adrenal gland

Dilates blood vessels in intestines

Sacral (5 segments)

Constricts blood vessels in skin

Dilates blood vessels in skin

Stimulates secretion of epinephrine and norepinephrine

Coccygeal (1 segment)

Sympathetic chain

Relaxes bladder

Contracts bladder

Ganglion

Stimulates ejaculation

Stimulates penile erection and clitoral engorgement

Cranial

Cervical

The sympathetic and parasympathetic projections use different neurotransmitters (see Chapter 4) and have opposing effects on the organs they innervate, allowing precise control.

Thoracic

Lumbar

Sacral

Coccygeal

Neurons releasing norepinephrine

Postganglionic

Axon terminal

Neurons releasing acetylcholine

Preganglionic

Cell body

Postganglionic

FIGURE 2.9 The Autonomic Nervous System

BOX 2.2
Three Customary Orientations for Viewing the Brain and Body

Because the nervous system is a three-dimensional structure, two-dimensional illustrations and diagrams cannot represent it completely. The brain is usually cut in one of three main planes to obtain a two-dimensional section from this three-dimensional object. The plane that bisects the body into right and left halves is called the **sagittal plane**. The plane that divides the body into a front (anterior) and a back (posterior) part is called the **coronal plane** (also known as the *frontal* or *transverse plane*). The third main plane, which divides the brain into upper and lower parts, is called the **horizontal plane**.

In addition, several directional terms are used. **Medial** means "toward the middle" and is contrasted with **lateral**, "toward the side." Relative to one location, a second location is **ipsilateral** if it is on the same side of the body and **contralateral** if on the opposite side of

the body. These terms are all relative, as are the terms **superior** ("above") and **inferior** ("below"); for example, the eye is lateral to the nose but medial to the ear, and the mouth is inferior to the nose but superior to the chin. The term **basal** simply means "toward the base" or "toward the bottom" of a structure.

The head end of the body, and therefore the front of the brain, is referred to as **anterior** or **rostral**; the tail end of the body and the back of the head are described as **posterior** or **caudal** (from the Latin *cauda*, "tail"). **Proximal** means "near the center," and **distal** means "toward the periphery" or "toward the end of a limb." We call an axon, tract, or nerve **afferent** if it carries information into a region that we're interested in,

and **efferent** if it carries information away from the region of interest (a handy way to remember this is that *ef*ferents *e*xit but *a*fferents *a*rrive, relative to the region of interest).

Dorsal means "toward or at the back," and **ventral** means "toward or at the belly." In four-legged animals, such as cats or rats, *dorsal* refers to both the back of the body and the top of the head and brain. For consistency in comparing brains among species, this term is also used to refer to the top of the brain of a human or of a chimpanzee, even though in such two-legged animals the top of the brain is not at the back of the body. Similarly, *ventral* is understood to designate the bottom of the brain of a two-legged as well as of a four-legged animal. (Photographs courtesy of S. Mark Williams and Dale Purves, Duke University Medical Center.)

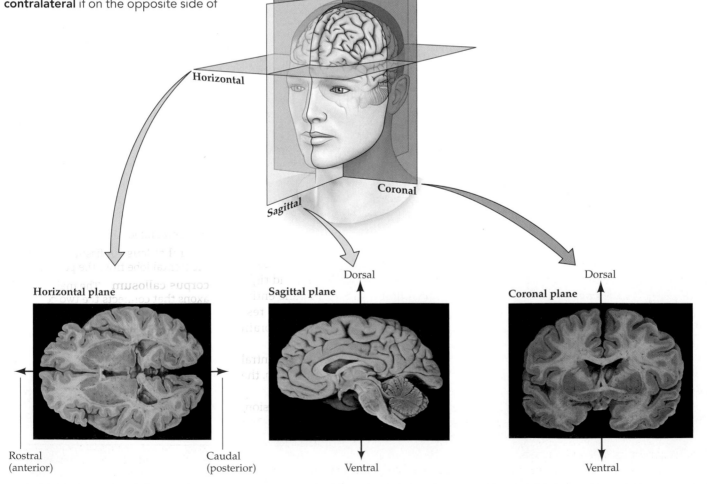

Horizontal

Sagittal

Coronal

Horizontal plane

Rostral (anterior)   Caudal (posterior)

Sagittal plane

Dorsal

Ventral

Coronal plane

Dorsal

Ventral

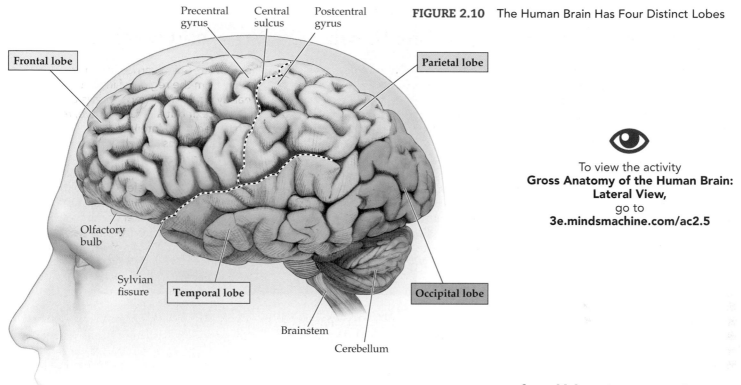

Precentral gyrus   Central sulcus   Postcentral gyrus

FIGURE 2.10 The Human Brain Has Four Distinct Lobes

Frontal lobe

Parietal lobe

Olfactory bulb

Sylvian fissure

Temporal lobe

Occipital lobe

Brainstem

Cerebellum

To view the activity
**Gross Anatomy of the Human Brain:
Lateral View,**
go to
3e.mindsmachine.com/ac2.5

Neuroscientists rely on a combination of landmarks and functions to distinguish among four major cortical regions of the cerebral hemispheres: the **frontal**, **parietal**, **temporal**, and **occipital lobes** (**FIGURE 2.10**). In some cases the boundaries between adjacent lobes are very clear; for example, the **Sylvian fissure** (or *lateral sulcus*) divides the temporal lobe from other regions of the hemisphere. The **central sulcus** provides a distinct landmark dividing the frontal and parietal lobes. The physical boundaries between the occipital lobe and the temporal and parietal lobes are less obvious, but the lobes are quite different with regard to the functions they perform.

The cortex is the seat of complex cognition. Depending on the specific regions affected, cortical damage can cause symptoms ranging from impairments of movement or body sensation; through speech errors, memory problems, and personality changes; to many kinds of visual impairments. In people with undamaged brains, the four lobes of the cortex are continually communicating and collaborating in order to produce the seamless control of complex behavior that distinguishes us as individuals. Furthermore, hundreds of millions of axons connect the left and right hemispheres via the **corpus callosum**, allowing the brain to act as a single entity during complex processing. Some life-sustaining functions—heart rate and respiration, reflexes, balance, and the like—are governed by lower, subcortical brain regions.

The sense of touch is mediated by a strip of parietal cortex just behind the central sulcus called the **postcentral gyrus** (see Figure 2.10). In front of the central sulcus, the **precentral gyrus** of the frontal lobe is crucial for motor control, organized like a map of the body (Penfield and Rasmussen, 1950). The occipital lobes are crucial for vision, and the temporal lobes receive auditory inputs and help in memory formation. But each lobe of the brain also performs a wide variety of other high-level functions. These will be major topics in later chapters.

Most people have heard brain tissue referred to as **gray matter**. When you cut into a brain, you see that the outer layers of the cortex have a darker grayish shade

frontal lobe   The most anterior portion of the cerebral cortex.

parietal lobe   The large region of cortex lying between the frontal and occipital lobes in each cerebral hemisphere.

temporal lobe   The large lateral region of cortex in each cerebral hemisphere. It is continuous with the parietal lobe posteriorly and separated from the frontal lobe by the Sylvian fissure.

occipital lobe   A large region of cortex that covers much of the posterior part of each cerebral hemisphere.

Sylvian fissure   Also called *lateral sulcus*. A deep fissure that demarcates the temporal lobe.

central sulcus   A fissure that divides the frontal lobe from the parietal lobe.

corpus callosum   The main band of axons that connects the two cerebral hemispheres.

postcentral gyrus   The strip of parietal cortex, just posterior to (behind) the central sulcus, that receives somatosensory information from the entire body.

precentral gyrus   The strip of frontal cortex, just anterior to (in front of) the central sulcus, that is crucial for motor control.

gray matter   Areas of the brain that are dominated by cell bodies and are devoid of myelin. Gray matter mostly receives and processes information.

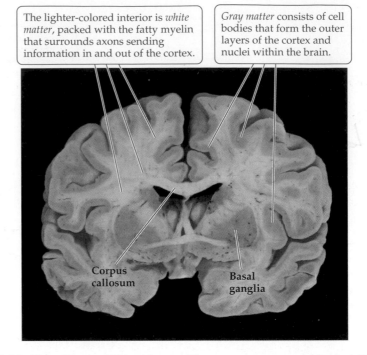

The lighter-colored interior is *white matter*, packed with the fatty myelin that surrounds axons sending information in and out of the cortex.

Gray matter consists of cell bodies that form the outer layers of the cortex and nuclei within the brain.

Corpus callosum

Basal ganglia

FIGURE 2.11 Gray Matter, White Matter (Photograph courtesy of S. Mark Williams and Dale Purves, Duke University Medical Center.)

white matter A light-colored layer of tissue, consisting mostly of myelin-sheathed axons, that lies underneath the gray matter of the cortex. White matter mostly transmits information.

neural tube An embryonic structure with subdivisions that correspond to the future forebrain, midbrain, and hindbrain.

forebrain The frontal division of the neural tube, containing the cerebral hemispheres, the thalamus, and the hypothalamus.

midbrain The middle division of the brain.

hindbrain The rear division of the brain, which in the mature vertebrate contains the cerebellum, pons, and medulla.

telencephalon The anterior part of the fetal forebrain, which will become the cerebral hemispheres in the adult brain.

diencephalon The posterior part of the fetal forebrain, which will become the thalamus and hypothalamus in the adult brain.

brainstem The region of the brain that consists of the midbrain, the pons, and the medulla.

nucleus Here, a collection of neuronal cell bodies within the central nervous system (e.g., the caudate nucleus).

tract A bundle of axons found within the central nervous system.

(**FIGURE 2.11**). This is because they contain a preponderance of neuronal cell bodies and dendrites. In contrast, the underlying **white matter** gets its snowy appearance from the whitish fatty myelin that insulates the axons of many neurons. So, a simple view is that gray matter mostly receives and processes information, while white matter mostly transmits information.

SUBDIVISIONS WITHIN THE BRAIN It can be difficult to understand some of the anatomical distinctions applied to the adult human brain. For example, part of the brain closest to the back of the head is anatomically identified as part of the forebrain. Why? The key to understanding this confusing terminology is to consider how the gross anatomy of the brain develops early in life.

In a very young embryo of any vertebrate, the CNS looks like a tube. The walls of this **neural tube** are made of cells, and the interior is filled with fluid. A few weeks after conception, the human neural tube begins to show three separate swellings at the head end (**FIGURE 2.12A**): the **forebrain**, the **midbrain**, and the **hindbrain**. By about 50 days, the fetal forebrain features two clear subdivisions. At the very front is the **telencephalon** (from the Greek *encephalon*, "brain"), which will become the cerebral hemispheres (consisting of cortex plus some deeper structures). The other part of the forebrain is the **diencephalon**, which will go on to become the thalamus and the hypothalamus, two of the many subcortical structures of the forebrain.

Similarly, the hindbrain further develops into several large structures: the cerebellum, pons, and medulla. The term **brainstem** usually refers to the midbrain, pons, and medulla combined (some scientists include the diencephalon too). **FIGURES 2.12B** and **C** show the positions of these structures and their relative sizes in the adult human brain. Even when the brain achieves its adult form, it is still a fluid-filled tube, but a tube of very complicated shape.

The main sections of the brain can be subdivided in turn. We can work our way from the largest, most general divisions of the nervous system on the left of the schematic in Figure 2.12B to more-specific ones on the right.

Within and between the major brain regions are collections of neurons called **nuclei** (singular *nucleus*) and bundles of axons called **tracts**. Recall that outside the CNS, collections of neurons are called *ganglia*, and bundles of axons are called *nerves*. Unfortunately, the same word *nucleus* can mean either "a collection of neurons in the CNS"

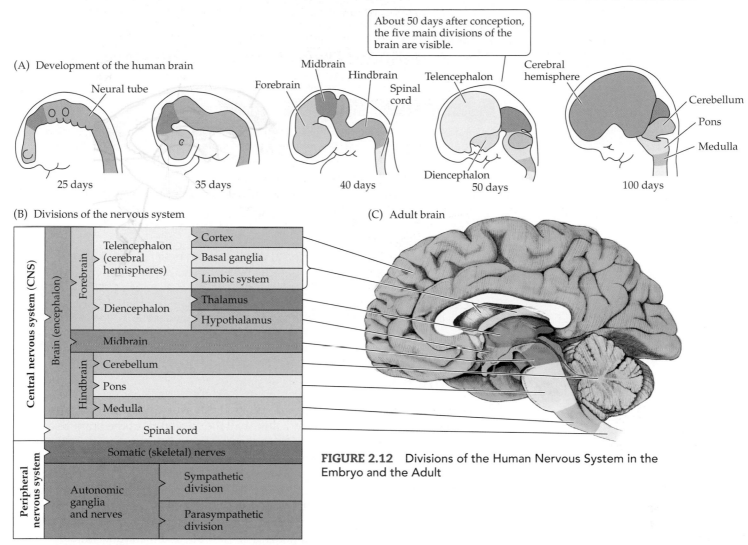

(A) Development of the human brain

About 50 days after conception, the five main divisions of the brain are visible.

Neural tube

Forebrain · Midbrain · Hindbrain · Spinal cord

Telencephalon · Cerebral hemisphere · Cerebellum · Pons · Medulla

Diencephalon

25 days   35 days   40 days   50 days   100 days

(B) Divisions of the nervous system

Central nervous system (CNS)

Brain (encephalon)

Forebrain
- Telencephalon (cerebral hemispheres)
  - Cortex
  - Basal ganglia
  - Limbic system
- Diencephalon
  - Thalamus
  - Hypothalamus

Midbrain

Hindbrain
- Cerebellum
- Pons
- Medulla

Spinal cord

Peripheral nervous system
- Somatic (skeletal) nerves
- Autonomic ganglia and nerves
  - Sympathetic division
  - Parasympathetic division

(C) Adult brain

FIGURE 2.12 Divisions of the Human Nervous System in the Embryo and the Adult

or "the spherical DNA-containing organelle within a single cell." You must rely on the context to understand which meaning is intended. Because brain tracts and nuclei are the same in different individuals, and often the same in different species, they have names too (many, many names).

You are probably more interested in the functions of all these parts of the brain than in their names, but as we noted earlier, each region serves more than one function, and our knowledge of the functional organization of the brain is continually being updated with new research findings. So, with that caution in mind, we'll briefly survey the functions of specific brain structures next, leaving the detailed discussion for later chapters.

HOW'S IT GOING ?

1. Name and briefly describe the major divisions of the peripheral nervous system. What general function does each part perform?
2. Briefly sketch and describe the anatomical organization of the cranial nerves. How many nerves are there? Now do the same for the spinal nerves.
3. Give some examples of how each division of the autonomic nervous system affects organs of the body.
4. Why does the cortex look so lumpy on the outside?
5. What is special about the pre- and postcentral gyri?
6. Review the fetal development of the brain, and the three major divisions of the brain that arise from the earlier fetal form of the nervous system.

To view the activity **The Developing Brain,** go to 3e.mindsmachine.com/ac2.6

To see the video **Brain Development,** go to 3e.mindsmachine.com/av2.3

pyramidal cell   A type of large nerve cell that has a roughly pyramid-shaped cell body and is found in the cerebral cortex.

cortical column   One of the vertical columns that constitute the basic organization of the cerebral cortex.

PART III
The Functional Organization of the Nervous System

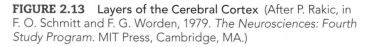 THE ROAD AHEAD

The final part of the chapter introduces functional neuroanatomy—the connection of behaviors to brain regions—and the support systems allow the brain to function. By the end of this section, you should be able to:

1. Describe the cellular organization of the cortex.
2. Distinguish between the basal ganglia, and the limbic system, and state some of the behavioral functions of each.
3. Name the major divisions of the brainstem and midbrain, and identify major functions performed by each.
4. Name and describe the meninges and ventricular system, and their clinical significance.
5. Give an outline of the vascular supply of the brain, and note the signs and symptoms of stroke.
6. Describe the major brain imaging technologies, highlighting their differing uses and limitations, and discuss the importance of the connectome.

The Brain Is Described in Terms of Both Structure and Function

Vertebrates are bilaterally symmetrical: our bodies have mirror-image left and right sides. The brain is no exception, and almost all the structures of the brain also come in twos. One important principle of the vertebrate brain is that each side of the brain generally controls the opposite (or contralateral; see Box 2.2) side of the body. The right side of the brain thus controls movement of the left side of the body and receives left-sided sensory information. Likewise the left side of the brain monitors and controls the right side of the body. In Chapter 15 we'll learn about how the two cerebral hemispheres interact, but for now let's review the various components of the brain and their functions.

The cerebral cortex performs complex cognitive processing

Neuroscientists are only just beginning to understand how the structures and functions of the cerebral cortex accomplish the feats of human cognition. If the human cortex were unfolded, it would occupy an area of about 2,000 square centimeters (315 square inches)—more than 3 times the area of this book's front cover. How are all those millions of cells arranged?

Cortical neurons make up six distinct layers, as shown in **FIGURE 2.13**. Each cortical layer has a unique appearance because it consists of either a band of similar neurons, or a particular pattern of dendrites or axons. For example, the outermost layer, layer I, is distinct because it has few cell bodies, while layers V and VI stand out because of their many neurons with large cell bodies. The most prominent kind of neuron in the cerebral cortex—the **pyramidal cell**—usually has its pyramid-shaped cell body in layer III or V.

In some regions of the cerebral cortex, neurons are organized into regular columns, perpendicular to the layers, that seem to serve as information-processing units (Horton and Adams, 2005). These **cortical columns**

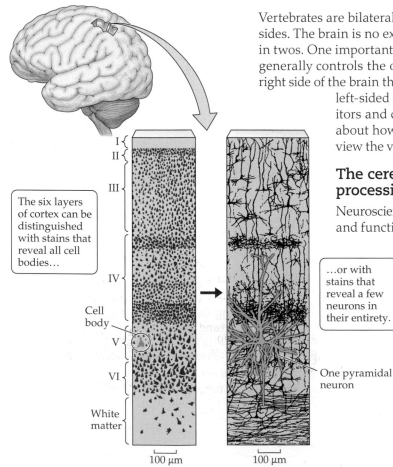

The six layers of cortex can be distinguished with stains that reveal all cell bodies…

…or with stains that reveal a few neurons in their entirety.

Cell body

One pyramidal neuron

White matter

100 μm   100 μm

FIGURE 2.13   Layers of the Cerebral Cortex (After P. Rakic, in F. O. Schmitt and F. G. Worden, 1979. *The Neurosciences: Fourth Study Program*. MIT Press, Cambridge, MA.)

(A) Basal ganglia

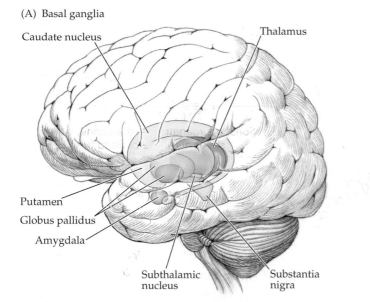

(B) Limbic system

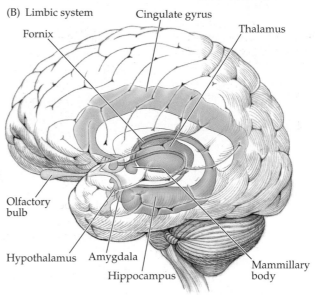

FIGURE 2.14 Two Important Brain Systems

extend through the entire thickness of the cortex, from the white matter to the surface. Within each column, most of the synaptic interconnections of neurons are vertical, although there are some horizontal connections as well (Mountcastle, 1979).

Important nuclei are hidden beneath the cerebral cortex

Buried within the cerebral hemispheres are several large gray matter structures, richly connected to each other and to other brain regions and contributing to a wide variety of behaviors. One prominent cluster—the **basal ganglia**, consisting primarily of the *caudate nucleus*, the *putamen*, and the *globus pallidus* (**FIGURE 2.14A**)—plays a critical role in the control of movement, which we will discuss in Chapter 5.

Overlapping and curled around the basal ganglia, the **limbic system** is a loosely defined, widespread network of structures (identified in **FIGURE 2.14B**) that are involved in emotion and learning: The **amygdala** consists of several subdivisions with quite diverse functions, including emotional regulation (see Chapter 11) and the perception of odor (see Chapter 6). The **hippocampus** and **fornix** are important for learning and memory (discussed in Chapter 13). Lying over the corpus callosum in each hemisphere is a strip of cortex called the **cingulate gyrus**, which is implicated in many cognitive functions, including the direction of attention (see Chapter 14). The **olfactory bulb** is involved in the sense of smell. Other limbic structures near the base of the brain, especially the hypothalamus, help to govern motivated behaviors, like sex and aggression, and to regulate the hormonal systems of the body.

Toward the medial (middle) and basal (bottom) aspects of the forebrain are found the **thalamus** and the **hypothalamus** (the latter means simply "under thalamus"). You can see both the hypothalamus and thalamus in Figures 2.14B and 2.15A. The thalamus is the brain's traffic cop, directing virtually all incoming sensory information to the appropriate regions of the cortex for further processing, and receiving instructions back from the cortex about which sensory information is to be transmitted. The small but mighty hypothalamus has a much different role: it is packed with discrete nuclei involved in many vital functions, such as hunger, thirst, temperature regulation, sex, and many more. Furthermore, because the hypothalamus also controls the pituitary gland, it serves as the brain's main interface with the hormonal systems of the body. We'll encounter the hypothalamus again in several later chapters.

The midbrain has sensory and motor components

Compared with the forebrain and hindbrain, the midbrain doesn't encompass a lot of tissue, but that doesn't mean its components are unimportant. The top part of the

To view the activities
The Basal Ganglia
and
The Limbic System,
go to
3e.mindsmachine.com/ac2.7
and **3e.mindsmachine.com/ac2.8**

basal ganglia   A group of forebrain nuclei, including the *caudate nucleus*, *globus pallidus*, and *putamen*, found deep within the cerebral hemispheres.

limbic system   A loosely defined, widespread group of brain nuclei that innervate each other and form a network.

amygdala   A group of nuclei in the medial anterior part of the temporal lobe.

hippocampus   A medial temporal lobe structure that is important for learning and memory.

fornix   A fiber tract that extends from the hippocampus to the mammillary body.

cingulate gyrus   A strip of cortex, found in the frontal and parietal midline, that is part of the limbic system and is implicated in many cognitive functions.

olfactory bulb   An anterior projection of the brain that terminates in the upper nasal passages and provides the primary inputs for the sense of smell.

thalamus   Paired structures to either side of the third ventricle that direct the flow of sensory information to and from the cortex.

hypothalamus   Part of the diencephalon, lying ventral to the thalamus.

tectum   The dorsal portion of the midbrain consisting of the inferior and superior colliculi.

superior colliculi   Paired gray matter structures of the dorsal midbrain that process visual information.

inferior colliculi   Paired gray matter structures of the dorsal midbrain that process auditory information.

tegmentum   The main body of the midbrain, containing the substantia nigra, periaqueductal gray, part of the reticular formation, and multiple fiber tracts.

substantia nigra   A brainstem structure that innervates the basal ganglia and is a major source of dopaminergic projections.

periaqueductal gray   A midbrain region involved in pain perception.

To view the activities
Gross Anatomy of the Human Brain: Midsaggital View
and
Gross Anatomy of the Human Brain: Basal View,
go to
3e.mindsmachine.com/ac2.9
and 3e.mindsmachine.com/ac2.10

midbrain, called the **tectum** (from the Latin for "roof," because it's atop the midbrain), features two pairs of bumps—one pair in each hemisphere—with specific roles in sensory processing. The more rostral bumps are called the **superior colliculi** (singular *colliculus*), and they have specific roles in visual processing. The more caudal bumps, called the **inferior colliculi** (see Figure 2.15A), process information about sound.

The main body of the midbrain is called the **tegmentum**, and it also contains several important structures. The **substantia nigra** is in many ways a part of the basal ganglia, and loss of its neurons (which normally release the neurotransmitter dopamine within the forebrain) leads to Parkinson's disease, discussed in Chapter 5. The **periaqueductal gray** is a midbrain structure implicated in the perception of pain (discussed in Chapter 4). The **reticular formation** (*reticular* means "netlike") is a loose collection of neurons that are important in a variety of behaviors, including sleep and arousal (see Chapter 10). Multiple large tracts of nerve fibers run in, out, and through the midbrain to connect the brain to the rest of the body.

The brainstem controls vital body functions

The midsagittal and basal views of the brain in **FIGURE 2.15** show the hemispheres of the **cerebellum**, which is tucked up under the posterior cortex and attached to the dorsal brainstem. Like the cerebral cortex, the cerebellum is highly convoluted, but it is made up of a simpler three-layered tissue instead of the six layers found in the cerebral cortex. The cerebellum has long been known to be crucial for motor coordination and control, but we now know that it also participates in certain aspects of cognition, including learning. The adjacent **pons** (from the Latin word for "bridge") contains many nerve fibers and important motor control and sensory nuclei; it is the point of origin for several cranial nerves. The reticular formation, which we first saw in the midbrain, stretches down through the pons and ends in the medulla.

The **medulla** marks the transition from the brain to the spinal cord. In addition to conveying all of the major motor and sensory fibers to and from the body, the medulla contains nuclei that drive such essential processes as respiration and heart rate, so brainstem injuries are often lethal. And like other parts of the brainstem, the medulla gives rise to several cranial nerves.

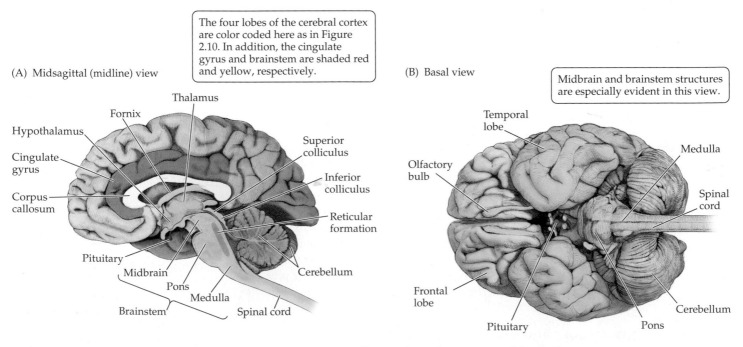

The four lobes of the cerebral cortex are color coded here as in Figure 2.10. In addition, the cingulate gyrus and brainstem are shaded red and yellow, respectively.

(A) Midsagittal (midline) view

Thalamus
Fornix
Hypothalamus
Cingulate gyrus
Corpus callosum
Pituitary
Midbrain
Pons
Medulla
Brainstem
Spinal cord
Superior colliculus
Inferior colliculus
Reticular formation
Cerebellum

(B) Basal view

Midbrain and brainstem structures are especially evident in this view.

Temporal lobe
Olfactory bulb
Frontal lobe
Pituitary
Medulla
Spinal cord
Cerebellum
Pons

FIGURE 2.15   Midline and Basal Structures of the Brain

Networks of connections between brain regions determine behavior

In order to understand the neural origins of our most complex behaviors and experiences—thought, language, music—it will be necessary to understand how different brain regions with distinct functions collaborate in larger-scale networks. This applies to functional units as small as the individual cortical columns we mentioned earlier and to much larger assemblages of millions of cells making up substantial parts of cortical lobes.

Cortical regions communicate with one another via tracts of axons looping through the underlying white matter. Some of these connections are short pathways to nearby cortical regions; others travel longer distances through and between the two cerebral hemispheres and subcortical structures like the basal ganglia. Understanding the "connectome" of the human brain—the network map that completely describes the functional connections within and between brain regions (Glasser et al., 2016)—is an area of intense research activity, involving large international collaborations (Huang and Luo, 2015). Dealing with the immense volume of data generated by such approaches, where connections are tracked from the level of individual synapses to large fiber pathways in the brain, is an additional technological challenge for the near future.

HOW'S IT GOING ?

1. How are the cells of the cerebral cortex organized?
2. Name the major components of the basal ganglia and the limbic system. What behaviors especially rely on these systems?
3. What functions are served by the thalamus and hypothalamus?
4. Name and describe the general functions of the major components of the midbrain and hindbrain.
5. Why are injuries to the medulla often fatal?
6. Define the connectome and discuss its significance for understanding the functioning of the brain.

Specialized Support Systems Protect and Nourish the Brain

The brain is relatively soft and easily damaged. It also needs a steady and substantial supply of fuel to maintain normal functioning, and thus keep us alive. Fortunately, the brain is equipped with systems that protect and cushion the brain and that provide a continual source of energy, nutrients, and important chemicals.

The brain floats within layers of membranes

Within the bony skull and vertebrae, the brain and spinal cord are swaddled by three protective membranes called **meninges** (see Figure 2.8). Between a tough outer sheet called the **dura mater** (in Latin, literally "tough mother") and the delicate **pia mater** ("tender mother") that adheres tightly to the surface of the brain, a webby substance called the **arachnoid** ("spiderweb-like") suspends the brain in a bath of a watery liquid called **cerebrospinal fluid (CSF)**. The meninges can become inflamed by infections, and because the inflammation ends up squeezing the brain, the resultant **meningitis** is a medical emergency. Sometimes large tumors called **meningiomas** can form in the meninges; these are usually classified as benign, because most do not invade the brain tissue, but in an enclosed space like the cranium, any mass that takes up space is far from harmless.

The brain relies on two fluids for survival

The brain essentially floats in cerebrospinal fluid, cushioning it from minor blows to the head. But CSF is also a source of important materials, such as nutrients and signaling chemicals. Inside the brain is a series of chambers called the *cerebral ventricles*,

reticular formation   An extensive region of the brainstem, extending from the medulla through the thalamus, that is involved in sleep and arousal.

cerebellum   A structure located at the back of the brain, dorsal to the pons, that is involved in the central regulation of movement and in some forms of learning.

pons   The portion of the brainstem that connects the midbrain to the medulla.

medulla   The posterior part of the hindbrain, continuous with the spinal cord.

meninges   The three protective membranes—dura mater, pia mater, and arachnoid—that surround the brain and spinal cord.

dura mater   The outermost of the three meninges that surround the brain and spinal cord.

pia mater   The innermost of the three meninges that surround the brain and spinal cord.

arachnoid   The thin covering (one of the three meninges) of the brain that lies between the dura mater and the pia mater.

cerebrospinal fluid (CSF)   The fluid that fills the cerebral ventricles.

meningitis   An acute inflammation of the meninges, usually caused by a viral or bacterial infection.

meningioma   A noninvasive tumor of the meninges.

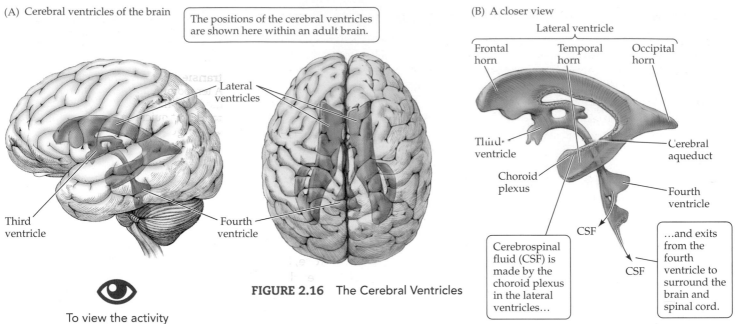

(A) Cerebral ventricles of the brain

The positions of the cerebral ventricles are shown here within an adult brain.

Lateral ventricles

Third ventricle

Fourth ventricle

(B) A closer view

Lateral ventricle

Frontal horn

Temporal horn

Occipital horn

Third ventricle

Choroid plexus

Cerebral aqueduct

Fourth ventricle

CSF

Cerebrospinal fluid (CSF) is made by the choroid plexus in the lateral ventricles…

CSF

…and exits from the fourth ventricle to surround the brain and spinal cord.

FIGURE 2.16   The Cerebral Ventricles

To view the activity
The Cerebral Ventricles,
go to
3e.mindsmachine.com/ac2.11

ventricular system   A system of fluid-filled cavities inside the brain.

lateral ventricle   A complex C-shaped lateral portion of the ventricular system within each hemisphere of the brain.

choroid plexus   A specialized membrane lining the ventricles that produces cerebrospinal fluid by filtering blood.

third ventricle   The midline ventricle that conducts cerebrospinal fluid from the lateral ventricles to the fourth ventricle.

fourth ventricle   The passageway within the pons that receives cerebrospinal fluid from the third ventricle and releases it to surround the brain and spinal cord.

hydrocephalus   A ballooning of the ventricles, at the expense of the surrounding brain, which may occur when the circulation of CSF is blocked.

glymphatic system   A lymphatic system in the brain that participates in removal of wastes and the movement of nutrients and signaling compounds.

cerebral arteries   The three pairs of large arteries within the skull that supply blood to the cerebral cortex.

blood-brain barrier   The mechanisms that make the movement of substances from blood vessels into brain cells more difficult than exchanges in other body organs, thus affording the brain greater protection from exposure to some substances found in the blood.

which are filled with CSF (**FIGURE 2.16**). These chambers comprise the **ventricular system**. Each hemisphere of the brain contains a **lateral ventricle** extending into all four lobes of the hemisphere. The lateral ventricles are lined with a specialized membrane called the **choroid plexus**, which produces CSF by filtering blood. The CSF flows from the lateral ventricles into a midline **third ventricle** (so named because it follows the two lateral ventricles) and continues down a narrow passage (the *cerebral aqueduct*) to the **fourth ventricle**, which lies between the cerebellum and the pons. Just below the cerebellum, three small openings allow CSF to exit the ventricular system and circulate over the outer surface of the brain and spinal cord. The CSF is absorbed back into the circulatory system through large veins beneath the top of the skull. A problem that blocks the flow of CSF through the ventricular system may result in **hydrocephalus**, a ballooning of the ventricles as they accumulate fluid, resulting in greatly varying symptoms. And although the brain had long been thought to lack the lymphatic system found in other tissues, the recently discovered **glymphatic system** (the name reflects the involvement of glial cells) provides for drainage of wastes in the brain as well as the distribution of various nutrients and signaling substances (Jessen et al., 2015).

The second crucial fluid for the brain is, of course, blood. Without a continual supply of a high volume of oxygen- and nutrient-rich blood, the tissue of the brain would swiftly die. That's because brain tissue is unusually needy: it accounts for only 2% of the average human body but consumes more than 20% of the body's energy. So the brain is critically dependent on a set of large blood vessels. Blood arrives in the brain via two pairs of arteries: the *carotid arteries* in the neck and the *vertebral arteries* that ascend within each side of the vertebrae of the neck. Inside the skull these arteries give rise to a set of three pairs of **cerebral arteries** that supply the cortex, plus a number of smaller vessels that penetrate and supply other regions of the brain. Fine vessels and capillaries branching off from the arteries deliver nutrients and other substances to brain cells and remove waste products. In contrast to capillaries in the rest of the body, capillaries in the brain are highly resistant to the passage of large molecules across their walls and into neighboring neurons. This **blood-brain barrier** probably evolved to help protect the brain from infections and blood-borne toxins, but it also makes the delivery of drugs to the brain more difficult. You can learn more about the brain's elaborate vascular system in **A STEP FURTHER 2.1**, on the website.

HOW'S IT GOING ❓

1. Name the three meninges, and describe how they're organized. Identify one special characteristic of each.
2. What is CSF? What function does it serve, where does it come from, and where does it go?
3. Describe the ventricular system of the brain.
4. What is the blood-brain barrier?

stroke Damage to a region of brain tissue that results from the blockage or rupture of vessels that supply blood to that region.

transient ischemic attack (TIA) A temporary blood restriction to part of the brain that causes stroke-like symptoms that quickly resolve, serving as a warning of elevated stroke risk.

SIGNS & SYMPTOMS

Stroke

The general term **stroke** applies to a situation in which a clot, a narrowing, or a rupture interrupts the supply of blood to a particular brain region, causing the affected region to stop functioning or die (**FIGURE 2.17A**). Although the exact effects of stroke depend on the region of the brain that is affected (**FIGURE 2.17B**), the five most common warning signs are sudden numbness or weakness, altered vision, dizziness, severe headache, and confusion or difficulty speaking. Effective treatments are available to help restore blood flow and minimize the long-term effects of a stroke, but only if the victim is treated immediately (Albers et al., 2018). Some people experience temporary stroke-like symptoms lasting for a few minutes. Caused by a brief interruption of blood supply to some part of the brain, this **transient ischemic attack** (from the Greek *ischemia*, "interrupted blood"), or **TIA**, is a serious warning sign that a major stroke may be imminent, and it should be treated as a medical emergency.

FIGURE 2.17 Stroke

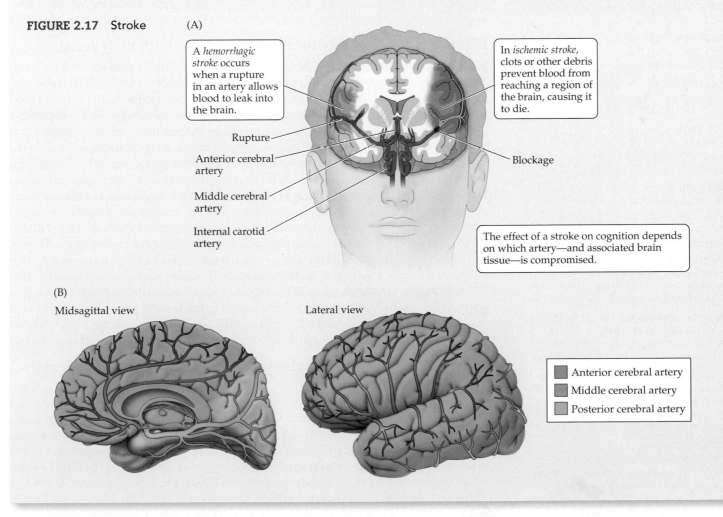

(A)

A *hemorrhagic stroke* occurs when a rupture in an artery allows blood to leak into the brain.

In *ischemic stroke*, clots or other debris prevent blood from reaching a region of the brain, causing it to die.

Rupture

Anterior cerebral artery

Middle cerebral artery

Internal carotid artery

Blockage

The effect of a stroke on cognition depends on which artery—and associated brain tissue—is compromised.

(B)

Midsagittal view

Lateral view

Anterior cerebral artery
Middle cerebral artery
Posterior cerebral artery

Brain-Imaging Techniques Reveal the Structure and Function of the Human Brain

Unlike older, more invasive techniques, modern brain imaging technology permits study of healthy humans too, revealing both fine structure and patterns of activity in the brain.

CT uses X-rays to reveal brain structure

In **computerized axial tomography** (**CAT** or **CT**), X-ray energy is used to generate images. In a CT scanner, an X-ray source is moved by steps in an arc around the head. At each point, detectors on the opposite side of the head measure the amount of X-ray radiation that is absorbed; this value is proportional to the density of the tissue through which the X-rays passed. When this process is repeated from many angles and the results are mathematically combined, an anatomical map of the brain based on tissue density can be generated by computer (**FIGURE 2.18A**). CT scans are medium-resolution images, useful for visualizing problems such as strokes, tumors, or cortical shrinkage.

Sam, whom we met at the beginning of the chapter, had developed a meningioma that was pressing on and deforming the motor cortex on the left side of his brain. The pressure caused abnormal firing—a seizure—that spread to adjacent areas, resulting in unconsciousness. The tumor subsequently impaired the functioning of regions of the motor cortex responsible for voluntary control of the muscles of Sam's right arm and the right side of his face, producing his alarming symptoms. Fortunately, his emergency CT scan was able to pinpoint the meningioma within Sam's skull, and later that evening a surgeon removed the tumor in pieces without damaging nearby tissue. Sam experienced immediate improvement and has been healthy ever since.

MRI maps density to deduce brain structure with high detail

Magnetic resonance imaging (**MRI**) provides higher-resolution images than CT, and because MRI uses magnetic fields and radio waves instead of X-rays, MRI also has fewer damaging effects than CT. When an MRI image of the brain is made, the person's head is first placed in an extremely powerful magnet that causes all the protons in the brain's tissues and fluids to line up in parallel, instead of in their usual random orientations (protons are found in the nuclei of atoms; in body tissues, most protons are found within water molecules). Next, the protons are knocked over by a powerful pulse of radio waves. When this pulse is turned off, the protons relax back to their original configuration, emitting radio waves as they go. Detectors surrounding the head measure those radio waves, which differ for tissues of varying densities. This density-based information is then used by a computer to create a detailed cross-sectional view of the brain (**FIGURE 2.18B**) that scientists use to evaluate the size and shape of distinct brain regions. Thanks to their high resolution, MRI images can also reveal subtle changes in the brain, such as the local loss of myelin that is characteristic of multiple sclerosis. A variant of MRI, called **diffusion tensor imaging** (**DTI**), exploits a signal associated with the diffusion of water within axons in order to visualize axonal fiber tracts within the brain. This kind of research, generally known as *tractography*, is helping us to learn how networks of brain structures work together in various forms of complex cognition and consciousness.

Functional MRI uses local changes in metabolism to identify active brain regions

Functional MRI (**fMRI**), which generates images of the brain's activity rather than details of its structure, has revolutionized cognitive neuroscience. Offering both reasonable speed (temporal resolution) and sharpness (spatial resolution) at the gross anatomical level, fMRI uses rapidly oscillating magnetic fields to detect regional changes in brain metabolism, particularly patterns of oxygen use and blood flow in the most active regions of the brain. Scientists can use fMRI data to create what are known as "difference images" of the specific activity of different parts of the brain while people engage in various experimental tasks. Although fMRI cannot resolve the fine cellular

To view the animation
Visualizing the Living Human Brain,
go to
3e.mindsmachine.com/av2.4

computerized axial tomography (CAT or CT) A noninvasive technique for examining brain structure through computer analysis of X-ray absorption at several positions around the head.

magnetic resonance imaging (MRI) A noninvasive brain-imaging technology that uses magnetism and radio-frequency energy to create images of the gross structure of the living brain.

diffusion tensor imaging (DTI) A modified form of MRI in which the diffusion of water in a confined space is exploited to produce images of axonal fiber tracts.

functional MRI (fMRI) Magnetic resonance imaging that detects changes in blood flow and therefore identifies regions of the brain that are particularly active during a given task.

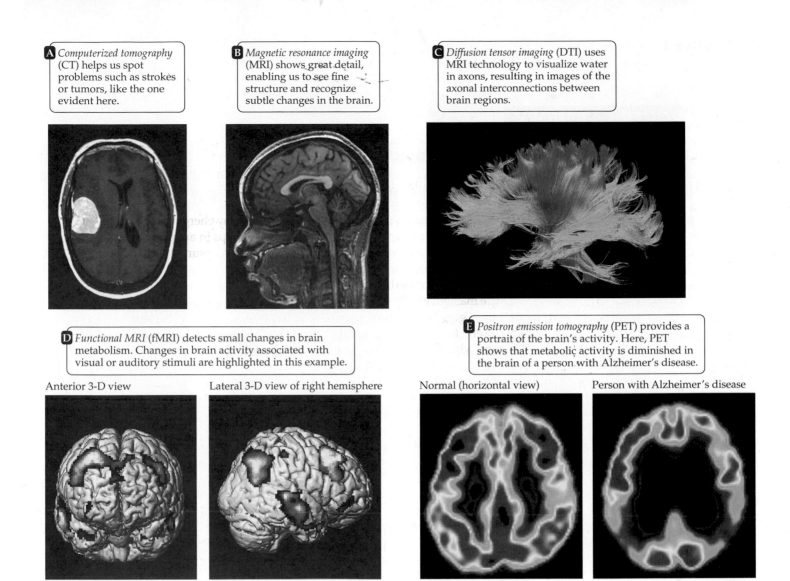

A *Computerized tomography* (CT) helps us spot problems such as strokes or tumors, like the one evident here.

B *Magnetic resonance imaging* (MRI) shows great detail, enabling us to see fine structure and recognize subtle changes in the brain.

C *Diffusion tensor imaging* (DTI) uses MRI technology to visualize water in axons, resulting in images of the axonal interconnections between brain regions.

D *Functional MRI* (fMRI) detects small changes in brain metabolism. Changes in brain activity associated with visual or auditory stimuli are highlighted in this example.

Anterior 3-D view   Lateral 3-D view of right hemisphere

E *Positron emission tomography* (PET) provides a portrait of the brain's activity. Here, PET shows that metabolic activity is diminished in the brain of a person with Alzheimer's disease.

Normal (horizontal view)   Person with Alzheimer's disease

FIGURE 2.18 Visualizing the Living Human Brain (A © Living Art Enterprises, LLC/Science Source; B © Guy Croft SciTech/ Alamy; C © Living Art Enterprises/Science Source; D courtesy of Samir Zeki; E © Science Source/Science Source.)

structure of the brain and is too slow to track rapid, moment-by-moment changes in the activity of networks of neurons, fMRI combined with conventional anatomical MRI has revealed many important clues about how networks of brain structures collaborate on complex cognitive processes (**FIGURES 2.18C** and **D**). An additional consideration is that, as in other imaging techniques, fMRI imagery is not photographic: it is created by a computer based on metabolic and structural assumptions. There is some concern that the computer algorithms used in this process may sometimes be misleading (Eklund et al., 2016; Poldrack et al., 2017).

PET tracks radioactive substances to produce images of brain activity

Like fMRI, **positron emission tomography** (PET) depicts the brain's activity during behavioral tasks. Short-lived radioactive chemicals are injected into the bloodstream, and radiation detectors encircling the head map the destination of these chemicals in the brain. A particularly effective strategy is to inject radioactively labeled glucose ("blood sugar") while the person is engaged in a cognitive task of interest to the researcher. Because the radioactive glucose is selectively taken up and used by the most active parts of the brain, a moment-to-moment color-coded portrait of brain activity can be created (**FIGURE 2.18E**) (P. E. Roland, 1993). Although PET can't match the detailed resolution of fMRI, it tends to be faster and thus better able to track quick changes in brain activity. Next we'll discuss how precise experimental methods allow researchers to identify brain regions that contribute to specific functions.

positron emission tomography (PET)
A brain-imaging technology that tracks the metabolism of injected radioactive substances in the brain, in order to map brain activity.

RESEARCHERS AT WORK

Subtractive analysis isolates specific brain activity

Modern brain imaging provides dramatic pictures showing the particular brain regions that are activated during specific cognitive processes; there are many such images in this book. But if you do a PET scan of a healthy person, you find that almost all of the brain is active at any given moment (showing that the old notion that "we use only 10% of our brain" is nonsense). How do researchers obtain these highly specific images of brain activity?

In order to associate specific brain regions with particular cognitive operations, researchers developed a sort of algebraic technique, in which activity during one behavioral condition is subtracted from activity during a different condition. So, for example, the data from a control PET scan made while a person was gazing at a blank wall might be subtracted from a PET scan collected while that person studied a complex visual stimulus. Averaged over enough trials, the specific regions that are almost always active during the processing task become apparent, even though, on casual inspection, a single experimental scan might not look much different from a single control scan (**FIGURE 2.19**). It is important to keep in mind that although functional brain images seem unambiguous and easy to label, they are subject to a variety of procedural and experimental limitations (Racine et al., 2005).

FIGURE 2.19   Isolating Specific Brain Activity (Courtesy of Marcus Raichle.)

■ Hypothesis

Brain regions engaged in a specific behavior can be isolated by algebraic means, subtracting resting scans from scans during activity.

■ Test

Participants are scanned twice—once while looking at a blank screen, and once while looking at test stimuli. The control scan is then subtracted from the test scan.

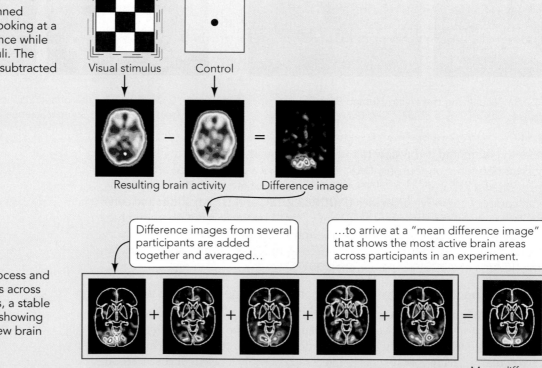

Visual stimulus   Control

Resulting brain activity   Difference image

Difference images from several participants are added together and averaged…

…to arrive at a "mean difference image" that shows the most active brain areas across participants in an experiment.

■ Result

By repeating the process and averaging the results across multiple participants, a stable "difference image" showing activation of just a few brain regions is formed.

Mean difference image

■ Conclusion

The activated brain regions in the difference image—in this case, in the occipital cortex—are selectively involved in the particular cognitive processing required by the stimulus.

Magnetism can be used to study the brain

It is a simple matter to pass magnetic fields into the brain. However, it is technically more challenging to project magnetic fields in a highly focused and precise manner. In **transcranial magnetic stimulation** (**TMS**) (**FIGURE 2.20**), focal magnetic currents are used to briefly stimulate the cortex of alert people directly, without any lasting physical alterations or surgery (Y. Noguchi et al., 2003). Using TMS allows experimenters to activate a discrete area of the brain while simultaneously tracking any resulting changes in behavior.

Not only can magnets stimulate neurons, but neurons also act as tiny electromagnets themselves! In **magnetoencephalography** (**MEG**), a large array of ultrasensitive detectors measures the minuscule magnetic fields produced by the electrical activity of cortical neurons. This information is used to construct real-time maps of brain activity during ongoing cognitive processing (**FIGURE 2.21**). Because MEG can track quick, moment-by-moment changes in brain activity, it is excellent for studying the rapidly shifting patterns of brain activity in cortical circuits that fMRI is too slow to track (Baillet, 2017). In the next chapter, we'll learn about electroencephalography (EEG), which measures ongoing electrical activity in the brain.

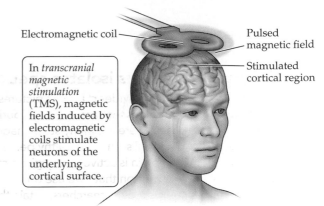

In *transcranial magnetic stimulation* (TMS), magnetic fields induced by electromagnetic coils stimulate neurons of the underlying cortical surface.

Electromagnetic coil

Pulsed magnetic field

Stimulated cortical region

FIGURE 2.20 Transcranial Magnetic Stimulation

HOW'S IT GOING ❓

1. Compare and contrast the main methods for producing still images of the structure of the brain. What do you think are some of the advantages and disadvantages of each method?
2. Compare and contrast the main functional-imaging technologies used for visualizing the activity of brain regions. What do you think are some of the advantages and disadvantages of each method?
3. Describe the process that neuroscientists can use to isolate brain activity associated with a specific behavior, as visualized by functional-imaging techniques.

transcranial magnetic stimulation (TMS) A noninvasive technique for examining brain function that applies strong magnetic fields to stimulate cortical neurons in order to identify discrete areas of the brain that are particularly active during specific behaviors.

magnetoencephalography (MEG) A noninvasive brain-imaging technology that creates maps of brain activity during cognitive tasks by measuring tiny magnetic fields produced by active neurons.

(A)

Face

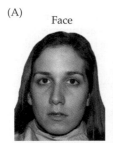

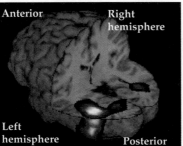

Anterior · Right hemisphere · Left hemisphere · Posterior

Magnetoencephalography (MEG) measures the minuscule magnetic fields given off by ensembles of cortical cells during specific behavioral functions. Here, MEG maps brain activity associated with viewing faces…

(B)

Object

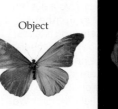

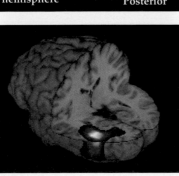

…versus viewing nonface objects.

FIGURE 2.21 Animal Magnetism (MEG images courtesy of Drs. Mario Liotti and Anthony Herdman, Simon Fraser University and Down Syndrome Research Foundation.)

Recommended Reading

Blumenfeld, H. (2010). *Neuroanatomy through Clinical Cases* (2nd ed.). Sunderland, MA: Oxford University Press/Sinauer.

Huettel, S. A., Song, A. W., and McCarthy, G. (2014). *Functional Magnetic Resonance Imaging* (3rd ed.). Sunderland, MA: Oxford University Press/Sinauer.

Papanicolau, A. C. (Ed.). (2017). *The Oxford Handbook of Functional Brain Imaging in Neuropsychology and Cognitive Neurosciences*. Oxford, UK: Oxford University Press.

Schoonover, C. (2010). *Portraits of the Mind: Visualizing the Brain from Antiquity to the 21st Century*. New York, NY: Abrams.

Swanson, L. W., Newman, E., Araque, A., and Dubinsky, J. M. (2017). *The Beautiful Brain: The Drawings of Santiago Ramón y Cajal*. New York, NY: Abrams.

2 ■ Visual Summary

3e.mindsmachine.com/vs2

You should be able to relate each summary to the adjacent illustration, including structures and processes. If you go to the website for our text (3e.mindsmachine.com), you can follow links to figures, animations, and activities that will help you consolidate the material.

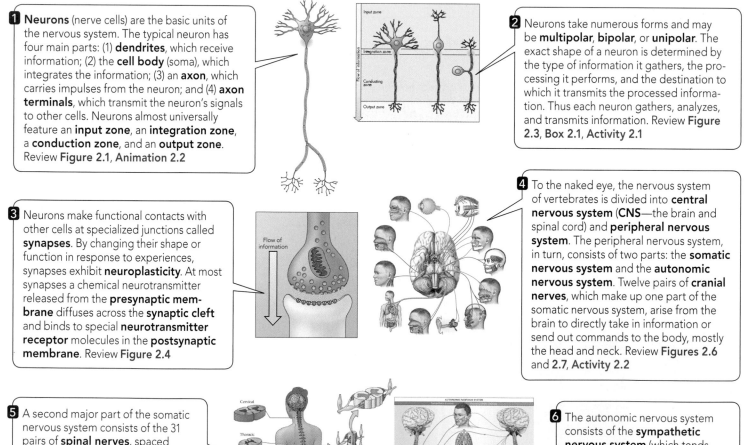

1 **Neurons** (nerve cells) are the basic units of the nervous system. The typical neuron has four main parts: (1) **dendrites**, which receive information; (2) the **cell body** (soma), which integrates the information; (3) an **axon**, which carries impulses from the neuron; and (4) **axon terminals**, which transmit the neuron's signals to other cells. Neurons almost universally feature an **input zone**, an **integration zone**, a **conduction zone**, and an **output zone**. Review **Figure 2.1, Animation 2.2**

2 Neurons take numerous forms and may be **multipolar**, **bipolar**, or **unipolar**. The exact shape of a neuron is determined by the type of information it gathers, the processing it performs, and the destination to which it transmits the processed information. Thus each neuron gathers, analyzes, and transmits information. Review **Figure 2.3, Box 2.1, Activity 2.1**

3 Neurons make functional contacts with other cells at specialized junctions called **synapses**. By changing their shape or function in response to experiences, synapses exhibit **neuroplasticity**. At most synapses a chemical neurotransmitter released from the **presynaptic membrane** diffuses across the **synaptic cleft** and binds to special **neurotransmitter receptor** molecules in the **postsynaptic membrane**. Review **Figure 2.4**

4 To the naked eye, the nervous system of vertebrates is divided into **central nervous system** (**CNS**—the brain and spinal cord) and **peripheral nervous system**. The peripheral nervous system, in turn, consists of two parts: the **somatic nervous system** and the **autonomic nervous system**. Twelve pairs of **cranial nerves**, which make up one part of the somatic nervous system, arise from the brain to directly take in information or send out commands to the body, mostly the head and neck. Review **Figures 2.6** and **2.7, Activity 2.2**

5 A second major part of the somatic nervous system consists of the 31 pairs of **spinal nerves**, spaced through the **cervical, thoracic, lumbar, sacral**, and **coccygeal segments** of the spinal cord. Review **Figure 2.8, Activity 2.3**

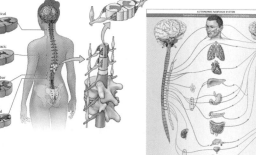

6 The autonomic nervous system consists of the **sympathetic nervous system** (which tends to ready the body for immediate action) and the **parasympathetic nervous system** (which tends to have an effect opposite to that of the sympathetic system). We cannot consciously control autonomic activity. Review **Figure 2.9, Activity 2.4**

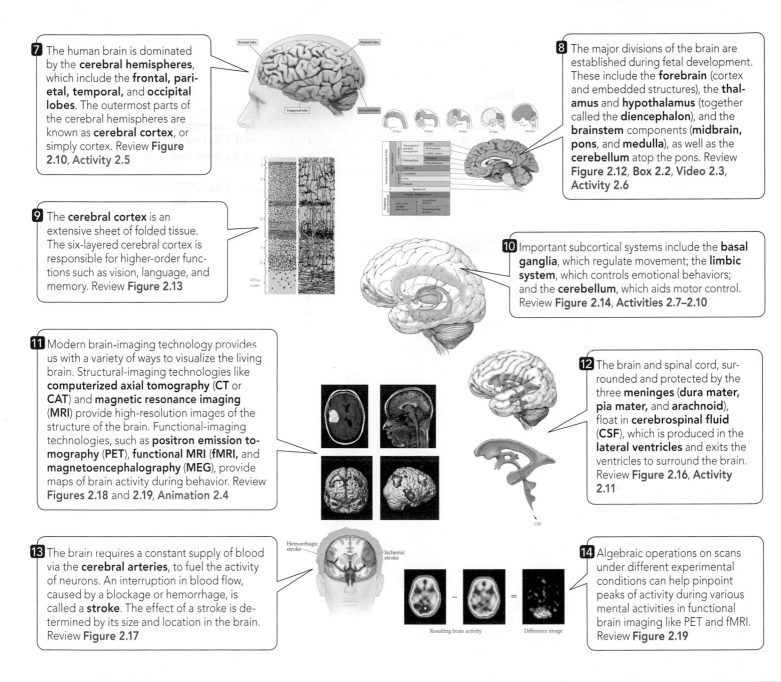

7 The human brain is dominated by the **cerebral hemispheres**, which include the **frontal, parietal, temporal,** and **occipital lobes**. The outermost parts of the cerebral hemispheres are known as **cerebral cortex**, or simply cortex. Review **Figure 2.10, Activity 2.5**

8 The major divisions of the brain are established during fetal development. These include the **forebrain** (cortex and embedded structures), the **thalamus** and **hypothalamus** (together called the **diencephalon**), and the **brainstem** components (**midbrain, pons,** and **medulla**), as well as the **cerebellum** atop the pons. Review **Figure 2.12, Box 2.2, Video 2.3, Activity 2.6**

9 The **cerebral cortex** is an extensive sheet of folded tissue. The six-layered cerebral cortex is responsible for higher-order functions such as vision, language, and memory. Review **Figure 2.13**

10 Important subcortical systems include the **basal ganglia**, which regulate movement; the **limbic system**, which controls emotional behaviors; and the **cerebellum**, which aids motor control. Review **Figure 2.14, Activities 2.7–2.10**

11 Modern brain-imaging technology provides us with a variety of ways to visualize the living brain. Structural-imaging technologies like **computerized axial tomography** (**CT** or **CAT**) and **magnetic resonance imaging** (**MRI**) provide high-resolution images of the structure of the brain. Functional-imaging technologies, such as **positron emission tomography** (**PET**), **functional MRI** (**fMRI**, and **magnetoencephalography** (**MEG**), provide maps of brain activity during behavior. Review **Figures 2.18** and **2.19, Animation 2.4**

12 The brain and spinal cord, surrounded and protected by the three **meninges** (**dura mater, pia mater,** and **arachnoid**), float in **cerebrospinal fluid** (**CSF**), which is produced in the **lateral ventricles** and exits the ventricles to surround the brain. Review **Figure 2.16, Activity 2.11**

13 The brain requires a constant supply of blood via the **cerebral arteries**, to fuel the activity of neurons. An interruption in blood flow, caused by a blockage or hemorrhage, is called a **stroke**. The effect of a stroke is determined by its size and location in the brain. Review **Figure 2.17**

14 Algebraic operations on scans under different experimental conditions can help pinpoint peaks of activity during various mental activities in functional brain imaging like PET and fMRI. Review **Figure 2.19**

Go to **3e.mindsmachine.com** for study questions, quizzes, flashcards, and other resources.

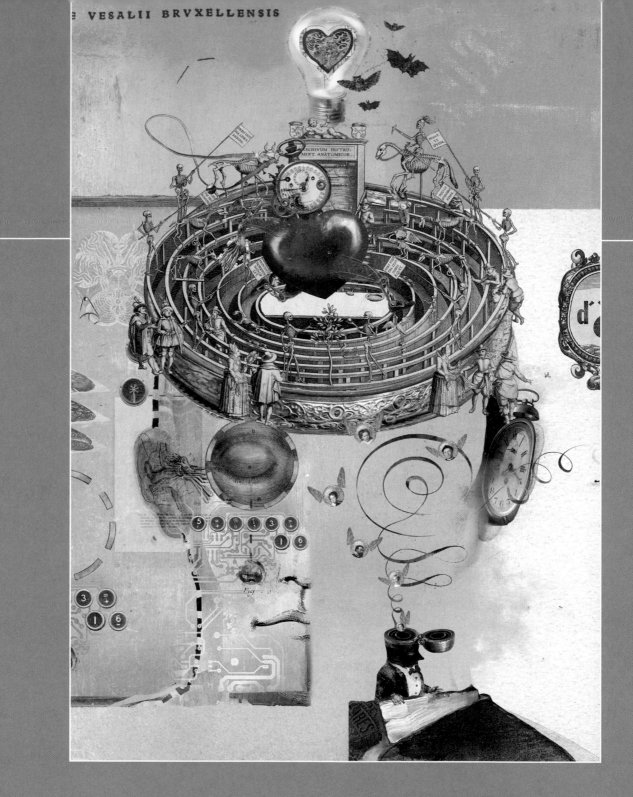

3
Neurophysiology
The Generation, Transmission, and Integration of Neural Signals

Stimulating Conversation

Perhaps the most dramatic neuroscience demonstration in history occurred in 1964 when Yale Professor José Delgado strolled into an arena in Spain to face an enraged bull trained to attack humans. Armed only with a remote control, Delgado watched the massive bull paw the earth, lower its head, and charge right at him. Just before the bull reached him, Delgado pressed a button on the remote control that caused a wire, called an *electrode*, in the bull's brain to deliver a tiny trickle of electricity. The bull stopped cold. When Delgado electrically stimulated another part of the bull's brain, the animal turned to the right and calmly trotted away. Repeated stimulations rendered the bull docile for several minutes (Marzullo, 2017). Other bulls responded differently to brain stimulation, depending on the brain region targeted. One animal produced a single "moo" for every button press—a hundred times in a row.

Delgado also electrically stimulated electrodes in the brains of people, in an attempt to pinpoint the cause of a neurological disorder. Depending on which part of the brain was stimulated, patients might suddenly become anxious or angry (Delgado, 1969). Maybe the creepiest response elicited by brain stimulation was in women who suddenly became romantically interested in the man interviewing them. Yet as soon as the electrical stimulation of their brains stopped, the women returned to their usual reserved behavior.

Why does a tiny bit of electrical stimulation in the brain produce such profound changes in mood and behavior? The reason is that neurons normally use electrical signals to sum up vast amounts of information. When Delgado electrically stimulated the brain, he was triggering those normal electrical signals in a very abnormal way, with sometimes startling results. To understand how even a tiny electrical charge to the brain can so dramatically affect the mind, we need to understand how electrical signaling works in the brain.

Neurophysiology is the study of the specialized life processes that allow neurons to use chemical and electrical signals to process and transmit information. In this chapter we'll study the electrical processes at work within a neuron; in the next chapter we'll look at the chemical signals that pass between neurons. We'll see that brain function is an alternating series of electrical signals within neurons and of chemical signals between neurons.

For example, a doctor may use a small rubber mallet to strike just below your knee and watch your leg kick upward in what is known as the *knee-jerk reflex*. Simple as it appears, a lot happens during this test. First, sensory neurons in the muscle detect the hammer tap and send a rapid electrical signal along their axons to your spinal cord. That rapid electrical signal along the axons from knee to spinal cord is called an *action potential*, which is a major topic in this chapter. When the action potential reaches the axon terminals, they

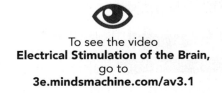

To see the video
Electrical Stimulation of the Brain,
go to
3e.mindsmachine.com/av3.1

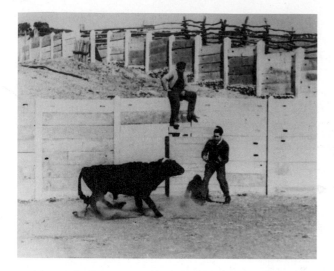

Hold It Right There! Dr. José Delgado stops a bull in the middle of a charge, using the remote control in his hand. (Courtesy of the Delgado estate and José Carlos Delgado.)

To view the
Brain Explorer,
go to
3e.mindsmachine.com/av3.2

neurophysiology The study of the life processes of neurons.

ion An atom or molecule that has acquired an electrical charge by gaining or losing one or more electrons.

anion A negatively charged ion, such as a protein or a chloride ion.

cation A positively charged ion, such as a potassium or sodium ion.

intracellular fluid Also called *cytoplasm*. The watery solution found within cells.

extracellular fluid The fluid in the spaces between cells (interstitial fluid).

cell membrane The lipid bilayer that encloses a cell.

microelectrode An especially small electrode used to record electrical potentials inside living cells.

release a chemical, called a *neurotransmitter*, to stimulate spinal motor neurons. In response to the neurotransmitter, the motor neurons send action potentials down their own axons to release yet another neurotransmitter onto muscles. In response to that neurotransmitter, the muscles contract, kicking your foot into the air. Problems in electrical or chemical signaling in this circuit might cause the kick to be stronger or weaker, faster or slower, than it should be.

So this "simple" behavior involves several rounds of signaling: first electrical (along sensory neuron axons), then chemical (sensory neurons to motor neurons), then electrical again (along motor neuron axons), and finally chemical again (motor neurons to muscle). This is the classic pattern of neural function: information flows *within* a neuron via electrical signals (action potentials) and passes *between* neurons through chemical signals (neurotransmitters). This sequence also reflects the organization of this chapter. First we explain how neurons produce action potentials and send them along their axons. Then we describe how the action potential causes axon terminals to release neurotransmitter into the synapse. Next we discuss how the neurotransmitter affects the electrical state of the neuron on the other side of the synapse. And we conclude the chapter by discussing how electrical probing of the brain revealed that the brain's surface reflects a map of the body. All this will prepare us for the next chapter, where we will learn more details about the chemical signals between neurons.

PART I
Electric Neurons

THE ROAD AHEAD

The first section of this chapter explains how neurons use electrical forces to process information. Reading this material should enable you to:

1. Identify the two physical forces that make neurons more negatively charged inside than outside.
2. Understand the changes in a neuron's membrane that produces a large electrical signal called an action potential.
3. Explain the changes in channels and movement of ions that underlie the action potential.
4. Understand how the action potential spreads along the length of an axon.
5. Understand how each neuron uses these electrical signals to integrate information from other neurons.

Electrical Signals Are the Vocabulary of the Nervous System

Like all living cells, neurons are more negative on the inside than on the outside, so we say they are *polarized*, meaning there is a difference in electrical charge between the inside and outside of the cell. Let's consider a neuron at rest, neither perturbed by other neurons nor producing its own signals. Of the many **ions** (electrically charged molecules) that a neuron contains, a majority are **anions** ("ANN-eye-ons"; negatively charged ions), especially large protein anions that cannot exit the cell. The rest are **cations** ("CAT-eye-ons"; positively charged ions). (It may help you to remember that the letter *t*, which occurs in the word *cation*, is shaped a bit like a plus sign, +.) All of these ions are dissolved in the **intracellular fluid** inside the cell and the **extracellular fluid** outside the **cell membrane**.

If we insert a fine **microelectrode** into the interior of a neuron and place another electrode in the extracellular fluid and take a reading (as in **FIGURE 3.1**), we find that the inside of the neuron is more negative than the fluid around it. Specifically,

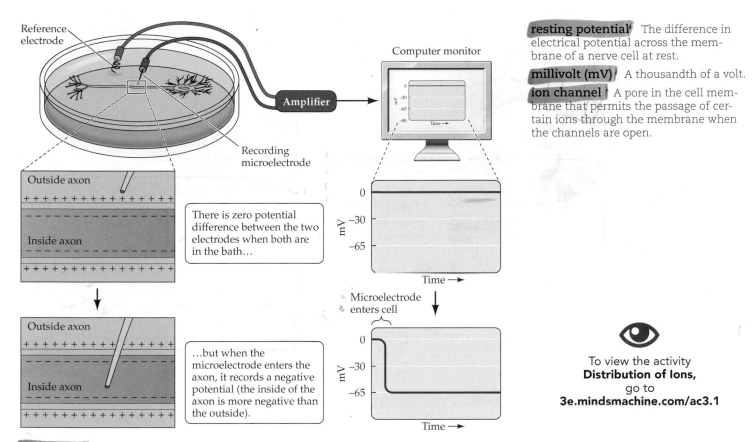

Reference electrode

Recording microelectrode

Amplifier

Computer monitor

Outside axon
+ + + + + + + + + + + + + +
Inside axon
+ + + + + + + + + + + + + +

There is zero potential difference between the two electrodes when both are in the bath…

Outside axon
+ + + + + + + + + + + + + +
Inside axon
+ + + + + + + + + + + + + +

…but when the microelectrode enters the axon, it records a negative potential (the inside of the axon is more negative than the outside).

Microelectrode enters cell

resting potential The difference in electrical potential across the membrane of a nerve cell at rest.

millivolt (mV) A thousandth of a volt.

ion channel A pore in the cell membrane that permits the passage of certain ions through the membrane when the channels are open.

To view the activity
Distribution of Ions,
go to
3e.mindsmachine.com/ac3.1

FIGURE 3.1 Measuring the Resting Potential

a neuron at rest exhibits a characteristic **resting potential** (an electrical difference across the membrane) of about −50 to −80 thousandths of a volt, or **milli-volts (mV)** (the negative sign indicates that the cell's interior is more negative than the outside). To understand how this negative membrane potential comes about, we have to consider some special properties of the cell membrane, as well as two forces that drive ions across it.

The cell membrane is a double layer of fatty molecules studded with many sorts of specialized proteins. One important type of membrane-spanning protein is the **ion channel**, a tubelike pore that allows ions of a specific type to pass through the membrane (**FIGURE 3.2**). As we'll see later, some types of ion channels are *gated*: they can open and close rapidly in response to various influences. But some ion channels leak, staying open all the time, and the cell membrane of a neuron contains many such channels that selectively allow

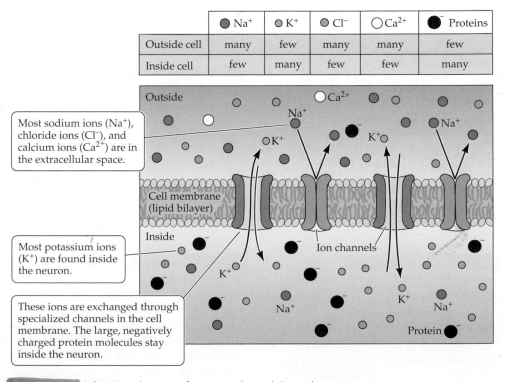

	Na⁺	K⁺	Cl⁻	Ca²⁺	Proteins
Outside cell	many	few	many	many	few
Inside cell	few	many	few	few	many

Most sodium ions (Na⁺), chloride ions (Cl⁻), and calcium ions (Ca²⁺) are in the extracellular space.

Cell membrane (lipid bilayer)

Most potassium ions (K⁺) are found inside the neuron.

These ions are exchanged through specialized channels in the cell membrane. The large, negatively charged protein molecules stay inside the neuron.

Outside

Inside

Ion channels

FIGURE 3.2 The Distribution of Ions Inside and Outside a Neuron

(A) Diffusion

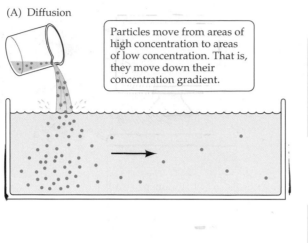

Particles move from areas of high concentration to areas of low concentration. That is, they move down their concentration gradient.

(B) Diffusion through semipermeable membranes

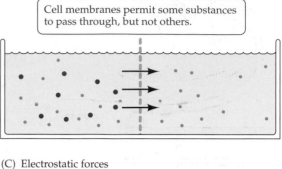

Cell membranes permit some substances to pass through, but not others.

(C) Electrostatic forces

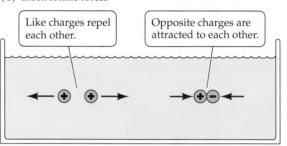

Like charges repel each other.

Opposite charges are attracted to each other.

FIGURE 3.3 Ionic Forces Underlying Electrical Signaling in Neurons

potassium ion (K⁺) A potassium atom that carries a positive charge.

sodium ion (Na⁺) A sodium atom that carries a positive charge.

selective permeability The property of a membrane that allows some substances to pass through, but not others.

diffusion The spontaneous spread of molecules from an area of high concentration to an area of low concentration.

electrostatic pressure The propensity of charged molecules or ions to move toward areas with the opposite charge.

sodium-potassium pump The energetically expensive mechanism that pushes sodium ions out of a cell, and potassium ions in.

equilibrium potential The point at which the movement of ions across the cell membrane is balanced, as the electrostatic pressure pulling ions in one direction is offset by the diffusion force pushing them in the opposite direction.

potassium ions (K⁺) to cross the membrane, but not sodium ions (Na⁺). Because it is studded with these K⁺ channels, we say that the cell membrane of a neuron exhibits selective permeability, allowing some things to pass through, but not others. The membrane allows K⁺ ions, but not Na⁺ ions, to enter or exit the cell fairly freely.

The resting potential of the neuron reflects a balancing act between two opposing processes that drive K⁺ ions in and out of the neuron. The first of these is diffusion (FIGURE 3.3A), which is the tendency of molecules of a substance to spread from regions of high concentration to regions of low concentration. For example, when placed in a glass of water, the molecules in a drop of food coloring will tend to spread from the drop out into the rest of the water, where they are less concentrated. So we say that molecules tend to "move down their concentration gradient" until they are evenly distributed. If a selectively permeable membrane divides the fluid, particles that can pass through the membrane, such as K⁺, will diffuse across until they are equally concentrated on both sides. Other ions, unable to cross the membrane, will remain concentrated on one side (FIGURE 3.3B).

The second force at work is electrostatic pressure, which arises from the distribution of electrical charges rather than the distribution of molecules. Charged particles exert electrical force on one another: like charges repel, and opposite charges attract (FIGURE 3.3C). Positively charged cations like K⁺ are thus attracted to the negatively charged interior of the cell; conversely, anions are repelled by the cell interior and so tend to exit to the extracellular fluid.

Now let's consider the situation across a neuron's cell membrane. Much of the energy consumed by a neuron goes into operating specialized membrane proteins called sodium-potassium pumps that pump three Na⁺ ions out of the cell for every two K⁺ ions pumped in (FIGURE 3.4A). This action results in a buildup of K⁺ ions inside the cell (and reduces Na⁺ inside the cell), but as we explained earlier, the membrane is selectively permeable to K⁺ ions (but not Na⁺ ions). Therefore, K⁺ ions can leave the interior, moving down their concentration gradient and causing a net buildup of negative charges inside the cell (FIGURE 3.4B). As negative charge builds up inside the cell, it begins to exert electrostatic pressure to pull positively charged K⁺ ions back inside. Eventually the opposing forces exerted by the K⁺ concentration gradient and by electrostatic pressure reach the equilibrium potential, the electrical charge that exactly balances

FIGURE 3.4 | The Ionic Basis of the Resting Potential

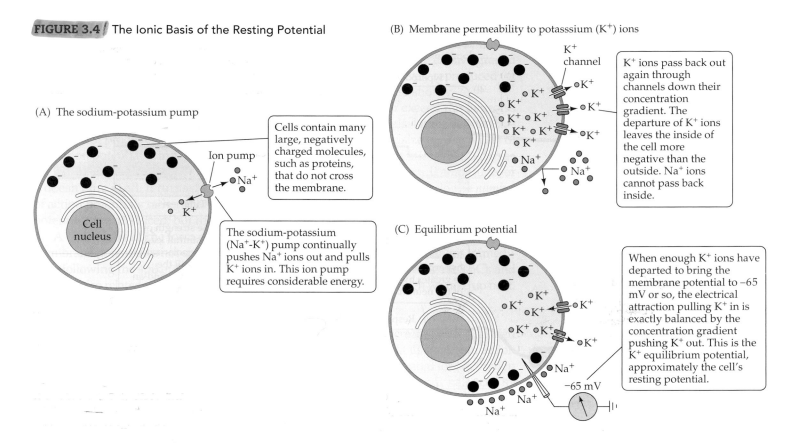

(A) The sodium-potassium pump

Cell nucleus

Ion pump

Cells contain many large, negatively charged molecules, such as proteins, that do not cross the membrane.

The sodium-potassium (Na⁺-K⁺) pump continually pushes Na⁺ ions out and pulls K⁺ ions in. This ion pump requires considerable energy.

(B) Membrane permeability to potasssium (K⁺) ions

K⁺ channel

K⁺ ions pass back out again through channels down their concentration gradient. The departure of K⁺ ions leaves the inside of the cell more negative than the outside. Na⁺ ions cannot pass back inside.

(C) Equilibrium potential

−65 mV

When enough K⁺ ions have departed to bring the membrane potential to −65 mV or so, the electrical attraction pulling K⁺ in is exactly balanced by the concentration gradient pushing K⁺ out. This is the K⁺ equilibrium potential, approximately the cell's resting potential.

the concentration gradient: any further movement of K⁺ ions into the cell (drawn by electrostatic attraction) is matched by the flow of K⁺ ions out of the cell (moving down their concentration gradient). This point approximates the cell's resting potential of about −65 mV (values may range between −50 and −80 mV), as **FIGURE 3.4C** depicts.

The resting potential of a neuron provides a baseline level of polarization found in all cells. But unlike most other cells, neurons routinely undergo a brief but radical *change* in polarization, sending an electrical signal from one end of the neuron to the other, as we'll discuss next.

A threshold amount of depolarization triggers an action potential

Action potentials are very brief but large changes in neuronal polarization that arise in the initial segment of the axon, just after the axon hillock (the cone-shaped region where the axon emerges from the cell body; see Figure 2.4A), and then move rapidly down the axon. The information that a neuron sends to other cells is encoded in patterns of these action potentials, so we need to understand their properties—where they come from, how they race down the axon, and how they send information across synapses to other cells. Let's turn first to the creation of the action potential.

Two concepts are central to understanding how action potentials are triggered. **Hyperpolarization** is an increase in membrane potential (i.e., the neuron becomes *even more negative* on the inside, relative to the outside). So if the neuron already has a resting potential of, say, −65 mV, hyperpolarization makes it even *farther from zero*, maybe −70 mV. **Depolarization** is the reverse, referring to a decrease in membrane potential. The depolarization of a neuron from a resting potential of −65 mV to, say, −50 mV makes the inside of the neuron more like the outside. In other words, depolarization of a neuron brings its membrane potential *closer to zero*.

Let's use an apparatus to apply hyperpolarizing and depolarizing stimuli to a neuron, via electrodes. (Later we'll talk about how synapses produce similar hyperpolarizations and depolarizations.) Applying a *hyperpolarizing* stimulus to the membrane

To view the animation
The Resting Membrane Potential,
go to
3e.mindsmachine.com/av3.3

axon hillock The cone-shaped area on the cell body from which the axon originates.

hyperpolarization An increase in membrane potential (the interior of the neuron becomes even more negative).

depolarization A decrease in membrane potential (the interior of the neuron becomes less negative).

TABLE 3.1 ■ Comparing Axons and Dendrites				
		Property		
	Size	Number per neuron	Information flow	Voltage changes
Axon	Thin, uniform	One (but may have branches)	Away from cell body	All-or-none
Dendrite	Thick, variable	Many	Into cell body	Graded, variable

membrane potential away from threshold—it decreases the probability that the neuron will fire an action potential—so it is called an inhibitory postsynaptic potential (IPSP).

Usually IPSPs result from the opening of channels that permit chloride ions (Cl⁻) to enter the cell. Because Cl⁻ ions are much more concentrated outside the cell than inside (see Figure 3.2), they rush into the cell, making its membrane potential more negative. What determines whether a synapse excites or inhibits the postsynaptic cell? One factor is the particular neurotransmitter released by the presynaptic cell. Some transmitters typically generate an EPSP in the postsynaptic cells; others typically generate an IPSP. Sometimes the same neurotransmitter can be excitatory at one synapse and inhibitory at another, depending on what sort of receptor the postsynaptic cell possesses. So in the end, whether a neuron fires an action potential at any given moment is decided by the balance between the number of excitatory and the number of inhibitory signals that it is receiving, and it receives many signals of both types at all times.

Now that you know more about the parts of neurons and how they communicate, we summarize the differences between axons (which send information via action potentials) and dendrites (which receive information from synapses) in **TABLE 3.1**.

Spatial summation and temporal summation integrate synaptic inputs

Synaptic transmission is an impressive process, but complex behavior requires more than the simple arrival of signals across synapses. Neurons must also be able to integrate the messages they receive. In other words, they perform *information processing*—by using a sort of neural algebra, in which each nerve cell adds and subtracts the many inputs it receives from other neurons. As we'll see next, this is possible because of the characteristics of synaptic inputs, the way in which the neuron integrates the postsynaptic potentials, and the trigger mechanism that determines whether a neuron will fire an action potential.

We've seen that postsynaptic potentials are caused by transmitter chemicals that can be either depolarizing (excitatory) or hyperpolarizing (inhibitory). From their points of origin on the dendrites and cell body, these graded EPSPs and IPSPs spread passively over the postsynaptic neuron, decreasing in strength over time and distance. Whether the postsynaptic neuron will fire depends on whether a depolarization exceeding threshold reaches the axon hillock, triggering an action potential. If many EPSPs are received, the axon may reach threshold and fire. But if both EPSPs and IPSPs arrive at the axon hillock, they partially cancel each other. Thus, the net effect is the *difference* between the two: the neuron subtracts the IPSPs from the EPSPs. Simple arithmetic, right?

Well, yes, summed EPSPs and IPSPs do tend to cancel each other out. But because postsynaptic potentials spread passively and dissipate as they cross the cell membrane, the resulting sum is also influenced by *distance*. For example, EPSPs from synapses close to the axon hillock will produce a larger effect there than will EPSPs from farther away. The summation of potentials originating from different physical locations across the cell body is called spatial summation. Only if the overall sum of *all* the potentials—both EPSPs and IPSPs—is sufficient to depolarize the cell to threshold at the axon hillock is an action potential triggered (**FIGURE 3.11A**). Usually it takes excitatory messages from many presynaptic neurons to cause a postsynaptic neuron to fire an action potential.

To view the animation
Spatial Summation,
go to
3e.mindsmachine.com/av3.6

inhibitory postsynaptic potential (IPSP)   A hyperpolarizing potential in a neuron. IPSPs decrease the probability that the postsynaptic neuron will fire an action potential.

chloride ion (Cl⁻)   A chlorine atom that carries a negative charge.

spatial summation   The summation of postsynaptic potentials that reach the axon hillock from different locations across the cell body. If this summation reaches threshold, an action potential is triggered.

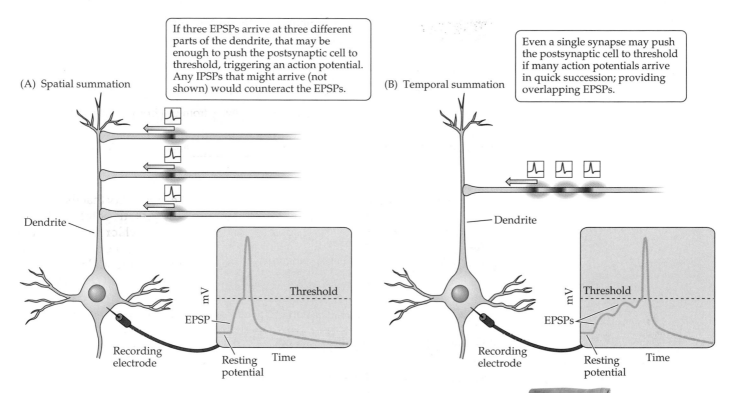

(A) Spatial summation

If three EPSPs arrive at three different parts of the dendrite, that may be enough to push the postsynaptic cell to threshold, triggering an action potential. Any IPSPs that might arrive (not shown) would counteract the EPSPs.

(B) Temporal summation

Even a single synapse may push the postsynaptic cell to threshold if many action potentials arrive in quick succession; providing overlapping EPSPs.

Dendrite

Dendrite

mV

Threshold

EPSP

Recording electrode

Resting potential

Time

mV

Threshold

EPSPs

Recording electrode

Resting potential

Time

FIGURE 3.11 Spatial versus Temporal Summation

Postsynaptic effects that are not absolutely simultaneous can also be summed, because the postsynaptic potentials last a few milliseconds before fading away. The closer they are in time, the greater is the overlap and the more complete is the summation, which in this case is called **temporal summation.** Temporal summation is easily understood if you imagine a neuron with only one input. If EPSPs arrive one right after the other, they sum and the postsynaptic cell eventually reaches threshold and produces an action potential (**FIGURE 3.11B**). But these graded potentials fade quickly, so if too much time passes between successive EPSPs, they will never sum and no action potentials will be triggered. **TABLE 3.2** summarizes the many properties of action potentials, EPSPs, and IPSPs, noting the similarities and differences among the three kinds of neural potentials.

It should now be clear that although action potentials are all-or-none phenomena, the postsynaptic effect they produce is graded in size and determined by the processing of many inputs occurring close together in time. The membrane potential at the axon hillock thus reflects the moment-to-moment integration of all the neuron's inputs, which the axon hillock encodes into action potentials.

temporal summation The summation of postsynaptic potentials that reach the axon hillock at different times. The closer in time the potentials occur, the greater the summation.

Type of signal	Signaling role	Typical duration (ms)	Amplitude	Character	Mode of propagation	Ion channel opening	Channel sensitive to:
Action potential	Conduction along an axon	1–2	Overshooting, 100 mV	All-or-none, digital	Actively propagated, regenerative	First Na⁺, then K⁺, in different channels	Voltage (depolarization)
Excitatory postsynaptic potential (EPSP)	Transmission between neurons	10–100	Depolarizing, from less than 1 to more than 20 mV	Graded, analog	Local, passive spread	Na⁺, K⁺	Chemical (neurotransmitter)
Inhibitory postsynaptic potential (IPSP)	Transmission between neurons	10–100	Hyperpolarizing, from less than 1 to about 15 mV	Graded, analog	Local, passive spread	Cl⁻, K⁺	Chemical (neurotransmitter)

TABLE 3.2 ■ Characteristics of Electrical Signals of Nerve Cells

Dendrites add to the story of neuronal integration. A vast number of synaptic inputs, arrayed across the dendrites and cell body, can induce postsynaptic potentials. So dendrites expand the receptive surface of the neuron and increase the amount of input the neuron can handle. All other things being equal, the farther out on a dendrite a potential occurs, the less effect it should have at the axon, because the potential decreases in size as it passively spreads. When the potential arises at a dendritic *spine* (see Figure 2.4), its effect is even smaller because it has to spread down the shaft of the spine. Thus, information arriving at various parts of the neuron is *weighted*, in terms of the distance to the axon hillock and the path resistance along the way.

HOW'S IT GOING ❓

1. What are EPSPs and IPSPs?
2. Compare and contrast spatial summation versus temporal summation.
3. Discuss the electrical properties of a neuron that allow it to process information.
4. Where does information enter a neuron, and how does a neuron send information to other cells?

PART II
Synaptic Transmission

THE ROAD AHEAD

This portion of the chapter explains how neurons release chemicals to signal one another. After reading this material you should be able to:

1. Identify the sequence of steps that take place when one neuron releases a chemical signal to affect another.
2. Understand how a variety of chemical signals enables a diversity of neuronal responses to other neurons.
3. Identify the interactions between neurons and muscles that underlie a simple reflex.

Synaptic Transmission Requires a Sequence of Events

The steps that take place during chemical synaptic transmission are summarized in **FIGURE 3.12**:

1. The action potential arrives at the presynaptic axon terminal.
2. Voltage-gated calcium channels in the membrane of the axon terminal open, allowing calcium ions (Ca^{2+}) to enter.
3. Ca^{2+} causes synaptic vesicles filled with neurotransmitter to fuse with the presynaptic membrane and rupture, releasing the transmitter molecules into the synaptic cleft.
4. Transmitter molecules bind to special receptor molecules in the postsynaptic membrane, leading—directly or indirectly—to the opening of ion channels in the postsynaptic membrane. The resulting flow of ions creates a local EPSP or IPSP in the postsynaptic neuron.
5. The IPSPs and EPSPs in the postsynaptic cell spread toward the axon hillock. (If the sum of all the EPSPs and IPSPs ultimately depolarizes the axon hillock enough to reach threshold, an action potential will arise.)
6. Synaptic transmission is rapidly stopped, so the message is brief and accurately reflects the activity of the presynaptic cell.
7. Synaptic transmitter may also activate presynaptic receptors, resulting in a decrease in transmitter release.

Let's look at these seven steps in a little more detail.

To view the animation
Synaptic Transmission,
go to
3e.mindsmachine.com/av3.7

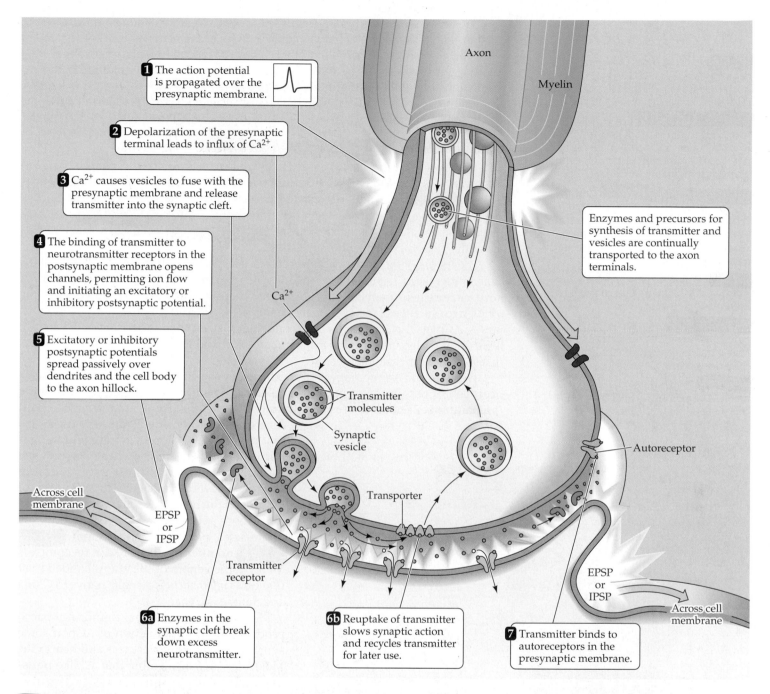

1 The action potential is propagated over the presynaptic membrane.

2 Depolarization of the presynaptic terminal leads to influx of Ca^{2+}.

3 Ca^{2+} causes vesicles to fuse with the presynaptic membrane and release transmitter into the synaptic cleft.

4 The binding of transmitter to neurotransmitter receptors in the postsynaptic membrane opens channels, permitting ion flow and initiating an excitatory or inhibitory postsynaptic potential.

5 Excitatory or inhibitory postsynaptic potentials spread passively over dendrites and the cell body to the axon hillock.

6a Enzymes in the synaptic cleft break down excess neurotransmitter.

6b Reuptake of transmitter slows synaptic action and recycles transmitter for later use.

7 Transmitter binds to autoreceptors in the presynaptic membrane.

Enzymes and precursors for synthesis of transmitter and vesicles are continually transported to the axon terminals.

Axon

Myelin

Ca^{2+}

Transmitter molecules

Synaptic vesicle

Autoreceptor

Transporter

Across cell membrane

EPSP or IPSP

EPSP or IPSP

Across cell membrane

Transmitter receptor

FIGURE 3.12   Steps in Transmission at a Chemical Synapse

Action potentials cause the release of transmitter molecules into the synaptic cleft

When an action potential reaches a presynaptic terminal, it causes hundreds of **synaptic vesicles** near the presynaptic membrane to fuse with the membrane and discharge their contents—molecules of neurotransmitter—into the **synaptic cleft** (the space between the presynaptic and postsynaptic membranes). The key event in this process is an influx of **calcium ions (Ca^{2+})**, rather than K^+ or Na^+, into the axon terminal. These ions enter through voltage-gated Ca^{2+} channels opening in response to the arrival of an action potential. **Synaptic delay** is the time needed for Ca^{2+} to enter the terminal, for the transmitter to diffuse across the synaptic cleft, and for transmitter molecules to interact with their receptors before the postsynaptic cell responds.

synaptic vesicle   A small, spherical structure that contains molecules of neurotransmitter.

synaptic cleft   The space between the presynaptic and postsynaptic cells at a synapse. This gap measures about 20–40 nm.

calcium ion (Ca^{2+})   A calcium atom that carries a double positive charge.

synaptic delay   The brief delay between the arrival of an action potential at the axon terminal and the creation of a postsynaptic potential.

ligand A substance that binds to receptor molecules, such as a neurotransmitter or drug that binds postsynaptic receptors.

acetylcholine (ACh) A neurotransmitter that is produced and released by parasympathetic postganglionic neurons, by motor neurons, and by many neurons in the brain.

neurotransmitter receptor Also called simply receptor. A specialized protein, embedded in the cell membrane, that selectively senses and reacts to molecules of a corresponding neurotransmitter.

curare A neurotoxin that causes paralysis by blocking acetylcholine receptors in muscle.

bungarotoxin A neurotoxin, isolated from the venom of the many-banded krait, that selectively blocks acetylcholine receptors.

agonist A substance that mimics or boosts the actions of a transmitter or other signaling molecule.

The presynaptic terminal normally produces and stores enough transmitter to ensure that it is ready for activity. Intense activity of the neuron reduces the number of available vesicles, but soon more vesicles are produced to replace those that were discharged. Neurons differ in their ability to keep pace with a rapid rate of incoming action potentials. Furthermore, the rate of making the transmitter is regulated by enzymes that are manufactured in the neuronal cell body and transported down the axons to the terminals.

Receptor molecules recognize transmitters

The action of a key in a lock is a good analogy for the action of a transmitter on a receptor protein. Just as a particular key can open a door, a molecule of the correct shape, called a **ligand** (see Chapter 4), can fit into a receptor protein and activate or block it. So, for example, at synapses where the transmitter is **acetylcholine (ACh)**, the ACh fits into areas called *ligand-binding sites* in **neurotransmitter receptor** molecules located in the postsynaptic membrane (**FIGURE 3.13**).

The nature of the postsynaptic receptors at a synapse determines the action of the transmitter (see Chapter 4). For example, ACh can function as either an inhibitory or an excitatory neurotransmitter, at different synapses. At excitatory synapses, binding of ACh to one type of receptor opens channels for Na$^+$ and K$^+$ ions. At inhibitory synapses, ACh may act on another type of receptor to open channels that allow Cl$^-$ ions to enter, thereby hyperpolarizing the membrane (i.e., making it more negative and so less likely to create an action potential).

The lock-and-key analogy is strengthened by the observation that various chemicals can fit onto receptor proteins and block the entrance of the key. Some of the preparations used in this research sound like the ingredients for a witches' brew. As an example, consider some potent poisons that block ACh receptors: curare and bungarotoxin. **Curare** is an arrowhead poison used by native South Americans. Extracted from a plant, it greatly increases the efficiency of hunting: if the hunter hits any part of the prey, the arrow's poison soon blocks ACh receptors on muscles, paralyzing the animal. **Bungarotoxin**, another blocker of ACh receptors, is found in the venom of the many-banded krait (*Bungarus multicinctus*), a snake native to China and Southeast Asia.

The chemical nicotine, found in tobacco products, mimics the action of ACh at some synapses, increasing alertness and heart rate. Molecules such as nicotine that act like transmitters at a receptor are called **agonists** (from the Greek *agon*, "contest" or "struggle") of that transmitter. Conversely, molecules that interfere with or prevent the action of a transmitter, like curare, are called **antagonists**.

Just as there are master keys that fit many different locks, there are submaster keys that fit a certain group of locks, as well as keys that fit only a single lock. Similarly, each chemical transmitter binds to several different receptor molecules. ACh acts on at least four subtypes of **cholinergic** receptors. Nicotinic cholinergic receptors are found at synapses on muscles and in autonomic ganglia; it is the blockade of these

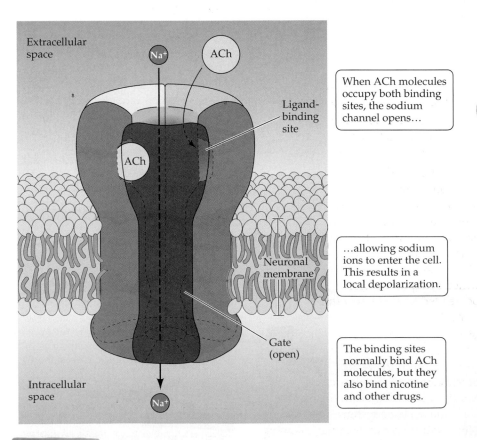

Extracellular space

Na$^+$

ACh

Ligand-binding site

ACh

Neuronal membrane

Gate (open)

Intracellular space

Na$^+$

When ACh molecules occupy both binding sites, the sodium channel opens…

…allowing sodium ions to enter the cell. This results in a local depolarization.

The binding sites normally bind ACh molecules, but they also bind nicotine and other drugs.

FIGURE 3.13 A Nicotinic Acetylcholine Receptor

receptors that causes paralysis brought on by curare and bungarotoxin. Most nicotinic sites are excitatory, but there are also inhibitory nicotinic synapses. The many types of receptors for each transmitter have evolved to enable a variety of actions in the nervous system.

The nicotinic ACh receptor resembles a lopsided dumbbell with a tube running down its central axis (see Figure 3.12). The handle of the dumbbell spans the cell membrane, with two sites on the outside that fit ACh molecules (Karlin, 2002). For the channel to open, both of the ACh-binding sites must be occupied. Receptors for some of the synaptic transmitter molecules that we will consider in later chapters, such as gamma-aminobutyric acid (GABA), glycine, and glutamate, are similar.

The coordination of different transmitter systems of the brain is incredibly complex. Each subtype of neurotransmitter receptor has a unique pattern of distribution within the brain. Different receptor systems become active at different times in fetal life. The number of any given type of receptor remains plastic in adulthood: not only are there seasonal variations, but many kinds of receptors show a regular daily variation of 50% or more in number, affecting the sensitivity of cells to that particular transmitter. Similarly, the numbers of some receptors have been found to vary with the use of drugs. We'll learn more about these properties of neurotransmitter receptors in Chapter 4.

The action of synaptic transmitters is stopped rapidly

When a chemical transmitter such as ACh is released into the synaptic cleft, its postsynaptic action is not only prompt but usually very brief as well. It is important that each activation of the synapse be brief in order to maximize how much information can be transmitted. Think of it this way: the worst doorbell in the world is one that, when the button is pushed, rings forever. Such a doorbell would be able to transmit only one piece of information, and only once. But a doorbell that could ring as fast as a thousand times per minute would be able to send a lot of information—Morse code maybe. Likewise, a synapse can signal over a thousand times per *second*, potentially sending a lot of information (but not by Morse code).

Two processes bring transmitter effects to a prompt halt:

1. *Degradation* Transmitter molecules can be rapidly broken down and thus inactivated by special enzymes—a process known as **degradation** (step 6a in Figure 3.12). For example, the enzyme that inactivates ACh is **acetylcholinesterase (AChE)**. AChE breaks down ACh very rapidly into products that are recycled (at least in part) to make more ACh in the axon terminal.

2. *Reuptake* Alternatively, transmitter molecules may be swiftly cleared from the synaptic cleft by being absorbed back into the axon terminal that released them—a process known as **reuptake** (step 6b in Figure 3.12). Norepinephrine, dopamine, and serotonin are examples of transmitters whose activity is terminated mainly by reuptake. In these cases, special receptors for the transmitter, called **transporters**, are located on the presynaptic axon terminal and bring the transmitter back inside. Once taken up into the presynaptic terminal, transmitter molecules may be repackaged into newly formed synaptic vesicles to await re-release, conserving the resources that would be needed to make new transmitter molecules. Malfunction of reuptake mechanisms is suspected to cause some kinds of mental illness, such as depression (see Chapter 12).

Neural circuits underlie reflexes

For simplicity, so far we have focused on the classic **axo-dendritic synapses** (from axon to dendrite) and **axo-somatic synapses** (from axon to cell body, or soma). But many nonclassic forms of chemical synapses exist in the nervous system. As the name implies, **axo-axonic synapses** form on axons, often near the axon terminal, allowing the presynaptic neuron to strongly facilitate or inhibit the activity of the postsynaptic

antagonist A substance that blocks or reduces the actions of a transmitter or other signaling molecule.

cholinergic Referring to cells that use acetylcholine as their synaptic transmitter.

degradation The chemical breakdown of a neurotransmitter into inactive metabolites.

acetylcholinesterase (AChE) An enzyme that inactivates the transmitter acetylcholine.

reuptake The process by which released synaptic transmitter molecules are taken up and reused by the presynaptic neuron, thus stopping synaptic activity.

transporter A specialized membrane component that returns transmitter molecules to the presynaptic neuron for reuse.

axo-dendritic synapse A synapse at which a presynaptic axon terminal synapses onto a dendrite of the postsynaptic neuron, either via a dendritic spine or directly onto the dendrite itself.

axo-somatic synapse A synapse at which a presynaptic axon terminal synapses onto the cell body (soma) of the postsynaptic neuron.

axo-axonic synapse A synapse at which a presynaptic axon terminal synapses onto the axon terminal of another neuron.

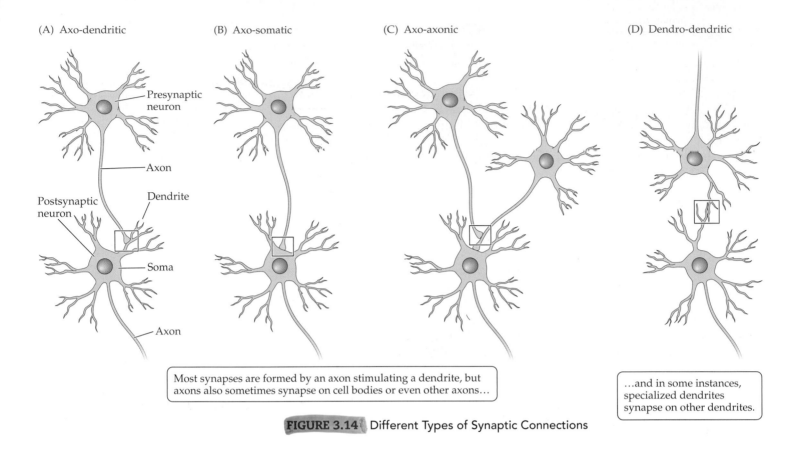

(A) Axo-dendritic

Presynaptic neuron

Axon

Postsynaptic neuron

Dendrite

Soma

Axon

(B) Axo-somatic

(C) Axo-axonic

(D) Dendro-dendritic

Most synapses are formed by an axon stimulating a dendrite, but axons also sometimes synapse on cell bodies or even other axons…

…and in some instances, specialized dendrites synapse on other dendrites.

FIGURE 3.14 Different Types of Synaptic Connections

axon terminal. Similarly, neurons may form **dendro-dendritic synapses**, allowing coordination of their activities (**FIGURE 3.14**).

Now that we know more about the electrical signaling that takes place *within* each neuron and the neurotransmitter signaling that goes on *between* neurons, we can revisit the **knee-jerk reflex** that we discussed at the start of the chapter (**FIGURE 3.15**). Note that this reflex is extremely fast: only about 40 milliseconds elapse between the hammer tap and the start of the kick. Several factors account for this speed: (1) both the sensory and the motor axons involved are myelinated and of large diameter, so they conduct action potentials rapidly; (2) the sensory cells synapse directly on the motor neurons; and (3) both the central synapse and the neuromuscular junction are fast synapses. We discuss other aspects of neural circuits in **A STEP FURTHER 3.2**, on the website.

We offered this reflex at the start of the chapter as an example of neural processing—electrical signaling within each neuron alternating with chemical signaling between neurons. The next chapter will explain how drugs can interfere with the chemical signaling between neurons. For the final part of this chapter, let's see how scientists exploit the electrical signaling within neurons to learn more about brain function.

HOW'S IT GOING ❓

1. Recount the seven steps in synaptic transmission, including processes that end the signal.
2. What ion must enter the axon terminal to trigger neurotransmitter release?
3. What are drug agonists and antagonists?
4. Describe how information is processed within neurons by electrical signals yet communicated to other neurons by chemical signals.

dendro-dendritic synapse A synapse at which a synaptic connection forms between the dendrites of two neurons.

knee-jerk reflex A variant of the stretch reflex in which stretching of the tendon beneath the knee leads to an upward kick of the leg.

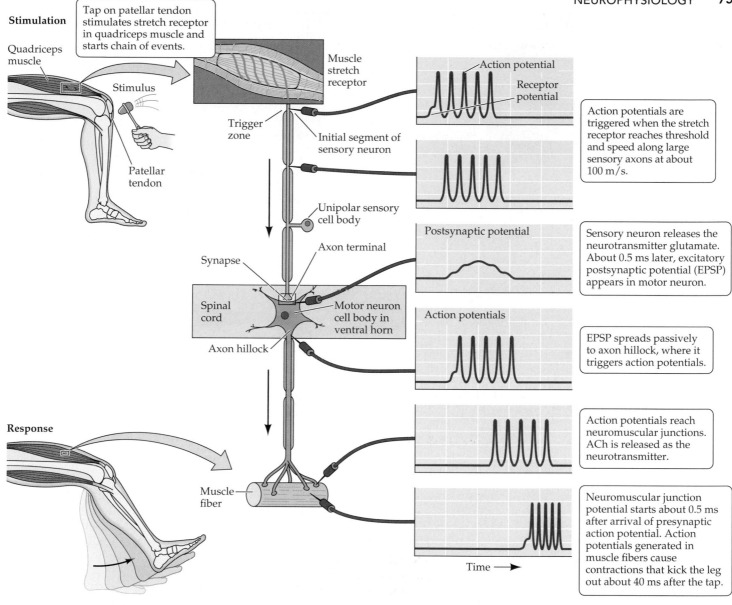

Stimulation

Tap on patellar tendon stimulates stretch receptor in quadriceps muscle and starts chain of events.

Quadriceps muscle

Stimulus

Patellar tendon

Muscle stretch receptor

Trigger zone

Initial segment of sensory neuron

Unipolar sensory cell body

Axon terminal

Synapse

Spinal cord

Motor neuron cell body in ventral horn

Axon hillock

Action potential

Receptor potential

Action potentials are triggered when the stretch receptor reaches threshold and speed along large sensory axons at about 100 m/s.

Postsynaptic potential

Sensory neuron releases the neurotransmitter glutamate. About 0.5 ms later, excitatory postsynaptic potential (EPSP) appears in motor neuron.

Action potentials

EPSP spreads passively to axon hillock, where it triggers action potentials.

Action potentials reach neuromuscular junctions. ACh is released as the neurotransmitter.

Response

Muscle fiber

Time ⟶

Neuromuscular junction potential starts about 0.5 ms after arrival of presynaptic action potential. Action potentials generated in muscle fibers cause contractions that kick the leg out about 40 ms after the tap.

FIGURE 3.15 The Knee-Jerk Reflex

PART III
Gross Potentials

THE ROAD AHEAD

The final section of the chapter explains how we can exploit electrical signals to monitor and understand brain function. Reading this section should allow you to:

1. Understand how electroencephalograms (EEGs) work.
2. Understand the electrical activity underlying the brain disorder called epilepsy.
3. Appreciate how neurosurgeons discovered important "maps" by electrically stimulating the brain.

EEGs Measure Gross Electrical Activity of the Human Brain

The electrical activity of millions of cells working together combines to produce electrical potentials large enough that we can detect them with electrodes applied to the surface of the scalp. Recordings of these spontaneous brain potentials (or *brain waves*),

(A) Multichannel EEG recording

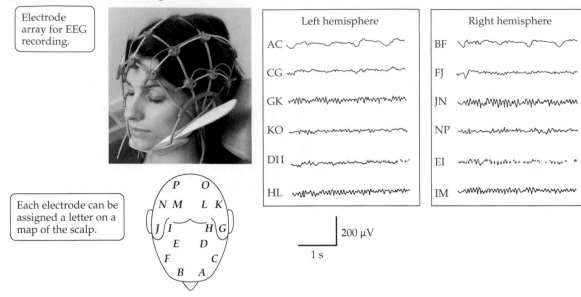

Electrode array for EEG recording.

Each electrode can be assigned a letter on a map of the scalp.

Left hemisphere

AC
CG
GK
KO
DII
HL

Right hemisphere

BF
FJ
JN
NP
EI
IM

Typical EEG recordings showing potential measured between various points on the scalp.

200 μV

1 s

(B) Event-related potentials (average of many stimulus presentations)

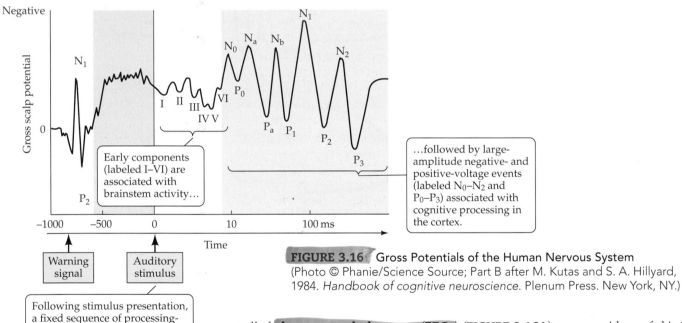

Negative

Gross scalp potential

N_1

N_0 N_a N_b

N_1

N_2

P_0

I   II   III   IV V   VI

P_a P_1

P_2

P_3

P_2

0

−1000   −500   0   10   100 ms

Time

Early components (labeled I–VI) are associated with brainstem activity…

…followed by large-amplitude negative- and positive-voltage events (labeled N_0–N_2 and P_0–P_3) associated with cognitive processing in the cortex.

Warning signal

Auditory stimulus

Following stimulus presentation, a fixed sequence of processing-related potentials is generated.

FIGURE 3.16 Gross Potentials of the Human Nervous System (Photo © Phanie/Science Source; Part B after M. Kutas and S. A. Hillyard, 1984. *Handbook of cognitive neuroscience*. Plenum Press. New York, NY.)

electroencephalogram (EEG)
A recording of gross electrical activity of the brain via large electrodes placed on the scalp.

event-related potential (ERP) Also called *evoked potential*. Averaged EEG recordings measuring brain responses to repeated presentations of a stimulus. Components of the ERP tend to be reliable because the background noise of the cortex has been averaged out.

epilepsy A brain disorder marked by major, sudden changes in the electrophysiological state of the brain that are referred to as seizures.

called **electroencephalograms (EEGs)** (**FIGURE 3.16A**), can provide useful information about the activity of brain regions during behavioral processes. As we will see in Chapter 10, EEG recordings can distinguish whether a person is asleep or awake. In many countries, EEG activity determines whether someone is legally dead.

Event-related potentials (ERPs) are EEG responses to a single stimulus, such as a flash of light or a loud sound. Typically, many ERP responses to the same stimulus are averaged to obtain a reliable estimate of brain activity (**FIGURE 3.16B**). ERPs have very distinctive characteristics of wave shape and time delay (or *latency*) that reflect the type of stimulus, the state of the participant, and the site of recording (Luck, 2005). ERPs can also be used to detect hearing problems in babies, evident as reduced or absent auditory ERPs in response to sounds. In Chapter 14 we'll learn how ERPs are used to study subtler psychological processes, such as attention.

EEG recordings can also provide vital information for diagnosing seizure disorders, as we discuss next.

Electrical storms in the brain can cause seizures

Since the dawn of civilization, people have pondered the causes of **epilepsy**, a disorder in which **seizures** lasting for a few seconds or minutes may produce dramatic

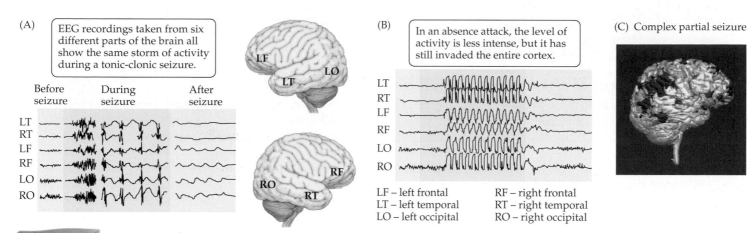

(A) EEG recordings taken from six different parts of the brain all show the same storm of activity during a tonic-clonic seizure.

LF
LT
LO

Before seizure   During seizure   After seizure

LT
RT
LF
RF
LO
RO

RF
RO
RT

(B) In an absence attack, the level of activity is less intense, but it has still invaded the entire cortex.

LT
RT
LF
RF
LO
RO

LF – left frontal   RF – right frontal
LT – left temporal   RT – right temporal
LO – left occipital   RO – right occipital

(C) Complex partial seizure

FIGURE 3.17 **Seizure Disorders** (Part C courtesy of Hal Blumenfeld, Rik Stokking, Susan Spencer, and George Zubal, Yale School of Medicine.)

behavioral changes such as alterations or loss of consciousness and rhythmic convulsions of the body. Worldwide, about 30 million people suffer from epilepsy, which we now know to be a disorder of electrical potentials in the brain.

In the normal, active brain, electrical activity tends to be desynchronized; that is, different brain regions carry on their functions more or less independently. In contrast, during a seizure there is widespread synchronization of electrical activity: broad stretches of the brain start firing in simultaneous waves, which are evident in the EEGs as an abnormal "spike-and-wave" pattern of brain activity. Many abnormalities of the brain, such as trauma, injury, or metabolic problems, can predispose brain tissue to produce such synchronized activity, which, once begun in one brain region, may readily spread to others.

There are several major categories of seizure disorders. The most severe, with loss of consciousness and rhythmic convulsions, are called **tonic-clonic seizures** (formerly known as *grand mal seizures*) and are accompanied by abnormal EEG activity all over the brain (**FIGURE 3.17A**). In the more subtle **simple partial seizures** (or *absence attacks*, formerly known as *petit mal seizures*), the characteristic spike-and-wave EEG activity is evident for 5–15 seconds at a time (**FIGURE 3.17B**), sometimes occurring many times per day. The person is unaware of the environment during these periods and later cannot recall events that occurred during the episodes. Behaviorally, people experiencing simple partial seizures show no unusual muscle activity; they just stop what they're doing and stare into space.

Complex partial seizures do not involve the entire brain and thus can produce a wide variety of symptoms, often preceded by an unusual sensation, or **aura**. In one example, a woman felt an unusual sensation in the abdomen, a sense of foreboding, and tingling in both hands before the seizure spread. At the height of the episode, she was unresponsive and rocked her body back and forth while speaking nonsensically, twisting her left arm, and looking toward the right. Of course, her seemingly random set of behavioral symptoms actually reflected the functions of the particular brain regions affected by the seizure (**FIGURE 3.17C**); others experiencing seizures would produce a completely different set of behaviors. In some individuals, complex partial seizures may be provoked by stimuli like loud noises or flashing lights.

Many seizure disorders can be effectively controlled with the aid of antiepileptic drugs. Although these drugs have a wide variety of neural targets, they tend to selectively reduce the excitability of neurons (Rogawski and Löscher, 2004). But some cases of epilepsy do not respond to medication, and if the seizures are severe, or happen very often, they may be life-threatening. Individuals suffering from such severe epilepsy may resort to the drastic step of having parts of the brain removed, as we'll see next.

seizure A wave of abnormally synchronous electrical activity in the brain.

tonic-clonic seizure Also called *grand mal seizure*. A type of generalized epileptic seizure in which nerve cells fire in high-frequency bursts, usually accompanied by involuntary rhythmic contractions of the body.

simple partial seizure Also called *absence attack*. A seizure that is characterized by a spike-and-wave EEG and often involves a loss of awareness and inability to recall events surrounding the seizure.

complex partial seizure A type of seizure that doesn't involve the entire brain and therefore can cause a wide variety of symptoms.

aura In epilepsy, the unusual sensations or premonition that may precede the beginning of a seizure.

RESEARCHERS AT WORK

Surgical probing of the brain revealed a map of the body

Usually the electrical activity causing seizures begins in one part of the brain and then spreads to others. So in the twentieth century, neurosurgeons began taking drastic measures to help people with severe epilepsy that did not respond to medication: surgical removal of the part of the brain where the seizures begin. The trick, of course, is to remove the part of the brain where the seizures begin, and *only* that part. Otherwise the patient might take the risks of surgery and still suffer from seizures, or might suffer impairment of a vital function, such as verbal or memory skills, if healthy tissue is removed. One way to locate the origin of the seizures is to compare EEG readings from different places on the skull (see Figure 3.17). But this approach gives only a rough idea of where the seizures begin, and it is problematic because the recording must be made when a seizure is actually starting.

To improve the success rate of such surgeries, Canadian neurosurgeon Wilder Penfield developed a procedure that,

nearly 90 years later, is still compelling (Foerster and Penfield, 1930). Using only local anesthesia to deaden the pain of cutting the scalp and opening up the skull, Penfield had patients remain awake and alert as he exposed the brain. Then he used electrodes to provide a tiny electrical stimulation to the surface of the cortex, asking the patient to report the results. One strategy for people whose epileptic seizures were preceded by an aura was to try to find the point where stimulation recreated the aura.

In one famous case of a woman whose seizures were preceded by the smell of burnt toast, Penfield was able to find a spot where stimulation caused her to smell burnt toast and, presuming that region was the origin of the seizures, surgically removed it. (The brain itself has no pain receptors, so cutting the cortex didn't hurt.) Using this refined technique, Penfield was able to cure about half of his patients, and seizures were reduced in another 25%. Later, José Delgado also stimulated patients' brains to seek the origin of seizures, as we discussed at the start of the chapter.

FIGURE 3.18   Mapping the Human Brain

■ Hypothesis

Sensory information from the body arrives in an organized fashion in the cortex.

■ Experiment

Electrically stimulate the surface of the cortex in alert patients, carefully recording the patient's experience with stimulation at each site. Compare these maps in various patients.

■ Result

Each side of the brain receives sensory information from the opposite side of the body, organized along the postcentral gyrus of the parietal lobe. Across the central sulcus, in the precentral gyrus, cortical regions control movement of that same part of the body, so that sensory and motor regions are aligned.

■ Conclusion

The maps of sensory cortex and motor cortex are remarkably consistent from one person to another.

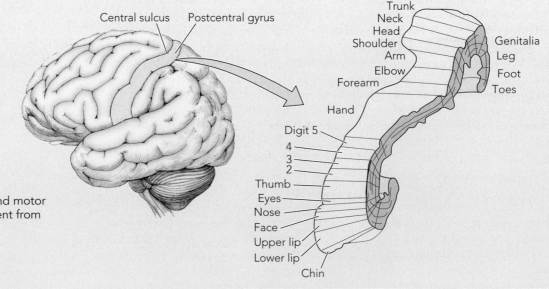

RESEARCHERS AT WORK   (continued)

Delgado altered the technique by implanting several electrodes temporarily, so the patient could walk around while doctors electrically stimulated different brain regions and observed the results. In Chapters 5 and 12 we'll learn that today electrodes are sometimes implanted in the brain as a treatment for other disorders.

In his pioneering work, Penfield did more than help his patients. He also made major discoveries about the organization of the human cortex (**FIGURE 3.18**). By carefully recording the effects of stimulating different regions of the brain, he found that stimulation of occipital cortex often caused the patient to "see" flashes of light. Stimulating another region might cause the person's thumb to tingle, while stimulation elsewhere might cause the patient's leg to move. Through these studies, Penfield confirmed that each side of the cortex receives information from, and sends commands to, the opposite side of the body. He found that stimulating the postcentral gyrus of the parietal cortex caused patients to experience sensations on various parts of the body in a way that was consistent from one person to another (see Figure 5.9). Just across the central sulcus from each site, in the precentral gyrus, stimulations caused that same part of the body to move (see Figure 5.22). These "maps" of how the various parts of the body are laid out on the cortex (Jasper and Penfield, 1954) have been reproduced in countless textbooks, providing the basis of what

is called the *homunculus*, the "little man" drawn on the surface of the cortex to depict Penfield's maps, as we will discuss further in Chapter 5.

These groundbreaking observations taught us that brain function is organized in a map that reproduces body parts. We also learned that the map is distorted, in the sense that parts of the body that are especially sensitive to touch, such as the lips or fingers, are monitored by a relatively large area of cortex compared with, say, the backs of the legs.

Penfield's studies also stimulated a rich store of speculation about the relationship between the workings of the brain and the mind. In a small minority of patients, electrical stimulation in some sites would sometimes elicit a memory of, for example, sitting on the porch step and hearing a relative's voice, or hearing a snatch of music. As we saw at the start of this chapter, other researchers would find that electrical stimulation of the brain could make people think they loved their examiner or could make an angry, murderous bull peaceful and calm. In another case, electrical stimulation of one part of her brain caused a young woman to find whatever was happening around her to be humorous (Fried et al., 1998).

These startling observations—showing that electrical stimulation of the brain triggers mental processes—remain a cornerstone of neuroscience, and a tantalizing demonstration that our mind is a result of physical processes at work in the machine we call the brain.

HOW'S IT GOING ?

1. What are EEGs and ERPs? How have these techniques been useful?
2. What are the three main categories of epileptic seizures, and what are the main characteristics of each type?
3. Describe Penfield's surgical procedure and what it revealed about organization of the brain.

Recommended Reading

Kandel, E. R., Schwartz, J. H., Jessell, T. M., Siegelbaum, S. A., and Hudspeth, A. J. (2013). *Principles of Neural Science* (5th ed.). New York, NY: McGraw-Hill.

Luck, S. J. (2005). *An Introduction to the Event-Related Potential Technique.* Cambridge, MA: MIT Press.

Nicholls, J. G., Martin, A. R., Fuchs, P. A., Brown, D. A., Diamond, M. E., and Weisblat, D. A. (2012). *From Neuron to Brain* (5th ed.). Sunderland, MA: Oxford University Press/Sinauer.

Purves, D., Augustine, G. J., Fitzpatrick, D., Hall, W. C., et al. (2017). *Neuroscience* (6th ed.). Sunderland, MA: Oxford University Press/Sinauer.

Valenstein, E. S. (2005). *The War of the Soups and the Sparks: The Discovery of Neurotransmitters and the Dispute over How Neurons Communicate.* New York, NY: Columbia University Press.

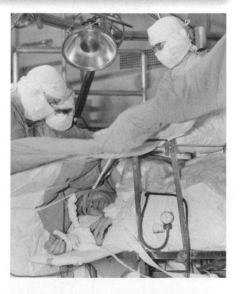

Brain Stimulation   Surgeon Wilder Penfield electrically stimulating the surface of the exposed brain in an awake patient. (Reproduced by permission of the Oster Library of the History of Medicine, McGill University.)

You should be able to relate each summary to the adjacent illustration, including structures and processes. If you go to the website for our text (3e.mindsmachine.com), you can follow links to figures, animations, and activities that will help you consolidate the material.

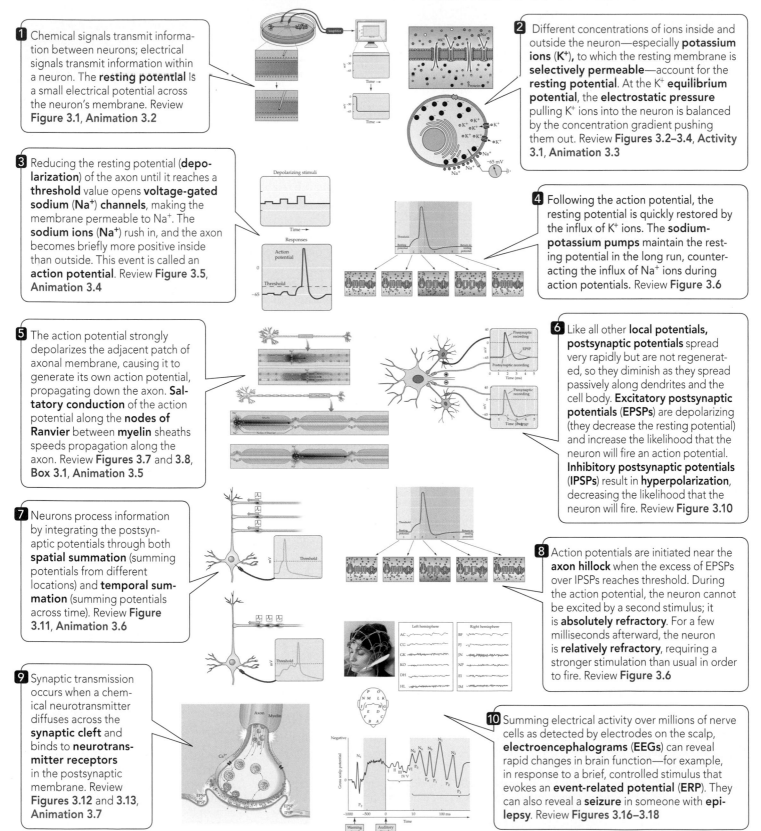

1 Chemical signals transmit information between neurons; electrical signals transmit information within a neuron. The **resting potential** is a small electrical potential across the neuron's membrane. Review **Figure 3.1, Animation 3.2**

2 Different concentrations of ions inside and outside the neuron—especially **potassium ions (K+)**, to which the resting membrane is **selectively permeable**—account for the **resting potential**. At the K+ **equilibrium potential**, the **electrostatic pressure** pulling K+ ions into the neuron is balanced by the concentration gradient pushing them out. Review **Figures 3.2–3.4, Activity 3.1, Animation 3.3**

3 Reducing the resting potential (**depolarization**) of the axon until it reaches a **threshold** value opens **voltage-gated sodium (Na+) channels**, making the membrane permeable to Na+. The **sodium ions (Na+)** rush in, and the axon becomes briefly more positive inside than outside. This event is called an **action potential**. Review **Figure 3.5, Animation 3.4**

4 Following the action potential, the resting potential is quickly restored by the influx of K+ ions. The **sodium-potassium pumps** maintain the resting potential in the long run, counteracting the influx of Na+ ions during action potentials. Review **Figure 3.6**

5 The action potential strongly depolarizes the adjacent patch of axonal membrane, causing it to generate its own action potential, propagating down the axon. **Saltatory conduction** of the action potential along the **nodes of Ranvier** between **myelin** sheaths speeds propagation along the axon. Review **Figures 3.7 and 3.8, Box 3.1, Animation 3.5**

6 Like all other **local potentials**, **postsynaptic potentials** spread very rapidly but are not regenerated, so they diminish as they spread passively along dendrites and the cell body. **Excitatory postsynaptic potentials (EPSPs)** are depolarizing (they decrease the resting potential) and increase the likelihood that the neuron will fire an action potential. **Inhibitory postsynaptic potentials (IPSPs)** result in **hyperpolarization**, decreasing the likelihood that the neuron will fire. Review **Figure 3.10**

7 Neurons process information by integrating the postsynaptic potentials through both **spatial summation** (summing potentials from different locations) and **temporal summation** (summing potentials across time). Review **Figure 3.11, Animation 3.6**

8 Action potentials are initiated near the **axon hillock** when the excess of EPSPs over IPSPs reaches threshold. During the action potential, the neuron cannot be excited by a second stimulus; it is **absolutely refractory**. For a few milliseconds afterward, the neuron is **relatively refractory**, requiring a stronger stimulation than usual in order to fire. Review **Figure 3.6**

9 Synaptic transmission occurs when a chemical neurotransmitter diffuses across the **synaptic cleft** and binds to **neurotransmitter receptors** in the postsynaptic membrane. Review **Figures 3.12 and 3.13, Animation 3.7**

10 Summing electrical activity over millions of nerve cells as detected by electrodes on the scalp, **electroencephalograms (EEGs)** can reveal rapid changes in brain function—for example, in response to a brief, controlled stimulus that evokes an **event-related potential (ERP)**. They can also reveal a **seizure** in someone with **epilepsy**. Review **Figures 3.16–3.18**

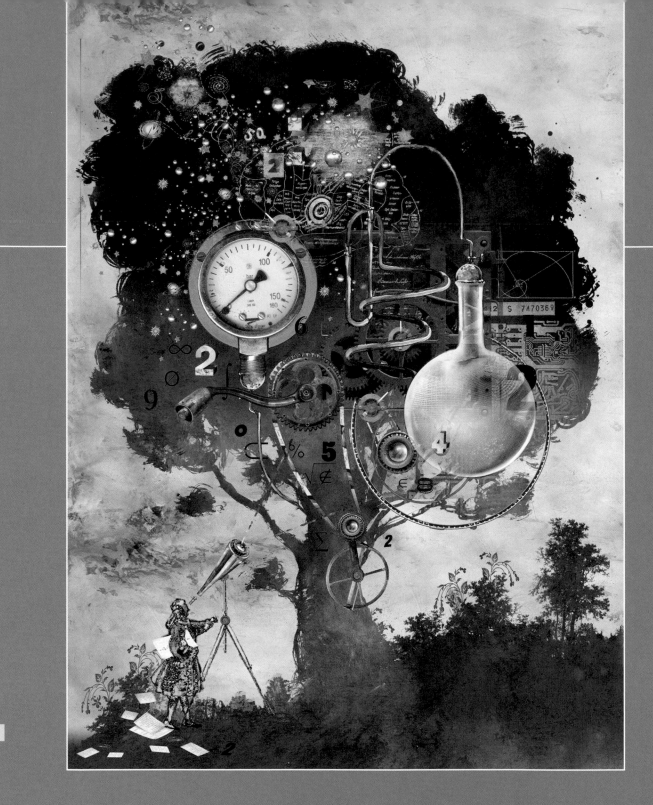

4

The Chemistry of Behavior
Neurotransmitters
and Neuropharmacology

A Dream of Soups and Sparks

As the twentieth century began, scientists knew that neurons were important for brain function, but there was a big controversy about how neurons communicated. What happened at those newly discovered synapses between one neuron and another? Did sparks of electricity pass from cell to cell? Or was some unknown chemical substance involved? Some scientists, nicknamed "sparks," favored the idea that electrical signals crossed synapses; other scientists, the "soups," thought neurons released a chemical that flowed across synapses. No one knew how to distinguish between these two possibilities.

Otto Loewi was so consumed with the question of neural communication that he even dreamed about it. One night he awoke suddenly, remembering a dream in which one experiment could provide a definitive answer to whether the "soups" or the "sparks" were right. He made a few notes and went back to sleep, only to discover the next day that he couldn't make any sense of the previous night's scribblings. So when he had the same dream again the following night, he got up and went straight to the lab to do the experiment while it was still fresh in his mind. The result was a discovery that would revolutionize the study of the brain.

Throughout the ages, people have experimented with **exogenous** substances (substances from outside the body) to try to change the functioning of their bodies and brains. Our ancestors sipped, swallowed, and smoked their way to euphoria, calmness, pain relief, and hallucination. They discovered deadly poisons in frogs, miraculous antibiotics in mold, powerful painkillers in poppies, and all the rest of a vast catalog of helpful and harmful substances. By studying the physiological actions of these substances, modern scientists have been able to unlock many mysteries of brain function.

The preceding chapters showed us that the brain is an electrochemical system. Today we know that, in general, each neuron *electrically* processes information received through many synapses, and then releases a *chemical* to pass the result of that information processing to the next cell. Specifically, a presynaptic neuron releases an **endogenous** substance (a substance from inside the body), a chemical called a *neurotransmitter*. The neurotransmitter then communicates with the postsynaptic cell. As you might have guessed, most drugs that affect behavior do so by affecting this chemical communication process at millions, or even billions, of synapses.

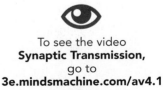

To see the video
Synaptic Transmission,
go to
3e.mindsmachine.com/av4.1

exogenous Arising from outside the body.

endogenous Produced inside the body.

To view the
Brain Explorer,
go to
3e.mindsmachine.com/av4.2

PART I
Chemical Neurotransmission

THE ROAD AHEAD

We open with a detailed look at the sequence of electrochemical events in synaptic transmission. After studying the first part of the chapter you should be able to:

1. Review the neuronal processes leading to the release of neurotransmitter into a synapse.

2. Explain how receptors capture, recognize, and respond to molecules of neurotransmitter.

3. Describe general properties shared by most neurotransmitters, and identify the major chemical families of transmitters.

4. Trace the neuroanatomical distribution of the major neurotransmitters, and briefly discuss some of their functional roles.

FIGURE 4.1 A Review of Synaptic Activity

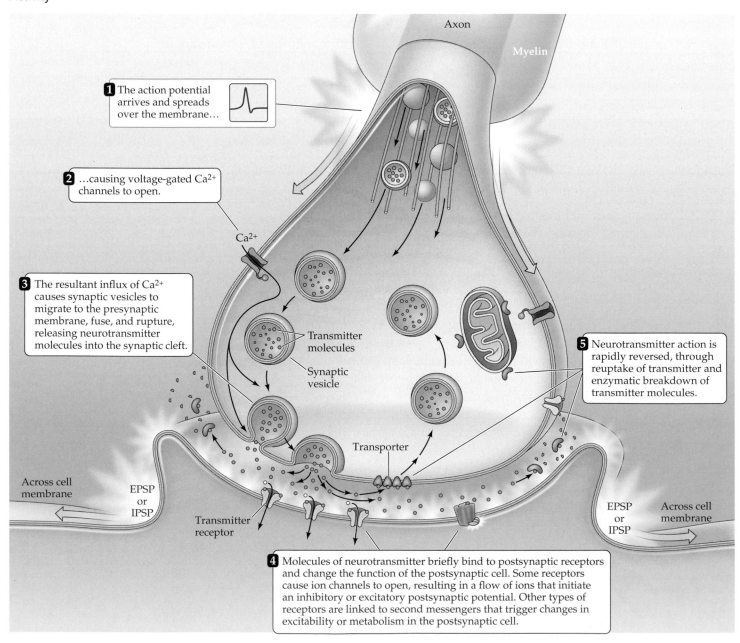

Synaptic Transmission Involves a Complex Electrochemical Process

As we learned in Chapter 3, the typical neuron integrates a variety of inputs and, if sufficiently excited (i.e., depolarized), fires a distinctive electrical signal called an *action potential* that rapidly sweeps down the axon toward the *axon terminals*, each of which forms the **presynaptic** side of a **synapse**. **FIGURE 4.1** recaps the events that follow the arrival of the action potential. First, the voltage change associated with the action potential induces voltage-gated calcium (Ca^{2+}) channels in the terminal membrane to open. The resulting inflow of Ca^{2+} ions drives the migration of synaptic vesicles to the nearby presynaptic membrane, where proteins on the walls of the vesicles and corresponding proteins on the synaptic membrane interact and cause the vesicles to release their cargo of molecules of **neurotransmitter** (or just *transmitter*) into the synaptic cleft (a process called *exocytosis*). In Chapter 3 we also saw that following their diffusion across the cleft, neurotransmitter molecules briefly bind to their corresponding **neurotransmitter receptors**—protein molecules embedded in the postsynaptic membrane that recognize a specific transmitter—which then mediate a response on the postsynaptic side. Eventually the neurotransmitter molecules are either (1) broken down by enzymes into simpler chemicals or (2) brought back into the presynaptic terminal in a process called **reuptake** (see Figure 4.1). Reuptake of transmitters relies on specialized proteins, called **transporters**, that bind molecules of neurotransmitter and conduct them back inside the presynaptic terminal. Once inside, the neurotransmitter molecules can be recycled.

Neurotransmitter receptors are very selective about the substances that they will respond to: as we saw in Chapter 3, the action of transmitters on receptors is often likened to a key opening a lock. Nevertheless, the various neurotransmitter receptors can all be categorized as belonging to one of two general kinds: ionotropic receptors or metabotropic receptors. **Ionotropic receptors** are just fancy ion channels; when bound by neurotransmitter molecules, they quickly change their shape to open or close the ion channel (**FIGURE 4.2**). The opening of the channel allows more (or fewer) of the channel's favored ions to flow into or out of the postsynaptic neuron, thus changing the local membrane potential. If that change in the postsynaptic membrane potential is a depolarization,

presynaptic   Located on the "transmitting" side of a synapse.

synapse   The cellular location at which information is transmitted from a neuron to another cell.

neurotransmitter   Also called simply *transmitter*. A signaling chemical, released by a presynaptic neuron, that diffuses across the synaptic cleft to alter the functioning of the postsynaptic neuron.

neurotransmitter receptor   Also called simply *receptor*. A specialized protein that is embedded in the cell membrane, allowing it to selectively sense and react to molecules of the corresponding neurotransmitter.

reuptake   The reabsorption of molecules of neurotransmitter by the neurons that released them, thereby ending the signaling activity of the transmitter molecules.

transporter   A specialized membrane component that returns transmitter molecules to the presynaptic neuron for reuse.

ionotropic receptor   Also called *ligand-gated ion channel*. A receptor protein containing an ion channel that opens when the receptor is bound by an agonist.

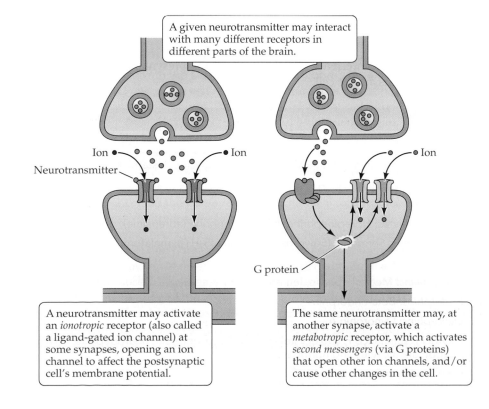

A given neurotransmitter may interact with many different receptors in different parts of the brain.

Ion

Neurotransmitter

Ion

Ion

G protein

A neurotransmitter may activate an *ionotropic* receptor (also called a ligand-gated ion channel) at some synapses, opening an ion channel to affect the postsynaptic cell's membrane potential.

The same neurotransmitter may, at another synapse, activate a *metabotropic* receptor, which activates *second messengers* (via G proteins) that open other ion channels, and/or cause other changes in the cell.

FIGURE 4.2   The Versatility of Neurotransmitters

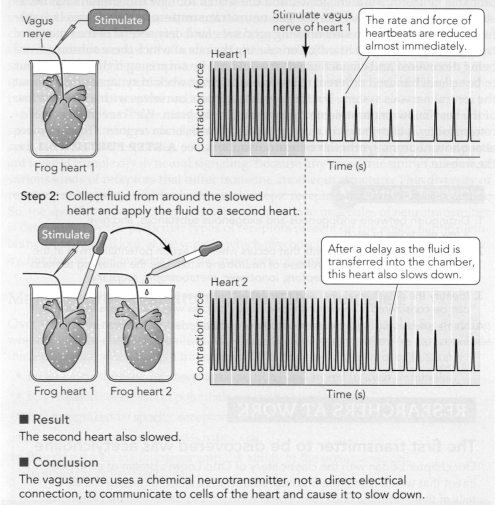

RESEARCHERS AT WORK   (continued)

FIGURE 4.3   "Soups" versus "Sparks": The First Neurotransmitter

■ **Question**

Do neurons release a chemical to communicate with other cells, or is the communication based on electrical signals?

■ **Experiment**

Step 1: Stimulate the vagus nerve to slow the heart.

Vagus nerve — Stimulate

Frog heart 1

Heart 1

Stimulate vagus nerve of heart 1

The rate and force of heartbeats are reduced almost immediately.

Contraction force

Time (s)

Step 2: Collect fluid from around the slowed heart and apply the fluid to a second heart.

Stimulate

Frog heart 1   Frog heart 2

Heart 2

After a delay as the fluid is transferred into the chamber, this heart also slows down.

Contraction force

Time (s)

■ **Result**

The second heart also slowed.

■ **Conclusion**

The vagus nerve uses a chemical neurotransmitter, not a direct electrical connection, to communicate to cells of the heart and cause it to slow down.

Neurotransmitter Systems Form a Complex Array in the Brain

The most common transmitters in the brain are amino acids, and of these, the two best studied are **glutamate**, the most widespread excitatory transmitter in the brain, and **gamma-aminobutyric acid** (**GABA**), the most widespread inhibitory transmitter. Both have wide-ranging effects at synapses throughout the central nervous system, and from an evolutionary perspective they are among the most ancient transmitters.

Glutamate interacts with several subtypes of receptors (**TABLE 4.2**). Activation of the ionotropic AMPA receptors, the most plentiful receptors in the brain, has rapid excitatory effects. NMDA receptors are another subtype of ionotropic glutamate receptors, with unique characteristics that suggest they play a central role in memory formation (discussed in Chapter 13 and on the website in **A STEP FURTHER 4.2**).

glutamate   An amino acid transmitter, the most common excitatory transmitter.

gamma-aminobutyric acid (GABA)   A widely distributed amino acid transmitter, the main inhibitory transmitter in the mammalian nervous system.

There are also several metabotropic glutamate receptors (mGluRs), which act more slowly because they work through second messengers.

Among the subtypes of receptors for GABA, the GABA$_A$ receptors have received decades of special scrutiny because of their relationship to anxiety relief. GABA$_A$ receptors are ionotropic; when activated, they allow more Cl$^-$ ions to flow into the postsynaptic cell, thus inhibiting that cell's activity. Substances that mimic this action of GABA$_A$ tend to be effective calming agents because they produce a widespread decrease in neural activity. In fact, drugs belonging to the family of *benzodiazepines*—examples include Xanax (alprazolam) and Ativan (lorazepam)—potently activate GABA$_A$ receptors and are widely used to treat anxiety and panic attacks, as well as to aid muscle relaxation, sleep induction, and the like.

Four amine neurotransmitters modulate brain activity

It is possible to stain brain tissue in such a way that only the neurons making a particular neurotransmitter end up being labeled (see Box 2.1). Studies of brain sections stained in this way have shown that transmitters are found in complex networks of neurons that extend throughout the brain. In **FIGURE 4.4**, this complicated anatomy is depicted for just four classical transmitters: acetylcholine, dopamine, serotonin, and norepinephrine. These amine transmitters—amines are nitrogen-containing compounds related to ammonia, often derived from an amino acid—have been implicated

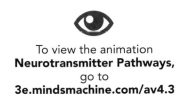

To view the animation **Neurotransmitter Pathways,** go to **3e.mindsmachine.com/av4.3**

FIGURE 4.4 Neurotransmitter Pathways in the Brain

In this midline view, the brain nuclei containing cell bodies of neurons that release four of the major transmitters are shown in different colors. Each system projects widely, but arises from a relatively small number of neurons, a vulnerability that accounts for loss of function in degenerative diseases like Parkinson's and Alzheimer's diseases. Although the projections may overlap, each neurotransmitter projects to a distinct set of brain targets.

Cholinergic

Basal forebrain to cortex, amygdala, and hippocampus

Dopaminergic

Mesolimbocortical pathway: ventral tegmental area (VTA) to nucleus accumbens and cortex

Mesostriatal pathway: substantia nigra to basal ganglia

Noradrenergic

Locus coeruleus to forebrain

Lateral tegmental area to brainstem and spinal cord

Serotonergic

Midbrain raphe nuclei to forebrain; brainstem raphe nuclei to spinal cord.

TABLE 4.2 ■ The Bewildering Multiplicity of Transmitter Receptor Subtypes

Transmitter	Known receptor subtypes	Function
Glutamate	AMPA, kainate, and NMDA receptors (ionotropic); mGluRs (*metabotropic glutamate receptors*)	Glutamate is the most abundant of all neurotransmitters and the most important excitatory transmitter. Glutamate receptors are crucial for excitatory signals, and NMDA receptors are especially implicated in learning and memory.
Gamma-aminobutyric acid (GABA)	GABA$_A$ (ionotropic)	GABA receptors mediate most of the brain's inhibitory activity, balancing the excitatory actions of glutamate. GABA$_A$ receptors are inhibitory in many brain regions, reducing excitability and preventing seizure activity.
	GABA$_B$ (metabotropic)	GABA$_B$ receptors are also inhibitory, by a different mechanism.
Acetylcholine (ACh)	Muscarinic receptors (metabotropic)	Both types of receptors are involved in cholinergic transmission in the cortex.
	Nicotinic receptors (ionotropic)	Nicotinic receptors are crucial for muscle contraction.
Dopamine (DA)	D$_1$ through D$_5$ receptors (all metabotropic)	DA receptors are found throughout the forebrain. DA receptors are involved in complex behaviors, including motor function, reward, and higher cognition.
Norepinephrine (NE)	α_1, α_2, β_1, β_2, and β_3 receptors (all metabotropic)	NE has multiple effects in visceral organs, important in sympathetic nervous system and fight-or-flight responses. In the brain, NE transmission provides an alerting and arousing function.
Serotonin	5-HT$_1$ receptor family (5 members)	Different subtypes differ in their distribution in the brain.
	5-HT$_2$ receptor family (3 members)	5-HT$_2$ receptors may be involved in mood, sleep, and higher cognition.
	5-HT$_3$ through 5-HT$_7$ receptors (All but one subtype [5-HT$_3$] metabotropic)	5-HT$_3$ receptors are particularly involved in nausea.
Miscellaneous peptides	Many specific receptors for peptides such as opiates (delta, kappa, and mu receptors), cholecystokinin (CCK), neurotensin, neuropeptide Y (NPY), and dozens more (all metabotropic)	Peptide transmitters have many different functions, depending on their anatomical localization. Some important examples include the control of feeding, sexual behaviors, and social functions.

in many categories of behavior and pathology, so amine neurotransmitter mechanisms are a major target for drug development. We'll be encountering them in many locations throughout the book.

The point to remember is that each of these amine neurotransmitters is carried by a different set of axons, and those axons project to different brain regions. Each type of neurotransmitter is talking to a distinct set of brain targets, and there may be overlap as two different transmitters arrive at the same target. How those targets respond depends on which neurotransmitter is being released, and which kind of receptors the target neurons possess. Despite its appearance, Figure 4.4 is a simplification; there are many more transmitters at work than the four we have shown here, and they are arranged in much more complicated networks. Furthermore, we now know that some neurons make and release more than one type of transmitter—a phenomenon known as neurotransmitter **co-localization**.

ACETYLCHOLINE   We now know that acetylcholine (ACh) plays a major role in neurotransmission in the forebrain. Many **cholinergic** (ACh-containing) neurons are found in nuclei within the **basal forebrain**. These cholinergic cells project widely in the brain, to sites such as the cerebral cortex, amygdala, and hippocampus (see Figure 4.4). Widespread loss of cholinergic neurons is associated with Alzheimer's disease, and experimental disruption of cholinergic pathways in rats interferes with learning and memory.

co-localization   The synthesis and release of more than one type of neurotransmitter by a given presynaptic neuron.

cholinergic   Referring to cells that use acetylcholine as their synaptic transmitter.

basal forebrain   A region, ventral to the basal ganglia, that is the major source of cholinergic projections in the brain.

DOPAMINE Of the more than 80 billion neurons in the human brain, only about a million synthesize **dopamine (DA)**, but they are critically important for many aspects of behavior. Figure 4.4 shows the paths of the major **dopaminergic** projections. One of these projections is called the *mesostriatal pathway* because it originates in the midbrain (mesencephalon) around the **substantia nigra** and projects axons to striatal cortex, specifically the basal ganglia. There aren't all that many neurons in the system—hundreds of thousands—but keep in mind that a single axon can divide to supply thousands of synapses. Those synapses play a crucial role in motor control. When people lose a significant number of mesostriatal dopaminergic neurons, from either exposure to toxins or just old age, they develop the profound movement problems of Parkinson's disease (described in Chapter 5), including tremors.

Another dopaminergic projection, called the *mesolimbocortical pathway*, also originates in the midbrain, in a region called the **ventral tegmental area (VTA)** (see Figure 4.4). From there, the pathway projects to various locations in the limbic system (see Chapter 2) and cortex. The mesolimbocortical system appears to be especially important for the processing of reward; it's probably where feelings of pleasure arise. Thus, it makes sense that the mesolimbocortical dopamine system is important for learning that is shaped by positive reinforcement (which usually involves a reward; see Chapter 13), especially via the D2 dopamine receptor subtype. Abnormalities in the mesolimbocortical pathway are associated with some of the symptoms of schizophrenia, as we discuss in Chapter 12. At the end of this chapter we'll look at the role of this pathway in addictive behaviors.

SEROTONIN Dopaminergic neurons may be scarce, but there are even fewer **serotonergic** neurons in the human brain—just 200,000 or so. Nevertheless, wide expanses of the brain are innervated by serotonergic fibers, originating from neurons sprinkled along the midline of the midbrain and brainstem in the **raphe nuclei** (*raphe* is pronounced "rafay") (see Figure 4.4).

Serotonin (**5-HT**, short for its chemical name, 5-hydroxytryptamine) participates in the control of all sorts of behaviors: mood, vision, sexual behavior, anxiety, sleep, and many other functions. As we'll see a little later, drugs that increase serotonergic activity are often prescribed for depression and anxiety. The precise behavioral actions of serotonergic drugs depend on which of the many 5-HT receptor subtypes are affected (see Table 4.2) (Gorzalka et al., 1990; Miczek et al., 2002).

NOREPINEPHRINE As Figure 4.4 shows, many of the brain's **noradrenergic** neurons (we use this term because **norepinephrine [NE]** is also known as *noradrenaline*) have their cell bodies in two regions of the brainstem and midbrain: the **locus coeruleus** ("blue spot") and the **lateral tegmental area**. Noradrenergic axons from these regions project broadly throughout the cerebrum, including the cerebral cortex, limbic system, and thalamic nuclei. They participate in the control of behaviors ranging from alertness to mood to sexual behavior (and many more).

Many peptides function as neurotransmitters

Peptides are very important signaling chemicals both in the brain and in the other organs of the body. Here are some examples of peptides that act as neurotransmitters:

- The **opioid peptides**, a group of endogenous substances with actions that resemble those of opiate drugs like morphine: some key opioids are met-enkephalin, leu-enkephalin, beta-endorphin, and dynorphin. As with morphine, these peptides reduce our perception of pain and have rewarding properties.
- A diverse group of peptides originally discovered in the periphery, and especially in the organs of the gut (which explains some of their names), that are also made by neurons in the spinal cord and brain: these peptides may act as synaptic transmitters, and they are often co-localized with classical transmitters. Examples

dopamine (DA) A monoamine transmitter found in the midbrain—especially the substantia nigra—and in the basal forebrain.

dopaminergic Referring to cells that use dopamine as their synaptic transmitter.

substantia nigra A brainstem structure that innervates the basal ganglia and is a major source of dopaminergic projections.

ventral tegmental area (VTA) A portion of the midbrain that projects dopaminergic fibers to the nucleus accumbens.

serotonergic Referring to cells that use serotonin as their synaptic transmitter.

raphe nuclei A string of nuclei in the midline of the midbrain and brainstem that contain most of the serotonergic neurons of the brain.

serotonin (5-HT) A synaptic transmitter that is produced in the raphe nuclei and is active in structures throughout the cerebral hemispheres.

noradrenergic Referring to cells using norepinephrine (noradrenaline) as a transmitter.

norepinephrine (NE) Also called *noradrenaline*. A neurotransmitter produced and released by sympathetic postganglionic neurons to accelerate organ activity.

locus coeruleus A small nucleus in the brainstem whose neurons produce norepinephrine and modulate large areas of the forebrain.

lateral tegmental area A brainstem region that provides some of the norepinephrine-containing projections of the brain.

opioid peptide A type of endogenous peptide that mimics the effects of morphine in binding to opioid receptors and producing marked analgesia and reward.

To view the activity
Families of Transmitters,
go to
3e.mindsmachine.com/ac4.1

subtypes can be, take another look at Table 4.2. For example, there are more than a dozen different subtypes of serotonin receptors. Some are inhibitory, some excitatory, some ionotropic, some metabotropic; in fact, the only thing they all really share is that they are normally stimulated by serotonin. They even differ in their anatomical distribution within the brain. This division of transmitter receptors into multiple subtypes presents us with an opportunity because, although the natural transmitter will act on *all* its receptor subtypes, we humans can craftily design drugs that single out just one or a few receptor subtypes. Selectively activating or blocking specific subtypes of receptors can produce diverse effects, some of which are beneficial. For example, treating someone with large doses of the neurotransmitter serotonin would necessarily activate *all* of her different subtypes of serotonin receptors, producing a confusing welter of different effects. But drugs that selectively block 5-HT$_3$ receptors while ignoring other subtypes of serotonin receptors produce a powerful and specific anti-nausea effect that brings relief to people undergoing cancer chemotherapy.

The effects of a drug depend on its dose

The tuning of drug molecules to receptor subtypes is not absolutely specific. In reality, a particular drug will generally bind strongly to one kind of receptor, more weakly to a few other types, and not at all to many others. This chemical attraction is known as **binding affinity** (or simply *affinity*). At low doses, when relatively few drug molecules are in circulation, drugs will preferentially bind to their highest-affinity receptors. At higher doses, enough molecules of the drug are available to bind both the highest-affinity receptors and some of the lower-affinity receptors. It's interesting to note that neurotransmitter molecules are low-affinity ligands: they bind only comparatively weakly to their receptors, so they can rapidly detach a moment later, allowing the synapse to reset in preparation for the next presynaptic signal.

Once it is bound to a receptor, the extent to which a drug molecule *activates* the receptor is termed its **efficacy** (or *intrinsic activity*). As you might guess, agonists have high efficacy: they tend to activate the receptors they bind to. Conversely, antagonists have low or no efficacy (see Figure 4.5). Partial agonists, unsurprisingly, have appreciable but submaximal efficacy. So it is a combination of affinity and efficacy—where it binds and what it does—that determines the overall action of a drug. For example, the classic antipsychotic drugs tend to have high affinity and low efficacy at the D$_2$ subtype of dopamine receptors; in other words, they are D$_2$ blockers. It's a topic we'll revisit later in this chapter and in Chapter 12.

Administering larger doses of a drug ultimately increases the proportion of receptors that are bound and affected by the drug. Within certain limits, this increase in receptor binding also increases the response to the drug; in other words, greater doses tend to produce greater effects. When plotted as a graph, the relationship between drug doses and observed effects is called a **dose-response curve** (**DRC**), typically taking the sigmoidal shape shown in **FIGURE 4.6A**. Careful analysis of DRCs reveals many aspects of a drug's activity, such as useful and safe dose ranges (**FIGURE 4.6B**), and it is one of the main tools for understanding the functional relationships between drugs and their targets.

Drugs are administered and eliminated in many different ways

Drug molecules aren't magic bullets; they don't somehow know where to go to find particular receptor molecules. Instead, drug molecules just spread widely throughout the body, binding to their selective receptors when they happen to encounter them. This binding triggers a chain of cellular events, but it is usually temporary, and when the drug (or transmitter) breaks away from the receptor, the receptor resumes its unbound shape and functioning.

The amount of a drug that gets to the brain, and how fast it gets there, depends in part on the drug's route of administration. Some routes, such as smoking or intravenous injection, rapidly ramp up the amount of drug that is **bioavailable** (free to act on the target tissue, and thus not in use elsewhere or in the process of being eliminated). With other routes, such as ingestion (swallowing), the concentration of drug builds up

binding affinity   Also called simply *affinity*. The propensity of molecules of a drug (or other ligand) to bind to receptors.

efficacy   Also called *intrinsic activity*. The extent to which a drug activates a response when it binds to a receptor.

dose-response curve (DRC)
A formal graph of a drug's effects (on the y-axis) versus the dose given (on the x-axis).

bioavailable   Referring to a substance, usually a drug, that is present in the body in a form that is able to interact with physiological mechanisms.

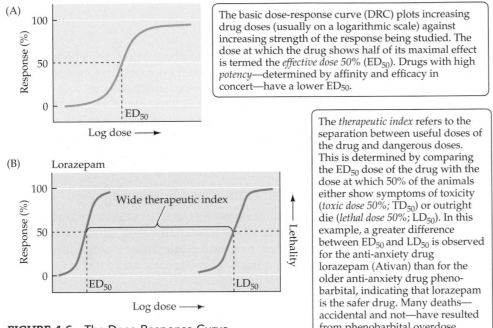

(A)

The basic dose-response curve (DRC) plots increasing drug doses (usually on a logarithmic scale) against increasing strength of the response being studied. The dose at which the drug shows half of its maximal effect is termed the *effective dose 50%* (ED_{50}). Drugs with high *potency*—determined by affinity and efficacy in concert—have a lower ED_{50}.

The *therapeutic index* refers to the separation between useful doses of the drug and dangerous doses. This is determined by comparing the ED_{50} dose of the drug with the dose at which 50% of the animals either show symptoms of toxicity (*toxic dose 50%*; TD_{50}) or outright die (*lethal dose 50%*; LD_{50}). In this example, a greater difference between ED_{50} and LD_{50} is observed for the anti-anxiety drug lorazepam (Ativan) than for the older anti-anxiety drug phenobarbital, indicating that lorazepam is the safer drug. Many deaths—accidental and not—have resulted from phenobarbital overdose.

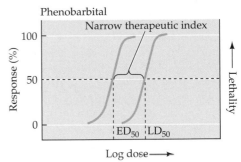

FIGURE 4.6 The Dose-Response Curve

more slowly over longer periods of time. The duration of a drug effect also depends on how the drug is metabolized and excreted from the body—via the kidneys, liver, lungs, or other routes. In some cases, the metabolites of drugs are themselves active; this **biotransformation** of drugs can produce substances with beneficial or harmful actions. The factors that affect the movement of a drug into, through, and out of the body are collectively referred to as **pharmacokinetics**.

Humans have devised a variety of ingenious techniques for introducing substances into the body; these are summarized in **TABLE 4.3**. In Chapter 2 we described how

biotransformation The process in which enzymes convert a drug into a metabolite that is itself active, possibly in ways that are substantially different from the actions of the original substance.

pharmacokinetics Collective name for all the factors that affect the movement of a drug into, through, and out of the body.

TABLE 4.3 ■ The Relationship between Routes of Administration and Effects of Drugs

Route of administration	Examples and mechanisms	Typical speed of effects
INGESTION Tablets and capsules Syrups Infusions and teas Suppositories	Many sorts of drugs and remedies: ingestion depends on absorption by the gut, which is somewhat slower than most other routes and affected by digestive factors such as acidity of the stomach and the presence of food.	Slow to moderate
INHALATION Smoking Nasal absorption (snorting) Inhaled gases, powders, and sprays	Nicotine, cocaine, organic solvents such as airplane glue and gasoline, other drugs of abuse, and a variety of prescription drugs and hormone treatments: inhalation methods take advantage of the rich vascularization of the nose and lungs to convey drugs directly into the bloodstream.	Moderate to fast
PERIPHERAL INJECTION Subcutaneous Intramuscular Intraperitoneal (abdominal) Intravenous	Many drugs: subcutaneous (under the skin) injections tend to have the slowest effects because they must diffuse into nearby tissue in order to reach the bloodstream; intravenous injections have very rapid effects because the drug is placed directly into circulation.	Moderate to fast
CENTRAL INJECTION Intracerebroventricular (into ventricular system) Intrathecal (into the cerebrospinal fluid of the spine) Epidural (under the dura mater) Intracerebral (directly into a brain region)	Central methods involve injection directly into the central nervous system and are used in order to circumvent the blood-brain barrier, to rule out peripheral effects, or to directly affect a discrete brain location.	Fast to very fast

tight junctions between the cells of the walls of blood vessels create a **blood-brain barrier** that inhibits the movement of larger molecules out of the bloodstream and into the brain. This barrier poses a major challenge for neuropharmacology because many drugs that might be useful are too large to cross the blood-brain barrier into the brain. To a limited extent this problem can be circumvented by administering the drugs directly into the brain, but that is a drastic step. Alternatively, some drugs can take advantage of active transport systems that normally move nutrients out of the bloodstream and into the brain.

Repeated treatments may reduce the effectiveness of drugs

Our bodies are well equipped to maintain a constant internal environment, optimized for cellular activities, and to counteract physiological challenges. In the case of drugs, this adaptation may result in the development of **drug tolerance**, where a drug's effectiveness diminishes over repeated treatments. Consequently, successively larger and larger doses of drug are needed to cause the same effect.

Drug tolerance can develop in several different ways. Some drugs provoke **metabolic tolerance**, in which the body (especially metabolic organs, such as the liver with its specialized enzymes) becomes more effective at eliminating the drug from the bloodstream before it can have an effect. Alternatively, the target tissue may change its sensitivity to the drug—a phenomenon called **functional tolerance**. One important way in which a cell develops functional tolerance is by changing how many receptors it has on its surface. So, for example, after repeated doses of an *agonist* drug, neurons may **down-regulate** their receptors (decrease the number of available receptors to which the drug can bind), thereby becoming less sensitive and countering the drug effect. If the drug is an *antagonist,* target neurons may instead **up-regulate** (increase) the number of receptors. Indeed, continual modification of receptor densities is a key feature of synapses and is crucial for neurotransmission and plasticity (Choquet and Triller, 2013).

Tolerance to a particular drug often generalizes to other drugs of the same chemical class; this effect is termed **cross-tolerance**. For example, people who have developed tolerance to heroin tend to exhibit a degree of tolerance to all the other drugs in the opiate category, including codeine, morphine, and methadone. This is because all those drugs act on the same family of receptors.

HOW'S IT GOING ?
---

1. Briefly explain agonist and antagonist actions of a ligand, with respect to effects on receptors.
2. What are receptor subtypes? What is their significance for drug development?
3. Briefly explain how dose-response curves are calculated and why they are useful to pharmacologists. Distinguish between a drug's binding affinity and its efficacy.
4. Provide a review of the different ways in which drugs can be administered, in particular noting some considerations that are taken into account when deciding on a route of administration. How does repeated exposure to a drug alter its effects? (*Hint*: Use the words *tolerance* and *regulate* in your answer.)

Drugs Affect Each Stage of Neural Conduction and Synaptic Transmission

As the saying goes, it takes two to tango. Synaptic transmission involves a complicated choreography of the two participating neurons, and drugs that affect the brain and behavior may act on either side of the synapse. Let's consider these two sites of action in turn.

blood-brain barrier   The protective property of cerebral blood vessels that impedes the movement of some harmful substances from the bloodstream into the brain.

drug tolerance   Also called simply *tolerance*. A condition in which, with repeated exposure to a drug, an individual becomes less responsive to a constant dose.

metabolic tolerance   The form of drug tolerance that arises when repeated exposure to the drug causes the metabolic machinery of the body to become more efficient at clearing the drug.

functional tolerance   The form of drug tolerance that arises when repeated exposure to the drug causes receptors to be up-regulated or down-regulated.

down-regulation   A compensatory decrease in receptor availability at the synapses of a neuron.

up-regulation   A compensatory increase in receptor availability at the synapses of a neuron.

cross-tolerance   A condition in which the development of tolerance for one drug causes an individual to develop tolerance for another drug.

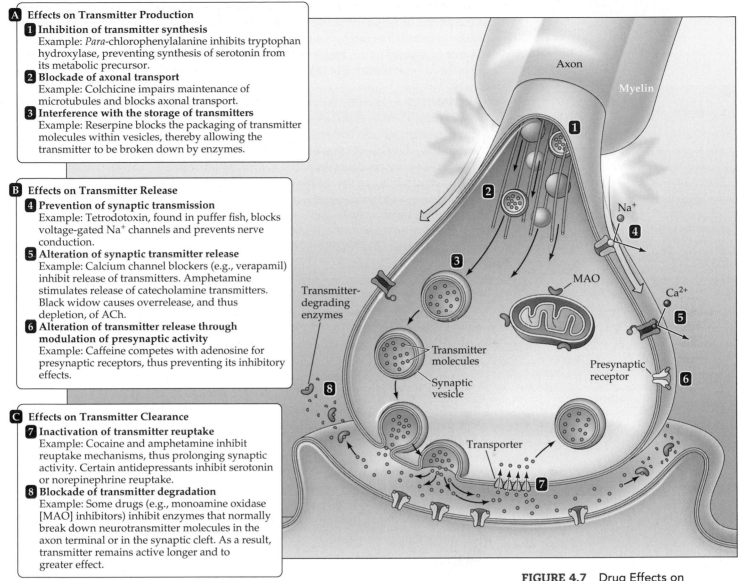

A Effects on Transmitter Production

1 Inhibition of transmitter synthesis
Example: *Para*-chlorophenylalanine inhibits tryptophan hydroxylase, preventing synthesis of serotonin from its metabolic precursor.

2 Blockade of axonal transport
Example: Colchicine impairs maintenance of microtubules and blocks axonal transport.

3 Interference with the storage of transmitters
Example: Reserpine blocks the packaging of transmitter molecules within vesicles, thereby allowing the transmitter to be broken down by enzymes.

B Effects on Transmitter Release

4 Prevention of synaptic transmission
Example: Tetrodotoxin, found in puffer fish, blocks voltage-gated Na^+ channels and prevents nerve conduction.

5 Alteration of synaptic transmitter release
Example: Calcium channel blockers (e.g., verapamil) inhibit release of transmitters. Amphetamine stimulates release of catecholamine transmitters. Black widow causes overrelease, and thus depletion, of ACh.

6 Alteration of transmitter release through modulation of presynaptic activity
Example: Caffeine competes with adenosine for presynaptic receptors, thus preventing its inhibitory effects.

C Effects on Transmitter Clearance

7 Inactivation of transmitter reuptake
Example: Cocaine and amphetamine inhibit reuptake mechanisms, thus prolonging synaptic activity. Certain antidepressants inhibit serotonin or norepinephrine reuptake.

8 Blockade of transmitter degradation
Example: Some drugs (e.g., monoamine oxidase [MAO] inhibitors) inhibit enzymes that normally break down neurotransmitter molecules in the axon terminal or in the synaptic cleft. As a result, transmitter remains active longer and to greater effect.

FIGURE 4.7 Drug Effects on Presynaptic Mechanisms, with Examples

Some drugs alter presynaptic processes

One of the ways that a drug may change synaptic transmission is by affecting the presynaptic neuron, changing the system that converts an electrical signal (an action potential) into a chemical signal (secretion of neurotransmitter). As **FIGURE 4.7** illustrates, the most common presynaptic drug effects can be grouped into three main categories: effects on transmitter *production*, effects on transmitter *release*, and effects on transmitter *clearance*.

TRANSMITTER PRODUCTION   In order for the presynaptic neuron to produce neurotransmitter, a steady supply of raw materials and enzymes must arrive at the axon terminals and carry out the needed reactions. Drugs are available that alter this process in various ways (**FIGURE 4.7A**). For example, a drug may inhibit an enzyme that neurons need in order to synthesize a particular neurotransmitter, resulting in depletion of that transmitter. Alternatively, drugs that block axonal transport prevent raw materials from reaching the axon terminals in the first place, which could also cause the presynaptic terminals to run out of neurotransmitter. In both cases, affected presynaptic neurons are prevented from having their usual effects on postsynaptic neurons, with sometimes profound effects on behavior. A third class of drug (e.g., reserpine) doesn't prevent the *production* of transmitter but instead interferes with the cell's ability to *store* the transmitter in synaptic vesicles for later release. The effect on behavior may be complicated, depending on how much transmitter is able to reach the postsynaptic cell.

TRANSMITTER RELEASE   As we saw in Chapter 3, transmitter is released when action potentials arrive at the axon terminal and trigger an inflow of calcium ions. But a number of drugs and toxins can block those action potentials from ever arriving. For example, compounds that block sodium channels (like the toxin that makes puffer fish a dangerous delicacy, called *tetrodotoxin*) prevent axons from firing action potentials, shutting down synaptic transmission with deadly results. And drugs called *calcium channel blockers* do exactly as their name suggests, blocking the calcium influx that normally drives the release of transmitter into the synapse (**FIGURE 4.7B**). The active ingredient in Botox—botulinum toxin—specifically blocks ACh release from axon terminals near the injection site. The resulting local paralysis of underlying muscles reduces wrinkling of the overlying skin, but it may also interfere with the ability to produce normal facial expressions.

A different way to alter transmitter release is to modify the systems that the neuron normally uses to monitor and regulate its own transmitter release. For example, presynaptic neurons often use **autoreceptors** to monitor how much transmitter they have released; it's a kind of feedback system. Drugs that stimulate these receptors provide a false feedback signal, prompting the presynaptic cell to release less transmitter. Drugs that instead *block* autoreceptors prevent the presynaptic neuron from receiving its normal feedback, tricking the cell into releasing more transmitter than usual. Worldwide, we drink more than 2.2 billion cups of coffee every day, and the **caffeine** we get from all that coffee blocks a type of autoreceptor called the *adenosine receptor*. Adenosine, which is classified as a *neuromodulator*, is coreleased with the neuron's transmitter and acts to reduce further transmitter release. So, blocking presynaptic adenosine receptors increases the amount of neurotransmitter released, which results in the overall increase in alertness for which coffee is renowned (McLellan et al., 2016). Interestingly, consuming caffeine after a period of studying may improve memory consolidation in humans for some, but not all, learning tasks (Borota et al., 2014; Hussain and Cole 2015), perhaps thanks to enhanced neural activity.

TRANSMITTER CLEARANCE   After action potentials have arrived at the axon terminals and prompted a release of transmitter substance, the transmitter is rapidly cleared from the synapse by several processes. Obviously, getting rid of the used transmitter is an important step, because until it is gone, new releases of transmitter from the presynaptic side won't be able to have much extra effect. However, researchers think that under certain circumstances, neurons may be *too* good at clearing the used transmitter and that a significant lack of transmitter in certain synapses may contribute to disorders such as depression. As we'll see shortly, some important psychiatric drugs, called *reuptake inhibitors*, work by blocking the presynaptic system that normally reabsorbs transmitter molecules after their release; this blocking action allows transmitter molecules to accumulate in the synaptic cleft and have a stronger effect on the postsynaptic cell. Other drugs achieve a similar result by blocking the enzymes that normally break up molecules of neurotransmitter into inactive metabolites, again allowing the transmitter to accumulate, having a greater effect on the postsynaptic cell (**FIGURE 4.7C**).

Some drugs alter postsynaptic processes

An alternate way for drugs to change synaptic transmission is by altering the postsynaptic systems that respond to the released neurotransmitter. This change may be

autoreceptor   A receptor for a synaptic transmitter that is located in the presynaptic membrane and tells the axon terminal how much transmitter has been released.

caffeine   A compound found in coffee and other plants that exerts a stimulant action by blocking adenosine receptors.

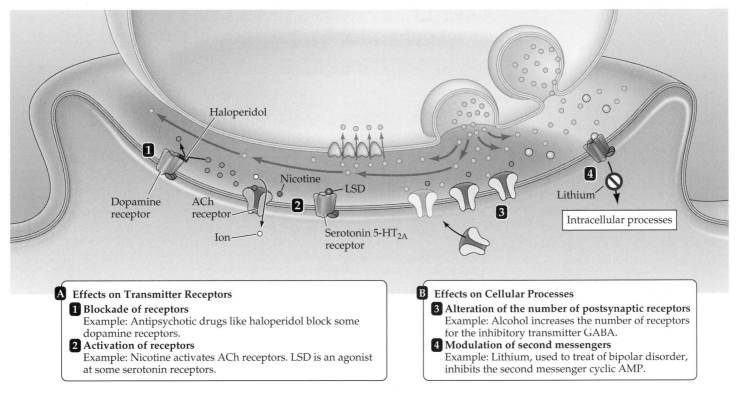

Haloperidol

1

Dopamine
receptor

ACh
receptor

Ion

Nicotine

2

LSD

Serotonin 5-HT$_{2A}$
receptor

3

4

Lithium

Intracellular processes

A **Effects on Transmitter Receptors**
1 **Blockade of receptors**
Example: Antipsychotic drugs like haloperidol block some
dopamine receptors.
2 **Activation of receptors**
Example: Nicotine activates ACh receptors. LSD is an agonist
at some serotonin receptors.

B **Effects on Cellular Processes**
3 **Alteration of the number of postsynaptic receptors**
Example: Alcohol increases the number of receptors
for the inhibitory transmitter GABA.
4 **Modulation of second messengers**
Example: Lithium, used to treat of bipolar disorder,
inhibits the second messenger cyclic AMP.

FIGURE 4.8 Drug Effects on
Postsynaptic Mechanisms

accomplished either by direct actions on the transmitter receptors of the postsynaptic
membrane or by indirect tinkering with other cellular processes within the postsynaptic cell, as illustrated in **FIGURE 4.8**.

TRANSMITTER RECEPTOR ACTIVATION   As we discussed earlier in the chapter, selective receptor antagonists bind directly to postsynaptic receptors and block them
from being activated by their neurotransmitter (**FIGURE 4.8A**). The results may be immediate and dramatic. Curare, for example, blocks the nicotinic ACh receptors found
on muscles, resulting in immediate paralysis of all skeletal muscles, including those
used for breathing (which is why curare is an effective arrow poison).

Selective receptor *agonists* bind to specific receptors and activate them, mimicking the natural neurotransmitter at those receptors. These drugs are often very
potent, with effects that vary depending on the particular types of receptors activated. LSD is an example, producing bizarre visual experiences through strong
stimulation of a subtype of serotonin receptors (namely, 5-HT$_{2A}$ receptors) found in
visual cortex.

POSTSYNAPTIC INTRACELLULAR PROCESSES   When they bind to their matching
receptors on postsynaptic membranes, neurotransmitters can stimulate a variety of
changes within the postsynaptic cells, such as the activation of second messengers,
the activation of genes, and the production of various proteins. These intracellular
processes present additional targets for drug action (**FIGURE 4.8B**). For example,
some drugs induce the postsynaptic cell to up-regulate its receptors, thus changing the sensitivity of the synapse. Other drugs cause a down-regulation in receptor
density. Some drugs, like lithium chloride, directly alter second-messenger systems,
with widespread effects in the brain. Future research will probably focus on drugs
to selectively activate, alter, or block targeted genes within the DNA of neurons.
These *genomic* effects could produce profound long-term changes in the structure
and function of neurons.

PART III
Psychopharmacology: Effects of Drugs on Behavior

THE ROAD AHEAD

The third part of the chapter looks at types of drugs that have been developed to treat mental illness. On completing this section you should be able to:

1. Discuss the historical development of drugs to treat schizophrenia, describe their most prominent actions in the brain, and distinguish between first-generation and second-generation antipsychotics.

2. Identify several categories of antidepressant medications and summarize their modes of action.

3. Describe the development of compounds to treat anxiety, and summarize the mode of action of the most prominent family of these drugs.

4. Summarize the major categories of opiates, and give a general account of their actions on the brain to control pain.

first-generation antipsychotics Also called *neuroleptics*. Any of a class of antipsychotic drugs that alleviate symptoms of schizophrenia, typically by blocking dopamine receptors.

second-generation antipsychotic An antipsychotic drug that has actions other than or in addition to the dopamine D_2 receptor antagonism that characterizes first-generation antipsychotics.

antidepressant A drug that relieves the symptoms of depression.

monoamine oxidase (MAO) An enzyme that breaks down monoamine transmitters, thereby inactivating them.

Some Neuroactive Drugs Ease the Symptoms of Psychiatric Illness

Mental disorders have bedeviled people across the centuries. Historical accounts of sorcery, strange visions, and possession by demons no doubt reflect their authors' misunderstanding of the symptoms of severe mental illness (the topic of Chapter 12) rather than the operation of a supernatural underworld. But where the historical response to psychiatric illness was to lock away the afflicted, neuroscience breakthroughs of the last 70 years have revolutionized psychiatry and liberated millions from the purgatory of institutionalized care. In the sections that follow, we will briefly review some of the major categories of psychoactive drugs, based on how they affect behavior.

Antipsychotics relieve symptoms of schizophrenia

It's hard to believe now, but prior to the 1950s about half of all hospital beds were taken up by psychiatric patients (Menninger, 1948), and, owing to its debilitating nature, a high proportion of these were people suffering from the delusions and hallucinations of schizophrenia. This awful situation was suddenly and dramatically improved by the development of a family of drugs now called **first-generation antipsychotics** (or *neuroleptics*). The first of these drugs, chlorpromazine (Thorazine), and successors like haloperidol (Haldol) and loxapine (Loxitane) all share one crucial feature: they act as selective antagonists of dopamine D_2 receptors in the brain. These drugs are so good at relieving the symptoms of schizophrenia that a dopaminergic model of the disease became dominant (see Chapter 12). More recently, **second-generation antipsychotics** have been developed that have both dopaminergic and additional, nondopaminergic actions, especially the blockade of certain serotonin receptors. These drugs may be helpful in relieving symptoms that are resistant to first-generation antipsychotics, but early hopes that these drugs would generally outperform first-generation antipsychotics have not been borne out (Kane and Correll, 2010). Emerging evidence that schizophrenia also involves transmitters other than the classic targets has since prompted an intense research effort aimed at developing third-generation antipsychotics, with novel targets like glutamate and oxytocin, but effective treatments remain elusive (Davis et al., 2014; O'Tuathaigh et al., 2017). So, although there has been progress in its treatment, schizophrenia remains a difficult, multifaceted disease and a major health problem.

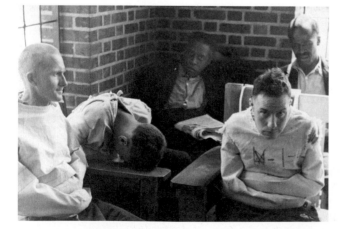

The Antipsychotic Revolution The introduction of antipsychotic drugs relieved the suffering of millions of patients who had previously required hospitalization in psychiatric institutions like this one. Antipsychotics dramatically curb the striking hallucinations and delusions that are symptomatic of schizophrenia. (© Alfred Eisenstadt/Time & Life Pictures/Getty Images.)

Antidepressants reduce chronic mood problems

Disturbances of mood called *affective disorders* are among the most common of all psychiatric complaints (World Health Organization, 2001). In contrast to the antipsychotic drugs, which reduce synaptic activity by blocking receptors, effective **antidepressant** drugs act to *increase* synaptic transmission. Some of the earliest antidepressants were the **monoamine oxidase** (**MAO**) inhibitors, which, as their name suggests, block the enzyme responsible for breaking down monoamine transmitters such as dopamine, serotonin, and norepinephrine. This action allows transmitter molecules to accumulate in the synapses (see Figure 4.7, step 8), with an associated improvement in mood. A second generation of drugs, called the **tricyclic antidepressants** (an example is imipramine), likewise promote an accumulation of synaptic transmitter, by blocking the reuptake of transmitter molecules into the presynaptic terminal (see Figure 4.7, step 7). More recent generations of antidepressants also increase synaptic transmitter availability, but they focus on specific transmitters: **selective serotonin reuptake inhibitors** (**SSRIs**) like fluoxetine (Prozac) and citalopram (Celexa) are so named because they act specifically to block reuptake at serotonergic synapses, whereas serotonin-norepinephrine reuptake inhibitors (SNRIs) like venlafaxine (Effexor) promote the accumulation of both serotonin and norepinephrine by blocking reuptake of both transmitters.

Anxiolytics combat anxiety

Severe anxiety, in the form of panic attacks, phobias (specific irrational fears), and generalized anxiety, can spiral out of control and become disabling; many millions of people suffer from anxiety disorders (see Chapter 12). Anything that reduces or *depresses* the excitability of neurons tends to counter these states, which explains some of the historical popularity of **depressants** like alcohol and opium. Unfortunately, these substances have a strong potential for intoxication and addiction, so they are not suitable for therapeutic use. **Barbiturate** drugs, such as phenobarbital, were originally developed to reduce anxiety, promote sleep, and avoid epileptic seizures. They are still used occasionally for those purposes, but they are also addictive and easy to overdose on, often fatally, as illustrated in Figure 4.6B.

Since the 1970s the most widely prescribed **anxiolytics** (antianxiety drugs) have been the **benzodiazepines**, which are both safer and more specific than the barbiturates (see Figure 4.6B), although they still carry some risk of addiction. Members of this class of drug, such as diazepam (Valium) and lorazepam (Ativan), bind to specific sites on $GABA_A$ receptors and enhance the activity of GABA (Walters et al., 2000). Because $GABA_A$ receptors are inhibitory, benzodiazepines help GABA to produce larger inhibitory postsynaptic potentials than GABA would produce alone. The net effect is a reduction in the excitability of neurons. The hunt for new antianxiety agents—both exogenous and endogenous—is an area of intense research effort. Hormones that interact with GABA receptors, as well as drugs that subtly alter serotonergic neurotransmission, are examples of these novel anxiolytics. Antidepressant drugs are often effective anxiolytics too.

Opiates have powerful painkilling effects

Opium, extracted from poppy flower seedpods, has been used by humans since at least the Stone Age. **Morphine**, the major active substance in opium, is a very effective **analgesic** (painkiller) that has brought relief from severe pain to many millions of people (see Chapter 5). Unfortunately, because it produces powerful feelings of euphoria, morphine also has a strong potential for addiction, as do close relatives like **heroin** (diacetylmorphine) and opiate painkillers like oxycodone (OxyContin) and fentanyl, a synthetic opiate that is 30 to 40 times stronger than heroin. Accidental opiate overdose is a rapidly

tricyclic antidepressant   An antidepressant that acts by increasing the synaptic accumulation of serotonin and norepinephrine.

selective serotonin reuptake inhibitor (SSRI)   An antidepressant drug that blocks the reuptake of transmitter at serotonergic synapses.

depressant   A drug that reduces the excitability of neurons.

barbiturate   An early anxiolytic drug and sleep aid that has depressant activity in the nervous system.

anxiolytic   A drug that is used to combat anxiety.

benzodiazepine   Any of a class of antianxiety drugs that are agonists of $GABA_A$ receptors in the central nervous system. One example is diazepam (Valium).

opium   An extract of the opium poppy, Papaver somniferum. Drugs based on opium are potent painkillers.

morphine   An opiate compound derived from the poppy flower.

analgesic   Having painkilling properties.

heroin   Diacetylmorphine, an artificially modified, very potent form of morphine.

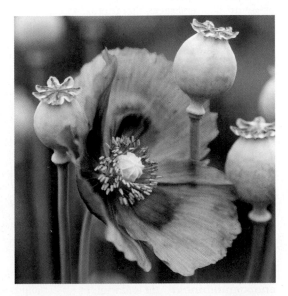

The Source of Opium and Morphine   The opium poppy has a distinctive flower and seedpod. The bitter flavor and brain actions of opium may provide the poppy plant a defense against being eaten. (© South West Images Scotland/Alamy.)

FIGURE 4.9 An Epidemic of Overdose Deaths (After NIDA [2017] based on data from Natl. Ctr. Hlth. Stat., CDC Wonder database, 2017.)

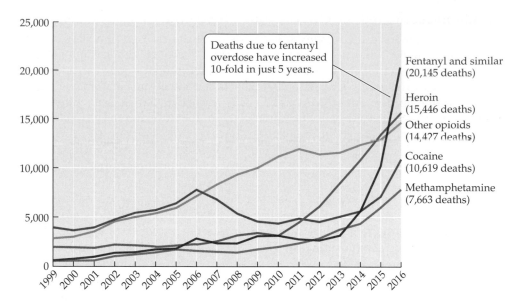

Deaths due to fentanyl overdose have increased 10-fold in just 5 years.

Fentanyl and similar (20,145 deaths)
Heroin (15,446 deaths)
Other opioids (14,427 deaths)
Cocaine (10,619 deaths)
Methamphetamine (7,663 deaths)

growing epidemic: the fatal fentanyl overdose of the musician Prince in 2016 was just one of many thousands every year (**FIGURE 4.9**).

Opiates like morphine, heroin, and codeine bind to specific receptors—**opioid receptors**—that are concentrated in various regions of the brain. An area within the midbrain called the **periaqueductal gray** (**FIGURE 4.10**) contains a very high density of opioid receptors and is an especially important target because it is here that opiates exert their painkilling effects (see Chapter 5).

As we mentioned earlier in the chapter, we now know that the brain makes its own morphine-like compounds, called **endogenous opioids**. Researchers have identified three major families of these potent peptides: the *enkephalins*, from the Greek *en*, "in," and *kephale*, "head" (Hughes et al., 1975); the *endorphins*, a contraction of *endogenous*

opioid receptor   A receptor that responds to endogenous opioids and/or exogenous opiates.

periaqueductal gray   A midbrain region involved in pain perception.

endogenous opioid   Any of a class of opium-like peptide transmitters that have been referred to as the body's own narcotics. The three kinds are enkephalins, endorphins, and dynorphins.

cannabis   Also known as *marijuana*, although this name is considered pejorative. A psychoactive plant containing numerous active compounds in varying proportions.

delta-9-tetrahydrocannabinol (THC)   The major active ingredient in cannabis.

cannabidiol (CBD)   One of the two major types of active compounds found in cannabis. The other is THC.

cannabinoid receptors   A receptor that responds to endogenous and/or exogenous cannabinoids.

endocannabinoid   An endogenous ligand of cannabinoid receptors, thus an analog of cannabis that is produced by the brain.

anandamide   An endogenous substance that binds the cannabinoid receptor molecule.

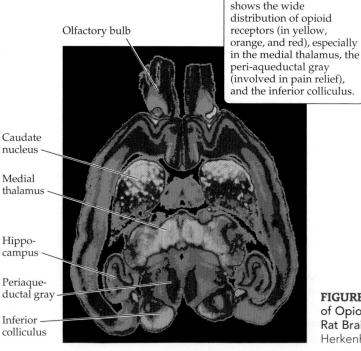

This horizontal section shows the wide distribution of opioid receptors (in yellow, orange, and red), especially in the medial thalamus, the peri-aqueductal gray (involved in pain relief), and the inferior colliculus.

Olfactory bulb
Caudate nucleus
Medial thalamus
Hippocampus
Periaqueductal gray
Inferior colliculus

FIGURE 4.10 The Distribution of Opioid Receptors in the Rat Brain (Courtesy of Miles Herkenham, Natl. Inst. Ment. Hlth.)

morphine; and the *dynorphins*, short for *dynamic endorphins*, in recognition of their potency and speed of action (see Table 4.1). There are also three main kinds of opioid receptors—delta (δ), kappa (κ), and mu (μ)—all of which are metabotropic receptors (see Table 4.2). Powerful drugs that block opioid receptors—naloxone (Narcan) is an example—can rapidly reverse the effects of opiates and rescue people from overdose. Opiate antagonists also block the rewarding aspects of drugs like heroin, so they can be helpful for treating addiction, as we discuss at the end of this chapter.

Some Neuroactive Drugs Are Used to Alter Conscious Experience

Whether to experience pleasurable sensations, to artificially increase vigor and wakefulness, or simply to satisfy curiosity, people have a long history of tinkering with their conscious experience of the world. Some of the most familiar types of drugs that modify consciousness include cannabinoids, stimulants, alcohol, and hallucinogens.

Cannabinoids have many effects

Cannabis and its related preparations, such as hashish, are derived from the *Cannabis sativa* plant, which has been widely cultivated and used by human societies for thousands of years (Russo, 2008). (The common alternative name *marijuana* is considered by some to have dubious, possibly racist origins; see Halperin, 2018.) Typically administered by smoking, by vaping, or via edible products such as cookies and candies, cannabis contains dozens of active ingredients, especially the compounds **delta-9-tetrahydrocannabinol** (**THC**) and **cannabidiol** (**CBD**). Cannabis use usually produces pleasant relaxation and mood alteration, although the drug can occasionally cause stimulation and paranoia instead.

Occasional use of cannabis seems to be mostly harmless, but as with other substances, heavy use can be harmful. For example, persistent heavy use (i.e., ongoing use of cannabis four or more times per week) may be associated with respiratory problems, addiction, cognitive decline, and psychiatric disorders (Meier et al., 2012). A particular concern is that adolescent use of cannabis may increase the risk of later developing schizophrenia (Marconi et al., 2016; Jones et al., 2018). However, it remains to be determined whether the cannabis use causes the illness, or conversely whether adolescents who are already experiencing symptoms of mental illness may be more drawn to cannabis use (Bourque et al., 2017).

As with opiates and benzodiazepines, researchers found that the brain contains specific **cannabinoid receptors** that mediate the effects of compounds like THC. Cannabinoid receptors are found in the substantia nigra, the hippocampus, the cerebellar cortex, and the cerebral cortex (**FIGURE 4.11**) (Devane et al., 1988). Later research revealed that the brain makes several THC-like endogenous ligands for these receptors. The most studied of these **endocannabinoids** is **anandamide** (from the Sanskrit *ananda*, "bliss") (Devane et al., 1992), which produces some of the most familiar physiological and psychological effects of cannabis use, such as mood improvement, pain relief, lowered blood pressure, relief from nausea, improvements in the eye disease glaucoma, and so on. Cannabinoids are thus targets of an intense research effort aimed at developing drugs with some of the specific beneficial effects of cannabis.

The documented use of cannabis for recreational and medicinal purposes spans over 6,000 years, but for most of the twentieth century it was subject to widespread legal prohibition. More recently, recreational sale and use of cannabis is being legalized in various U.S. states, Canada, and other countries. Possession of cannabis

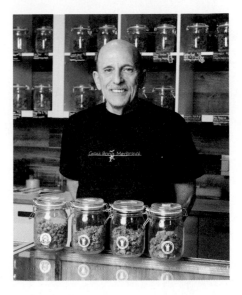

Relaxation Cannabis laws are being relaxed in many jurisdictions. Legal access through licensed shops, like this one in Canada, acknowledges existing widespread use of cannabis for recreational and medicinal purposes, and is expected to reduce criminal activity, but health risks remain for adolescents and heavy users. (David Buzzard/Alamy Stock Photo.)

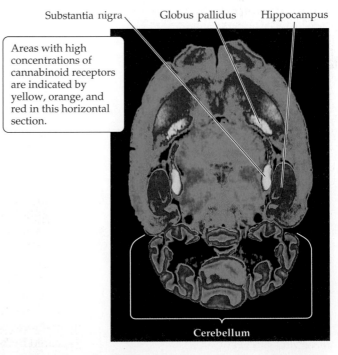

Substantia nigra   Globus pallidus   Hippocampus

Areas with high concentrations of cannabinoid receptors are indicated by yellow, orange, and red in this horizontal section.

Cerebellum

FIGURE 4.11 The Distribution of Cannabinoid Receptors in the Rat Brain (Courtesy of Miles Herkenham, Natl. Inst. Ment. Hlth.)

for recreational or medical purposes has been "decriminalized" (i.e., tolerated while technically illegal) in many other jurisdictions. It seems likely that the relaxation of cannabis laws will continue, so a fuller understanding of the beneficial and adverse effects of cannabis, and potential for cannabis addiction, is a high priority for researchers (Curran et al., 2016).

Stimulants increase neural activity

Proper functioning of the nervous system involves a fine balance between excitatory and inhibitory influences. A **stimulant** is a drug that tips the balance toward the excitatory side, with an overall alerting, activating effect. Some stimulants act directly by increasing excitatory synaptic potentials. Others act by blocking normal inhibitory processes: we've already seen that caffeine acts as a stimulant by blocking presynaptic adenosine receptors that normally inhibit transmitter release. The stimulants therefore form a diverse class of drugs that range from mild, commonplace substances like coffee to powerfully addictive and harmful substances such as nicotine, cocaine, and methamphetamine.

NICOTINE Tobacco is native to the Americas, where European explorers first encountered smoking; these explorers brought tobacco back to Europe with them. Tobacco use became much more widespread following technological innovations that made it easier to smoke, in the form of cigarettes (W. Bennett, 1983). Delivered to the large surface of the lungs, the **nicotine** from conventional or e-cigarettes enters the blood and brain much more rapidly than does nicotine from other tobacco products. Nicotine acts as a stimulant, increasing heart rate, blood pressure, digestive action, and alertness. In the short run, these effects make tobacco use pleasurable. But these alterations of body function, quite apart from the effects of tobacco tar on the lungs, make prolonged exposure to nicotine unhealthful. Smoking and nicotine exposure in adolescence has a lasting impact on attention and cognitive development, due to changes in the pubertal development of cholinergic and glutamatergic systems, and possible long-lasting epigenetic modifications of neural function (Counotte et al., 2011; Yuan et al., 2015).

The *nicotinic* ACh receptors didn't get their name by coincidence; it is through these receptors that the nicotine from tobacco exerts most of its effects in the body. Nicotinic receptors drive the contraction of skeletal muscles, and the activation of various visceral organs, but they are also found in high concentrations in the brain, including the cortex. This is one way in which nicotine enhances some aspects of cognitive performance. Nicotine also stimulates the ventral tegmental area to exert its rewarding/addicting effects (Maskos et al., 2005). (We will discuss the ventral tegmental area in more detail when we discuss positive reward models later in this chapter.)

COCAINE For hundreds of years, people in Bolivia, Colombia, and Peru have used the leaves of the coca shrub—either chewed or brewed as a tea—to increase endurance, alleviate hunger, and promote a sense of well-being. The use of coca leaves in this manner does not seem to cause problems. But processing and concentrating an extract from this plant produces a much more potent and dangerous compound: **cocaine**.

First isolated in 1859, cocaine was added to beverages (such as Coca-Cola) and tonics for its stimulant qualities, and subsequently it was used as a local anesthetic (it is in the same chemical family as procaine) and as an antidepressant. But people soon discovered that the rapid hit resulting from snorting cocaine (see Table 4.3) has a stimulant effect that is powerful and pleasurable. Crack, a smokable form of cocaine that appeared in the mid-1980s, enters the blood and the brain even more rapidly and thus is even more addictive than cocaine powder. However it is taken, cocaine is highly addictive. Furthermore, heavy cocaine use raises the risk of serious side effects like stroke, psychosis, loss of gray matter, and severe mood disturbances (Franklin et al.,

stimulant A drug that enhances the excitability of neurons.

nicotine A compound found in plants, including tobacco, that acts as an agonist on a large class of cholinergic receptors.

cocaine A drug of abuse, derived from the coca plant, that acts by enhancing catecholamine neurotransmission.

In this coronal image, brain regions with high degrees of cocaine binding are shown in orange and yellow. Cocaine acts in these areas to cause an accumulation of norepinephrine and dopamine.

FIGURE 4.12 Cocaine Action in the Monkey Brain (Courtesy of Bertha K. Madras and Marc J. Kaufman.)

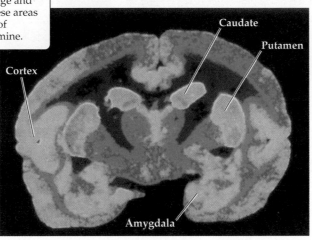

Caudate

Putamen

Cortex

Amygdala

amphetamine A molecule that resembles the structure of the catecholamine transmitters and enhances their activity.

2002). Cocaine causes changes in the structure and function of many regions of the brain (Hanlon et al., 2013), which contribute to high rates of relapse in people attempting to quit cocaine use. Cocaine exerts its stimulant effects by blocking the reuptake of monoamine transmitters—especially dopamine and norepinephrine—from synapses. This action causes transmitters to accumulate in synapses throughout much of the brain (**FIGURE 4.12**), therefore boosting their effects.

AMPHETAMINE The synthetic stimulant **amphetamine** ("speed") and its potent relatives, like methamphetamine ("meth"), have a mode of action that superficially resembles that of cocaine, inducing an accumulation of the synaptic transmitters norepinephrine and dopamine. However, the mechanics of amphetamine's actions, involving two steps, are quite different from those of cocaine. First, amphetamine acts within axon terminals to cause a larger-than-normal release of neurotransmitter when the synapse is activated. Second, amphetamine then interferes with the clearance of the released transmitter by blocking its reuptake. The result is that the affected synapses become unnaturally potent, having strong effects on behavior.

Over the short term, amphetamine causes increased vigor and stamina, wakefulness, decreased appetite, and feelings of euphoria. For these reasons, amphetamine has historically been used in military applications and other settings where intense sustained effort is required. However, the quality of the work being performed may suffer, and the costs of amphetamine use soon outweigh the benefits. Addiction and tolerance to amphetamine and methamphetamine develop rapidly, requiring ever-larger doses that lead to sleeplessness, severe weight loss, and general deterioration of mental and physical condition.

Prolonged use of amphetamine or methamphetamine may lead to symptoms that resemble those of schizophrenia: compulsive, agitated behavior and irrational suspiciousness. Users may neglect their diet and basic hygiene, aging rapidly. Users also experience a variety of peripheral effects, like high blood pressure, tremor, dizziness, sweating, rapid breathing, and nausea. And worst of all, people who chronically abuse amphetamine often display symptoms of brain damage long after they quit using the drug (Ernst et al., 2000). As we'll discuss a little later in the chapter, increased activation of

Faces of Meth These before and after photos, taken just 2½ years apart, testify to the heavy toll taken by chronic methamphetamine abuse. Meth causes multiple severe problems such as motor disorders, cognitive impairment, psychosis, rapid changes in appearance due to accelerated tooth decay ("meth mouth"), skin pathology, and excessive weight loss. (Mug shots courtesy of the Multnomah County Sheriff's Office and the Faces of Meth™ program.)

FIGURE 4.13 Abnormal Brain Development in Fetal Alcohol Syndrome (Courtesy of E. Riley.)

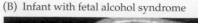

(A) Healthy infant   Corpus callosum   (B) Infant with fetal alcohol syndrome

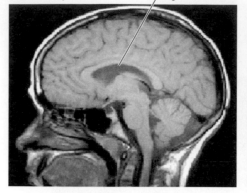 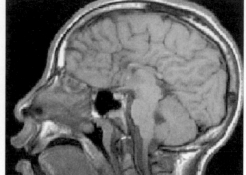

Compared to MRI images of a healthy infant's brain…

…the MRI of an infant affected by fetal alcohol syndrome—caused by heavy consumption of alcohol by the mother during pregnancy—shows extensive abnormality, including reduced gray matter, complete absence of the corpus callosum, abnormal organization of the brain, and characteristic deformities of the head and face.

the mesolimbocortical dopaminergic reward system of the brain appears to be crucial for the rewarding aspects of drug use.

Amphetamine-like stimulants called *cathinones* are released when the African shrub **khat** (or *qat*, pronounced "cot") is chewed. Many types of synthetic cathinones—known collectively as "bath salts"—have been developed and marketed in recent years (often via the internet). These new designer drugs, especially *mephedrone* ("plant food" or "meow meow"), have shown rapid growth in popularity (Kelly, 2011; Zawilska, 2014).

Alcohol acts as both a stimulant and a depressant

The most widely consumed psychoactive drug, alcohol, is easily produced by the fermentation of fruit or grains. Taken in moderation (perhaps one or two drinks per day at most), alcohol is harmless or even beneficial to the health of adults, but *excessive* alcohol consumption is very damaging and linked to a multitude of serious diseases (Mukamal et al., 2003; O'Keefe et al., 2014).

Alcohol has a biphasic effect on the nervous system: at first it acts as a stimulant, and then it has a more prolonged depressant phase. (Remember, the word *depressant* relates to a depression or inhibition of neural activity, not an effect on mood.) Like the anxiety-reducing benzodiazepines we discussed earlier, alcohol inhibits postsynaptic activity via an action on GABA receptors, resulting in the social disinhibition, poor motor control, and sensory disturbances that we call *drunkenness*. Alcohol additionally activates dopamine-mediated reward systems of the brain, accounting for some of the pleasurable aspects of drinking.

Chronic abuse of alcohol damages or destroys nerve cells in many regions of the brain. Alcohol abuse by expectant mothers can cause grievous permanent damage to the developing fetus, termed **fetal alcohol spectrum disorder** (**FASD**), which in the most severe cases is characterized by facial deformities and stunted brain growth, sometimes including the absence of the corpus callosum that normally connects the two hemispheres of the brain (**FIGURE 4.13**). Concerns remain that even modest intake of alcohol during pregnancy may have a damaging effect on the fetus, depending on a variety of physical and behavioral characteristics of the mother (May and Gossage, 2011), and the CDC currently advises that there is no known safe level of alcohol use in pregnancy (Centers for Disease Control and Prevention, 2016). In adults, the frontal lobes are especially affected by chronic alcohol use (Kril et al., 1997). Happily, some of the anatomical changes associated with chronic alcoholism may be reversible with abstinence. In humans suffering from alcoholism, MRI studies show an increase in the volume of cortical

khat   Also spelled *qat*. An African shrub that, when chewed, acts as a stimulant.

fetal alcohol spectrum disorder (FASD)   A family of developmental disorders that vary in severity, resulting from fetal exposure to alcohol consumed by the mother. Severe cases, associated with high levels of alcohol abuse by the mother, include characteristic intellectual disability and facial abnormalities.

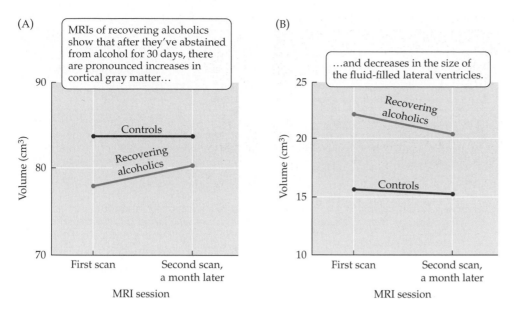

(A)

MRIs of recovering alcoholics show that after they've abstained from alcohol for 30 days, there are pronounced increases in cortical gray matter…

Controls

Recovering alcoholics

Volume (cm³)

First scan   Second scan, a month later

MRI session

(B)

…and decreases in the size of the fluid-filled lateral ventricles.

Recovering alcoholics

Controls

Volume (cm³)

First scan   Second scan, a month later

MRI session

FIGURE 4.14 The Effects of Alcoholism on the Structure of the Brain (After A. Pfefferbaum et al., 1995. *Alcohol. Clin. Exp. Res.* 19: 1177.)

gray matter and an associated reduction in ventricular volume within weeks of giving up alcohol (**FIGURE 4.14**) (Pfefferbaum et al., 1995). Even in the absence of clear-cut alcoholism, periodic binge drinking (generally, five or more drinks on a single occasion, a common mode of alcohol use in young people) can harm the brains and alter the behavior of adolescents in ways that last into adulthood (Crews et al., 2016).

Hallucinogens alter sensory perceptions

Humans have long prized **hallucinogens**, substances that produce powerful sensory alterations, often believing the resultant experiences to have deep spiritual or psychological meaning. Dozens of such hallucinogens are found in nature—psilocybin and muscarine (from "magic" mushrooms), mescaline (from the peyote plant), and bufotenine (from toads) are a few examples. But the term *hallucinogen* is really a misnomer because, whereas a hallucination is a novel perception that takes place in the absence of sensory stimulation (hearing voices, or seeing something that isn't there), the drugs in this category mostly alter or distort *existing* perceptions (mainly visual in nature). Users may see fantastic images (**FIGURE 4.15**), often with intense colors, but often they are aware that these strangely altered perceptions are not real events.

Hallucinogenic agents are diverse in their neural actions. Whereas muscarine affects the ACh system, mescaline acts via noradrenergic and serotonergic systems. The

hallucinogen A drug that alters sensory perception and produces peculiar experiences.

These images are portraits produced by a professional artist just after taking LSD (leftmost drawing) and then at three successive time points as the drug took effect. The model for all four drawings is the same man (the researcher, in fact).

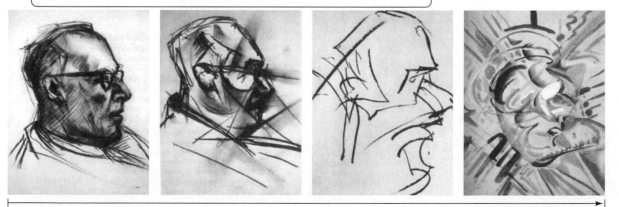

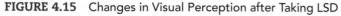

20 minutes   Time   3 hours

FIGURE 4.15 Changes in Visual Perception after Taking LSD

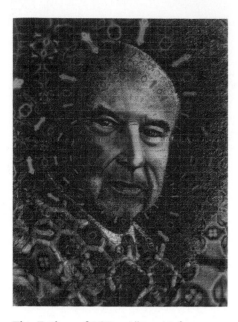

The Father of LSD   Albert Hofmann discovered LSD by accidentally taking some in 1943, and he devoted the rest of his career to studying it. A prohibited drug in most jurisdictions, LSD is distributed on colorful blotter paper. This example, picturing Hofmann and the LSD molecule, is made up of 1,036 individual doses, or "hits." (Art by Wes Black, courtesy of www.blotterart.com.)

TABLE 4.4 ■ Possible Clinical Applications for Hallucinogens	
Drug name and date of discovery	Action in brain
Psilocybin/psilocin (*Psilocybe* mushroom) (according to archaeological evidence, used in prehistory)	Is a partial agonist of 5-HT receptors, especially 5-HT$_{2A}$ receptors that occur in high density in visual cortex. Modifies activity of frontal and occipital cortex.
Lysergic acid diethylamide (LSD) (1938)	Activates many subtypes of monoamine receptors, especially DA and 5-HT, resulting in heightened activity in many cortical regions, especially frontal, cingulate, and occipital cortex.
Ketamine (1962)	Has widespread effects in the brain, especially blockade of NMDA receptors, and stimulates opioid and ACh receptors.
3,4-Methylenedioxymeth-amphetamine (MDMA) (1912/1970s)	Stimulates release of monoamine transmitters and the prosocial hormone oxytocin.

LSD · Also called *acid*. Lysergic acid diethylamide, a hallucinogenic drug.

MDMA   Also called *Ecstasy* or *Molly*. 3,4-Methylenedioxymethamphetamine, a drug of abuse.

herb *Salvia divinorum* is unusual among hallucinogens because it acts on the opioid kappa receptor. But research with LSD and related drugs suggests that perhaps the most important shared neural action of hallucinogens is the stimulation of serotonin receptors. Discovered by Albert Hofmann in the 1940s, **LSD** (lysergic acid diethylamide, or more simply *acid*) structurally resembles serotonin. Even in tiny doses, LSD strongly activates serotonin 5-HT$_{2A}$ receptors that are found in especially heavy concentrations in the visual cortex. Other hallucinogens, such as mescaline and psilocybin, share this action. Research with psilocybin has also demonstrated disinhibition of emotion-processing regions in the limbic system (Carhart-Harris et al., 2012), perhaps accounting for some of the drug's emotional, mystical qualities. In addition to their impressive perceptual effects, LSD, psilocybin, and other hallucinogens can produce mood changes, introspective states, and feelings of creativity that have led to renewed interest in the possibility of using hallucinogens to treat specific psychiatric disorders, including depression, anxiety, and obsessive-compulsive disorder (Kyzar et al., 2017).

Ketamine (known as Special K) is a drug that is already in widespread use in medical settings as a component of anesthesia but that also has pronounced hallucinogenic properties. Acting principally (but not exclusively) to block NMDA receptors, ketamine increases activity in prefrontal cortex and hippocampus and produces feelings of depersonalization and detachment from reality. Ketamine increases activity in the prefrontal cortex (Breier et al., 1997; Zorumski et al., 2016), and while high doses produce transient hallucinogenic effects and occasional psychotic symptoms in volunteers, low doses have a potent and rapid antidepressant effect that may help ease symptoms in resistant cases (Carlson et al., 2013; Williams and Schatzberg, 2016).

Like LSD, the hallucinogenic amphetamine derivative **MDMA** (3,4-methylenedioxymethamphetamine, known as *Molly* or *Ecstasy*) stimulates visual cortical 5-HT$_{2A}$ receptors, but it also changes the levels of dopamine and certain hormones, such as prolactin. Exactly how these activities account for the subjective effects of MDMA—positive emotions, empathy, euphoria, a sense of well-being, and colorful visual phenomena—remains uncertain.

Complications due to hallucinogen use are quite varied. The major hallucinogens seem to have comparatively low addiction potential. LSD has relatively few negative side effects (although some users report long-lasting visual changes). Long-term MDMA use may cause problems with mood and cognitive performance (Sumnall and Cole, 2005; Parrott, 2013) and long-lasting changes in patterns of brain activation,

Recreational use	Possible clinical application
Users of "shrooms" often report spiritual experiences and feelings of transcendence, along with intense visual experiences and alterations in the perception of time. The exact effects are strongly influenced by the expectations and surroundings of the user.	Recent studies suggest that psilocybin—administered in controlled settings—can offer substantial and enduring improvements in the symptoms of obsessive-compulsive disorder (OCD), cluster headache (a type of migraine), treatment-resistant depression, and debilitating anxiety and anguish (as in a sample of terminal cancer patients) (Grob et al., 2011; E. A. Schindler et al., 2015; Carhart-Harris et al., 2016).
"Acid" produces pronounced perceptual changes that resemble hallucinations. Intense colors in geometric patterns, novel visual objects, and an altered sense of time are common.	LSD may be an effective treatment for alcoholism and other addictions and may also be an effective treatment for some types of debilitating anxiety (Bogenschutz and Johnson, 2016; Gasser et al., 2014).
"Special K" creates a detached, trancelike state, in keeping with its routine medical use as an anesthetic. It may also produce hallucinogenic perceptual alterations.	Recent experiments have revealed a potent antidepressant effect of ketamine at lower doses, even in cases that resist other types of treatments (Williams and Schatzberg, 2016).
Users of "Ecstasy" experience intense visual phenomena, empathy, strongly prosocial feelings, and euphoria.	MDMA treatment may reduce symptoms of post-traumatic stress disorder (PTSD), especially in combination with conventional psychotherapy, but concerns remain regarding drug safety (Parrott, 2014; Sessa, 2017).

even at low doses (de Win et al., 2008). However, short-term MDMA treatment is also being investigated as a possible treatment for persistent post-traumatic stress disorder (Mithoefer et al., 2013). The neural actions, recreational properties, and possible psychiatric uses of some of the major hallucinogens are summarized in **TABLE 4.4**.

HOW'S IT GOING ?

1. Compare and contrast the three major categories of presynaptic effects of psychoactive drugs. Give examples of each kind of action. (*Hint*: The words *production*, *release*, and *clearance* will be important for your discussion.)
2. Compare and contrast the main postsynaptic actions of psychotropic drugs, with examples. Be sure to distinguish between actions at receptors and actions within the postsynaptic neuron.
3. At least four general categories of psychoactive drugs are used to relieve disorders. Describe these categories, and give some examples of each class of drugs. Be sure to discuss the modes of action of the drugs you cite.
4. Identify and discuss the major categories of drugs that people use to alter their consciousness. In what ways are the major categories similar, and in what ways do they differ? What are some of the threats to health that these compounds present?
5. Discuss the renewed scientific interest in the therapeutic use of hallucinogens. How might they help in psychiatric disorders?

Substance Abuse and Addiction Are Global Social Problems

The habitual use of drugs to alter consciousness can be costly to the user and to society. Governments attempt to minimize these costs by controlling (or preventing) the production and distribution of designated drugs, but the division of drugs into licit and illicit categories is largely a matter of historical accident. Some classes of drugs—the opiates, for example—span both categories, being both useful medicines and harmful drugs of abuse. And some substances, like tobacco, are legal only because they have been cultivated for centuries and are backed by powerful economic interests. In terms of illness, death, lost productivity, and sheer human misery, some of the legal drugs may be the worst offenders. Just one example reveals the extent of the problem: in the

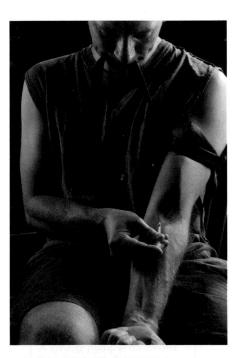

"The Needle and the Damage Done" Addiction has a powerful grip, inducing people to go to sometimes extreme lengths to obtain larger and more frequent doses. (© ejwhite/Shutterstock.)

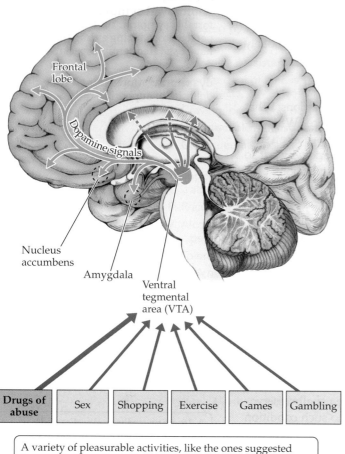

A variety of pleasurable activities, like the ones suggested here, probably activate the dopaminergic pathway that produces rewarding sensations. Drugs of abuse powerfully activate this system and may eclipse other sources of pleasure.

FIGURE 4.17   A Neural Pathway Implicated in Drug Abuse (After H. O. Pettit and J. B. Justice, Jr., 1991. *Brain Res.* 539: 94.)

nucleus accumbens   A region of the forebrain that receives dopaminergic innervation from the ventral tegmental area, often associated with reward and pleasurable sensations.

insula   A region of cortex lying below the surface, within the lateral sulcus, of the frontal, temporal, and parietal lobes.

will perform for a single dose, or the smaller the dose that will support the lever-pressing behavior, the more rewarding and addictive the drug must be. For example, it turns out that animals will self-administer doses of morphine that are so low that no signs of physical dependence ever develop (Schuster, 1970). Animals will also furiously press a lever to self-administer tiny doses of cocaine and other stimulants (Pickens and Thompson, 1968; Koob, 1995; Tanda et al., 2000). In fact, cocaine supports some of the highest rates of lever pressing ever recorded.

Experiments using drug self-administration suggest that, by itself, the physical dependence model is inadequate to explain drug addiction, although physical dependence and tolerance may contribute to drug hunger. The more comprehensive view of drug self-administration interprets it as a behavior controlled by a powerful pattern of positive and negative rewards (a variant of operant conditioning theory; see Chapter 13), without the need to implicate a disease process.

Many—but not all—addictive drugs cause the release of dopamine in the **nucleus accumbens**, just as occurs with more conventional rewards, such as food, sex, and gambling (Nutt et al., 2015; Volkow et al., 2017). As we mentioned previously, dopamine released from axons originating in the ventral tegmental area (VTA), part of the mesolimbocortical dopaminergic pathway illustrated in Figure 4.4, has been widely implicated in the perception of reward (**FIGURE 4.17**). If the dopaminergic pathway from the VTA to the nucleus accumbens serves as a reward system for a wide variety of experiences, then the addictive power of drugs may come from their extra strong stimulation of this pathway. When the drug activates this system, providing an abnormally powerful reward, the user learns to associate the drug-taking behavior with that pleasure and begins seeking out drugs more and more until life's other pleasures fade into the background. If natural activities like conversation, food, and even sex no longer provide appreciable reward, addicts may seek drugs as the only source of pleasure available to them.

Intriguingly, people suffering damage to a brain region tucked within the frontal cortex, called the **insula** (Latin for *island*), are reportedly able to effortlessly quit smoking (Naqvi et al., 2007), indicating that this brain region is also involved in addiction. The reciprocal connections between the VTA and the insula (Oades and Halliday, 1987) suggest that these two regions may normally interact to mediate addiction.

Not everyone who uses an addictive drug becomes addicted. For example, very, very few hospitalized patients treated with opiates for pain relief go on to abuse opiates after leaving the hospital (Brownlee and Schrof, 1997). However, prescription painkillers are highly effective at activating the dopamine reward system, so the use of these drugs outside of medical contexts carries a high risk of addiction. The individual and environmental factors that account for differential susceptibility are the subject of active investigation (Karch, 2006). Some of the major risk factors include biological factors (being male; heritable tendencies to addiction), poor family life, personality factors (poor emotional control), and environmental factors (living in a neighborhood with high rates of addiction). Simply returning to a neighborhood where drugs were previously used can trigger drug craving in an addict (Ciccocioppo et al., 2004); this *cue-induced drug use* is thought to rely on long-lasting associations that involve remodeling of the brain's reward circuitry (Wolf, 2016).

Medical Interventions for Substance Abuse

Some people can overcome their dependence on substances by themselves. For example, the great majority of ex-smokers, and about half of ex-alcoholics, appear to have quit on their own (S. Cohen et al., 1989; Institute of Medicine, 1990). Many others have benefited from counseling and social interventions such as the 12-step program developed by Alcoholics Anonymous in the 1930s. However, However, overcoming addiction may require stronger measures in some cases, especially for the most powerfully addictive substances. An intensive research effort has identified a variety of medicines that can help lessen the grip of addiction through the following strategies:

- *Lessening the discomfort of withdrawal and drug craving.* Benzodiazepines and other sedatives, anti-nausea medications, and drugs that promote sleep all help reduce withdrawal symptoms. Other medications help reduce uncomfortable cravings for the abused substance; for example, acamprosate (trade name Campral) eases alcohol- associated withdrawal symptoms. And preliminary evidence suggests that noninvasive stimulation of regions of prefrontal cortex using rTMS (repetitive transcranial magnetic stimulation; see Chapter 2) may potently reduce drug hunger and relapse rates in addicted individuals (Diana et al., 2017).

- *Providing an alternative to the addictive drug.* Agonist or partial agonist analogs of the addictive drug weakly activate the same mechanisms as the addictive drug, to help wean the individual. For example, the opioid receptor agonist methadone reduces heroin appetite; nicotine patches work in a similar fashion to reduce cravings for cigarettes.

- *Directly blocking the actions of the addictive drug.* Specific receptor antagonists can prevent an abused drug from interacting with its receptors. For example, the opiate receptor antagonist naloxone (Narcan) blocks heroin's actions, but it also may produce harsh withdrawal symptoms.

- *Altering metabolism of the addictive drug.* Changing the breakdown of a drug can reduce or reverse its rewarding properties. Disulfiram (Antabuse) changes alcohol metabolism such that a nausea-inducing metabolite (acetaldehyde) accumulates.

- *Blocking the brain's reward circuitry.* When a person takes drugs (e.g., dopamine receptor blockers) that blunt the activity of the mesolimbocortical dopamine reward system, the addictive drugs lose their pleasurable qualities (but at the cost of a general loss of pleasurable feelings called anhedonia).

- *Immunization to render the drug ineffective.* Vaccines against such drugs as cocaine, heroin, and methamphetamine have been developed and are being tested (Hicks et al., 2011; Nguyen et al., 2017). Here the strategy is to prompt the individual's immune system to produce antibodies that remove the targeted drugs from circulation before they ever reach the brain (**FIGURE 4.18**).

No single approach appears to be uniformly effective, and rates of relapse remain high. Research breakthroughs are therefore badly needed.

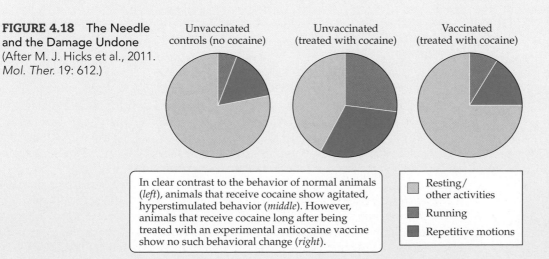

FIGURE 4.18 **The Needle and the Damage Undone** (After M. J. Hicks et al., 2011. *Mol. Ther.* 19: 612.)

Unvaccinated controls (no cocaine)

Unvaccinated (treated with cocaine)

Vaccinated (treated with cocaine)

In clear contrast to the behavior of normal animals (*left*), animals that receive cocaine show agitated, hyperstimulated behavior (*middle*). However, animals that receive cocaine long after being treated with an experimental anticocaine vaccine show no such behavioral change (*right*).

- Resting/ other activities
- Running
- Repetitive motions

HOW'S IT GOING ?

1. Define substance abuse. How prevalent is drug abuse in the population?
2. Summarize the major models of drug abuse and addiction, highlighting the strengths and shortcomings of each perspective.
3. Describe an experimental setup for measuring the rewarding properties of a drug.
4. Provide a survey of the anatomical system that mediates reward. What happens when this system is activated? What are some triggers that can activate the system, and how does activity of the reward system relate to drug addiction?
5. Provide a thorough overview of medical approaches and interventions in substance abuse.

Recommended Reading

Advokat, C. D., Comaty, J. E., and Julien, R. M. (2014). *Julien's Primer of Drug Action* (13th ed.). New York, NY: Worth.

Grilly, D. M., and Salamone, J. (2011). *Drugs, Brain and Behavior* (6th ed.). Boston, MA: Allyn & Bacon.

Karch, S. B., and Drummer, O. (2015). *Karch's Pathology of Drug Abuse* (5th ed.). Boca Raton, FL: CRC Press.

Meyer, J. S., and Quenzer, L. F. (2013). *Psychopharmacology: Drugs, the Brain, and Behavior* (2nd ed.). Sunderland, MA: Oxford University Press/Sinauer.

Nestler, E., Hyman, S., and Malenka, R. (2014). *Molecular Neuropharmacology* (3rd ed.). New York, NY: McGraw-Hill.

Nutt, D. (2012). *Drugs without the Hot Air*. Cambridge, UK: UIT Cambridge.

Schatzberg, A. F., and Nemeroff, C. B. (Eds.). (2013). *Essentials of Clinical Psychopharmacology*. Arlington, VA: American Psychiatric Publishing.

Thombs, D. L., and Osborn, C. J. (2013). *Introduction to Addictive Behaviors* (4th ed.). New York, NY: Guilford Press.

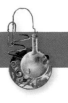

You should be able to relate each summary to the adjacent illustration, including structures and processes. If you go to the website for this text (3e.mindsmachine.com), you can follow links to figures, animations, and activities that will help you consolidate the material.

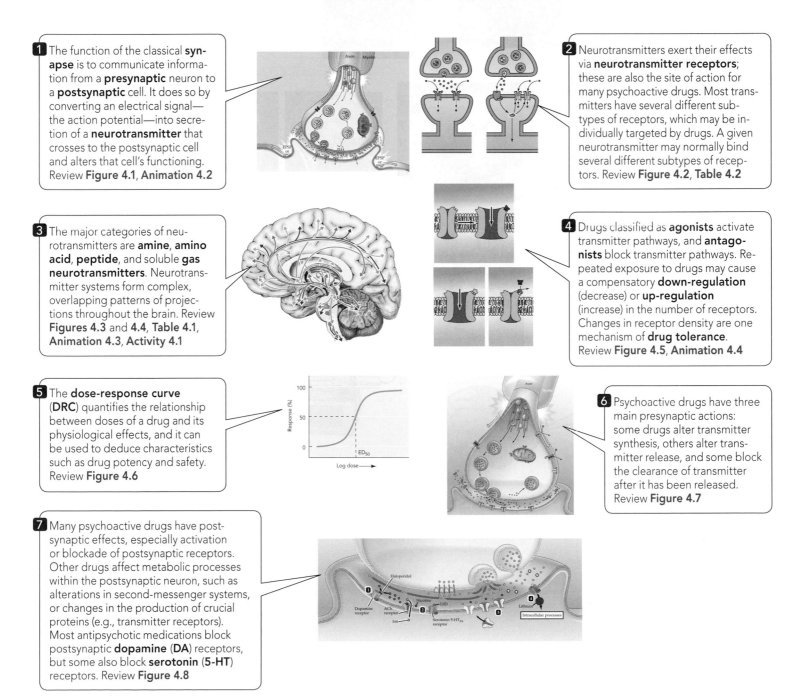

1 The function of the classical **synapse** is to communicate information from a **presynaptic** neuron to a **postsynaptic** cell. It does so by converting an electrical signal— the action potential—into secretion of a **neurotransmitter** that crosses to the postsynaptic cell and alters that cell's functioning. Review **Figure 4.1**, **Animation 4.2**

2 Neurotransmitters exert their effects via **neurotransmitter receptors**; these are also the site of action for many psychoactive drugs. Most transmitters have several different subtypes of receptors, which may be individually targeted by drugs. A given neurotransmitter may normally bind several different subtypes of receptors. Review **Figure 4.2**, **Table 4.2**

3 The major categories of neurotransmitters are **amine, amino acid, peptide,** and soluble **gas neurotransmitters**. Neurotransmitter systems form complex, overlapping patterns of projections throughout the brain. Review **Figures 4.3** and **4.4**, **Table 4.1**, **Animation 4.3**, **Activity 4.1**

4 Drugs classified as **agonists** activate transmitter pathways, and **antagonists** block transmitter pathways. Repeated exposure to drugs may cause a compensatory **down-regulation** (decrease) or **up-regulation** (increase) in the number of receptors. Changes in receptor density are one mechanism of **drug tolerance**. Review **Figure 4.5**, **Animation 4.4**

5 The **dose-response curve (DRC)** quantifies the relationship between doses of a drug and its physiological effects, and it can be used to deduce characteristics such as drug potency and safety. Review **Figure 4.6**

6 Psychoactive drugs have three main presynaptic actions: some drugs alter transmitter synthesis, others alter transmitter release, and some block the clearance of transmitter after it has been released. Review **Figure 4.7**

7 Many psychoactive drugs have postsynaptic effects, especially activation or blockade of postsynaptic receptors. Other drugs affect metabolic processes within the postsynaptic neuron, such as alterations in second-messenger systems, or changes in the production of crucial proteins (e.g., transmitter receptors). Most antipsychotic medications block postsynaptic **dopamine (DA)** receptors, but some also block **serotonin (5-HT)** receptors. Review **Figure 4.8**

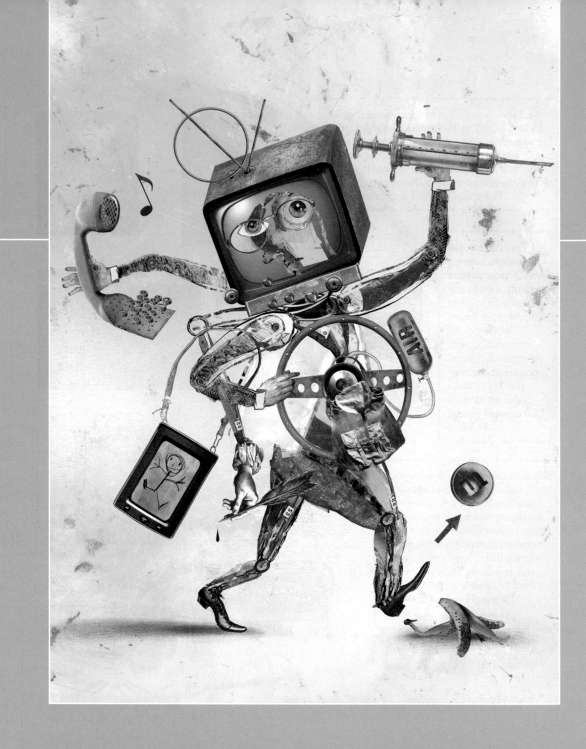

5

The Sensorimotor System

What You See Is What You Get

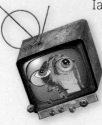

Ian Waterman had a perfectly ordinary life until he caught a viral infection at age 19. For reasons no one understands, the infection targeted a very specific set of nerves sending information from his body to his brain. Ian can still feel pain or deep pressure, as well as warm and cool surfaces on his skin, but he has no sensation of light touch below his neck. What's more, although Ian can still move all of his muscles, he receives no information about muscle activity or body position (Cole, 1995). You might think this deficiency wouldn't cause any problem, because you've probably never thought much about your "body sense"; it's not even one of the five senses that people talk about, is it?

In fact, however, the loss of this information was devastating. Ian couldn't walk across a room without falling down, and he couldn't walk up or down stairs. The few other people suffering a loss like this have spent the rest of their lives in wheelchairs. But Ian was a young and determined person, so he started teaching himself how to walk using another source of feedback about his body: his vision. Now, as long as the lights are on, Ian can carefully watch his moving body to judge which motor commands to send out to keep walking. If the lights go out, however, he collapses, and he has learned that in that circumstance he just has to lie where he is until the lights come on again. He has so finely honed this ability to guide movements with vision that if asked to point repeatedly to the same location in the air, he does so more accurately than control participants do. Still, it's a mental drain to have to watch and attend constantly to his body just to do everyday tasks.

Today Ian has a good job and an active, independent life, but he is always vigilant. Lying in bed, he has to be very careful to remain calm, tethering his limbs with the covers to prevent them from flailing about. And the lights are always on at Ian's house.

Every species, including our own, is surrounded by forms of environmental energy that may signal life-or-death events. Molecules in the air are sensed as odors—of food, or mates, or smoke. Vibrations traveling through air are perceived as sounds, ranging from infant cries to the roar of a predator (or a waterfall). Light particles reflected from surfaces present a visual representation of the world.

We open this chapter by considering basic principles of sensory processing, using the sense of touch to illustrate some of the major concepts. In Part II, we take a closer look at an unpleasant but crucial sense: pain. And in Part III of the chapter, we turn our attention to the integration of sensory inputs and motor control mechanisms: the streamlined system that allows us to interact with our environment.

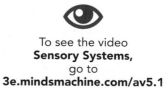

To see the video
Sensory Systems,
go to
3e.mindsmachine.com/av5.1

To view the
Brain Explorer,
go to
3e.mindsmachine.com/av5.2

PART I
Sensory Processing and the Somatosensory System

THE ROAD AHEAD

The first section of this chapter covers the general principles that apply to all sensory systems. Reading this material should allow you to:

1. Understand the concepts of labeled lines and sensory transduction.
2. Describe several different types of receptors in the skin and the stimuli they detect.
3. Relate the concepts of receptive fields and sensory adaptation.
4. Describe the neural pathway for the system reporting touch information from the body.

Sensory Systems Detect Various Forms of Energy

Because species differ in the environmental features they must sense for survival, evolution has endowed each species with its own unique set of capabilities. Bats are specially equipped to detect their own ultrasonic cries, which we humans are unable to hear. Some snakes have infrared-sensing organs in their faces that allow them to "see" heat sources (like a warm, tasty mouse) in the dark. Some of the impressive array of sensory modalities that animals may possess are listed in **TABLE 5.1**.

All animals have sensory organs containing **receptor cells** that sense some forms of energy—called **stimuli**—but not others. So in a way, receptor cells act as filters, ignoring the environmental background and converting the key stimuli into the language of the nervous system: electrical signals. Information from sensory receptors floods the brain in an unending barrage of action potentials traveling along millions of axons, and our brains must make sense of it all. What type of stimulus was that, where did it come from, how intense was it, etc. Of course, different kinds of energy—light, sound, touch, and so on—need different sensory organs to convert them into neural activity, just as taking a photograph requires a camera, not a microphone. There is tremendous diversity in sensory organs across the animal

receptor cell   A specialized cell that responds to a particular energy or substance in the internal or external environment and converts this energy into a change in the electrical potential across its membrane.

stimulus   A physical event that triggers a sensory response.

TABLE 5.1 ■ Classification of Sensory Systems		
System type	Modality	Sensed stimuli
Mechanical	Touch	Contact with body surface
	Hearing	Sound vibrations in air or water
	Vestibular	Head movement and orientation
	Joint	Position and movement
	Muscle	Tension
Photic	Vision	Photons, from light sources or reflected from surface
Thermal	Cold	Decrease in skin temperature
	Warmth	Increase in skin temperature
Chemical	Smell	Odorant chemicals in air
	Taste	Substances in contact with the tongue or other taste receptor
	Vomeronasal	Pheromones in air or water
Electrical	Electroreception	Differences in density of electrical currents
Magnetic	Magnetoreception	Magnetic fields for orientation

FIGURE 5.1 **Do You Hear What I Hear?** (After R. R. Fay, 1988. *Hearing in vertebrates: A psychophysics databook.* Hill-Fay Associates. Winnetka, IL. Courtesy of Dr. Richard Fay and the Fay Foundation.)

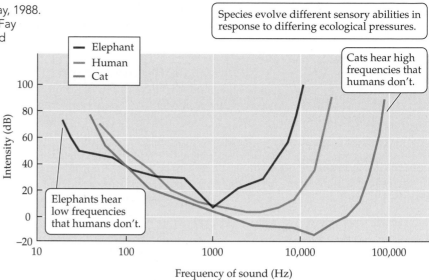

Species evolve different sensory abilities in response to differing ecological pressures.

Cats hear high frequencies that humans don't.

Elephants hear low frequencies that humans don't.

kingdom; for example, the eye is just one type of sensory organ, yet it is found in a dazzling array of sizes, shapes, and forms, reflecting the varying survival needs of different animals. Likewise, the specific auditory abilities of species reflect their unique ecological pressures (**FIGURE 5.1**).

Although the end product of sensory receptors—action potentials—is the same for all the different sensory modalities, the brain recognizes the modalities as separate and distinct because the action potentials for each sense are carried in separate nerve tracts. This is the concept of **labeled lines**: particular neurons that are, right from the outset, labeled for distinctive sensory experiences. Action potentials in one line signal a sound, activity in another line signals a smell, and activity in other lines signals touch. And there are labeled lines within general sensory categories too; for example, we can distinguish different types of touch because our skin contains a variety of receptors and uses some lines to signal light touch, others to signal vibration, and yet other lines to signal stretching of the skin (**FIGURE 5.2**).

labeled lines The concept that each nerve input to the brain reports only a particular type of information.

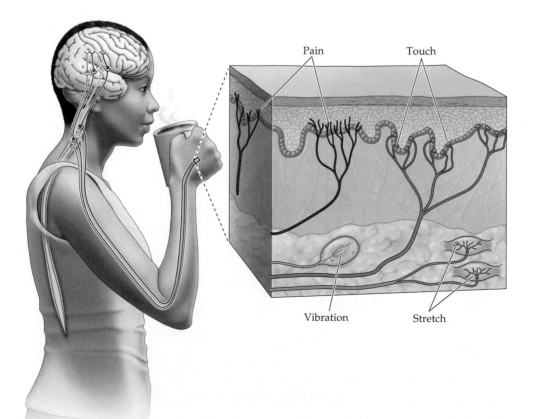

FIGURE 5.2 Labeled Lines

Receptor Cells Convert Sensory Signals into Electrical Activity

The structure of a receptor cell determines the particular kind of energy or chemical to which it will respond. And although a wide variety of cellular mechanisms are used to detect different stimuli, the outcome is always the same: an electrical change in the receptor, called a **generator potential**, that resembles the excitatory postsynaptic potentials we discussed in Chapter 3. Converting the signal in this way—from environmental stimuli into action potentials that our brain can understand—is called **sensory transduction**.

Our skin contains a rich array of receptors that transduce different forms of energy to provide our sense of touch. But touch is not just touch. Careful studies of skin sensations reveal qualitatively different sensory experiences: pressure, vibration, tickle, "pins and needles," and more-complex dimensions, such as smoothness or wetness—all recorded by the receptors in the skin (**FIGURE 5.3**), then transmitted along separate axons to the brain.

A skin receptor that provides a clear example of the process of sensory transduction is the **Pacinian corpuscle** (or *lamellated corpuscle*) (Loewenstein, 1971), a tiny onion-like structure embedded in the innermost layer of the skin that selectively responds to vibration and pressure. Acting as a filter, the corpuscle allows only vibrations of more than about 200 cycles per second to stimulate the sensory nerve ending inside it; this type of stimulation is what's created when we feel a texture against our skin (see Figure 5.3). By stretching the membrane of the sensory nerve ending, stimuli cause mechanically gated sodium channels to pop open, creating a graded generator potential (**FIGURE 5.4**). The amplitude (size) of this generator potential is directly proportional to the strength of the stimulus that was received. If the generator potential exceeds the firing **threshold**, action potentials are generated that travel via sensory nerves to the spinal cord.

Other dimensions of the sense of touch are mediated by their own unique sensory receptors. In contrast to the texture sensitivity of Pacinian corpuscles, **Meissner's corpuscles** (also known as *tactile corpuscles*) and **Merkel's discs** mediate most of our

generator potential A local change in the resting potential of a receptor cell in response to stimuli, which may initiate an action potential.

sensory transduction The process in which a receptor cell converts the energy in a stimulus into a change in the electrical potential across its membrane.

Pacinian corpuscle Also called *lamellated corpuscle*. A skin receptor cell type that detects vibration and pressure.

threshold Here, the stimulus intensity that is just adequate to trigger an action potential in a sensory cell.

Meissner's corpuscle Also called *tactile corpuscle*. A skin receptor cell type that detects light touch, responding especially to changes in stimuli.

Merkel's disc A skin receptor cell type that detects light touch, responding especially to edges and isolated points on a surface.

To view the activity
Receptors in Skin,
go to
3e.mindsmachine.com/ac5.1

FIGURE 5.3 Receptors in Skin

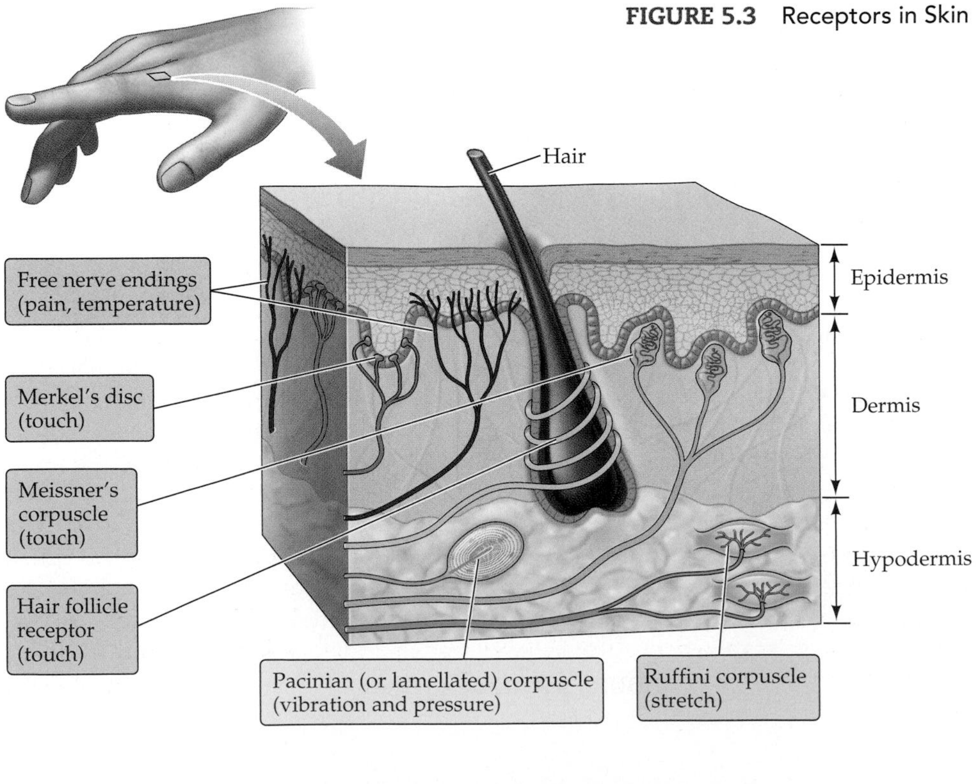

Hair

Free nerve endings (pain, temperature)

Merkel's disc (touch)

Meissner's corpuscle (touch)

Hair follicle receptor (touch)

Pacinian (or lamellated) corpuscle (vibration and pressure)

Ruffini corpuscle (stretch)

Epidermis

Dermis

Hypodermis

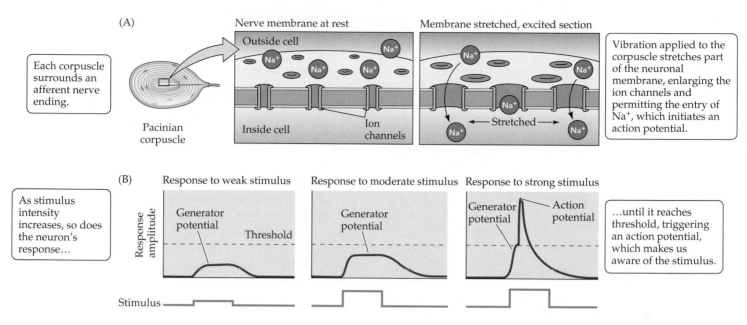

FIGURE 5.4 The Structure and Function of the Pacinian Corpuscle

ability to perceive the forms of objects we touch. While Merkel's discs are especially responsive to edges and to isolated *points* on a surface, the more numerous Meissner's corpuscles seem to respond to *changes* in stimuli, allowing them to detect localized movement between the skin and a surface (Heidenreich et al., 2011). **Ruffini corpuscles**, which are only sparsely distributed in the skin (Pare et al., 2003), detect stretching of patches of the skin when we move fingers or limbs (Johansson and Flanagan, 2009). Finally, pain, heat, and cold stimuli are detected by **free nerve endings** in the skin (see Figure 5.3), which we'll return to a little later in the chapter. All of these sensory receptors are found in their highest concentrations in regions of the skin where our sense of touch is finest (fingertips, tongue, and lips).

— HOW'S IT GOING ?

1. Discuss the relationship between the ecology of a species and its sensory capabilities.
2. What are labeled lines? What do they transmit?
3. Give a general explanation of sensory transduction. What is a generator potential?
4. Identify and describe four sensory receptors found in the skin.

Sensory Information Processing Is Selective and Analytical

Many people assume that the sensory systems simply capture an accurate snapshot of stimulation and transmit it to the brain—in other words, that the sensory systems provide an uncolored window on the world. But neuroscientists realize that the sensory organs and pathways convey only limited—*even distorted*—information to the brain. A good deal of selection and analysis takes place along sensory pathways, before the information ever reaches the brain. So the brain ultimately receives a highly filtered representation of the external world, in which stimuli that are critical for survival are strongly emphasized at the expense of less important stimuli. This processing and filtering is seen in several aspects of sensory transduction, including stimulus coding and processing across receptive fields, as well as in adaptation and active suppression by the brain, which we discuss next.

Ruffini corpuscle A skin receptor cell type that detects stretching of the skin.

free nerve ending An axon that terminates in the skin and has no specialized cell associated with it. Free nerve endings detect pain and/or changes in temperature.

Sensory events are encoded as streams of action potentials

We've already seen that the nervous system uses labeled lines to identify the *type* of stimulus that is encountered. But how do sensory neurons tell the brain about the *intensity* or *location* of a stimulus? Because the action potentials produced by a sensory neuron always have the same size and duration, the other characteristics of a sensory stimulus must be *encoded* in the number and frequency of the action potentials, the rhythm in which clusters of action potentials occur, and so on.

We can respond to amazingly small differences in stimulus intensity, over a wide range of intensities. Although a single sensory receptor neuron could simply encode the intensity of a stimulus in the frequency of action potentials that the cell produces, only a very limited range of intensities could be represented this way, because neurons can fire only so fast (up to maybe 1,200 action potentials per second, and probably less in most nerves). Some sensory systems solve this problem by employing multiple sensory receptor cells, each specializing in just one part of the overall range of intensities, to cover the whole range. As the strength of a stimulus increases, additional sensory neurons sensitive to the higher intensities are "recruited"; thus, intensity of a stimulus can be represented by the number and thresholds of activated cells.

The position of a stimulus, either outside or inside the body, is likewise an important piece of information. Some sensory systems—the **somatosensory system** ("body sensation" system), for example—reveal this information by the position of receptors on the sensory surface. Thanks to labeled lines that uniquely convey spatial information, we can directly encode which patch of skin that darn mosquito is biting, in order to know exactly where to aim the slap. Similarly, in the visual system an object's spatial location determines which receptors in the eye are stimulated. In bilateral receptor systems—the two eyes, two ears, and two nostrils—differences in stimulation of the left and right receptors are encoded, providing the brain with additional cues to the location of the stimulus (this type of processing is discussed in more detail in Chapter 6).

Neurons at all levels of the visual and the touch pathways—from the surface sheet of receptors all the way up to the cerebral cortex—are arranged in an orderly, maplike manner. The map at each level is not exact, but it does reflect both spatial positions

To view the animation
Somatosensory Receptive Fields,
go to
3e.mindsmachine.com/av5.3

somatosensory system   A set of specialized receptors and neural mechanisms responsible for body sensations such as touch and pain.

FIGURE 5.5 Identifying Somatosensory Receptive Fields

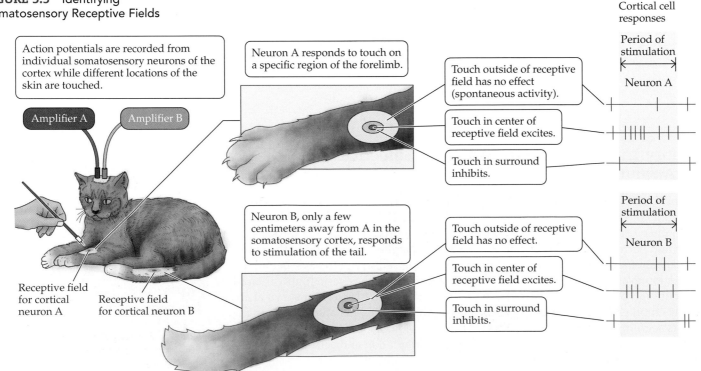

Action potentials are recorded from individual somatosensory neurons of the cortex while different locations of the skin are touched.

Amplifier A   Amplifier B

Receptive field for cortical neuron A

Receptive field for cortical neuron B

Neuron A responds to touch on a specific region of the forelimb.

Touch outside of receptive field has no effect (spontaneous activity).

Touch in center of receptive field excites.

Touch in surround inhibits.

Neuron B, only a few centimeters away from A in the somatosensory cortex, responds to stimulation of the tail.

Touch outside of receptive field has no effect.

Touch in center of receptive field excites.

Touch in surround inhibits.

Cortical cell responses

Period of stimulation

Neuron A

Period of stimulation

Neuron B

and receptor density. More cells are allocated to the spatial representation of sensitive, densely innervated sites, like the lips, than to sites that are less sensitive, such as the skin of the back. Each cell in the sensory map thus preferentially responds to a particular type of stimulus occurring in a particular place, as we'll see next.

Sensory neurons respond to stimuli falling in their receptive fields

The **receptive field** of a sensory neuron consists of a region of space in which a stimulus will alter that neuron's firing rate. To determine this receptive field, investigators record the neuron's electrical responses to a variety of stimuli to see what makes the activity of the cell change from its resting rate. For example, which patch of skin must we stimulate to change the activity of one particular touch receptor? Experiments show that these somatosensory receptive fields are shaped like doughnuts, with either an excitatory center and an inhibitory surround (**FIGURE 5.5**), or an inhibitory center and an excitatory surround. The somatosensory receptive fields make it easier to detect edges on the objects we feel. Receptive fields differ in size and shape, and in the quality of stimulation that activates them. For example, some neurons respond preferentially to light touch, while others fire most rapidly in response to painful stimuli, and still others respond to cooling.

Experiments tracing sensory information along the pathway from the receptor cell to the brain show that neurons at every level will respond to particular stimuli, so each of these cells has its own receptive field. But as each successive neuron performs additional processing, the receptive fields change considerably, as we will see later in this chapter and in later chapters.

Receptors may show adaptation to unchanging stimuli

Sensory adaptation is the progressive decrease in a receptor's response to sustained stimulation (**FIGURE 5.6**). This process allows us to ignore unimportant events. By not noticing the touch of our clothes on our skin, the buzz of overhead lights, and other stimuli that are unchanging, our sensory systems avoid overload and can remain vigilant for critical events. Neuroscientists distinguish between **phasic receptors**, which display this sort of adaptation, and **tonic receptors**, which show little or no adaptation and thus can signal the duration of a stimulus. (As each of us knows all too well, pain sensors are often tonic receptors, maintaining a high level of activity to help us avoid further injury.)

The process of adaptation illustrates the principle we referred to earlier in our discussion of selection and analysis: sensory systems often shift *away from accurate*

receptive field   The stimulus region and features that affect the activity of a cell in a sensory system.

sensory adaptation   The progressive loss of receptor response as stimulation is maintained.

phasic receptor   A receptor in which the frequency of action potentials drops rapidly as stimulation is maintained.

tonic receptor   A receptor in which the frequency of action potentials declines slowly or not at all as stimulation is maintained.

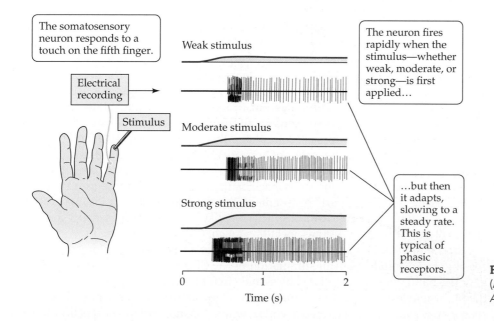

The somatosensory neuron responds to a touch on the fifth finger.

Electrical recording

Stimulus

Weak stimulus

Moderate stimulus

Strong stimulus

The neuron fires rapidly when the stimulus—whether weak, moderate, or strong—is first applied…

…but then it adapts, slowing to a steady rate. This is typical of phasic receptors.

Time (s)

FIGURE 5.6   Sensory Adaptation (After M. Knibestol and A. B. Valbo, 1970. *Acta Physiol. Scand.* 80: 178.)

central modulation of sensory information The process in which higher brain centers, such as the cortex and thalamus, suppress some sources of sensory information and amplify others.

dorsal column system A somatosensory system that delivers most touch stimuli via the dorsal columns of spinal white matter to the brain.

dermatome A strip of skin innervated by a particular spinal nerve.

portrayal of the external world. In some mechanical receptors, such as the Pacinian corpuscle described earlier, adaptation develops from the elasticity of the receptor cell itself. When the corpuscle (which is a separate, accessory structure) is removed, the uncovered sensory nerve fiber does not adapt, but continues discharging action potentials in response to a constant stimulus.

Sometimes we need receptors to be quiet

We've already noted that survival depends more on sensitivity to important *changes* than on exact reporting of stimuli. To maintain such sensitivity, we need to suppress unneeded or unimportant sensory activity. As we just discussed, adaptation is one way in which sensory activity is controlled, and we are equipped with two additional suppression systems.

One way to suppress sensory activity is simply to physically prevent the stimuli from reaching the sensors. Closing the eyelids provides this function in the visual system; in the auditory system, tiny middle-ear muscles reduce the intensity of sounds that reach the inner ear. A second kind of suppression of sensory inputs is entirely neural in nature. In many sensory and pain pathways, reciprocal neural connections descend from the brain to synapse on lower sensory levels, where they can then actively inhibit activity in the ascending sensory axons. This **central modulation of sensory information**, whereby the brain actively controls the information it receives, is a feature of many sensory and pain pathways. Such modulation helps the brain attend to some stimuli more than others.

HOW'S IT GOING ?

1. In general terms, explain how a sensory event is encoded in action potentials in sensory fibers.
2. Why do some receptor cells respond only to strong stimuli?
3. Describe receptive fields and how scientists detect them.
4. Name and briefly describe a couple of processes that change a sensory neuron's response to stimuli.

Successive Levels of the CNS Process Sensory Information

Sensory information travels from the sensory surface to the highest levels of the brain, and each sensory system—such as touch, vision, or hearing—has its own distinctive pathway from the periphery to successively higher levels of the spinal cord and/or brain. For example, the somatosensory touch receptors that we've been discussing send their axons—eventually bundled into sensory nerves—from the skin to the dorsal (rear) part of the spinal cord. On entering the cord, the somatosensory projections ascend as part of the spinal cord's **dorsal column system**, a large wedge of white matter in the dorsal spinal cord (**FIGURE 5.7**). These axons go all the way up to the brainstem, where they synapse onto neurons that project contralaterally (to the opposite side) and then go to the thalamus. From there, the incoming sensory information is directed to cortex. At all levels, the inputs are organized according to a somatosensory map in which the body surface is divided into discrete bands. Each band, called a **dermatome** (from the Greek *derma*, "skin," and *tome*, "part" or "segment"), is the strip of skin that is innervated by a particular spinal nerve (**FIGURE 5.8**). This maplike organization of sensory inputs is a feature of several sensory systems, including touch, vision, and hearing.

Each station in a sensory pathway accomplishes a basic aspect of information processing. For example, painful stimulation of the finger leads to reflexive withdrawal of the hand, which is mediated by spinal circuits before we even feel any pain. At the brainstem level, other circuits turn the head toward the source of pain. Eventually, sensory pathways reach the cerebral cortex, where the most complex aspects of sensory

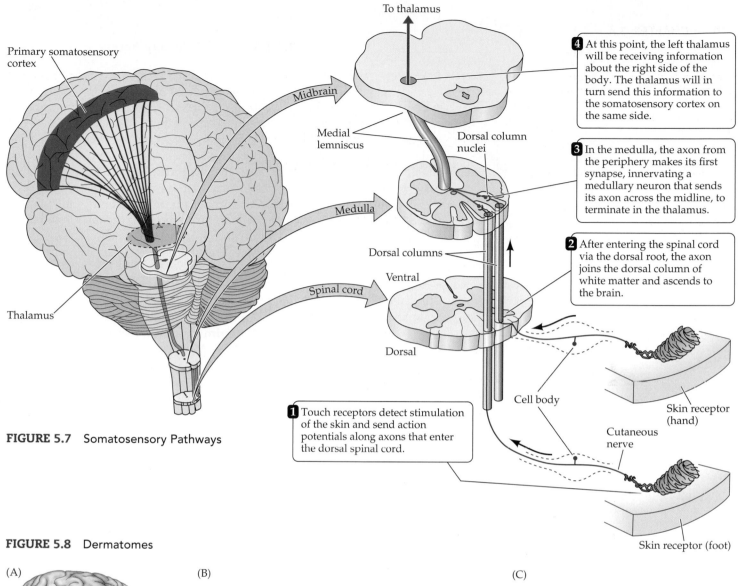

Primary somatosensory cortex

Thalamus

Midbrain

Medulla

Spinal cord

Ventral

Dorsal

To thalamus

Medial lemniscus

Dorsal column nuclei

Dorsal columns

Cell body

Skin receptor (hand)

Cutaneous nerve

Skin receptor (foot)

4 At this point, the left thalamus will be receiving information about the right side of the body. The thalamus will in turn send this information to the somatosensory cortex on the same side.

3 In the medulla, the axon from the periphery makes its first synapse, innervating a medullary neuron that sends its axon across the midline, to terminate in the thalamus.

2 After entering the spinal cord via the dorsal root, the axon joins the dorsal column of white matter and ascends to the brain.

1 Touch receptors detect stimulation of the skin and send action potentials along axons that enter the dorsal spinal cord.

FIGURE 5.7 Somatosensory Pathways

FIGURE 5.8 Dermatomes

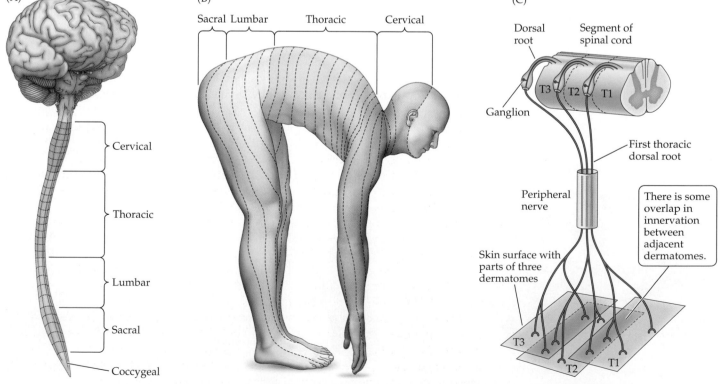

(A)

Cervical

Thoracic

Lumbar

Sacral

Coccygeal

(B)

Sacral   Lumbar   Thoracic   Cervical

(C)

Dorsal root

Segment of spinal cord

T3   T2   T1

Ganglion

First thoracic dorsal root

Peripheral nerve

Skin surface with parts of three dermatomes

There is some overlap in innervation between adjacent dermatomes.

T3   T2   T1

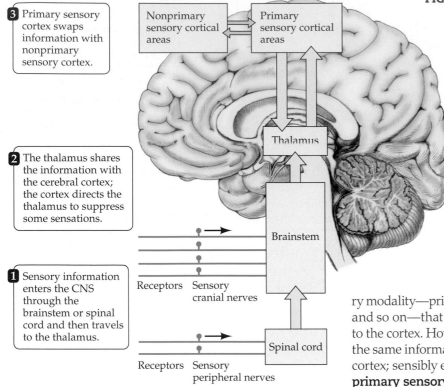

3 Primary sensory cortex swaps information with nonprimary sensory cortex.

2 The thalamus shares the information with the cerebral cortex; the cortex directs the thalamus to suppress some sensations.

1 Sensory information enters the CNS through the brainstem or spinal cord and then travels to the thalamus.

FIGURE 5.9 Levels of Sensory Processing

processing take place, perhaps consciously identifying the source of the pain (darn, another sliver!) and planning a response (where did I leave those tweezers?). For most senses, information reaches the **thalamus** before being relayed to the cortex (**FIGURE 5.9**). Information about each sensory modality is sent to a separate division of the thalamus. One way for the brain to suppress particular stimuli is for the cortex to direct the thalamus to emphasize some sensory information and suppress other information.

Sensory cortex is highly organized

Researchers have identified a region designated as **primary sensory cortex** for each sensory modality—primary somatosensory cortex, primary auditory cortex, and so on—that is generally the initial destination of sensory inputs to the cortex. However, other cortical regions may receive and process the same information, often in collaboration with the primary sensory cortex; sensibly enough (pardon the pun), we call these regions **nonprimary sensory cortex** (see Figure 5.9). Each cortical sensory region processes different aspects of our perceptual experiences.

Primary somatosensory cortex (also called *somatosensory 1* or *S1*) of each hemisphere is located in the postcentral gyrus, the long strip of tissue that lies just posterior to the central sulcus dividing the parietal lobe from the frontal lobe (**FIGURE 5.10A**). S1 receives touch information from the opposite side of the body. The cells in S1 are arranged as a map of the body (**FIGURE 5.10B**), but it is a very unusual map: it is distorted so that the size of each region on the map is proportional to the density of sensory receptors found in that region of the skin. Parts of the body where we are especially sensitive to touch (like the hand and fingers) have large representations in S1 compared with less sensitive areas (like the shoulder). This proportional mapping is illustrated in the strange-looking character in **FIGURE 5.10C**, called a *sensory homunculus*, in whom the

thalamus   The brain regions at the top of the brainstem that trade information with the cortex.

primary sensory cortex   For a given sensory modality, the region of cortex that receives most of the information about that modality from the thalamus (or, in the case of olfaction, directly from the secondary sensory neurons).

FIGURE 5.10 Representation of the Body Surface in Somatosensory Cortex

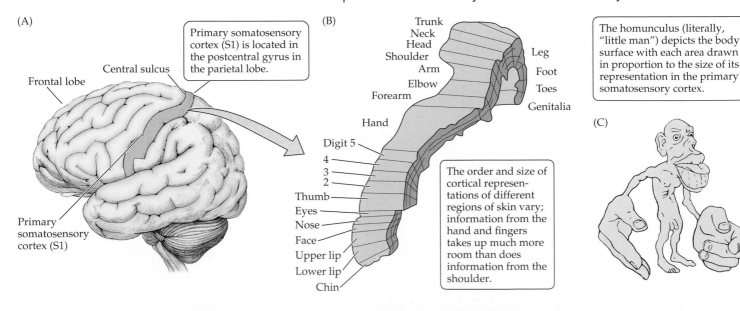

size of each body part reflects the proportion of S1 devoted to that part. We discuss other aspects of cortical organization in **A STEP FURTHER 5.1**, on the website.

Sensory brain regions influence one another and change over time

Often the use of one sensory system influences perception from another sensory system. For example, humans detect a visual signal more accurately if it is accompanied by a sound from the same part of space (McDonald et al., 2000).

Many sensory areas in the brain—called *association areas*—process a mixture of inputs from different modalities. Some "visual" cells, for instance, also respond to auditory or touch stimuli. The convergence of information from different sensory systems on these **polymodal neurons** allows different sensory systems to interact (B. E. Stein and Stanford, 2008). And for a few people, a stimulus in one sensory modality may evoke an additional perception in another sensory modality, as when seeing a number evokes a color, or music literally becomes a matter of taste, where each note has both a sound and a flavor (Beeli et al., 2005). This condition is known as **synesthesia**. For more information and an example of synesthesia, see **A STEP FURTHER 5.2**, on the website.

At one time, most researchers thought that sensory regions of cortex were fixed early in life. Now, however, we know that cortical maps are highly plastic, changing considerably as a result of experience (D. T. Blake et al., 2006). For example, professional musicians who play stringed instruments have expanded cortical representations of their left fingers, presumably because they use these fingers to depress the strings for precisely the right note (Elbert et al., 1995; Münte et al., 2002). Brain imaging also reveals cortical reorganization in people who lose a hand in adulthood (**FIGURE 5.11**). One man received a transplanted hand (from an accident victim) 35 years after losing his own. Despite the length of time that had passed, his brain reorganized in just a few months to receive sensation from the hand in the appropriate part of S1 (Frey et al., 2008). Some changes in cortical maps occur after weeks or months of use or disuse; they may arise from the growth of new synapses and dendrites (Florence et al., 1998; Hickmott and Steen, 2005) or from the loss of others.

nonprimary sensory cortex Also called *secondary sensory cortex*. For a given sensory modality, the cortical regions receiving direct projections from primary sensory cortex for that modality.

primary somatosensory cortex Also called *somatosensory 1* or *S1*. Primarily the postcentral gyrus of the parietal lobe, where sensory inputs from the body surface are mapped.

polymodal neuron A neuron upon which information from more than one sensory system converges.

synesthesia A condition in which stimuli in one modality evoke the involuntary experience of an additional sensation in another modality.

HOW'S IT GOING ?

1. Name the main somatosensory pathway to the brain, describe its organization, and name its main components.
2. Where is the primary somatosensory cortex located? How is it organized?
3. Discuss interactions between sensory modalities—for example, effects of auditory inputs on visual perception.

(A)

Normally, the hand region of S1 lies between the regions representing the upper arm and the face.

(B)

After the loss of one hand, the cortical regions representing the upper arm and face expand, taking over the cortical region previously representing the missing hand.

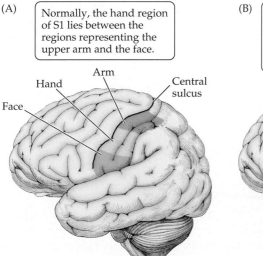

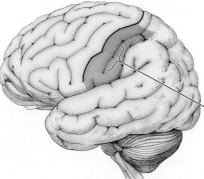

Region formerly stimulated by receptors in the hand now responds to touch on face or arm.

FIGURE 5.11 Plasticity in Somatosensory Cortex (After T. T. Yang et al., 1994. *NeuroReport* 5: 701.)

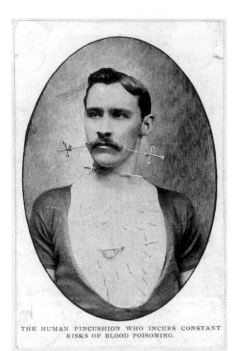

THE HUMAN PINCUSHION WHO INCURS CONSTANT
RISKS OF BLOOD POISONING.

Doesn't That Hurt?   Although it might seem like a blessing, people with congenital insensitivity to pain, like the "Human Pincushion" pictured here (Dearborn, 1932), tend to die young as a consequence of repeated body injuries. (Photograph by Culver Pictures, Inc.)

PART II
Pain: The Body's Emergency Signaling System

THE ROAD AHEAD

This next section describes the system bringing us the unpleasant but adaptive sensation of pain. Studying this material should enable you to:

1. List and describe the three separate components of pain experience.
2. Describe the neuronal receptor cells that detect painful stimuli and the molecular receptor proteins they use.
3. Trace the neuronal pathway that transmits pain information from the periphery to the brain, as well as the neuronal pathway by which the brain can modulate pain.
4. Discuss the various methods for controlling pain, including the advantages and disadvantages of each.

Human Pain Varies in Several Dimensions

One important aspect of body sensation is at best a mixed blessing. The International Association for the Study of Pain defines **pain** as "an unpleasant sensory and emotional experience associated with actual or potential tissue damage, or described in terms of such damage." Pain forcefully guides our behavior in several ways that minimize the risk to our bodies (Dennis and Melzack, 1983). Immediate, short-term pain causes us to withdraw from the source, often reflexively, thus preventing further damage. Longer-lasting pain encourages behaviors, such as sleep, inactivity, grooming, feeding, and drinking, that promote recuperation. And the pain-related social communication—grimacing, groaning, shrieking, and the rest of the miserable line-up—provides a warning to kin and elicits caregiving behaviors from them, including grooming, defending, and feeding.

Learning, experience, emotion, and culture all affect our perception of pain in striking ways, and these factors may strongly influence people's descriptions of pain, ranging from an apparent absence of pain in badly injured soldiers and athletes, to the anguish of a child with a paper cut. A widely used quantitative measure of pain perception—the McGill Pain Questionnaire (Melzack, 1984)—asks people to select words that tap three different dimensions of pain:

1. The *sensory-discriminative* dimension (e.g., throbbing, gnawing, shooting)
2. The *motivational-affective* (emotional) dimension (e.g., tiring, sickening, fearful)
3. An overall *cognitive-evaluative* dimension (e.g., no pain, mild, excruciating)

Researchers found that people use different constellations of descriptors in various forms of pain: tooth pain is described differently from arthritic pain, which in turn is described differently from menstrual pain. This more detailed analysis provides better information for the diagnosis and treatment of illness.

A Discrete Pain Pathway Projects from Body to Brain

Most tissues of the body (but not all) contain receptors specialized for detecting painful stimuli. These receptors are particularly well studied in the skin; in this section we discuss some features of these receptors, along with the peripheral and CNS pathways that mediate pain.

Peripheral receptors get the initial message

When tissue is injured, the affected cells release chemicals that activate nearby pain receptors, called **nociceptors**, on *free nerve endings* specialized to detect damage, as well as causing inflammation (**FIGURE 5.12**). Many different substances in injured

pain   The discomfort normally associated with tissue damage.

nociceptor   A receptor that responds to stimuli that produce tissue damage or pose the threat of damage.

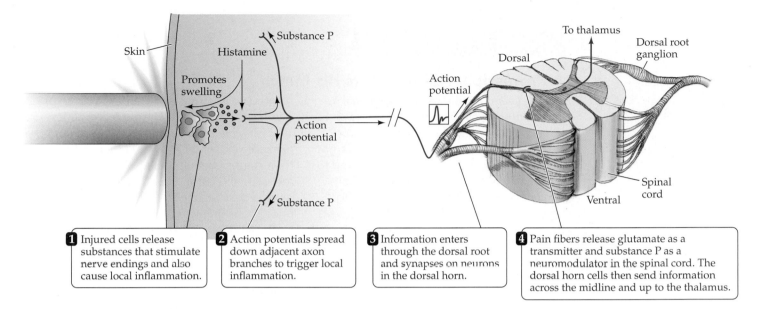

1. Injured cells release substances that stimulate nerve endings and also cause local inflammation.

2. Action potentials spread down adjacent axon branches to trigger local inflammation.

3. Information enters through the dorsal root and synapses on neurons in the dorsal horn.

4. Pain fibers release glutamate as a transmitter and substance P as a neuromodulator in the spinal cord. The dorsal horn cells then send information across the midline and up to the thalamus.

FIGURE 5.12 Peripheral Mediation of Pain

tissue—serotonin, histamine, and various enzymes and peptides, to name just a few—can stimulate these nociceptors. Different nociceptors respond to various stimuli, such as pain and/or changes in temperature.

Identification of the nociceptor that detects *physical* damage was aided through careful study of the family of a Pakistani boy who died in tragic circumstances—performing dangerous pranks because he could feel no pain. Scientists isolated a mutation in a gene (called *SCN9A*) that appears to be responsible for his congenital insensitivity to pain (CIP). Children with CIP require constant monitoring to prevent them from poking out their eyes or pulling out their teeth (Oppenheim, 2006). The *SCN9A* gene encodes a sodium channel expressed in free nerve endings that serve as nociceptors (Cox et al., 2006), offering a new target for developing high-potency pain medication.

Some free nerve endings detect temperature changes. Studies of capsaicin, the chemical that makes chili peppers spicy hot, helped reveal the receptor that signals sudden increases in temperature (this action is the reason spicy food seems to *burn*) (Caterina et al., 1997). This receptor, with the not-so-spicy name *transient receptor potential vanilloid type 1* (*TRPV1*, or just *vanilloid receptor 1*), belongs to a larger family of proteins called *transient receptor potential (TRP) ion channels*. Mice lacking the gene for TRPV1 still respond to mechanosensory pain, but not to mild heat or capsaicin (Caterina et al., 2000).

TRPV1's normal job is to report a rise in temperature to warn us of danger, so chili peppers cleverly evolved capsaicin to ward off mammalian predators—by falsely signaling burning heat. A related receptor, **transient receptor potential type M3 (TRPM3)**, detects even higher temperatures than does TRPV1, but it does *not* respond to capsaicin (Vriens and Voets, 2018). TRPM3 receptors are found on **A delta (Aδ) fibers**, which are large-diameter, myelinated axons. Because of the relatively large axon diameter and myelination, action potentials in these fibers reach the spinal cord very quickly. In contrast, the nerve fibers that possess TRPV1 receptors consist of thin, unmyelinated fibers called **C fibers**. So, when you burn your hand on that hot pan, the initial sharp pain you feel is conducted by the fat A delta fibers activated by their TRPM3 receptors, and the long-lasting dull ache that follows arises from slower C fibers and their TRPV1 receptors. Other members of the TRP family of receptors detect coolness as well as constituents of spices like oregano, cloves, garlic, and wasabi (Jordt et al., 2004; Bautista et al., 2007; Salazar et al., 2008), but their relation to pain receptors remains a delicious mystery (sorry). Stimulating your TRPV1 receptor too much can be hazardous to your health, as we see in Signs & Symptoms next.

transient receptor potential type M3 (TRPM3)   A receptor, found in some free nerve endings, that opens its channel in response to rising temperatures.

A delta (Aδ) fiber   A moderately large, myelinated, and therefore fast-conducting axon that usually transmits pain information.

C fiber   A small, unmyelinated axon that conducts pain information slowly and adapts slowly.

SIGNS & SYMPTOMS

A Professional Eater Meets His Match

The 34-year-old man was a professional eater, entering contests to see how quickly he could down huge quantities of food. He'd been moderately successful in this pursuit, but a chili pepper contest proved to be too much. After eating an entire "Carolina Reaper" pepper, purposely bred to be 6 times hotter than a habanero pepper, the man suffered dry heaves and pain in his neck followed by a series of thunderclap headaches: excruciating, sudden-onset headaches that peak in a minute before subsiding, only to return (Boddhula et al., 2018). MRI scans of the man's brain showed no abnormalities, but a CAT scan of blood vessels revealed that several arteries supplying his brain had narrowed to a remarkable extent (**FIGURE 5.13A**), which may have caused the headaches. Over the next few days, the man suffered several more thunderclap headaches lasting a few seconds. Once the headaches had stopped, the CAT scan showed that the arteries supplying his brain had expanded to a more normal size (**FIGURE 5.13B**). The gentleman may have gotten off lightly. People have suffered severe, even fatal, heart attacks after eating super-hot chili peppers (Davis, 2018).

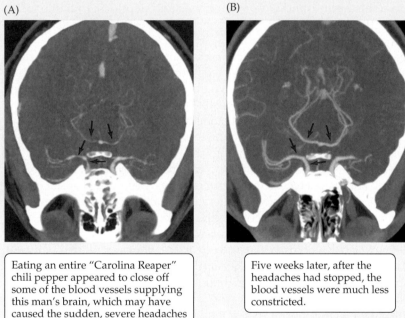

(A) Eating an entire "Carolina Reaper" chili pepper appeared to close off some of the blood vessels supplying this man's brain, which may have caused the sudden, severe headaches he suffered.

(B) Five weeks later, after the headaches had stopped, the blood vessels were much less constricted.

FIGURE 5.13   Thunderclap Headache (From S. K. Boddhula et al., 2018. *BMJ Case Reports*. Courtesy of Kulothungan Gunasekaran.)

Special neural pathways carry pain information to the brain

Nerve fibers carrying information about pain and temperature send their axons to enter the dorsal horns of the spinal cord, where they synapse onto spinal neurons that project across the midline to the opposite side and then up toward the thalamus of the brain (via several brainstem sites), forming the **anterolateral system** (or *spinothalamic system*) (**FIGURE 5.14**). This projection is distinct from the somatosensory system that we discussed earlier (the dorsal column system; see Figure 5.7), but as in that system, each hemisphere receives its inputs from the contralateral side of the body. Within the

anterolateral system   Also called *spinothalamic system*. A somatosensory system that carries most of the pain information from the body to the brain.

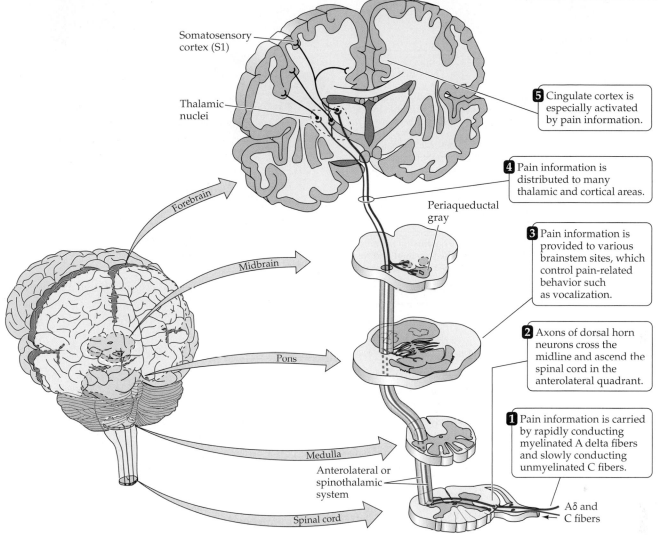

Somatosensory
cortex (S1)

Thalamic
nuclei

5 Cingulate cortex is
especially activated
by pain information.

4 Pain information is
distributed to many
thalamic and cortical areas.

Periaqueductal
gray

3 Pain information is
provided to various
brainstem sites, which
control pain-related
behavior such
as vocalization.

2 Axons of dorsal horn
neurons cross the
midline and ascend the
spinal cord in the
anterolateral quadrant.

1 Pain information is carried
by rapidly conducting
myelinated A delta fibers
and slowly conducting
unmyelinated C fibers.

Forebrain

Midbrain

Pons

Medulla

Anterolateral or
spinothalamic
system

Spinal cord

Aδ and
C fibers

FIGURE 5.14   Ascending Pain Pathways in the CNS Pain sensation travels from its origin to the brain via the anterolateral (spinothalamic) system, crossing the midline in the spinal cord.

spinal cord, the arriving pain fibers release the excitatory transmitter glutamate along with a peptide, **substance P**, that selectively boosts pain signals and remodels pain pathway neurons (Mantyh et al., 1997). Mice lacking substance P cannot feel intense pain, but they still feel mild pain (Cao et al., 1998; De Felipe et al., 1998).

Pain information is eventually integrated in the **cingulate cortex**, part of the limbic system we mentioned in Chapter 2 (see Figure 2.14.B). The extent of activation in the cingulate (as well as in somatosensory) cortex correlates with how much discomfort different people report in response to the same mildly painful stimulus (Coghill et al., 2003). Different subregions of the cingulate cortex seem to mediate emotional versus sensory aspects of pain (Vogt, 2005); one part of the cingulate cortex becomes active even when we just empathize with a loved one experiencing pain (T. Singer et al., 2004).

Sometimes pain persists long after the injury that started it has healed. This **neuropathic pain** is a disagreeable example of neuroplasticity, where neurons continue to directly signal pain, and indeed *amplify* the pain signal, in the absence of any tissue damage (Woolf and Salter, 2000). In one example of neuropathic pain called *phantom limb pain*, patients experience great pain that seems to come from an amputated limb. It is notoriously difficult to treat. One approach that has met with some success involves using a mirror to trick the brain into believing it is controlling the missing limb (**FIGURE 5.15**) (Ramachandran and Rogers-Ramachandran, 2000); apparently, visual feedback (even if false) allows the brain to recalibrate the pain signal.

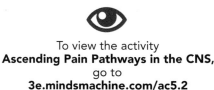

To view the activity
Ascending Pain Pathways in the CNS,
go to
3e.mindsmachine.com/ac5.2

substance P   A peptide transmitter that is involved in pain transmission.

cingulate cortex   Also called *cingulum*. A region of medial cerebral cortex that lies dorsal to the corpus callosum.

neuropathic pain   Pain that persists long after the injury that started it has healed.

FIGURE 5.15 Using a Visual Illusion to Relieve Phantom Limb Pain (After V. S. Ramachandran and D. Rogers-Ramachandran, 2000. *Arch. Neurol.* 57: 317.)

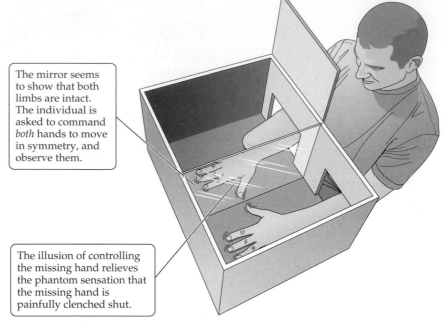

The mirror seems to show that both limbs are intact. The individual is asked to command *both* hands to move in symmetry, and observe them.

The illusion of controlling the missing hand relieves the phantom sensation that the missing hand is painfully clenched shut.

HOW'S IT GOING ?

1. Define *pain*. Why should it be viewed as a positive adaptation?
2. Provide a general explanation of the way pain receptors work. How do pain receptors differ from touch receptors?
3. Name and distinguish between the two sizes of fibers that carry pain information from the periphery to the spinal cord.
4. Sketch the pain pathways from the periphery to the cortex.

Pain Control Can Be Difficult

Throughout history, suffering humans have sought remedies to reduce their experience of pain. It's not easy; even cutting nerves may provide only temporary relief, until the pain system finds a way to restore its signal to the brain. A dominant model of pain transmission, called the *gate control theory*, hypothesizes that spinal "gates"—modulation sites at which pain can be facilitated or blocked—control the signal that gets through to the brain (Melzack and Wall, 1965). If this theory is right, effective pain relief may depend on finding ways to keep the gates closed, cutting off the pain signal. Popular strategies for **analgesia** (absence of pain; from the Greek *an*, "not," and *algesis*, "feeling of pain") fall into four general categories, which we'll discuss next.

Analgesic drugs are highly effective

The opiates (opium-related drugs, like morphine) have been known for centuries to relieve pain sensations. Along with brain-derived painkillers such as the **endorphins** and other endogenous opioids, opiate drugs bind to specific receptors in the brain to reduce pain (see Chapter 4). Researchers have found that this action is especially pronounced in the brainstem region called the *periaqueductal gray* (see Figure 5.14); one possibility is that the brainstem system activates the pain-gating mechanism of the spinal cord via descending projections, thereby blocking the transmission of pain signals. Similar benefits can be obtained by (carefully!) injecting opiates directly into the spinal cord; this is called an *epidural* or *intrathecal* injection.

Although people sometimes do become addicted to painkillers, that is usually not true of people who are using them to treat severe pain; in fact, the danger of addiction from the use of morphine to relieve surgical pain has been vastly exaggerated (Melzack, 1990) and is estimated to be less than 1% (Brownlee and Schrof, 1997).

analgesia   Absence of or reduction in pain.

endorphin   One of three kinds of endogenous opioids.

Unfortunately, those few who do become addicted face a very real danger of death by overdose (Volkow et al., 2018), an epidemic made worse by the development of extremely potent opioids such as OxyContin and fentanyl.

Of course, there are other painkilling drugs, but none are as effective as the opiates. Over-the-counter medications like aspirin and acetaminophen (Tylenol) act via non-opiate mechanisms (especially the cyclooxygenase enzymes COX-1 and COX-2) to reduce pain and inflammation. Cannabis reduces pain by stimulating endogenous cannabinoid receptors (CB_1 receptors) in the spinal cord and in the brain (Agarwal et al., 2007; Pernía-Andrade et al., 2009).

Electrical stimulation can sometimes relieve pain

In **transcutaneous electrical nerve stimulation** (**TENS**), mild electrical stimulation is applied to nerves around the injury sites to relieve pain. The exact mechanism of this pain relief is not clear, but one possibility is that TENS closes the spinal "gate" for pain that Melzack and Wall (1965) described. Recall, for example, the last time you stubbed your toe. In addition to expelling a string of expletives, you may have vigorously rubbed the injured area, bringing a little relief. TENS is a more efficient way of stimulating those adjacent nerves, and it may bring dramatic relief lasting for hours (Vance et al., 2014). We know that TENS acts at least in part by releasing endogenous opioids, because administration of **naloxone**, an opioid antagonist, partially blocks this analgesic action (Gonçalves et al., 2014).

Placebos effectively control pain in some people, but not all

In some people, simply believing that they are receiving a proven treatment can effectively relieve pain. In a striking example of this **placebo effect**, when participants who had just had their wisdom teeth extracted were given morphine or a placebo, fully a third of those receiving the placebo experienced pain relief (J. D. Levine et al., 1978). But when the placebo was coadministered with a drug that blocks opioid receptors (naloxone), the participants did not experience the benefits of the placebo effect. This latter finding strongly implies that placebos work by activating the brain's endogenous opioid system. In fact, functional brain imaging indicates that opioids and placebos activate the same brain regions (Petrovic et al., 2002; D. J. Scott et al., 2008). For reasons unknown, some people consistently experience relief from placebos while others do not (**FIGURE 5.16**).

Activation of endogenous opioids relieves pain

Although the ancient pain-relieving technique **acupuncture** remains very popular, only a minority of people using acupuncture achieve lasting relief from chronic pain. In those people for whom acupuncture is effective, a release of endorphins may be an important part of the process, since treatment with naloxone blocks acupuncture's effectiveness (N. M. Tang et al., 1997). Acupuncture thus resembles placebos in this regard. Although many rules govern needle placement in acupuncture, systematic research indicates that the placement of the needles actually has little to do with its effects on pain (Linde et al., 2009). The *expectation* that the needles will relieve pain appears to be the important factor, presumably inducing a release of endogenous opioids.

Likewise, stressful life events can produce significant analgesia; for example, tales abound of gravely wounded soldiers who feel no pain for some time after their injuries occur (Bowman, 1997). Research in animals indicates that stress activates both an opioid-dependent form of analgesia, which can be blocked by naloxone, and another, non-opioid analgesia system that has not yet been characterized (but may rely on endocannabinoids) (A. G. Hohmann et al., 2005). These endogenous analgesic systems allow a wounded individual to fight or escape rather than be overwhelmed with pain.

transcutaneous electrical nerve stimulation (TENS)   The delivery of electrical pulses through electrodes attached to the skin, which excite nerves that supply the region to which pain is referred.

naloxone   A potent antagonist of opiates that is often administered to people who have taken drug overdoses. It blocks receptors for endogenous opioids.

placebo effect   Relief of a symptom, such as pain, that results following a treatment that is known to be ineffective or inert.

acupuncture   The insertion of needles at designated points on the skin to alleviate pain or neurological malfunction.

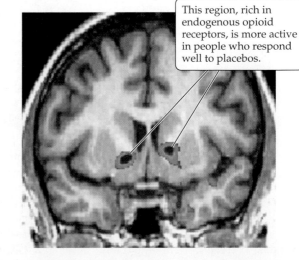

This region, rich in endogenous opioid receptors, is more active in people who respond well to placebos.

FIGURE 5.16   Placebos Affect Opioid Systems in the Brain (From D. J. Scott et al., 2008. *Arch. Gen. Psychiatry* 65: 220. Courtesy of Jon-Kar Zubieta.)

TABLE 5.2 ■ Types of Pain Relief

Type	Mechanism
PSYCHOGENIC	
Placebo	May activate endorphin-mediated pain control system
Hypnosis	Alters brain's perception of pain
Stress	Uses both opioid and non-opioid mechanisms
Cognitive (learning, coping strategies)	May activate endorphin-mediated pain control system
PHARMACOLOGICAL	
Opiates	Bind to opioid receptors in periaqueductal gray and spinal cord
Spinal block	Blocks pain signals in spinal cord
Anti-inflammatory drugs	Block chemical inflammatory signals at the site of injury (see Figure 5.12)
Cannabinoids	Act in spinal cord and on nociceptor endings
STIMULATION	
TENS/mechanical	On large fibers, blocks or alters pain signal to brain
Acupuncture	Activates endogenous opioids and/or placebo-like effect, possibly modulating effect on activity of peripheral pain pathways
Central gray	Electrically activates endorphin-mediated pain-control systems, blocking pain signal in spinal cord

Pain relief remains a major challenge for neuroscience research. Chronic pain can have dramatic effects on the brain: for example, the prefrontal cortex in people with chronic back pain shrinks much faster than normal, as if the patients are rapidly aging (Apkarian et al., 2004). The wide range of pain relief strategies (summarized in **TABLE 5.2**), some of which reflect desperation in the face of great anguish, testifies to the elusive nature of pain. As we learn more about how the brain controls pain, we can hope for better, safer analgesics in the future.

─── HOW'S IT GOING ? ───

1. What is the most effective pharmacological method of pain control? How and where do these drugs work in the brain?
2. How is TENS thought to work to control pain?
3. Compare and contrast placebos and acupuncture for pain. Discuss the possibility that they act on the same neural system.

PART III
Movement and the Motor System

THE ROAD AHEAD

This final section concerns the system by which the brain moves the body, allowing us to interact with the world. Learning this information means you can:

1. Discuss the importance of motor planning and sensory feedback in controlling behavior.
2. Trace the pathways by which the brain sends commands to individual muscles.
3. Distinguish between the two main types of sensory feedback from muscles to the nervous system.
4. Discuss the interaction of various cortical and subcortical brain regions in regulating behavior.
5. Describe the behavioral symptoms and underlying pathology of two major motor disorders.

Behavior Requires Movements That Are Precisely Programmed and Monitored

Our apparently effortless adult motor abilities—such as reaching out and picking up an object, walking across the room, sipping a cup of coffee—require complex muscular systems with constant feedback from the body. Ian, whom we met at the beginning of the chapter, knows this all too well. Our survey of motor control starts with a discussion of a theoretical framework for studying motor behavior, followed by a tour of the anatomy and pathology of movement.

When you think about it, *all* behavior must involve **movements**—contractions of muscles that provide our sole means of interacting with the world around us. Centuries of research focused on the organization of motor behavior as both an engineering problem (how is movement programmed?) and a physiological system (how is movement produced?). Early discoveries suggested that **reflexes**—simple, unvarying, and unlearned responses to sensory stimuli such as touch, pressure, and pain—might be the basic units of behavior. It was thought that more-complex behaviors, or **acts**, such as getting dressed, walking, or speaking a sentence, might result from simply connecting together different reflexes, the sensation from one reflex triggering the next.

The flaws of this perspective soon became apparent: for most acts we have a *plan* in which several units (arm movements, leg movements, speech sounds) are placed in a larger pattern (the intended complete act), and they are not always produced in the same (or even the correct) order. So, researchers realized that acts require a **motor plan** (or *motor program*), a complex set of commands to muscles that is established *before* an act occurs. Feedback from movements informs and fine-tunes the motor program as the execution is unfolding, but the basic sequence of movements is planned. Examples of behaviors that exhibit this kind of internal plan range from highly skilled acts, such as piano playing, to the simple escape behaviors of animals such as crayfish.

Researchers can track the simple movements that make up an act by recording the electrical activity of muscles as they contract—a technique called **electromyography** (**EMG**)—and the moment-to-moment positions of the body. The EMG recordings in **FIGURE 5.17** show that a person pulling a lever will adjust his legs just before moving his arm—an example of motor planning. Motor plans resemble engineering concepts that are applied to the operation of machines. In designing machines, engineers commonly have two goals: (1) accuracy, to prevent or minimize error; and (2) speed, to complete a task quickly and efficiently. Improvements in one goal usually come at some cost to the other goal; in other words, there is a trade-off between speed and accuracy, and this trade-off is also apparent in motor planning by the nervous system.

The neuromuscular system consists of the muscles of the body plus a collection of brain mechanisms and nerves that prepare and execute motor plans and obtain feedback information from the sensory system for use in error correction. The system is organized according to a distinct hierarchy:

1. The *skeletal system* and the muscles attached to it determine which movements are possible.

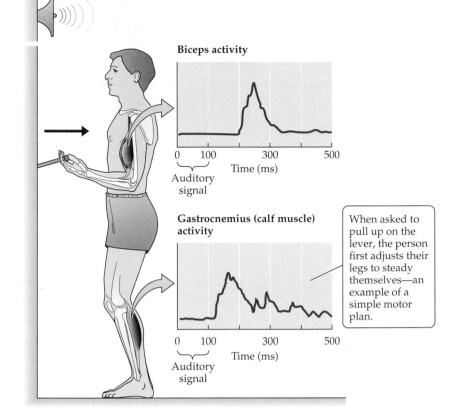

FIGURE 5.17 Elecromyography (After D. Purves et al., 2001. *Neuroscience* [2nd ed.]. Oxford University Press/Sinauer. Sunderland, MA.)

movement A single relocation of a body part, usually resulting from a brief muscle contraction. It is less complex than an act.

reflex A simple, highly stereotyped, and unlearned response to a particular stimulus (e.g., an eye blink in response to a puff of air).

act Complex behavior, as distinct from a simple movement.

motor plan Also called *motor program*. A plan for a series of muscular contractions, established in the nervous system prior to its execution.

electromyography (EMG) The electrical recording of muscle activity.

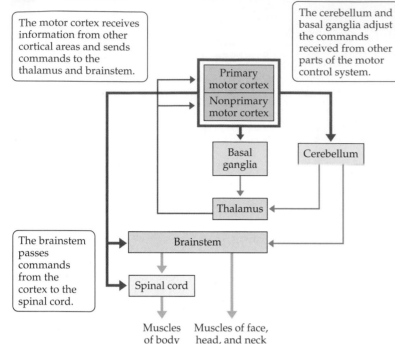

The motor cortex receives information from other cortical areas and sends commands to the thalamus and brainstem.

The cerebellum and basal ganglia adjust the commands received from other parts of the motor control system.

The brainstem passes commands from the cortex to the spinal cord.

Primary motor cortex
Nonprimary motor cortex
Basal ganglia
Cerebellum
Thalamus
Brainstem
Spinal cord
Muscles of body
Muscles of face, head, and neck

FIGURE 5.18 The Hierarchy of Movement Control

2. The *spinal cord* controls skeletal muscles in response to motor commands from the brain or, in the case of simple reflexes, in direct response to sensory inputs.

3. The *brainstem* integrates motor commands from higher levels of the brain and transmits them to the spinal cord. It also relays sensory information about the body from the spinal cord to the forebrain.

4. Some of the main commands for action are initiated in the *primary motor cortex*.

5. Areas adjacent to the primary motor cortex, *nonprimary motor cortex*, provide an additional source of motor commands, acting indirectly via primary motor cortex and through direct connections to lower levels of the motor hierarchy. At the very top of the movement hierarchy is the prefrontal cortex, which is crucial to the conscious formulation of behavioral plans.

6. Other brain regions—the *cerebellum* and *basal ganglia*, via the *thalamus*—modulate the activities of the other parts of the control system.

Through the remainder of the chapter we'll look at the elements of this hierarchy, as outlined in **FIGURE 5.18**, in a bit more detail.

HOW'S IT GOING ?

1. Distinguish among reflexes, movements, and acts.
2. Discuss the importance of sensory feedback for the control of movements. How are speed and accuracy related, in the context of movement control?
3. What is a motor plan?
4. Identify the six major levels of the motor control hierarchy.

A Complex Neural System Controls Muscles to Create Behavior

So much processing power is devoted to movement that the range of possible behaviors and their speed of execution can be astonishing. One of the primary factors in determining the range of movements of a species is the type and arrangement of its muscles around joints, so we begin there and then work our way up through the central nervous system.

Muscles and the skeleton work together to move the body

Our skeleton, like those of other species with bones, is articulated with joints that vary in their planes of movement—ranging from "universal" joints, like the hip or shoulder, to joints that act more like hinges and move mostly in one direction, such as the elbow or knee. Around a joint, different muscles, connected to the bones by tendons, are arranged in a reciprocal fashion such that when one muscle group contracts, it stretches the other group; that is, the muscles are **antagonists**. Some groups of muscles, called **synergists**, may work together to move a limb in one direction. A simple example of muscle action around a joint is shown in **FIGURE 5.19**. The movement of a limb is determined by the degree and rate of contraction in some muscles and relaxation in others, or we can lock a limb in position by contracting opposing muscles simultaneously.

The muscles that we use for movement of the skeleton are called *skeletal muscles*. Because they have a striped appearance on microscopic examination, due to overlapping layers of contractile proteins called *myosin* and *actin*, skeletal muscles are said to be made of *striate muscle*. (*Smooth muscle*, which has a different appearance and is found

antagonist   A muscle that counteracts the effect of another muscle.

synergist   A muscle that acts together with another muscle.

motor neuron   Also called *motoneuron*. A neuron that transmits neural messages to muscles (or glands).

neuromuscular junction   The region where the motor neuron terminal meets its target muscle fiber. It is the point where the nerve transmits its message to the muscle fiber.

acetylcholine (ACh)   A neurotransmitter that is produced and released by the autonomic nervous system, by motor neurons, and by neurons throughout the brain.

in visceral organs and blood vessels, is not generally involved in voluntary behavior, so we will not concern ourselves with it here.) Contraction of the muscle increases the overlap of the actin and myosin filaments within *muscle fibers*, and as these filaments slide past each other, the muscle fiber shortens. Most muscles consist of a specific mixture of two types of fibers: *slow-twitch fibers* that contract with relatively low intensity but fatigue slowly, and *fast-twitch fibers* that contract strongly but fatigue quickly. Through training, endurance athletes enhance the slow-twitch properties of their muscles (Putman et al., 2004).

Muscles contract because **motor neurons** (or *motoneurons*) of the spinal cord and brainstem (see Figures 2.7 and 2.8) send action potentials along their axons and axon collaterals to terminate at specialized synapses, called **neuromuscular junctions**, that are found on muscle fibers (**FIGURE 5.20**). The production of an action potential by a motor neuron triggers a release of the neurotransmitter **acetylcholine** (**ACh**) at all of the motor neuron's axon terminals. The motor neuron, together with all of the muscle fibers it innervates, is known as a *motor unit*; the fibers respond to the release of ACh by triggering the molecular events that cause actin and myosin to produce contraction (see Figure 5.20).

Some large motor units—where motor neurons innervate thigh muscle, for example—may involve hundreds or

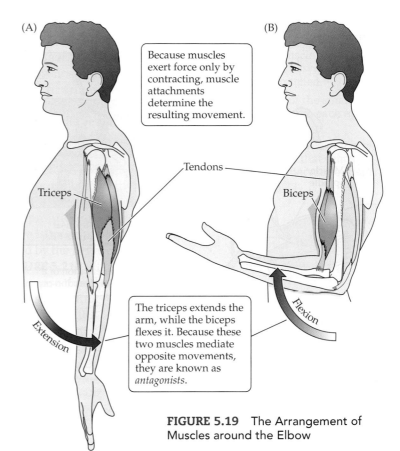

(A)

(B)

Because muscles exert force only by contracting, muscle attachments determine the resulting movement.

Tendons

Triceps

Biceps

Extension

Flexion

The triceps extends the arm, while the biceps flexes it. Because these two muscles mediate opposite movements, they are known as *antagonists*.

FIGURE 5.19   The Arrangement of Muscles around the Elbow

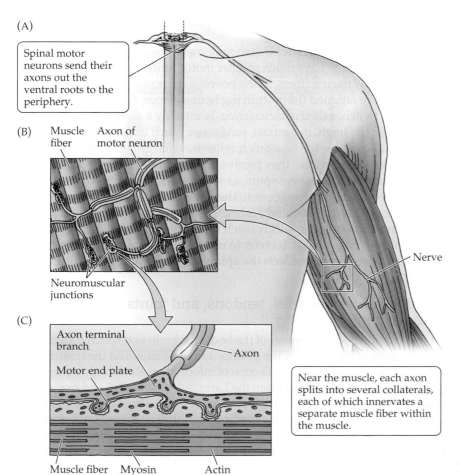

(A)

Spinal motor neurons send their axons out the ventral roots to the periphery.

(B)   Muscle fiber   Axon of motor neuron

Neuromuscular junctions

(C)

Axon terminal branch

Motor end plate

Axon

Nerve

Near the muscle, each axon splits into several collaterals, each of which innervates a separate muscle fiber within the muscle.

Muscle fiber   Myosin   Actin

FIGURE 5.20   The Innervation of Muscle

FIGURE 5.23   The Stretch Reflex Circuit

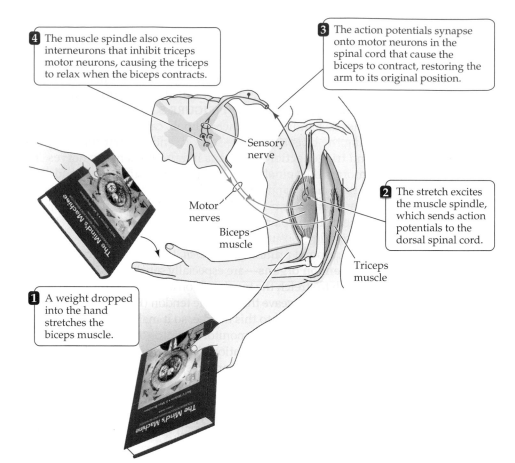

4 The muscle spindle also excites interneurons that inhibit triceps motor neurons, causing the triceps to relax when the biceps contracts.

3 The action potentials synapse onto motor neurons in the spinal cord that cause the biceps to contract, restoring the arm to its original position.

2 The stretch excites the muscle spindle, which sends action potentials to the dorsal spinal cord.

1 A weight dropped into the hand stretches the biceps muscle.

Sensory nerve

Motor nerves

Biceps muscle

Triceps muscle

To view the animation
The Stretch Reflex Circuit,
go to
3e.mindsmachine.com/av5.4

if the good arm is restrained, the animal soon learns to use the affected arm, and indeed it can become quite dexterous (Taub, 1976). Monkeys manage to do this the same way Ian does, by guiding their movements with visual feedback about how the arm is moving. In fact, we all supplement our proprioceptive information with feedback from other sensory channels, like vision.

The spinal cord mediates "automatic" responses and receives inputs from the brain

To really understand the physiology of movement, we need to understand how the "final common pathway" is controlled by the CNS. The lowest level of this hierarchy is the spinal cord, where relatively simple circuits produce reflexive behavioral responses to sensory stimuli. A straightforward example is the **stretch reflex**, illustrated in **FIGURE 5.23**, that can be elicited by stretching any muscle. In this case, dropping a load into the outstretched hand causes a sudden stretch of the biceps muscle, which is detected by muscle spindles. In the spinal cord, the incoming sensory information from the spindles has two immediate effects: it stimulates motor neurons of the biceps, causing a contraction, and it simultaneously inhibits the antagonistic motor neurons that connect to the triceps muscle on the back of the arm. The reflex thus generates a compensatory movement to bring the hand and arm back to their intended position. Not all spinal circuits are quite this simple; for example, the rhythmic movements of walking are governed by spinal circuits that may involve many neurons across multiple spinal segments.

Although muscles of the head are controlled *directly* by the brain, via the cranial nerves (see Figure 2.7), the muscles of the rest of the body are ultimately controlled by commands from the brain via the spinal cord. The brain sends these commands to the spinal cord through two major pathways: the pyramidal system and the extrapyramidal system. The **pyramidal system** (or *corticospinal system*) consists of neuronal cell bodies within the frontal cortex and their axons, which pass through the brainstem, forming the pyramidal tract to the spinal cord (**FIGURE 5.24A**). In a cross section of the medulla, the tract is a wedge-shaped anterior protuberance (pyramid) on each side of the midline.

stretch reflex   The contraction of a muscle in response to stretch of that muscle.

pyramidal system   Also called *corticospinal system*. The motor system that includes neurons within the cerebral cortex and their axons, which form the pyramidal tract.

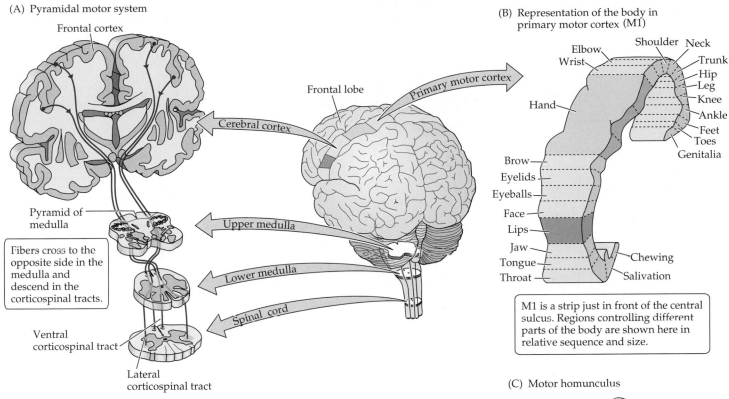

(A) Pyramidal motor system

Frontal cortex

Frontal lobe

Primary motor cortex

Cerebral cortex

Pyramid of medulla

Upper medulla

Fibers cross to the opposite side in the medulla and descend in the corticospinal tracts.

Lower medulla

Spinal cord

Ventral corticospinal tract

Lateral corticospinal tract

(B) Representation of the body in primary motor cortex (M1)

Elbow · Shoulder · Neck · Wrist · Trunk · Hip · Leg · Knee · Ankle · Feet · Toes · Genitalia

Hand

Brow · Eyelids · Eyeballs · Face · Lips · Jaw · Tongue · Throat · Chewing · Salivation

M1 is a strip just in front of the central sulcus. Regions controlling different parts of the body are shown here in relative sequence and size.

FIGURE 5.24 The Pyramidal System and Primary Motor Cortex (Part B after C. N. Prudente et al., 2015. *J. Neurosci.* 35: 9163.)

(C) Motor homunculus

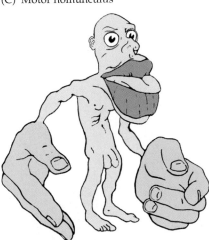

Here, the figure's body parts are proportional to the amount of motor cortex devoted to the corresponding muscles, although this sort of mapping oversimplifies the organization of the motor cortex.

Because the left and right pyramidal tracts each cross over to the other side, the right cortex controls the left side of the body while the left cortex controls the right. Lesions anywhere in the pyramidal tract will cause paralysis in the muscle targets of the damaged axons. Many of the axons of the pyramidal tract originate from neurons in the primary motor cortex (M1), which consists mainly of the precentral gyrus, just anterior to the central sulcus (**FIGURE 5.24B**). We will return to the topic of motor cortex a little later.

Many other axon pathways run from the forebrain to the brainstem and spinal cord. Because these tracts are outside the pyramids of the medulla, they and their connections are lumped together as the **extrapyramidal system**. In general, lesions of the extrapyramidal system do not prevent the movement of individual joints and limbs, but they do interfere with spinal reflexes, usually exaggerating them, and with systems that regulate and fine-tune motor behavior. Many of these extrapyramidal projections pass to the spinal cord via specialized motor regions (the reticular formation and red nucleus) of the midbrain and brainstem; as we'll see shortly, the basal ganglia are an important point of origin for extrapyramidal projections.

Spinal injuries due to vehicular accidents, violence, falls, and sports injuries are all too common, and they often cause heartbreaking disabilities. Because the spinal cord carries all of the instructions from the brain to the muscles, an injury that completely severs the cord results in immediate and permanent paralysis below the level of injury. Depending on the extent of destruction of the spinal cord below the injury site, spinal reflexes may or may not be lost as well (in fact, reflexes may become *stronger* because of the loss of descending inhibition from the brain). An estimated 250,000–400,000 individuals in the United States have spinal cord injuries, and thousands more occur each year, mostly in young people. Although much remains to be discovered, the hope of reconnecting the injured spinal cord no longer seems far-fetched, as discussed in **A STEP FURTHER 5.3**, on the website.

extrapyramidal system A motor system that includes the basal ganglia and some closely related brainstem structures. Axons of this system pass into the spinal cord outside the pyramids of the medulla.

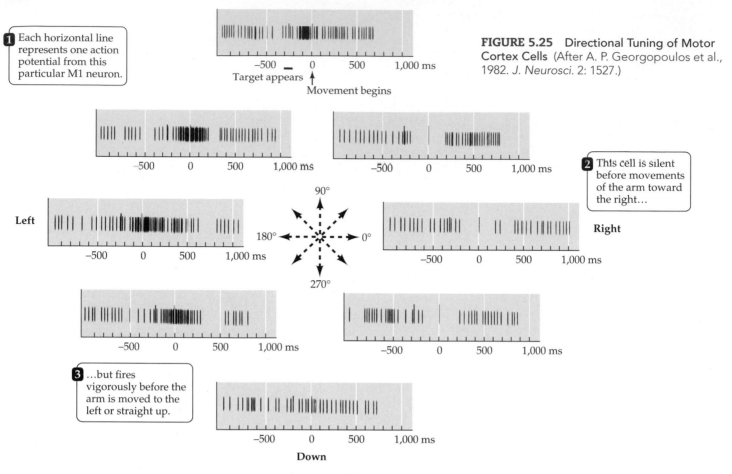

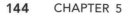

1 Each horizontal line represents one action potential from this particular M1 neuron.

FIGURE 5.25   Directional Tuning of Motor Cortex Cells (After A. P. Georgopoulos et al., 1982. *J. Neurosci.* 2: 1527.)

2 This cell is silent before movements of the arm toward the right...

3 ...but fires vigorously before the arm is moved to the left or straight up.

Motor cortex plans and executes movements—and more

The **primary motor cortex** of humans—**M1**—is a major source of axons forming the pyramidal tract. Like S1, the primary somatosensory cortex that we discussed earlier in the chapter, M1 occupies a single large cortical gyrus: the **precentral gyrus**, located immediately in front of the central sulcus (M1 is thus a part of the frontal lobe; see Figure 5.23B). And like S1, M1 is organized as a map of the contralateral side of the body. So, electrical stimulation of a discrete region of the left M1 will cause movement in the corresponding region of the right side of the body. Once again, the map is distorted, in the sense that the parts of the body that we control most precisely—hands, lips, tongue—are overrepresented in M1. **FIGURE 5.24C** shows the *motor homunculus*, a figure drawn using the body proportions represented in M1. But although the M1 map helps us understand the basic organization of motor cortex, recent research indicates that the map is really an oversimplification. The mapping of individual body regions in M1 isn't nearly as clear-cut and discrete as traditional M1 maps suggest. In fact, there is a fair bit of intermingling of body regions in the map, because many body parts coordinate with one another across regions of M1 (Schieber and Hibbard, 1993; Rathelot and Strick, 2006).

By recording from M1 neurons in monkeys making arm movements (Georgopoulos et al., 1993), we can eavesdrop on the commands originating there (**FIGURE 5.25**). Many M1 cells change their firing rates according to the direction of the movement, but for any one cell, discharge rates are highest in one particular direction. Only by averaging the activity of hundreds of M1 neurons at once can we predict the direction of arm movements with reasonable accuracy. But of course, *millions* of M1 neurons are available, so in principle a larger sampling would provide a more accurate prediction.

Motor representations in M1 are not static; they change as a result of training. For example, M1 is wider in piano players, especially in the hand area, than in nonmusicians. The younger the musician was at the start of musical training, the larger the gyrus is in

primary motor cortex (M1) The apparent executive region for the initiation of movement. It is primarily the precentral gyrus.

precentral gyrus   The strip of frontal cortex, just in front of the central sulcus, that is crucial for motor control.

(A) Before training

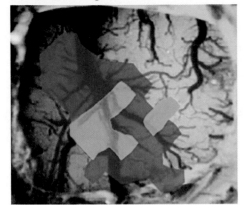

This map illustrates forelimb control in a rat's motor cortex, prior to training.

(B) After training

☐ Digits and wrist
☐ Shoulder and elbow

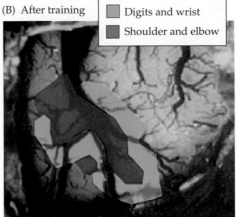

After 10 days of training on a task requiring precise reaching and grasping, the representation of the digits and wrist (green) has expanded into areas previously associated with the shoulder and elbow (blue).

FIGURE 5.26 Motor Learning Causes Remapping of Motor Cortex (From M. H. Monfils et al., 2005. *Neuroscientist* 11: 471. Courtesy of J. Kleim.)

adulthood (Amunts et al., 1997), so this expansion of M1 seems to be in response to the experience of musical training. Studies using transcranial magnetic stimulation (TMS) (see Chapter 2) to noninvasively stimulate cortical neurons have shown that the movements produced by a patch of M1 may change with repeated use (Classen et al., 1998) or as a result of motor learning. In rats, this cortical plasticity associated with motor learning has been directly observed by means of sophisticated mapping of the motor cortex before and after extended training of a new skill (Monfils et al., 2005) (**FIGURE 5.26**).

Just anterior to M1 are cortical regions, collectively known as **nonprimary motor cortex**, that make additional crucial contributions to motor control. Nonprimary motor systems can contribute to behavior directly, through communication with lower levels of the motor hierarchy in the brainstem and spinal cord systems, as well as indirectly, through M1. The traditional account of nonprimary motor cortex emphasizes two main regions: the **supplementary motor area** (**SMA**), which lies mainly on the medial aspect of the hemisphere, and the **premotor cortex**, which is anterior to the primary motor cortex (**FIGURE 5.27**).

The SMA seems important for the *initiation* of movement sequences, especially when they're being executed according to an internal preprogrammed plan (Tanji, 2001). In contrast, the premotor cortex seems to be activated when motor sequences are guided by *external* events (Halsband et al., 1994; Larsson et al., 1996). However, evidence is mounting that premotor cortex is not a single system, but really a mosaic of different units, controlling groups of motor behaviors that cluster together into major categories: defensive movements, feeding behavior, and so on (Graziano, 2006; Graziano and Aflalo, 2007). This organization suggests that motor and premotor areas mostly map *behaviors*, rather than mapping specific *movements*, as in M1.

nonprimary motor cortex   Frontal lobe regions adjacent to the primary motor cortex that contribute to motor control and modulate the activity of the primary motor cortex.

supplementary motor area (SMA)   A region of nonprimary motor cortex that receives input from the basal ganglia and modulates the activity of the primary motor cortex.

premotor cortex   A region of nonprimary motor cortex just anterior to the primary motor cortex.

FIGURE 5.27   Human Motor Cortical Areas

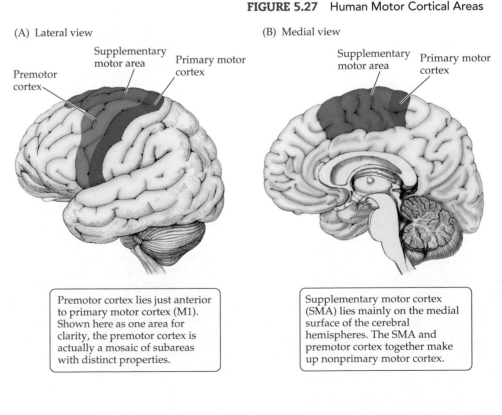

(A) Lateral view

Premotor cortex
Supplementary motor area
Primary motor cortex

Premotor cortex lies just anterior to primary motor cortex (M1). Shown here as one area for clarity, the premotor cortex is actually a mosaic of subareas with distinct properties.

(B) Medial view

Supplementary motor area
Primary motor cortex

Supplementary motor cortex (SMA) lies mainly on the medial surface of the cerebral hemispheres. The SMA and premotor cortex together make up nonprimary motor cortex.

plegia   Paralysis; the loss of the ability to move.

paresis   Muscular weakness, often the result of damage to motor cortex.

apraxia   An impairment in the ability to carry out complex movements, even though there is no muscle paralysis.

mirror neuron   A neuron that is active both when an individual makes a particular movement and when that individual sees another individual make the same movement.

Strokes or other injuries in motor areas of the cortex tend to result in **plegia** (paralysis) or **paresis** (weakness) of voluntary movements, usually on the contralateral side of the body (*hemiplegia* or *hemiparesis*). Damage to nonmotor zones of the cerebral cortex, such as some regions of parietal or frontal association cortex, produces more-complicated changes in motor control, such as **apraxia** (from the Greek *a*, "not," and *praxis*, "action"), the inability to carry out complex movements even though paralysis or weakness is not evident and language comprehension and motivation are intact. There are several subtypes of apraxia, but in general it's as though the patient is unable to work out the sequence of movements required to perform a desired behavior—a high-level motor-programming problem.

HOW'S IT GOING ❓

1. Describe the arrangement of muscles and joints that allows movement.
2. Briefly describe the main components of a motor unit.
3. Define *proprioception*. Explain how two specialized sensors in muscle provide feedback about the muscle's current state.
4. Provide a summary of the path taken by motor fibers innervating the skeletal musculature—from the level of the brain, through the spinal cord, to the muscle targets.
5. Where is primary motor cortex located, and how is it organized?
6. Distinguish between the pyramidal and extrapyramidal systems.
7. What are some of the contributions of nonprimary motor cortex?

RESEARCHERS AT WORK

Mirror neurons in premotor cortex track movements in others

A subregion of premotor cortex (called *F5*) may contain a population of remarkable neurons that seem to fulfill two functions. These neurons fire shortly before a monkey makes a very particular movement of the hand and arm to reach for an object; different neurons fire during different reaching movements. The data thus suggest that these neurons trigger specific movements. But these neurons also seem to fire whenever the monkey sees *another* monkey (or a human) make that same movement (**FIGURE 5.28**). These cells are called **mirror neurons** because they fire as though the monkey were imagining doing the same thing as the other individual. Mirror neurons are also found in adult humans (Buccino et al., 2004) and children (Lepage and Theoret, 2006), both in the premotor cortex and in other cortical locations.

Because the activity of these neurons suggests that they are important in the understanding of other individuals' actions (Rizzolatti and Craighero, 2004), an intriguing notion is that mirror neurons could be part of a neural system for empathy. Thus, there has been a great deal of speculation about the function of mirror neurons in the imitating behavior of human infants, the evolution of language, and other behavior (Gallese and Sinigaglia, 2011). Some have speculated that people with autism spectrum disorder, which is characterized by a failure to anticipate other people's thinking and actions, may have a deficit in mirror neuron activity (J. H. Williams et al., 2006). Note, however, that the specific functions ascribed to mirror neurons remain somewhat controversial (Caramazza et al., 2014).

RESEARCHERS AT WORK (continued)

FIGURE 5.28 Mirror Neurons (After M. A. Umilta et al., 2001. *Neuron* 31: 155.)

■ Question
The researchers hypothesized that neurons of the premotor cortex, in a ventral subregion called F5, encode specific and detailed movements rather than muscle contractions.

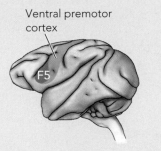

Ventral premotor cortex

F5

■ Experiment
The activity of single F5 neurons was recorded while the monkey made reaching movements.

■ Result
The neurons fired shortly before the monkey made a specific movement, in accordance with the initial hypothesis. But to the experimenters' surprise, the neurons also became active when the monkey simply watched an experimenter perform the same movement, as if the monkey was *imagining* making the movement.

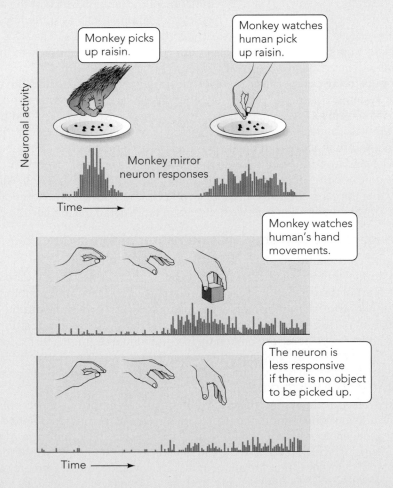

Monkey picks up raisin.

Monkey watches human pick up raisin.

Neuronal activity

Monkey mirror neuron responses

Time

Monkey watches human's hand movements.

The neuron is less responsive if there is no object to be picked up.

Time

■ Conclusion
These "mirror neurons" may be part of a system for analyzing the behavior of others (Umilta et al., 2001).

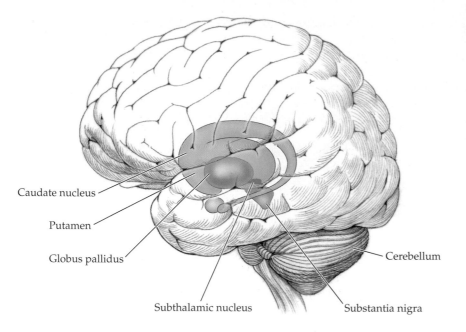

Caudate nucleus

Putamen

Globus pallidus

Cerebellum

Subthalamic nucleus

Substantia nigra

FIGURE 5.29 Subcortical Systems Involved in Movement

To view the activity
**Subcortical Systems
Involved in Movement,**
go to
3e.mindsmachine.com/ac5.3

basal ganglia A group of forebrain nuclei, including caudate nucleus, globus pallidus, and putamen, found deep within the cerebral hemispheres.

cerebellum A structure located at the back of the brain, dorsal to the pons, that is involved in the central regulation of movement and in some forms of learning.

ataxia A loss of movement coordination, often caused by disease of the cerebellum.

decomposition of movement
Difficulty of movement in which gestures are broken up into individual segments instead of being executed smoothly; it is a symptom of cerebellar lesions.

Parkinson's disease A degenerative neurological disorder, characterized by tremors at rest, muscular rigidity, and reduction in voluntary movement, caused by loss of the dopaminergic neurons of the substantia nigra.

substantia nigra A brainstem structure that is a major source of dopaminergic projections to the basal ganglia.

Extrapyramidal systems regulate and fine-tune motor commands

Earlier we noted that extrapyramidal projections—the motor fibers outside the pyramidal tracts—are especially important in modulation and ongoing control of movement. Two of the most important sources of extrapyramidal fibers are the basal ganglia and the cerebellum.

As we saw in Chapter 2, the **basal ganglia** are a group of several interconnected forebrain nuclei (especially the caudate nucleus, putamen, and globus pallidus), with strong inputs from the substantia nigra and the subthalamic nucleus. The basal ganglia receive inputs from wide expanses of the cortex via the thalamus, forming a loop from the cortex through the basal ganglia and thalamus and back to the cortex (**FIGURE 5.29**). The basal ganglia help control the amplitude and direction of movement, and changes in activity in regions of the basal ganglia appear to be important for the initiation of movement. Much of the motor function of the basal ganglia appears to be the modulation of activity started by other brain circuits, such as the motor pathways of the cortex (see Figure 5.24). The basal ganglia are especially important for movements performed by memory, in contrast to those guided by sensory control (Graybiel et al., 1994).

Inputs to the **cerebellum** come both from sensory sources and from other brain motor systems. Sensory inputs include the muscle and joint receptors and the vestibular, somatosensory, visual, and auditory systems. Both pyramidal and nonpyramidal pathways contribute inputs to the cerebellum and in turn receive outputs—all of which are inhibitory—from the deep nuclei of the cerebellum. The cerebellum helps establish and fine-tune neural programs for *skilled* movements, especially the kinds of rapid, repeated movements that become automatic (Y. Liu et al., 1999). Also, we now know that the cerebellum is crucial for a wide variety of motor and nonmotor learning (Katz and Steinmetz, 2002), as we'll discuss in more detail in Chapter 13.

Damage to extrapyramidal systems impairs movement

Different constellations of symptoms are associated with damage to the various extrapyramidal motor structures. The exact consequences of cerebellar damage depend on the part of the cerebellum that has been damaged, but common motor symptoms include characteristic abnormalities of gait and posture, especially **ataxia** (loss of coordination) of the legs. Other cerebellar lesions may cause **decomposition of movement** (in which gestures are broken up into individual segments instead of being executed smoothly) or difficulties with gaze and visual tracking of objects. The anatomy of the cerebellum and the symptomatology of cerebellar disease are discussed in more detail in **A STEP FURTHER 5.4**, on the website.

Two diseases that target the basal ganglia reveal important aspects of extrapyramidal contributions to motor control. Patients with **Parkinson's disease** show progressive degeneration of dopamine-containing cells in the **substantia nigra**. Loss of these neurons, which project to the caudate nucleus and putamen, is associated with a cluster of symptoms that are all too familiar: slow movement, tremors of the hands and face while at rest, a rigid bearing, and diminished facial expressions. Patients who have Parkinson's show few spontaneous actions and have great difficulty in all motor efforts, no matter how routine.

Whereas damage to the basal ganglia in Parkinson's disease *slows* movement, other kinds of basal ganglia disorders cause *excessive* movement. The first symptoms of **Huntington's disease** are subtle behavioral changes: clumsiness, and twitches in the fingers and face. Subtlety is rapidly lost as the illness progresses; a continuing stream of involuntary jerks engulfs the entire body. Aimless movements of the eyes, jerky leg movements, and writhing of the body make even routine activity a major challenge, exacerbated in later stages of the disease by intellectual deterioration. The neuroanatomical basis of this disorder is the progressive destruction of the basal ganglia, especially the caudate nucleus and the putamen, as well as impairment of the cerebral cortex.

Although much remains to be discovered, there is more reason than ever to look forward to the introduction of effective treatments for motor disorders. Scientists are learning more and more about what goes wrong in Parkinson's and Huntington's diseases, and their continuing research efforts may pave the way to new therapies.

Huntington's disease   A genetic disorder, with onset in middle age, in which the destruction of basal ganglia results in a syndrome of abrupt, involuntary writhing movements and changes in mental functioning.

─ HOW'S IT GOING ❓ ──────────────────────

1. What are mirror neurons, and what is their significance?
2. What are the symptoms of Parkinson's disease, and what brain changes cause it?
3. What are the symptoms of Huntington's disease, and what brain changes cause it?
4. Children of people with Huntington's disease have a fifty-fifty chance of inheriting the gene causing it. If you had a parent with Huntington's, would you want to take the test to see if you carry the disease?

Recommended Reading

Basbaum, A. I., and Bushnell, M. C. (2008). *Science of Pain.* New York, NY: Academic Press.

Cytowic, R. E., and Eagleman, D. M. (2009). *Wednesday Is Indigo Blue.* Cambridge, MA: MIT Press.

Lumpkin, E. A., and Caterina, M. J. (2007). "Mechanisms of Sensory Transduction in the Skin." *Nature, 445,* 858–865.

McMahon, C., Koltzenberg, M., Tracey, I., and Turk, D. C. (2013). *Wall and Melzack's Textbook of Pain* (6th ed.). Philadelphia, PA: Saunders.

Purves, D., Augustine, G. J., Fitzpatrick, D., Hall, W. et al. (Eds.). (2017). *Neuroscience* (6th ed.). Sunderland, MA: Oxford University Press/Sinauer. (See Unit III: "Movement and Its Central Control," Chapters 16–21.)

Rathmell, J. P., Ballantyne, J. C., and Fishman, S. M. (Eds.). (2018). *Bonica's Management of Pain* (5th ed.). Philadelphia, PA: Lippincott.

Wolfe, J. M., Kluender, J. R., Levi, D. M., Bartoshuk, L. M. et al. (2018). *Sensation & Perception* (5th ed.). Sunderland, MA: Oxford University Press/Sinauer.

You should be able to relate each summary to the adjacent illustration, including structures and processes. If you go to the website for our text (3e.mindsmachine.com), you can follow links to figures, animations, and activities that will help you consolidate the material.

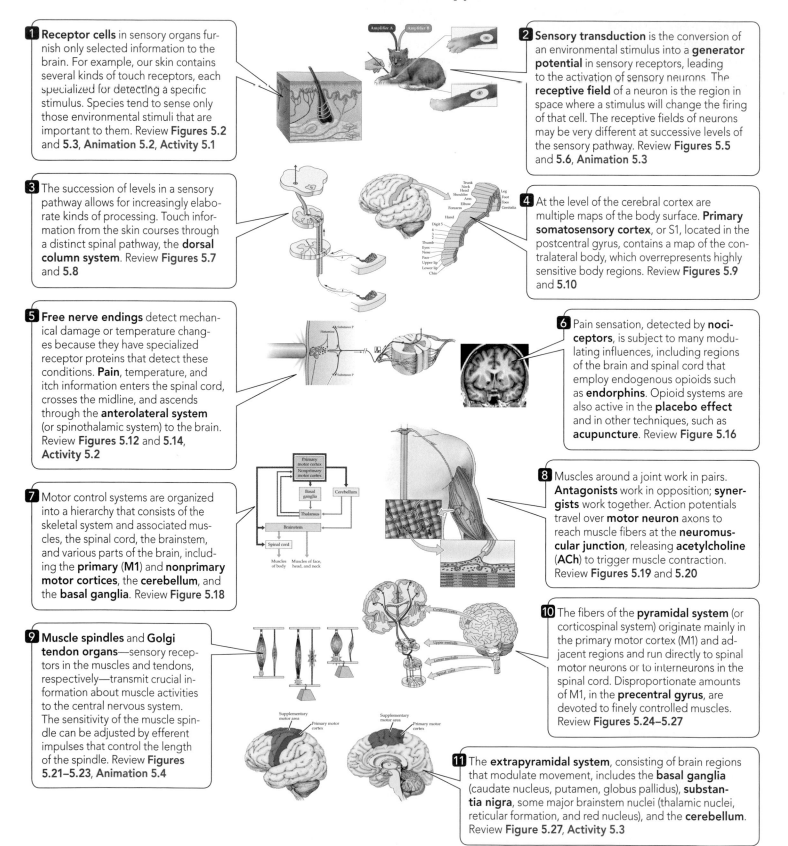

1 **Receptor cells** in sensory organs furnish only selected information to the brain. For example, our skin contains several kinds of touch receptors, each specialized for detecting a specific stimulus. Species tend to sense only those environmental stimuli that are important to them. Review **Figures 5.2** and **5.3**, **Animation 5.2**, **Activity 5.1**

2 **Sensory transduction** is the conversion of an environmental stimulus into a **generator potential** in sensory receptors, leading to the activation of sensory neurons. The **receptive field** of a neuron is the region in space where a stimulus will change the firing of that cell. The receptive fields of neurons may be very different at successive levels of the sensory pathway. Review **Figures 5.5** and **5.6**, **Animation 5.3**

3 The succession of levels in a sensory pathway allows for increasingly elaborate kinds of processing. Touch information from the skin courses through a distinct spinal pathway, the **dorsal column system**. Review **Figures 5.7** and **5.8**

4 At the level of the cerebral cortex are multiple maps of the body surface. **Primary somatosensory cortex**, or S1, located in the postcentral gyrus, contains a map of the contralateral body, which overrepresents highly sensitive body regions. Review **Figures 5.9** and **5.10**

5 **Free nerve endings** detect mechanical damage or temperature changes because they have specialized receptor proteins that detect these conditions. **Pain**, temperature, and itch information enters the spinal cord, crosses the midline, and ascends through the **anterolateral system** (or spinothalamic system) to the brain. Review **Figures 5.12** and **5.14**, **Activity 5.2**

6 Pain sensation, detected by **nociceptors**, is subject to many modulating influences, including regions of the brain and spinal cord that employ endogenous opioids such as **endorphins**. Opioid systems are also active in the **placebo effect** and in other techniques, such as **acupuncture**. Review **Figure 5.16**

7 Motor control systems are organized into a hierarchy that consists of the skeletal system and associated muscles, the spinal cord, the brainstem, and various parts of the brain, including the **primary (M1)** and **nonprimary motor cortices**, the **cerebellum**, and the **basal ganglia**. Review **Figure 5.18**

8 Muscles around a joint work in pairs. **Antagonists** work in opposition; **synergists** work together. Action potentials travel over **motor neuron** axons to reach muscle fibers at the **neuromuscular junction**, releasing **acetylcholine** (**ACh**) to trigger muscle contraction. Review **Figures 5.19** and **5.20**

9 **Muscle spindles** and **Golgi tendon organs**—sensory receptors in the muscles and tendons, respectively—transmit crucial information about muscle activities to the central nervous system. The sensitivity of the muscle spindle can be adjusted by efferent impulses that control the length of the spindle. Review **Figures 5.21–5.23**, **Animation 5.4**

10 The fibers of the **pyramidal system** (or corticospinal system) originate mainly in the primary motor cortex (M1) and adjacent regions and run directly to spinal motor neurons or to interneurons in the spinal cord. Disproportionate amounts of M1, in the **precentral gyrus**, are devoted to finely controlled muscles. Review **Figures 5.24–5.27**

11 The **extrapyramidal system**, consisting of brain regions that modulate movement, includes the **basal ganglia** (caudate nucleus, putamen, globus pallidus), **substantia nigra**, some major brainstem nuclei (thalamic nuclei, reticular formation, and red nucleus), and the **cerebellum**. Review **Figure 5.27**, **Activity 5.3**

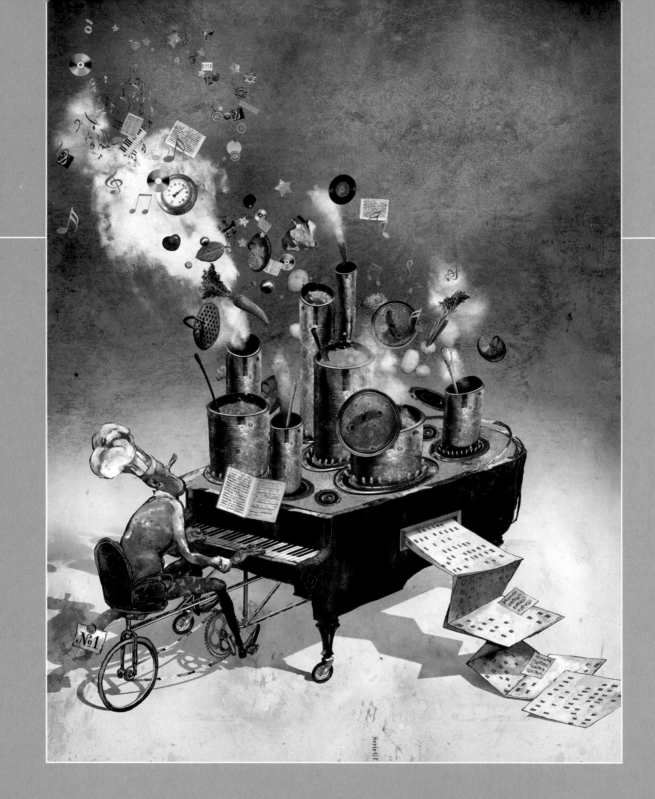

6

Hearing, Balance, Taste, and Smell

Hold the Phone

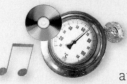

It's like a classic horror movie scene: a scientist using amazing technology in an attempt to reanimate parts of dead bodies, seeking out nature's secrets. But when the young Hungarian engineer Georg von Békésy started experimenting with cadavers in the 1920s, he was not trying to create life. He was seeking an answer to a practical question: Why are human ears so much more sensitive than most microphones? Békésy thought that learning how the human ear works might allow him to make a better microphone for his employer, the Hungarian phone company. He gathered cadavers from local hospitals and came up with a clever dissection that would reveal the inner ear without destroying it. (His work was not always appreciated by his fellow engineers; they didn't like finding their drill press full of human bone dust in the morning.)

Bringing his background in physics to bear on the question, Békésy devised exquisitely precise physical models and biophysical experiments that let him measure extremely brief, minuscule movements in the inner ear. His subsequent discoveries provided us with the key to understanding how we translate a stream of auditory data—sounds—into neural activity that the brain can understand.

In the end, Békésy did not come up with a better microphone, but his discoveries have helped restore hearing to thousands of people who once were deaf, as we'll see in this chapter.

Your existence is directly attributable to the keen senses possessed by your distant ancestors—senses that enabled them to find food and mates and to avoid predators and other dangers. In this chapter we consider some of the incredible sensors that let us monitor important signals from distant sources, especially sounds (by audition) and smells (by olfaction). We also discuss related systems for detecting position and movement of the body (the vestibular system, related to the auditory system) and tastes of foods (the gustatory or taste sense, which like olfaction is a chemical sense). We begin with hearing, because audition evolved from special mechanical receptors related to the touch system that we discussed in Chapter 5.

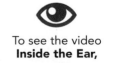

To see the video
Inside the Ear,
go to
3e.mindsmachine.com/av6.1

To view the
Brain Explorer,
go to
3e.mindsmachine.com/av6.2

PART I
Hearing and Balance

THE ROAD AHEAD

The first part of the chapter is concerned with the structure and function of the ear, especially the inner ear, which gives us our senses of hearing and balance. By the end of the section, you should be able to:

1. Name and describe the components of the auditory system and explain how they convert sound into neural activity.
2. Sketch the auditory projections in the brain and discuss the mechanisms by which we sense the pitch and point of origin of sounds.
3. Discuss the perception of higher order sound, like music and speech, and the main forms of hearing loss.
4. Describe the structure and function of the vestibular system, drawing parallels to the functioning of the auditory system.

Pressure Waves in the Air Are Perceived as Sound

Hearing is vital for the survival of many animals. Humans can produce an impressive variety of vocalizations—from barely audible murmurs to soaring flights of song—but we especially rely on speech sounds for our social relations and for the

The Ears Have It   The external ears, or pinnae, of mammals come in a variety of shapes, each adapted to a particular ecological niche. Many mammals can move their ears to direct them toward a particular sound. In such cases, the brain must account for the position of the ear to judge where a particular sound came from. (Top left © iStock.com/wrangel; top right © A.S. Floro/Shutterstock; bottom left © iStock.com/Ken-Canning; bottom right © bierchen/Shutterstock.)

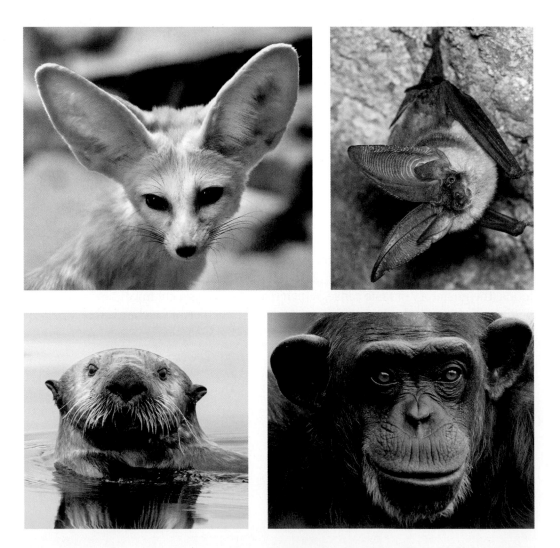

decibel (dB)   A measure of sound intensity, perceived as loudness.

hertz (Hz)   Cycles per second, as of an auditory stimulus. Hertz is a measure of frequency.

transmission of knowledge between individuals. Across the animal kingdom, species produce and perceive sounds in wildly different ways, shaped by their unique adaptive needs. Birds sing and crickets chirp in order to attract mates; monkeys grunt and screech and burble to signal comfort, danger, and pleasure; and owls and bats exploit the directional property of sound to locate prey and avoid obstacles in the dark.

How do small vibrations in air become the speech, music, and other sounds we hear? Your auditory system detects changes in the vibration of air molecules that are caused by sound sources, sensing both the *intensity* of sounds (measured in **decibels [dB]** and perceived as *loudness*) and their *frequency* (measured in cycles per second, or **hertz [Hz]**, and perceived as *pitch*). **BOX 6.1** describes some of the basic properties of sound. The outer ear directs sound into the inner parts of the ear, where the mechanical force of sound is **transduced** into neural activity: the action potentials that inform the brain. Your ears are incredibly sensitive organs; in fact, one of the main jobs of your powers of attention is to filter out the constant barrage of unimportant little noises that your ears detect (see Chapter 14).

transduction   The conversion of one form of energy to another.

pure tone   A tone with a single frequency of vibration.

amplitude   Also called *intensity*. The force that sound exerts per unit area, which we experience as loudness.

frequency   The number of cycles per second in a sound wave, measured in hertz.

fundamental   The predominant frequency of an auditory tone.

harmonic   A multiple of a particular frequency called the fundamental.

timbre   The characteristic sound quality of a musical instrument, as determined by the relative intensities of its various harmonics.

BOX 6.1
The Basics of Sound

We perceive a repetitive pattern of local increases and decreases in air pressure as sound. Usually this oscillation is caused by a vibrating object, such as a loudspeaker or a person's larynx during speaking. A single alternation of compression and expansion of air is called one *cycle*.

The figure illustrates the oscillations in pressure produced by a vibrating loudspeaker. Because the sound produced by the loudspeaker here has only one frequency of vibration, it is called a **pure tone** and can be represented by a sine wave. A pure tone is described physically in terms of two measures:

Amplitude   Also called *intensity*, this is usually measured as sound pressure in dynes per square centimeter (dyn/cm^2). Our perception of amplitude is termed *loudness*, expressed as decibels (dB). The decibel scale is logarithmic: one decibel is the threshold for human hearing, a whisper is about 20 dB, and a departing jetliner a couple of hundred feet overhead—a sound a million times as intense—is about 120 dB.

Frequency   This is the number of cycles per second, measured in hertz (Hz). So, middle A on a piano has a frequency of 440 Hz. Our perception of frequency is termed *pitch*.

Most sounds are more complicated than a pure tone. For example, a sound made by a musical instrument contains a fundamental frequency and harmonics. The **fundamental** is the basic frequency, and the **harmonics** are multiples of the fundamental. For example, if the fundamental is 440 Hz, the harmonics are 880 Hz, 1,320 Hz, 1,760 Hz, and so on. When different instruments play the same note, the notes differ in the relative intensities of the various harmonics and there are subtle qualitative differences between instruments in the way they commence, shape, and sustain the sound; these differences are what give each instrument its characteristic voice, or **timbre**.

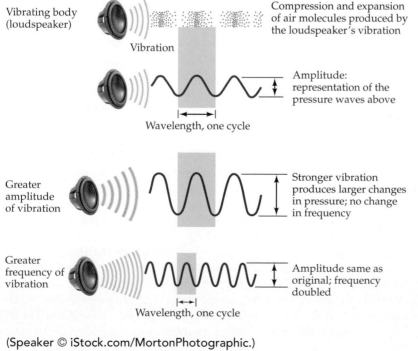

Amplitude and frequency of sound waves

Vibrating body (loudspeaker)

Vibration

Compression and expansion of air molecules produced by the loudspeaker's vibration

Amplitude: representation of the pressure waves above

Wavelength, one cycle

Greater amplitude of vibration

Stronger vibration produces larger changes in pressure; no change in frequency

Greater frequency of vibration

Amplitude same as original; frequency doubled

Wavelength, one cycle

(Speaker © iStock.com/MortonPhotographic.)

pinna The external part of the ear.

ear canal Also called *auditory canal*. The tube leading from the pinna to the tympanic membrane.

inner ear The cochlea and vestibular apparatus.

middle ear The cavity between the tympanic membrane and the cochlea.

tympanic membrane Also called *eardrum*. The partition between the external ear and the middle ear.

ossicles Three small bones (*incus, malleus*, and *stapes*) that transmit vibration across the middle ear, from the tympanic membrane to the oval window.

oval window The opening from the middle ear to the inner ear.

cochlea A snail-shaped structure in the inner ear canal that contains the primary receptor cells for hearing.

scala vestibuli Also called *vestibular canal*. One of three principal canals running along the length of the cochlea.

scala media Also called *middle canal*. The central of the three spiraling canals inside the cochlea, situated between the vestibular canal and the tympanic canal.

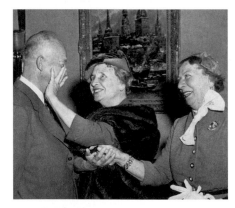

A Touching Moment Helen Keller, who was both blind and deaf, said, "Blindness deprives you of contact with things; deafness deprives you of contact with people"—a poignant reminder of the importance of speech for our social lives. Here, Keller (center, accompanied by her aide and interpreter, Polly Thompson) communicates with U.S. President Dwight Eisenhower by feeling Eisenhower's face as he speaks and makes facial expressions. Rather than living in sensory and social isolation, Keller honed her intact senses to such a degree that she was able to become a noted teacher and writer. (© MPI/Stringer/Getty Images.)

The external ear captures, focuses, and filters sound

The oddly shaped fleshy objects that most people call *ears* are properly known as **pinnae** (singular *pinna*). Aside from their occasional utility as handles and jewelry hangers, the pinnae funnel sound waves into the second part of the external ear: the **ear canal** (or *auditory canal*). The pinna is a distinctly mammalian characteristic, and mammals show a wide array of ear shapes and sizes. Furthermore, although only a minority of humans can move their ears, and even then only enough to entertain children, many other mammals deftly shape and swivel their pinnae to help determine the source of a sound. Animals with exceptional auditory localization abilities, such as bats, may have especially mobile ears.

The "ridges and valleys" of the pinna modify the character of sound that reaches the middle ear. Some frequencies of sound are enhanced; others are suppressed. For example, the shape of the human ear especially increases the reception of sounds between 2,000 and 5,000 Hz—a frequency range that is important for speech perception. The shape of the external ear—and, in many species, the direction in which it is being pointed—provides additional cues about the direction and distance of the source of a sound, as we will discuss later in this chapter.

The middle ear concentrates sound energies

A collection of tiny structures made of membrane, muscle, and bone—essentially a tiny biological microphone—links the ear canal to the neural receptor cells of the **inner ear** (**FIGURE 6.1A**). This **middle ear** (**FIGURE 6.1B**) consists of the taut **tympanic membrane** (*eardrum*) sealing the end of the ear canal plus a chain of tiny bones, called **ossicles**, that mechanically couple the tympanic membrane to the inner ear at a specialized patch of membrane called the **oval window**. These ossicles, the smallest bones in the body, are called the *malleus* (Latin for "hammer"), the *incus* (Latin for "anvil"), and the *stapes* (Latin for "stirrup").

Sound waves in the air strike the tympanic membrane and cause it to vibrate with the same frequency as the sound; as a result, the ossicles start moving too. Because of how they are attached to the eardrum, the ossicles concentrate and amplify the vibrations, focusing the pressures collected from the relatively large tympanic membrane onto the small oval window. This amplification is crucial for converting vibrations in air into movements of fluid in the inner ear, as we'll see shortly.

The middle ear is equipped with the equivalent of a volume control, which helps protect against the damaging forces of extremely loud noises. Two tiny muscles—the tensor tympani and the stapedius (see Figure 6.1B)—attach to the ends of the chain of ossicles. Within 200 milliseconds of the arrival of a loud sound, the brain signals the muscles to contract, which stiffens the chain of ossicles and reduces the effectiveness of the sounds. Interestingly, the middle-ear muscles activate just before we produce self-made sounds like speech or coughing, which is why we don't perceive our own sounds as distractingly loud.

The cochlea converts vibrational energy into neural activity

The part of the inner ear that ultimately converts vibrations from sound into neural activity—the coiled, fluid-filled **cochlea** (from the Greek *kochlos*, "snail")—is a marvel of miniaturization (**FIGURES 6.1C** and **D**). In an adult, the cochlea measures only about 9 millimeters in diameter at its widest point—roughly the size of a pea. Fully unrolled, the cochlea would be about 35–40 millimeters long.

The cochlea is a coil of three parallel canals: (1) the **scala vestibuli** (also called the *vestibular canal*), (2) the **scala media** (*middle canal*), and (3) the **scala tympani** (*tympanic canal*). The scala media contains the receptor system, called the **organ of Corti**, that converts vibration (from sound) into neural activity (see Figure 6.1D). It consists of three main structures: (1) the auditory sensory cells, called **hair cells (FIGURE 6.1E)**, which are embedded in the **basilar membrane**; (2) an elaborate framework

(A) Structures of the ear

FIGURE 6.1   External and Internal Structures of the Human Ear

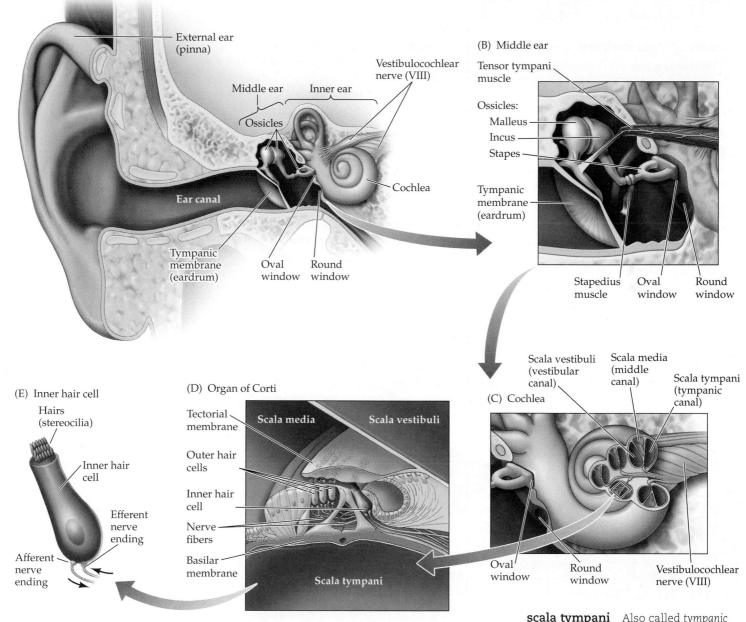

scala tympani   Also called *tympanic canal*. One of three principal canals running along the length of the cochlea.

organ of Corti   A structure in the inner ear that lies on the basilar membrane of the cochlea and contains the hair cells and terminations of the auditory nerve.

hair cell   One of the receptor cells for hearing in the cochlea, named for the stereocilia that protrude from the top of the cell and transduce vibrational energy in the cochlea into neural activity.

basilar membrane   A membrane in the cochlea that contains the principal structures involved in auditory transduction.

of supporting cells; and (3) the auditory nerve terminals that transmit neural signals to and from the brain.

When the ossicles transmit vibrations from the tympanic membrane to the oval window, waves or ripples are created in the fluid of the scala vestibuli, which in turn cause the basilar membrane to ripple, like shaking out a rug. A crucial feature of the basilar membrane is that it is tapered—it's much wider at the apex of the cochlea than at the base. Thanks to this taper, each successive location along the basilar membrane responds most strongly to a different frequency of sound. High frequencies thus produce their greatest effects near the base, where the membrane is narrow and comparatively stiff; low-frequency sounds produce a larger response near the apex, where the membrane is wider and floppier (Ashmore, 1994).

RESEARCHERS AT WORK

Georg von Békésy and the cochlear wave

The discovery of the mechanics of the basilar membrane garnered a Nobel Prize for Georg von Békésy in 1961 (**FIGURE 6.2**).

To view the animation
Sound Transduction,
go to
3e.mindsmachine.com/av6.3

FIGURE 6.2   Deformation of the Basilar Membrane Encodes Sound Frequencies

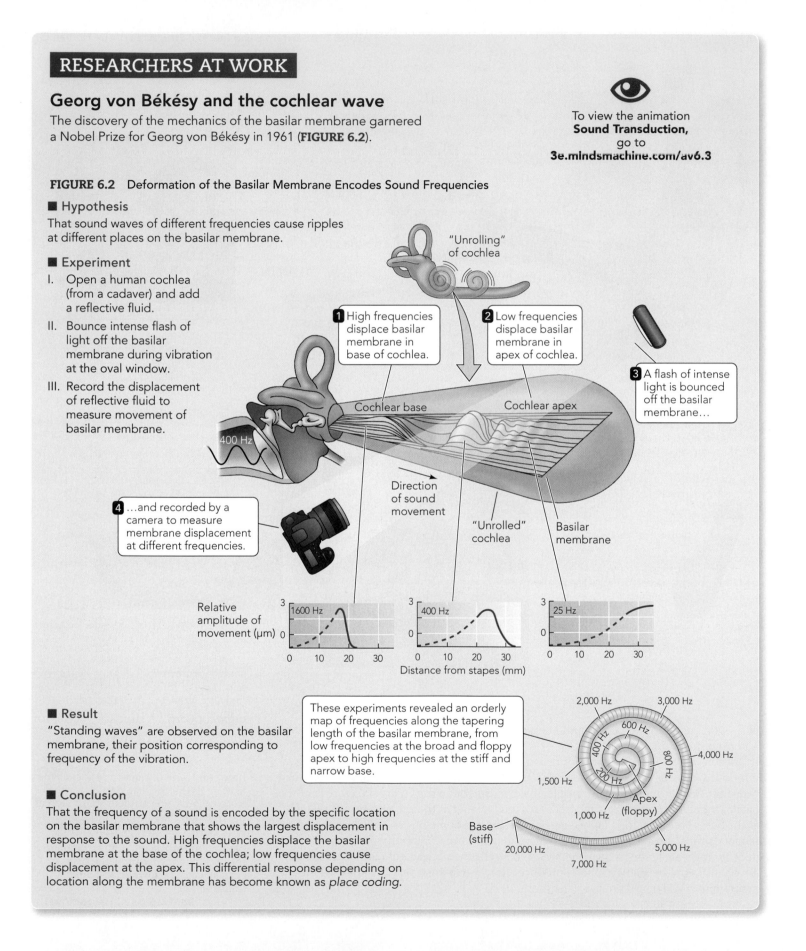

■ **Hypothesis**

That sound waves of different frequencies cause ripples at different places on the basilar membrane.

■ **Experiment**

I.   Open a human cochlea (from a cadaver) and add a reflective fluid.

II. Bounce intense flash of light off the basilar membrane during vibration at the oval window.

III. Record the displacement of reflective fluid to measure movement of basilar membrane.

"Unrolling" of cochlea

1 High frequencies displace basilar membrane in base of cochlea.

2 Low frequencies displace basilar membrane in apex of cochlea.

3 A flash of intense light is bounced off the basilar membrane…

400 Hz

Cochlear base

Cochlear apex

Direction of sound movement

4 …and recorded by a camera to measure membrane displacement at different frequencies.

"Unrolled" cochlea

Basilar membrane

Relative amplitude of movement (μm)

1600 Hz

400 Hz

25 Hz

Distance from stapes (mm)

■ **Result**

"Standing waves" are observed on the basilar membrane, their position corresponding to frequency of the vibration.

These experiments revealed an orderly map of frequencies along the tapering length of the basilar membrane, from low frequencies at the broad and floppy apex to high frequencies at the stiff and narrow base.

2,000 Hz   3,000 Hz
600 Hz
400 Hz
1,500 Hz
200 Hz   800 Hz
4,000 Hz
Apex (floppy)
1,000 Hz
Base (stiff)
20,000 Hz   5,000 Hz
7,000 Hz

■ **Conclusion**

That the frequency of a sound is encoded by the specific location on the basilar membrane that shows the largest displacement in response to the sound. High frequencies displace the basilar membrane at the base of the cochlea; low frequencies cause displacement at the apex. This differential response depending on location along the membrane has become known as *place coding*.

The hair cells transduce movements of the basilar membrane into electrical signals

The rippling of the basilar membrane is converted into neural activity through the actions of the hair cells. Each hair cell features a sloping brush of minuscule hairs called **stereocilia** (singular *stereocilium*) on its upper surface. In Figure 6.1D you'll notice that, although the bases of hair cells are implanted in the basilar membrane, the stereocilia nestle into hollows in the tectorial membrane that lies above. The hair cells—and especially the stereocilia themselves—thus form a mechanical bridge between the two membranes, and they are forced to bend when sounds cause the basilar membrane to ripple.

Even a tiny deflection of stereocilia produces a large and rapid depolarization of the hair cells. This depolarization results from the operation of a special type of large and nonselective ion channel found on stereocilia. Like spring-loaded trapdoors, these channels are mechanically popped open as stereocilia bend (Hudspeth et al., 2000), allowing an inrush of potassium (K^+) and calcium (Ca^{2+}) ions. Just as we saw in neurons (in Chapter 3), this depolarization leads to a rapid influx of Ca^{2+} at the base of the hair cell, which in turn causes synaptic vesicles there to fuse with the presynaptic membrane and release neurotransmitter, stimulating adjacent nerve fibers (Goutman et al., 2015). The stereocilia channels snap shut again in a fraction of a millisecond as the hair cell sways back. This ability to rapidly switch on and off allows hair cells to accurately track the rapid oscillations of the basilar membrane with exquisite sensitivity.

In the human cochlea, the hair cells are organized into a single row of about 3,500 **inner hair cells** (**IHCs**, called *inner* because they are closer to the central axis of the coiled cochlea) and about 12,000 **outer hair cells** (**OHCs**) in three rows (see Figure 6.1D). Fibers of the **vestibulocochlear nerve** (cranial nerve VIII) contact the bases of the hair cells (see Figure 6.1E). Some of these fibers do indeed convey sound information to the brain, but the neural connections of the cochlea are a little more complicated than this. In fact, there are four kinds of neural connections with hair cells, each relying on a different neurotransmitter (Eybalin, 1993), as you can see in **FIGURE 6.3**.

The fibers are distinguished as follows:

1. *IHC afferents* convey to the brain the action potentials that provide the perception of sounds. IHC afferents make up about 95% of the fibers leading to the brain.

2. *IHC efferents* lead from the brain to the IHCs—through which the brain can control the responsiveness of IHCs.

3. *OHC afferents* convey information to the brain about the mechanical state of the basilar membrane, but not the perception of sounds themselves.

4. *OHC efferents* from the brain enable it to activate a remarkable property of OHCs, making them change their length almost instantaneously (Zheng et al., 2000; He et al., 2014). Through

stereocilium A tiny bristle that protrudes from a hair cell in the auditory or vestibular system.

inner hair cell (IHC) One of the two types of receptor cells for hearing in the cochlea. Compared with outer hair cells, IHCs are positioned closer to the central axis of the coiled cochlea.

outer hair cell (OHC) One of the two types of receptor cells for hearing in the cochlea. Compared with inner hair cells, OHCs are positioned farther from the central axis of the coiled cochlea.

vestibulocochlear nerve Cranial nerve VIII, which runs from the cochlea to the brainstem auditory nuclei.

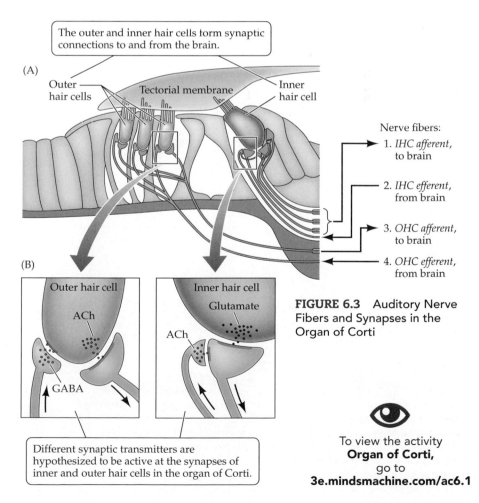

FIGURE 6.3 Auditory Nerve Fibers and Synapses in the Organ of Corti

To view the activity **Organ of Corti,** go to 3e.mindsmachine.com/ac6.1

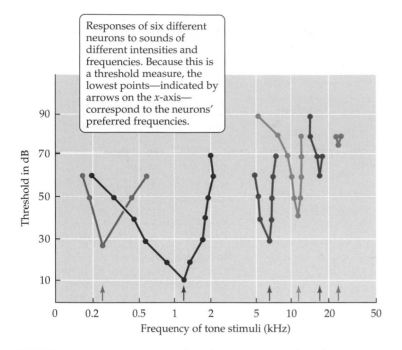

Responses of six different neurons to sounds of different intensities and frequencies. Because this is a threshold measure, the lowest points—indicated by arrows on the *x*-axis—correspond to the neurons' preferred frequencies.

FIGURE 6.4 Tuning Curves of Auditory Nerve Cells (After N. Y-S. Kiang et al., 1965. *Discharge patterns of single fibers in the cat's auditory nerve.* MIT Press. Cambridge, MA.)

cochlear nuclei Brainstem nuclei that receive input from auditory hair cells and send output to the superior olivary nuclei.

this electromechanical action, the brain continually modifies the stiffness of regions of the basilar membrane, resulting in both sharpened tuning and pronounced amplification (Hudspeth, 2014).

Now that the inner ear has transduced the vibrations from sound into trains of action potentials, the auditory signals must leave the cochlea and enter the brain.

Auditory Signals Run from Cochlea to Cortex

On each side of your head, about 30,000–50,000 auditory fibers from the cochlea make up the auditory part of the vestibulocochlear nerve (cranial nerve VIII), and most of these afferent fibers carry information from the IHCs (each of which stimulates several nerve fibers) to the brain. If we record from these IHC afferents, we find that each one has a maximum sensitivity to sound of a particular frequency but will also respond to neighboring frequencies if the sound is loud enough. For example, the auditory neuron whose responses are shown in red in **FIGURE 6.4** has its best frequency at 1,200 Hz (1.2 kHz)—that is, it is sensitive to even a very weak tone at 1,200 Hz—but for sounds that are 20 dB louder, the cell will respond to frequencies from 500 to 1,800 Hz. We call this the cell's tuning curve. If the brain received a signal from only one such fiber, it would not be able to tell whether the stimulus was a weak tone of 1,200 Hz or a stronger tone of 500 or 1,800 Hz, or any frequency in between. Instead, the brain analyzes the activity from thousands of such units simultaneously to calculate the intensity and frequency of each sound.

Within the brain, the auditory inputs are distributed via the ascending network shown in **FIGURE 6.5**. First, the auditory fibers terminate in the (sensibly named) **cochlear nuclei**, where some initial processing occurs. Output from the cochlear nuclei

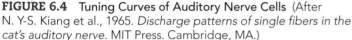

FIGURE 6.5 Auditory Pathways of the Human Brain

Auditory cortex

Medial geniculate nucleus

Inferior colliculus

Superior olivary nucleus

Cochlear nucleus

Cochlea

Brainstem

L   R

Binaural (two-ear) interactions commence in the brainstem superior olivary nucleus. Most (but not all) of the information from each ear projects to the cortex on the opposite side of the brain, depicted by the blended colors in this schematic.

primarily projects to the **superior olivary nuclei**, each of which receives inputs from both right and left cochlear nuclei. This bilateral input makes the superior olivary nucleus the first brain site at which binaural (two-ear) processing occurs. As you might expect, this mechanism plays a key role in localizing sounds by comparing the two ears, as we'll discuss shortly.

The superior olivary nuclei pass information derived from both ears to the **inferior colliculi**, which are the primary auditory centers of the midbrain. Outputs of the inferior colliculi go to the **medial geniculate nuclei** of the thalamus. Pathways from the medial geniculate nuclei extend to several auditory cortical areas.

At every level of the auditory system, from cochlea to auditory cortex, auditory pathways display **tonotopic organization**; that is, the pathways for the different tones are spatially arranged like a topographic map (*topos* is Greek for "place") from low frequency (sounds that we perceive as lower-pitched or "bass") to high frequency (perceived as higher-pitched or "treble"). Furthermore, at the higher levels of the auditory system, auditory neurons are not only excited by specific frequencies, but also inhibited by neighboring frequencies, resulting in much sharper tuning of the frequency responses of these cells. This precision helps us discriminate tiny differences in the frequencies of sounds.

Brain-imaging studies in humans have confirmed that many sounds (tones, noises, and so on) activate the **primary auditory cortex** (**A1**), which is located on the upper surface of the temporal lobes (**FIGURE 6.6A**). Speech sounds produce similar activation, but they also activate other, more specialized auditory areas (**FIGURE 6.6B**). Interestingly, at least some of these regions are activated when hearing people try to lip-read—that is, to understand someone by watching that person's lips without auditory cues (Calvert et al., 1997; L. E. Bernstein et al., 2002). This suggests that the auditory cortex integrates other, nonauditory, information with sounds. (The organization of auditory cortical areas in other species is described in **A STEP FURTHER 6.1**, on the website.)

superior olivary nuclei Brainstem nuclei that receive input from both right and left cochlear nuclei and provide the first binaural analysis of auditory information.

inferior colliculi Paired gray matter structures of the dorsal midbrain that process auditory information.

medial geniculate nucleus Either of two nuclei—left and right—in the thalamus that receive input from the inferior colliculi and send output to the auditory cortex.

tonotopic organization The organization of auditory neurons according to an orderly map of stimulus frequency, from low to high.

primary auditory cortex Also called A1. The cortical region, located on the superior surface of the temporal lobe, that processes complex sounds transmitted from lower auditory pathways.

To view the animation
Mapping Auditory Frequencies,
go to
3e.mindsmachine.com/av6.4

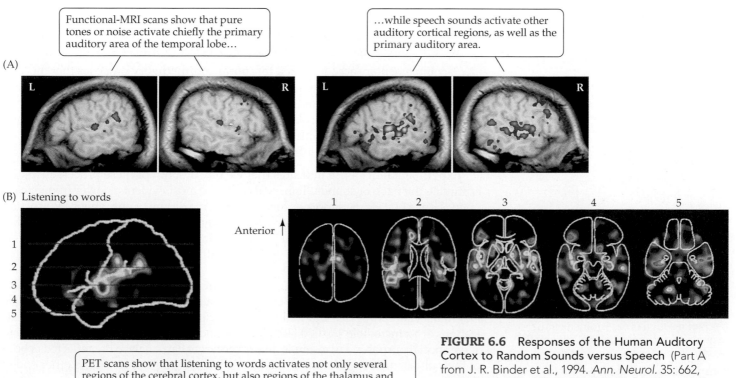

(A)

> Functional-MRI scans show that pure tones or noise activate chiefly the primary auditory area of the temporal lobe…

> …while speech sounds activate other auditory cortical regions, as well as the primary auditory area.

(B) Listening to words

Anterior

> PET scans show that listening to words activates not only several regions of the cerebral cortex, but also regions of the thalamus and the cerebellum. The numbered horizontal lines in the left panel correspond to the levels of the horizontal sections in the panel at right.

FIGURE 6.6 Responses of the Human Auditory Cortex to Random Sounds versus Speech (Part A from J. R. Binder et al., 1994. *Ann. Neurol.* 35: 662, courtesy of Jeffrey Binder; B from M. I. Posner and M. E. Raichle, 1994. *Images of mind.* Scientific American Library. New York, NY, courtesy of Marcus Raichle.)

HOW'S IT GOING ?

1. Identify the major components of the external ear. What does the external ear do?
2. Identify the three ossicles, and explain their function. To what structures do the ossicles connect, and how is their action moderated?
3. Provide a brief description of the organ of Corti, naming the components that are most important for the perception of sound.
4. Explain how the movement of hair cells transduces sound waves into action potentials. Compare and contrast the functions of inner hair cells and outer hair cells.
5. Sketch the major anatomical components of the auditory projections in the brain. Where does binaural processing first occur? What is tonotopic organization? What kind of processing does auditory cortex perform?

Our Sense of Pitch Relies on Two Signals from the Cochlea

At least when we're young, most of us can hear sounds ranging from 20 Hz to about 20,000 Hz, and within this range we can distinguish between sounds that differ by just a few hertz. Differences in frequency are important for our sense of pitch, but *pitch* and *frequency* are not synonymous. *Frequency* describes a *physical* property of sounds (see Box 6.1), but *pitch* relates solely to our subjective *perception* of those sounds. This is an important distinction because frequency is not the sole determinant of perceived pitch; at some frequencies, higher-intensity sounds may seem higher-pitched, and changes in pitch do not precisely parallel changes in frequency.

How do we distinguish pitches? Two signals from the cochlea appear to inform the brain about the pitch of sounds:

1. According to **place coding theory**, the pitch of a sound is determined by the location of activated hair cells along the length of the basilar membrane, as we discussed in this chapter's "Researchers at Work" feature. So, activation of receptors near the base of the cochlea (which is narrow and stiff and responds to high frequencies) signals *treble*, and activation of receptors nearer the apex (which is wide and floppy and responds to low frequencies) signals *bass*.

2. A complementary account called **temporal coding theory** proposes that the frequency of auditory stimuli is encoded in the rate of firing of auditory neurons. For example, a 500 Hz sound might cause some auditory neurons to fire 500 action potentials per second. *Volleys* of action potentials being produced at this rate, by a number of neurons with similar tunings, provide the brain with a reliable additional source of pitch information.

Experimental evidence indicates that we rely on both of these processes to discriminate the pitch of sounds. Temporal coding is most evident at lower frequencies, up to about 4,000 Hz: auditory neurons can fire a maximum of only about 1,000 action potentials per second, but to a limited extent they can encode sound frequencies that are multiples of the action potential frequency. Beyond about 4,000 Hz, however, this encoding becomes impossible, and pitch discrimination relies on place coding of pitch along the basilar membrane.

Mammalian species employ a huge range of frequencies in their vocalizations, from infrasound (less than 10 Hz) in elephants and whales to ultrasound (greater than 20,000 Hz) in bats and porpoises and many other species (the ghost-faced bat emits vocalizations at an incredible 160,000 Hz). These sounds have been shaped by evolution to serve special purposes. For example, many species of bats analyze the reflected echoes of their ultrasonic vocalizations to navigate and hunt in the dark. At the other end of the spectrum, elephants emit ultra-low-frequency alarm calls that are so powerful that they travel partly through the ground and are detected seismically by other elephants

place coding theory   Theory that the pitch of a sound is determined by the location of activated hair cells along the length of the basilar membrane.

temporal coding theory   Theory that the pitch of a sound is determined by the rate of firing of auditory neurons.

(O'Connell-Rodwell, 2007; Herbst et al., 2012) and yet are so nuanced that the elephants can distinguish human-related threats from bee-related threats (Soltis et al., 2014).

Brainstem Systems Compare the Ears to Localize Sounds

Being able to quickly identify where a sound is coming from—whether it is the crack of a twig under a predator's foot, or the sweet tones of a would-be mate—is a matter of great evolutionary significance. So it's no surprise that we are remarkably good at locating a sound source (our accuracy is about ±1 degree horizontally around the head, and many animals are even better). The auditory system accomplishes this feat by analyzing two kinds of binaural cues that signal the location of a sound source:

1. **Interaural intensity differences** (IIDs) are differences in *loudness* at the two ears (*interaural* means "between the two ears"). Depending on the species—and the placement and characteristics of their pinnae—intensity differences occur because one ear is pointed more directly toward the sound source or because the head casts a sound shadow (**FIGURE 6.7A**), preventing sounds originating on one side (called *off-axis sounds*) from reaching both ears with equal loudness. The head shadow (or sound shadow) effect is most pronounced for higher-frequency sounds (**FIGURE 6.7B**).

2. **Interaural temporal differences** (ITDs) are differences between the two ears in the *time of arrival* of sounds. They arise because one ear is always a little closer to an off-axis sound than the other ear is. Two kinds of temporal (time) differences are present in a sound: *onset disparity*, which is the difference between the two ears in hearing the beginning of the sound; and *ongoing phase disparity*, which is the continuing mismatch between the two ears in the arrival of all the peaks and troughs that make up the sound wave. These cues are illustrated in **FIGURE 6.7C**.

Both types of cues are employed in sound localization. At low frequencies, though, no matter where sounds are presented horizontally around the head, there are virtually no intensity differences between the ears. For these frequencies, differences in times of arrival are the principal cues for sound localization (and at very low

interaural intensity difference (IID) A perceived difference in loudness between the two ears, which the nervous system can use to localize a sound source.

interaural temporal difference (ITD) A difference between the two ears in the time of arrival of a sound, which the nervous system can use to localize a sound source.

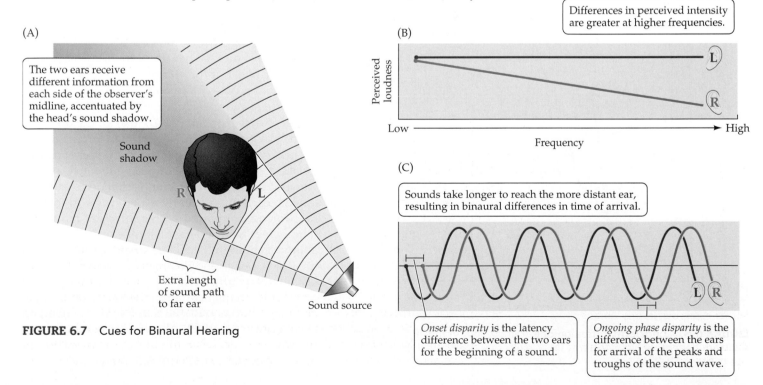

(A)

The two ears receive different information from each side of the observer's midline, accentuated by the head's sound shadow.

Sound shadow

R   L

Extra length of sound path to far ear

Sound source

FIGURE 6.7 Cues for Binaural Hearing

(B)

Differences in perceived intensity are greater at higher frequencies.

Perceived loudness

Low ———————————————→ High

Frequency

L

R

(C)

Sounds take longer to reach the more distant ear, resulting in binaural differences in time of arrival.

L R

Onset disparity is the latency difference between the two ears for the beginning of a sound.

Ongoing phase disparity is the difference between the ears for arrival of the peaks and troughs of the sound wave.

frequencies, neither cue is much help; this is why you can place the subwoofer of an audio system anywhere you want within a room). At higher frequencies, however, the sound shadow cast by the head produces significant binaural intensity differences. Of course, we can't perceive which types of processing we're relying on for any given sound; in general, we are aware of the results of neural processing but not the processing itself. (You can learn about brain mechanisms of auditory localization in **A STEP FURTHER 6.2**, on the website.)

The structure of the external ear provides yet another localization cue. As we mentioned earlier, the hills and valleys of the external ear selectively reinforce some frequencies in a complex sound and diminish others. This process is known as **spectral filtering**, and the frequencies that are affected depend on the angle at which the sound arrives at those peaks and valleys (Kulkarni and Colburn, 1998). That angle varies, of course, depending on where the sound came from; these spectral cues provide critical information about the vertical localization (or elevation) of a sound source. Without them, you would have a hard time knowing whether a sound from straight in front of you came from the ground or from the treetops. The various binaural and spectral cues used for sound localization converge and are integrated in the inferior colliculus (Slee and Young, 2014).

The Auditory Cortex Processes Complex Sound

In some sensory areas of the brain, lesions cause the loss of basic perceptions. For example, lesions of visual cortex result in blind spots, as we will discuss in Chapter 7. But the auditory cortex is different: researchers have long known that simple pure tones can be heard even after the entire auditory cortex has been surgically removed (Rosenzweig, 1946; Neff and Casseday, 1977). So if the auditory cortex is not involved in basic auditory perception, then what does it do? The auditory cortex seems to be specialized for the detection of more-complex "biologically relevant" sounds, of the sort we mentioned earlier—vocalizations of animals, footsteps, snaps, crackles, and pops—containing many frequencies and complex patterns (Theunissen and Elie, 2014). In other words, the auditory cortex evolved to process the sounds of everyday life.

The unique capabilities of the auditory cortex result from a sensitivity that is fine-tuned by experience as we grow (Kandler et al., 2009). Human infants have diverse hearing capabilities at birth, but their hearing for complex speech sounds in particular becomes more precise and rapid through exposure to the speech of their families and other people. Newborns can distinguish all the different sounds that are made in any human language. But as they develop, they get better and better at distinguishing sounds in the language(s) they hear, and worse at distinguishing sounds that occur in other languages. Similarly, early experience with binaural hearing, compared with equivalent monaural (one-eared) hearing, has a significant effect on the ability of children to localize sound sources later in life (W. D. Beggs and Foreman, 1980). Studies with lab animals confirm that experience with sounds of a particular frequency can cause a rapid retuning of auditory neurons (**FIGURE 6.8**) (N. M. Weinberger, 1998; Fritz et al., 2003). You can learn more about the role of experience in auditory localization in owls in **A STEP FURTHER 6.3**, on the website.

spectral filtering The process by which the hills and valleys of the external ear alter the amplitude of some, but not all, frequencies in a sound.

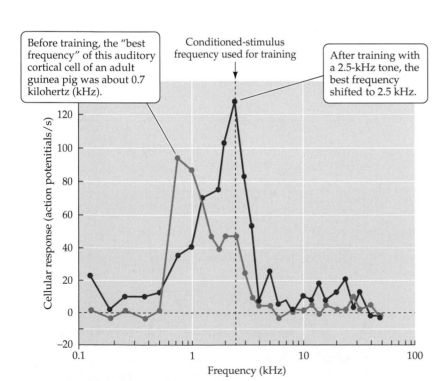

Before training, the "best frequency" of this auditory cortical cell of an adult guinea pig was about 0.7 kilohertz (kHz).

Conditioned-stimulus frequency used for training

After training with a 2.5-kHz tone, the best frequency shifted to 2.5 kHz.

FIGURE 6.8 Long-Term Retention of a Trained Shift in the Tuning of an Auditory Receptive Field (After N. M. Weinberger, 1998. *Neurobiol. of Learn. Mem.* 70: 226.)

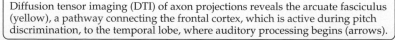

Diffusion tensor imaging (DTI) of axon projections reveals the arcuate fasciculus (yellow), a pathway connecting the frontal cortex, which is active during pitch discrimination, to the temporal lobe, where auditory processing begins (arrows).

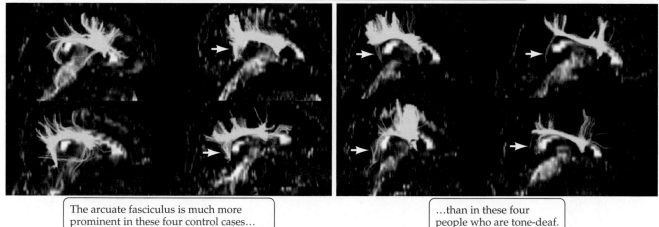

The arcuate fasciculus is much more prominent in these four control cases...

...than in these four people who are tone-deaf.

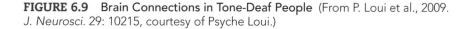

FIGURE 6.9 Brain Connections in Tone-Deaf People (From P. Loui et al., 2009. *J. Neurosci.* 29: 10215, courtesy of Psyche Loui.)

Music also shapes the responses of auditory cortex. It might not surprise you to learn that the auditory cortex of trained musicians shows a bigger response to musical sounds than does the same cortex in nonmusicians. After all, when two people differ in any skill, their brains must be different in some way, and maybe people born with brains that are more responsive to complex sounds are also more likely to become musicians. The surprising part is that the extent to which a musician's brain is extra sensitive to musical notes is correlated with the age at which they began their serious training in music: the earlier the training began, the bigger the difference in auditory cortex in adulthood (Pantev et al., 1998). This finding indicates that intensive musical experience in development alters the functioning of auditory cortex later in life. By adulthood, the portion of primary auditory cortex where music is first processed, called *Heschl's gyrus*, is more than twice as large in professional musicians as in nonmusicians, and more than twice as strongly activated by music (P. Schneider et al., 2002). As we've discussed, at least part of this difference is attributable to early experience with music. Furthermore, cortical regions that process music are reportedly influenced by the brain's mesolimbic reward system (see Chapter 4) to attach a reward value to music that is new to us (Salimpoor et al., 2015).

So, to what extent is music perception innate? Some people show a lifelong inability to discern tunes or sing, called **amusia**. Amusia is associated with subtly abnormal function in the right frontal lobe and impoverished connectivity between frontal and temporal cortex (**FIGURE 6.9**) (K. L. Hyde et al., 2006; Loui et al., 2009). The result is an inability to consciously access pitch information, even though cortical pitch-processing systems are intact (Zendel et al., 2015). Interestingly, studies of people with amusia indicate that when listening to music, we process pitch and rhythm quite separately (K. L. Hyde and Peretz, 2004). If you're worried about your own ability to carry a tune, the National Institutes of Health (NIH) provides an online test of pitch perception at www.nidcd.nih.gov/tunestest/test-your-sense-pitch.

Hearing Loss Is a Widespread Problem

Disorders of hearing, including **hearing loss** (defined as a moderate to severe decrease in sensitivity to sound) and **deafness** (defined as hearing loss so profound that speech cannot be perceived even with the use of hearing aids), affect some 37.5 million people in the United States alone (Blackwell et al., 2014). By now, you may have anticipated that there are three kinds of problems that can prevent sound waves in the air from

amusia A disorder characterized by the inability to discern tunes accurately or to sing.

hearing loss Decreased sensitivity to sound, in varying degrees.

deafness Hearing loss so profound that speech perception is lost.

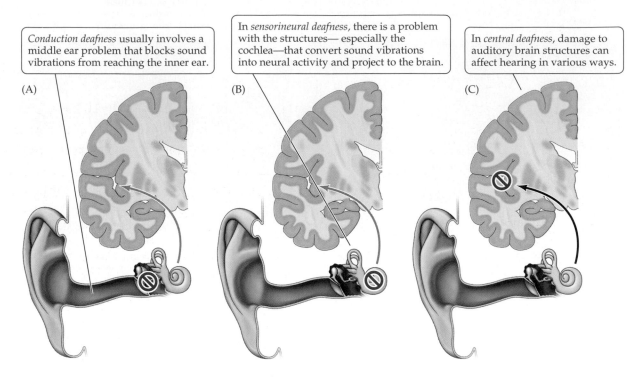

Conduction deafness usually involves a middle ear problem that blocks sound vibrations from reaching the inner ear.

In *sensorineural deafness*, there is a problem with the structures— especially the cochlea—that convert sound vibrations into neural activity and project to the brain.

In *central deafness*, damage to auditory brain structures can affect hearing in various ways.

(A)   (B)   (C)

FIGURE 6.10   Types of Hearing Loss

conduction deafness   A hearing impairment in which the ears fail to convert sound vibrations in air into waves of fluid in the cochlea. It is associated with defects of the external ear or middle ear.

sensorineural deafness   A hearing impairment most often caused by the permanent damage or destruction of hair cells or by interruption of the vestibulocochlear nerve that carries auditory information to the brain.

tinnitus   A sensation of noises or ringing in the ears not caused by external sound.

central deafness   A hearing impairment in which the auditory areas of the brain fail to process and interpret action potentials from sound stimuli in meaningful ways, usually as a consequence of damage in auditory brain areas.

word deafness   A form of central deafness that is characterized by the specific inability to hear words although other sounds can be detected.

cortical deafness   A form of central deafness, caused by damage to both sides of the auditory cortex, that is characterized by difficulty in recognizing all complex sounds, whether verbal or nonverbal.

being transformed into conscious auditory perceptions: a problem with sound waves reaching the cochlea, trouble converting sound waves into action potentials, and dysfunction of brain mechanisms that process sound (**FIGURE 6.10**):

1. Before anything even happens in the nervous system, the ear may fail to convert the sound vibrations in air into waves of fluid within the cochlea. This form of hearing loss, called **conduction deafness** (**FIGURE 6.10A**), often comes about when the ossicles of the middle ear become fused together and vibrations of the eardrum can no longer be conveyed to the oval window of the cochlea.

2. Even if the vibration is successfully conducted to the cochlea, the sensory apparatus of the cochlea—the hair cells—may fail to respond to the ripples created in the basilar membrane and thus fail to create the action potentials to inform the brain about sounds. This form of hearing loss, termed **sensorineural deafness** (**FIGURE 6.10B**), is most often due to the permanent damage or destruction of hair cells by any of a variety of causes (**FIGURE 6.11**). Some people are born with genetic abnormalities that interfere with the function of hair cells (Petit and Richardson, 2009). Many more people acquire sensorineural deafness during their lives as a result of being exposed to extremely loud sounds—overamplified music, nearby gunshots, and industrial noise are important examples—or because of medical problems such as infections and adverse drug effects (certain antibiotics, such as streptomycin, are particularly *ototoxic*). If you don't think it can happen to you, think again. Anyone listening to something for more than 5 hours per week at 89 dB or louder is already exceeding workplace limits for hearing safety (SCENIHR, 2008), yet many personal music players and music at concerts and clubs exceed 100 dB. Fortunately, earplugs are available that attenuate all frequencies equally, making concerts a little quieter without muffling the music. Various sound sources are compared in **FIGURE 6.12**; if you are concerned about your own exposure, excellent sound

(A) Normal cochlea

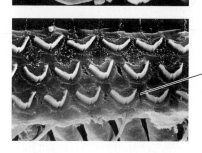

> In a normal cochlea, hair cells line the organ of Corti throughout its length, but exposure to excessively loud sounds can have rapid destructive effects. After exposure to excessive noise, a long section of the sound-damaged cochlea is completely missing its hair cells, resulting in deafness from the corresponding frequencies.

(B) Severe noise damage

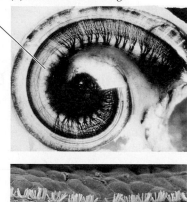

> Electron microscopy reveals that the orderly rows of stereocilia found in the organ of Corti in a normal cochlea are crushed and flattened by excessive noise exposure, like trees blown down in a windstorm.

FIGURE 6.11 The Destructive Effects of Loud Noise (Micrographs by H. Engstrom and B. Engstrom, courtesy of Widex.)

level meter apps for smartphones are available at little or no cost. Long-term exposure to loud sounds can cause hearing problems such as **tinnitus**—persistent ringing in the ears—and/or a profound loss of hearing for the frequencies being listened to at such high volumes.

3. For the action potentials sent from the cochlea to be of any use, the auditory areas of the brain must process and interpret them in meaningful ways. **Central deafness** (**FIGURE 6.10C**) occurs when auditory brain areas are damaged by, for example, strokes, tumors, or traumatic injuries. As you might expect from our earlier discussion of auditory processing in the brain, this type of deafness almost never involves a simple loss of auditory sensitivity. Afflicted individuals can often hear a normal range of pure tones but are impaired in the perception of complex, behaviorally relevant sounds. An example in humans is **word deafness**: selective trouble with speech sounds despite normal speech and normal hearing for nonverbal sounds. In **cortical deafness**—a rare syndrome involving bilateral lesions of auditory cortex—patients have more-complete impairment, struggling to recognize all complex sounds, whether verbal or nonverbal.

> Because the decibel scale is logarithmic, a noise that is 10 dB greater is actually 100 times louder.

> Possible hearing loss in as little as 30 minutes.

> Extended exposure to sounds over 90 dB may be harmful. As little as 30 minutes of exposure to sounds over 110 dB can harm hearing.

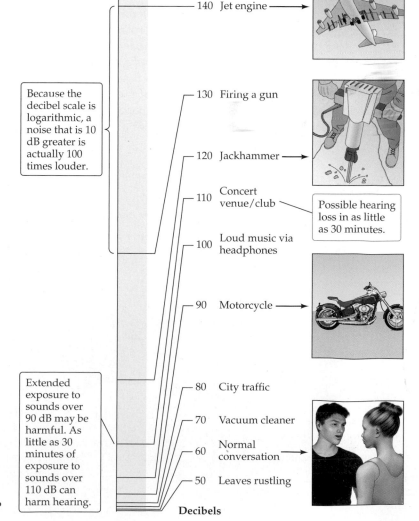

- 140 Jet engine
- 130 Firing a gun
- 120 Jackhammer
- 110 Concert venue/club
- 100 Loud music via headphones
- 90 Motorcycle
- 80 City traffic
- 70 Vacuum cleaner
- 60 Normal conversation
- 50 Leaves rustling

Decibels

FIGURE 6.12 How Loud Is Too Loud?

SIGNS & SYMPTOMS

Restoring Auditory Stimulation in Deafness

Although treatments for deafness have been greatly refined in the last few decades, they generally offer only partial restoration of the lost hearing. In cases of conduction deafness, it is sometimes possible to surgically free up the fused ossicles or replace them with Teflon prosthetics and thus restore the transmission of sound vibrations to the cochlea. But sensorineural deafness presents a much thornier problem because neural elements have been destroyed (or were absent from birth). Can new hair cells be grown? Fishes and amphibians produce new hair cells throughout life, but mammals historically have been viewed as incapable of regenerating hair cells. This conclusion may have been too hasty, however (Brigande and Heller, 2009). Using several different strategies, researchers have succeeded in inducing the birth of new hair cells in cochlear tissues of lab animals (Izumikawa et al., 2005; Koehler et al., 2013), so there is reason to hope that an effective restorative therapy for deafness may be available someday.

For now, treatments for deafness focus on the use of prostheses. Traditional hearing aids detect and amplify sounds to provide extra stimulation to an impaired—but still functional—auditory system. More recently, implantable devices called **cochlear implants** have been used to directly stimulate the auditory nerve fibers of the cochlea, bypassing the ossicles and hair cells altogether and offering partial restoration of hearing even in cases of complete deafness (**FIGURE 6.13**) (Loeb, 1990; J. M. Miller and Spelman, 1990). You may have had doubts about the value of Békésy's work with cadavers that we described at the start of this chapter. If so, consider this: the cochlear implants that have brought hearing to thousands of deaf people work by reproducing the phenomena Békésy discovered. In other words, the device sends information about low frequencies to electrodes stimulating nerves at the apex of the cochlea and sends information about high frequencies to electrodes stimulating nerves at the base. As you might predict from our discussion of the importance of experience in shaping auditory responsiveness, the earlier in life these devices are implanted, the better the person will be able to understand complex sounds, especially speech (Geers et al., 2017). So in a sense, the success of these implants is due in part to the cleverness of the brain.

Within the Deaf community, the use of cochlear implants is the subject of a lively controversy. While many hearing people might assume that deaf people would automatically want to have their hearing restored, some Deaf advocates are concerned that cochlear implants threaten a vibrant Deaf culture. The solution may lie in ensuring through education that a child with cochlear implants retains a sense of belonging in both the hearing and Deaf communities, rather than being forced to identify with one or the other.

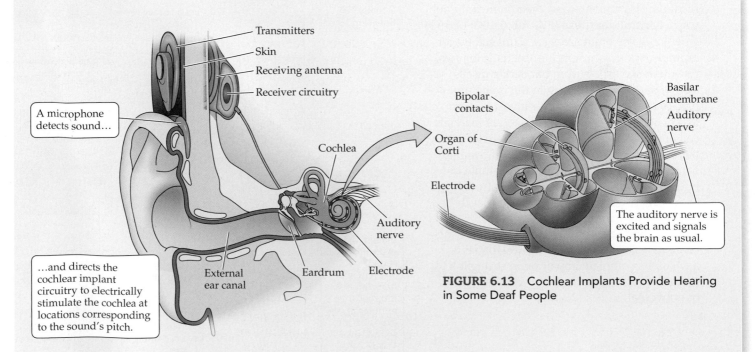

FIGURE 6.13 Cochlear Implants Provide Hearing in Some Deaf People

1. Compare and contrast the two important signals about pitch that the brain receives from the cochlea: place coding and temporal coding. How do they work together to give us our sense of pitch?
2. Discuss the sensory capabilities of different species as adaptations shaped by natural selection.
3. Provide an account of sound localization, identifying the several sources of information that we use to determine the source of a sound.
4. Discuss the types of processing that are performed by primary auditory cortex. Is experience with sound important for development of cortical auditory systems?
5. Name and describe the three major forms of deafness.

The Inner Ear Provides Our Sense of Balance

Without our sense of balance, it would be a challenge to simply stand on two feet. When you use an elevator, you clearly sense that your body is rising or falling, despite the sameness of your surroundings. When you turn your head, take a tight curve in your car, or bounce through the seas in a boat, your continual awareness of motion allows you to plan further movements and anticipate changes in perception due to movement of your head. And of course, too much of this sort of stimulation can make you lose your lunch.

Like hearing, our sense of balance is the product of the inner ear, relying on several small structures that adjoin the cochlea and are known collectively as the **vestibular system** (from the Latin *vestibulum*, "entrance hall," reflecting the fact that the system lies in hollow spaces in the temporal bone). In fact, it is generally accepted that the auditory organ evolved from the vestibular system, although the ossicles probably evolved from parts of the jaw. The most obvious components of the vestibular system are the three fluid-filled **semicircular canals**, plus two bulbs called the *saccule* and the *utricle* that are located near the ends of the semicircular canals (**FIGURE 6.14A**). Notice that the three canals are oriented in the three different planes in which the head can rotate (**FIGURE 6.14B**)—nodding up and down (technically known as *pitch*), shaking from side to side (*yaw*), and tilting left or right (*roll*).

The receptors of the vestibular system are hair cells—just like the ones in the cochlea—whose bending ultimately produces action potentials. The cilia of these hair cells are embedded in a gelatinous mass inside an enlarged chamber called the **ampulla** (plural *ampullae*) that lies at the base of the semicircular canals (see Figure 6.14B). Movement of the head in one axis sets up a flow of the fluid in the semicircular canal that lies in the same plane, deflecting the stereocilia in the ampulla and signaling the brain that the head has moved. Working together, the three semicircular canals accurately track the rotation of the head. The utricle and saccule each contain an otolithic membrane (a gelatinous sheet studded with tiny crystals; *otolith* literally means "ear stone") which, thanks to its mass, lags slightly when the head moves. This bends nearby hair cells, stimulating them to track straight-line acceleration and deceleration—the final signals that the brain needs in order to calculate the position and movement of the body in three-dimensional space.

Vestibular information is crucial for planning body movements, maintaining balance against gravity, and smoothly directing sensory organs like the eyes and ears toward specific locations, and the nerve pathways from the vestibular system have strong connections to brain regions responsible for the planning and control of movement. On entering the brainstem, many of the vestibular fibers of the vestibulocochlear nerve (cranial nerve VIII) terminate in the **vestibular nuclei**, while some fibers project directly to the cerebellum to aid in motor programming there. Outputs from the vestibular nuclei project in a complex manner to motor areas throughout the brain, including motor nuclei of the eye muscles, the thalamus, and the cerebral cortex.

cochlear implant   An electromechanical device that detects sounds and selectively stimulates nerves in different regions of the cochlea via surgically implanted electrodes.

vestibular system   The sensory system that detects balance. It consists of several small inner-ear structures that adjoin the cochlea.

semicircular canal   Any one of the three fluid-filled tubes in the inner ear that are part of the vestibular system. Each of the tubes, which are at right angles to each other, detects angular acceleration in a particular direction.

ampulla   An enlarged region of each semicircular canal that contains the receptor cells (hair cells) of the vestibular system.

vestibular nuclei   Brainstem nuclei that receive information from the vestibular organs through cranial nerve VIII (the vestibulocochlear nerve).

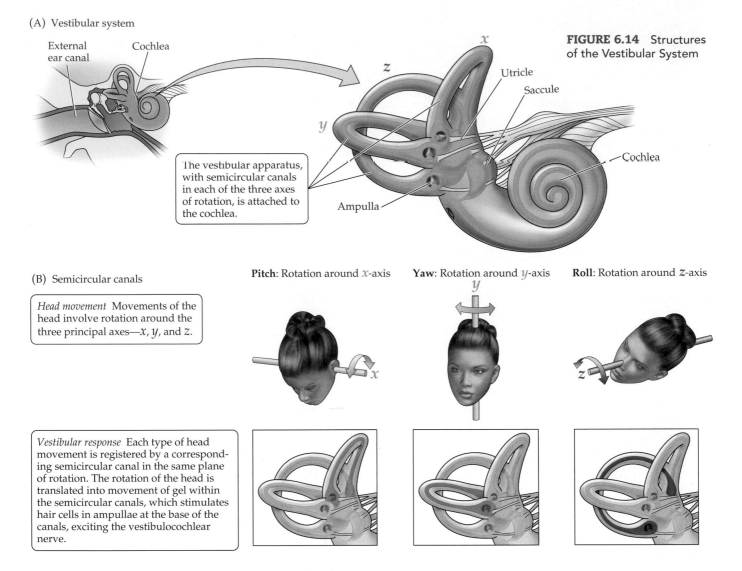

FIGURE 6.14 Structures of the Vestibular System

(A) Vestibular system

External ear canal

Cochlea

x

z

Utricle

Saccule

y

The vestibular apparatus, with semicircular canals in each of the three axes of rotation, is attached to the cochlea.

Cochlea

Ampulla

(B) Semicircular canals

Head movement Movements of the head involve rotation around the three principal axes—*x*, *y*, and *z*.

Pitch: Rotation around *x*-axis   **Yaw**: Rotation around *y*-axis   **Roll**: Rotation around *z*-axis

x   *y*   *z*

Vestibular response Each type of head movement is registered by a corresponding semicircular canal in the same plane of rotation. The rotation of the head is translated into movement of gel within the semicircular canals, which stimulates hair cells in ampullae at the base of the canals, exciting the vestibulocochlear nerve.

To view the animation
The Vestibular System,
go to
3e.mindsmachine.com/av6.5

motion sickness The experience of nausea brought on by unnatural passive movement, as may occur in a car or boat.

Some Forms of Vestibular Excitation Produce Motion Sickness

There is one aspect of vestibular activation that many of us would gladly do without. Too much strong vestibular stimulation—think of boats and roller coasters—can produce the misery of **motion sickness**. Motion sickness is caused by movements of the body that we cannot control. For example, passengers in a car are more likely to suffer from motion sickness than is the driver.

Why do we experience motion sickness? According to the *sensory conflict theory*, we feel bad when we receive contradictory sensory messages, especially a discrepancy between vestibular and visual information. When an airplane bounces around in turbulence, for instance, the vestibular system signals that various changes in direction and accelerations are occurring, but as far as the visual system is concerned, nothing is happening; the plane's interior is a constant. One hypothesis is that the stimulation is activating a system that originally evolved to rid the body of swallowed poison (M. Treisman, 1977). According to this hypothesis, discrepancies in sensory information might normally signal a dangerous neurological problem, triggering dizziness and vomiting to get rid of potentially toxic food. However, there is little objective evidence to support the "poison hypothesis," and overall the evolutionary origins of motion sickness remain a mystery (Oman, 2012). The observation that virtual reality devices frequently induce motion sickness, and that susceptibility to this sickness is associated with individual differences in pre-test body sway, has been interpreted as evidence that motion sickness results from postural instability rather than sensory conflict (Munafo et al., 2017).

flavor The sense of taste combined with the sense of smell.

taste Any of the five basic sensations detected by the tongue: sweet, salty, sour, bitter, and umami.

HOW'S IT GOING ?

1. Use a diagram to explain how the general layout of the vestibular system allows it to track movement in three axes. Where are the receptors for head movement located? Do they resemble other types of sensory receptors?
2. Where are the vestibular nuclei located? What nerve provides inputs to these nuclei?
3. How is vestibular information used in ongoing behavior?
4. Discuss the role of the vestibular system in motion sickness.

PART II
The Chemical Senses: Taste and Smell

THE ROAD AHEAD

The second part of the chapter is an exploration of the specialized senses that rely on chemical signals in the environment. After studying this material you should be able to:

1. Name the 5 basic tastes, discuss the ecological importance of each type of taste, and distinguish taste from flavor.
2. Describe the structure of the tongue, the cells that give rise to taste sensations, and the specialized cellular sensors for each type of basic taste.
3. Describe the organization of the principle olfactory structures in the nose and brain, and explain how olfactory receptor neurons sense odorants.
4. Discuss the perception of pheromones in humans and nonhuman animals.

Chemicals in Our Food Are Perceived as Five Basic Tastes

Delicious foods, poisons, dangerous adversaries, and fertile mates—these are just a few of the sources of chemical signals in the environment. Being able to detect these signals is vital for survival and reproduction throughout the animal kingdom.

Most people derive great pleasure from eating delicious food, and because we recognize many substances by their distinct flavors, we tend to think that we can discriminate many tastes. In reality, though, humans detect only a small number of basic tastes; the huge variety of sensations aroused by different foods are actually **flavors** rather than simple tastes, and they rely on the sense of smell as well as taste. (To appreciate the importance of smell to flavor, block your nose while eating first a little bit of raw potato and then some apple: without smell, you can't tell them apart!)

Scientists are in broad agreement that we possess five basic **tastes**: salty, sour, sweet, bitter, and umami. (*Umami*, Japanese for "delicious taste," is the term for the savory, meaty taste that is characteristic of gravy or soy sauce.) These tastes are determined genetically, as we will see shortly, but there is considerable genetic variation across the globe in both the strength and pleasurable qualities of the basic tastes (Pirastu et al., 2016). Further, the hunt continues for additional basic tastes. For example, studies suggest that humans may possess a primary fat taste (Mattes, 2011); another candidate, called *kokumi*, is described as the full-bodied, thick, mouth-filling quality of some foods (Brennan et al., 2014). But no matter how many basic tastes we are eventually shown to possess, it is clear that evolution shaped them to help us find nutritious food and avoid toxins.

FIGURE 6.15   A Cross Section of the **Tongue** (© Science Photo Library/Alamy Stock Photo.)

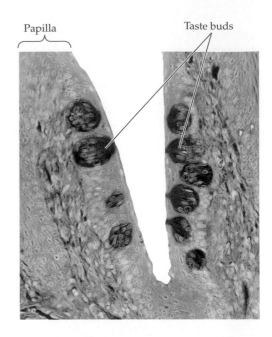

Papilla   Taste buds

Tastes excite specialized receptor cells on the tongue

Many people think that the myriad little bumps on their tongues are **taste buds**, but they aren't. They are actually **papillae** (singular *papilla*) (**FIGURE 6.15**), tiny lumps of tissue that increase the surface area of the tongue. There are three kinds of papillae—*circumvallate*, *foliate*, and *fungiform* papillae—occurring in different locations on the tongue (**FIGURE 6.16C**).

Taste buds, each consisting of a cluster of 50–150 taste receptor cells (**FIGURE 6.16A**), are found buried within the walls of the papillae (a single papilla may house several such taste buds; see Figure 6.15). Fine fibers, called *microvilli*, extend from the taste receptor cells into a tiny pore, where they can come into contact with substances that can be tasted, called *tastants* (**FIGURE 6.16B**). Each taste cell is sensitive to just one of the five basic tastes, and with a life span of only 10–14 days, taste cells are constantly being replaced. But as our varied experience with hot drinks, frozen flagpoles, or spicy foods informs us, taste is not the only sensory capability of the tongue. It also possesses sensory cells for pain, touch, and temperature.

Many books show a map of the tongue indicating that each taste is perceived mainly in one region (sweet at the tip of the tongue, bitter at the back, and so on), but this map is an enduring myth. All five basic tastes can be perceived anywhere on the tongue where there are taste receptors (Chandrashekar et al., 2006). Those areas do not differ greatly in the strength of taste sensations that they mediate (**FIGURE 6.16D**).

The five basic tastes are signaled by specific sensors on taste cells

The tastes salty and sour are evoked when taste cells are stimulated by simple ions acting on ion channels in the membranes of the taste cells. Sweet and bitter tastes are perceived by specialized receptor molecules and communicated by second messengers. And at least two types of receptors may be involved in the perception of umami.

SALTY   The transduction of the taste of salt (NaCl) is perhaps the easiest to understand because it relies mostly on ion channels of the sort we have seen in previous chapters. Sodium ions (Na^+) from salty food enter taste cells via sodium channels in the cell membrane, causing a depolarization of the cell and release of neurotransmitter. We know that this is a crucial mechanism for perceiving saltiness, because blocking the sodium channels with a drug greatly reduces—but does not eliminate—our ability to taste salt (Schiffman et al., 1986). The rest of our ability to taste salt comes from a second salt sensor, a variant of a receptor called *TRPV1* (*transient receptor*

taste bud   A cluster of 50–150 cells that detects tastes. Taste buds are found in papillae.

papilla   A small bump that projects from the surface of the tongue. Papillae contain most of the taste receptor cells.

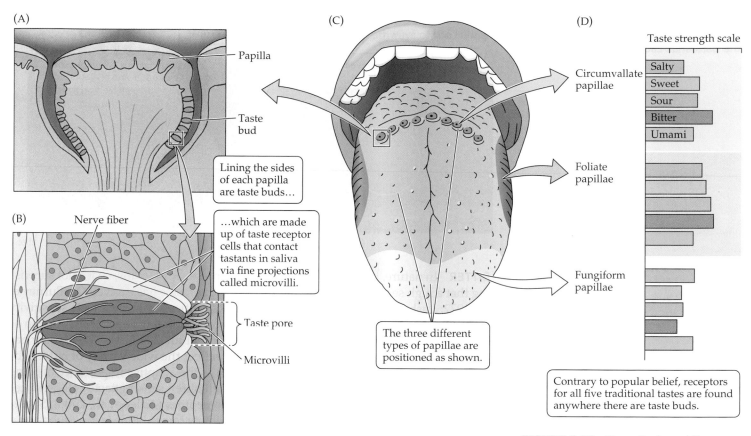

(A)

Papilla

Taste bud

Lining the sides of each papilla are taste buds…

…which are made up of taste receptor cells that contact tastants in saliva via fine projections called microvilli.

(B)

Nerve fiber

Taste pore

Microvilli

(C)

Circumvallate papillae

Foliate papillae

Fungiform papillae

The three different types of papillae are positioned as shown.

(D)

Taste strength scale

Salty
Sweet
Sour
Bitter
Umami

Contrary to popular belief, receptors for all five traditional tastes are found anywhere there are taste buds.

FIGURE 6.16 Taste Buds and Taste Receptor Cells (Part A after S. K. McLaughlin et al., 1994. *Physiol. Behav.* 56: 1157; C after L. M. Bartoshuk in D. Chadwick et al., 1993. *The Molecular Basis of Smell and Taste Transduction.* Wiley. New York and J. Chandrashekar et al., 2006. *Nature* 444: 288.)

To view the activity
Taste Buds and Taste Receptor Cells,
go to
3e.mindsmachine.com/ac6.2

potential vanilloid type 1), that not only gives us a bit of extra sensitivity to Na^+, but also detects the positively charged ions (cations) of other salts in food, such as potassium (K^+) (Treesukosol et al., 2007). Depolarization of the salt-sensitive taste cells causes them to release neurotransmitters that stimulate afferent neurons that relay the information to the brain.

SOUR   Acids in food taste sour—the more acidic the food, the more sour it tastes—but no one knows exactly how sour tastants are detected. Researchers think that the protons (H^+, also called *hydrogen ions*) that all acids release may interact with special acid-sensing ion channels (like the ionotropic receptors in Chapters 3 and 4) to change the polarity of taste cells and alter transmitter release. It seems that all sour-sensitive taste cells contain a particular type of ion channel protein and share an inward flow of protons that depolarizes the cell (Huang et al., 2006; Bushman et al., 2015). Interestingly, the same sensor appears to detect the sensation and taste of carbonation in drinks (Chandrashekar et al., 2009).

SWEET   The receptors for sweet, bitter, and umami tastes are more like metabotropic receptors than ionotropic receptors (see Figure 4.2) because tastant molecules bind to a complex receptor protein on the taste cell's surface that activates a second messenger within the cell. These receptors are made up of simpler proteins belonging to two families—designated **T1R** and **T2R**—that are combined in various ways.

     When two members of the T1R family—T1R2 and T1R3—combine (*heterodimerize*), they make a receptor that selectively detects sweet tastants (Nelson et al., 2001). Mice engineered to lack either T1R2 or T1R3 are insensitive to sweet tastes (Zhao et al., 2003). And if you've spent any time around cats, you may be aware that they couldn't care less about sweets. It turns out that in all cats, from tabbies to tigers, the gene that encodes T1R2 is disabled, so their sweet receptors don't work (X. Li et al., 2009).

T1R   A family of taste receptor proteins that, when particular members bind together, form taste receptors for sweet flavors and umami flavors.

T2R   A family of bitter taste receptors.

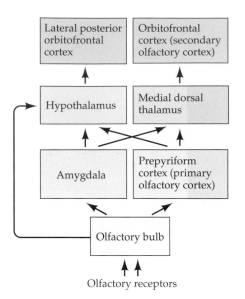

FIGURE 6.21 Components of the Brain's Olfactory System

pheromone A chemical signal that is released outside the body of an animal and affects other members of the same species.

vomeronasal system A specialized sensory system that detects pheromones and transmits information to the brain.

vomeronasal organ (VNO) A collection of specialized receptor cells, near to but separate from the olfactory epithelium, that detect pheromones and send electrical signals to the accessory olfactory bulb in the brain.

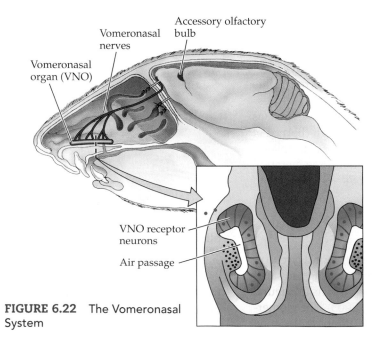

FIGURE 6.22 The Vomeronasal System

of smells, with neighboring glomeruli receiving inputs from receptors that are closely related. And, as Figure 6.20 shows, the spatial organization of glomeruli within the olfactory bulbs reflects the segregation of the four receptor protein subfamilies in the olfactory epithelium (Mori et al., 1999). This glomerular organization is established during a critical period in early life, after which it becomes fixed (Tsai and Barnea, 2014), resulting in an "olfactotopic" map that is maintained within the olfactory projections throughout the brain.

Olfactory information is conveyed to the brain via the axons of mitral cells (see Figure 6.19), which extend from the glomeruli in the olfactory bulbs to various regions of the forebrain; smell is the only sensory modality that synapses directly in the cortex rather than having to pass through the thalamus. Important targets for olfactory inputs include the hypothalamus, the amygdala, and the prepyriform cortex (**FIGURE 6.21**). These limbic structures are closely involved in memory and emotion, which may help explain the potency of odors in evoking nostalgic memories of childhood (M. Larsson and Willander, 2009).

Many vertebrates possess a vomeronasal system

Though many perfumers have tried to create one, there is no perfume for humans that is as alluring as the natural scents that other species use to find possible mates. The majority of terrestrial vertebrates—mammals, amphibians, and reptiles—possess a secondary chemical detection system that is specialized for detecting such **pheromones**. The system is called the **vomeronasal system** (**FIGURE 6.22**), and its receptors are found in the **vomeronasal organ** (**VNO**), near the olfactory epithelium.

In rodents, the sensory neurons of the VNO make hundreds of different vomeronasal receptor proteins, belonging to two large families called *V1R* and *V2R* (Dulac and Torello, 2003). These receptors are extremely sensitive, able to detect very low levels of the pheromone signals—such as sex hormone metabolites and signals of genetic relatedness—that are released by other individuals (Leinders-Zufall et al., 2000; Loconto et al., 2003). From the VNO, information is transmitted to the accessory olfactory bulb (adjacent to the main olfactory bulb), which projects to the medial amygdala and hypothalamus, structures that play crucial roles in governing emotional and sexual behaviors and in regulating hormone secretion. Hamsters and mice can distinguish relatives from nonrelatives just by smell (Mateo and Johnston, 2000; Isles et al., 2001), allowing these animals to optimize their reproductive activities. In parallel, dedicated mechanisms in olfactory cortex activate fear in response to predator odor signals, with immediate and obvious benefit (Kondoh et al., 2016).

Do humans communicate via pheromones? Studies reporting pheromone-like phenomena in humans attract plenty of media attention because of the apparent link to our evolutionary past. Well-known examples include the report that simple exposure to each other's bodily odors can cause women's menstrual cycles to synchronize (Stern and McClintock, 1998) and a report that exposure to female tears causes reductions in testosterone and sexual arousal in men (Gelstein et al., 2011). However, the VNO is either vestigial or absent in humans, and almost all of our V1R and V2R receptor genes have become nonfunctional "pseudogenes" over evolutionary time (Lübke and Pause, 2015). So, if humans do use olfactory communication, it is most likely accomplished using the main olfactory epithelium, and not the VNO. In mice, receptors in the main olfactory epithelium called **TAARs** (for **trace amine–associated receptors**) reportedly respond to sex-specific pheromones instead of odorants (Liberles and Buck, 2006), and mice with their TAAR genes knocked out stop reacting to certain urinary odor signals, even in the urine of predators (Dewan et al., 2013). Thus it seems the old notion that the olfactory epithelium detects odors while the VNO detects pheromones is an oversimplification, even in rodents. And because TAARs are also found in the human olfactory epithelium (Liberles, 2009), behavioral evidence indicating that humans respond to pheromones no longer presents a paradox. If rodents can detect pheromones through the olfactory epithelium, using TAARs or other yet-unknown mechanisms, then perhaps we can too. Whatever the details of the mechanism may be, evidence is rapidly accumulating that odor is an ecologically important channel for human social communication (de Groot et al., 2017).

trace amine–associated receptor (TAAR)   Any one of a family of probable pheromone receptors produced by neurons in the main olfactory epithelium.

HOW'S IT GOING ?

1. Discuss odor sensitivity in humans. How do we compare with other species?
2. Provide a brief sketch of the olfactory epithelium, showing the major cell types and their relationships to the brain.
3. Discuss the genetics of odor receptors, as well as their spatial organization in the nose and olfactory bulbs. What is a glomerulus?
4. Which regions of the brain receive strong olfactory inputs? What is the significance of this arrangement for an animal's behavior?
5. Discuss the structures and receptors associated with pheromone sensitivity, and speculate about the ecological importance of pheromone sensitivity in humans and other animals. Are humans sensitive to pheromones?

Recommended Reading

Doty, R. L. (2015). *Handbook of Olfaction and Gustation* (3rd ed.). New York, NY: Wiley-Blackwell.

Horowitz, S. S. (2012). *The Universal Sense: How Hearing Shapes the Mind*. London, UK: Bloomsbury.

Menini, A. (2009). *The Neurobiology of Olfaction*. Boca Raton, FL: CRC Press.

Musiek, F. E., and Baran, J. A. (2018). *The Auditory System: Anatomy, Physiology, and Clinical Correlates* (2nd ed.). San Diego, CA: Plural.

Palmer, A., and Rees, A. (2010). *Oxford Handbook of Auditory Science*. Oxford, UK: Oxford University Press.

Wolfe, J. M., Kluender, K. R., Levi, D. M., Bartoshuk, L. M. et al. (2017). *Sensation & Perception* (5th ed.). Sunderland, MA: Oxford University Press/Sinauer.

Wyatt, T. D. (2014). *Pheromones and Animal Behavior: Chemical Signals and Signatures* (2nd ed.). Cambridge, UK: Cambridge University Press.

Yost, W. A. (2013). *Fundamentals of Hearing* (5th ed.). San Diego, CA: Academic Press.

You should be able to relate each summary to the adjacent illustration, including structures and processes. If you go to the website for our text (3e.mindsmachine.com), you can follow links to figures, animations, and activities that will help you consolidate the material.

1 The **pinna** (external ear) captures, focuses, and filters sound. The sound arriving at the **tympanic membrane** (eardrum) is focused by the three **ossicles** of the **middle ear** onto the **oval window** to stimulate the fluid-filled **inner ear** (specifically, the cochlea). Review **Figure 6.1**, **Animations 6.2** and **6.3**

2 Sound arriving at the oval window causes traveling waves to sweep along the **basilar membrane** of the **cochlea**. For sounds of high **frequency**, the largest displacement of the basilar membrane is at the base of the cochlea, near the oval window; for low-frequency sounds, the largest amplitude is near the apex of the cochlea. Review **Figure 6.2**, **Box 6.1**

3 Movement of the **stereocilia** of **the hair** cells causes the opening and closing of ion channels, thereby **transducing** mechanical movement into changes in electrical potential. These changes in potential stimulate the nerve cell endings that contact the hair cells. Review **Figure 6.3**

4 The **organ of Corti** has both **inner hair cells** (IHCs, about 3,500 in humans) and **outer hair cells** (OHCs, about 12,000 in humans). The inner hair cells convey most of the information about sounds. The outer hair cells change their length under the control of the brain, amplifying the movements of the basilar membrane in response to sound and sharpening the frequency tuning of the cochlea. Review **Figure 6.3**, **Activity 6.1**

5 Afferents from the inner hair cells transmit auditory information to the **cochlear nuclei** of the brainstem. Cochlear neurons project bilaterally to the **superior olivary nucleus**, which in turn innervates the **inferior colliculus**. From there auditory information is relayed to the **medial geniculate nucleus** and then the **primary auditory cortex** in the temporal lobe. Review **Figure 6.5**, **Animation 6.4**

6 Auditory localization depends on differences in the sounds arriving at the two ears. For low-frequency sounds, **interaural temporal differences** (differences in time of arrival at the two ears) are especially important. For high-frequency sounds, **interaural intensity differences** are especially important, and **spectral filtering** provides cues about elevation. Review **Figure 6.7**

7 Primary auditory cortex is specialized for processing complex, biologically important sounds, rather than **pure tones**. Experiences with sound early in life can influence later auditory localization and the responses of neurons in auditory pathways. Experiences later in life can also lead to changes in the responses of auditory neurons. Review **Figures 6.8** and **6.9**

8 **Conduction deafness** consists of impairments in the transmission of sound through the external or middle ear to the cochlea. **Sensorineural deafness** arises in the cochlea, often because of the destruction of hair cells, or in the auditory nerve. **Central deafness** stems from brain damage. Review **Figure 6.10**

9 Some forms of deafness may be alleviated by direct electrical stimulation of the auditory nerve by a **cochlear implant**. Genetic manipulations can induce new hair cell growth in laboratory animals, raising hope of a gene therapy for sensorineural deafness. Review **Figure 6.13**

10 The receptors of the **vestibular system** that detect movement of the head lie within the inner ear next to the cochlea. In mammals the vestibular system consists of three **semicircular canals** plus the utricle and the saccule. The semicircular canals use hair cells to detect rotation of the body in three planes, and the utricle and saccule sense static positions and linear accelerations. Review **Figure 6.14**, **Animation 6.5**

11 Humans detect only five main **tastes**—salty, sour, sweet, bitter, and **umami**—using taste receptor cells located in clusters called **taste buds**. Taste cells extend fine filaments into the taste pore of each bud, where tastants come into contact with them. The taste buds are situated on small projections from the surface of the tongue called **papillae**. The tastes of salty and sour are evoked primarily by the action of simple ions on ion channels in the membranes of taste cells. Sweet, umami, and bitter tastes are perceived by specialized receptor molecules belonging to the **T1R** and **T2R** families, which are coupled to G proteins. Review **Figure 6.16**, **Activity 6.2**

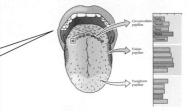

12 Each taste cell transmits information via cranial nerves to brainstem nuclei. This **gustatory system** extends from the taste receptor cells through brainstem nuclei to the thalamus and then to the cerebral cortex. Each taste axon responds most strongly to one category of tastes, providing a labeled line to the brain. Review **Figure 6.18**

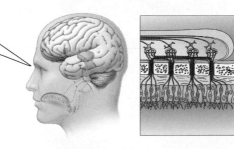

13 In contrast to being able to detect only a few tastes, humans can detect a huge number of different **odors**. Olfactory receptor neurons extend dendrites in the **olfactory epithelium** that express olfactory receptor proteins. The fine, unmyelinated axons of olfactory neurons project to the **olfactory bulbs** and synapse within **glomeruli**. If an olfactory receptor cell dies, an adjacent cell will replace it. Review **Figure 6.19**, **Animation 6.6**

14 There is a large family of odor receptor molecules, each of which utilizes G proteins and second messengers. Large subfamilies of receptors are synthesized in distinct bands of the olfactory epithelium. Review **Figure 6.20**

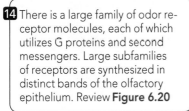

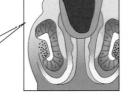

15 Outputs from the olfactory bulb extend to prepyriform cortex, amygdala, and hypothalamus, among other brain regions. Olfactory projections to the cortex maintain a stereotyped olfactory map of slightly overlapping projections from the glomeruli. Review **Figure 6.21**

16 The **vomeronasal organ** (**VNO**) contains receptors to detect pheromones released from other individuals of the species. These receptors transmit signals to the accessory olfactory bulb, which in turn communicates with the amygdala. **Pheromones** can also be detected by specialized receptors in the main olfactory epithelium. Review **Figure 6.22**

Go to **3e.mindsmachine.com** for study questions, quizzes, flashcards, and other resources.

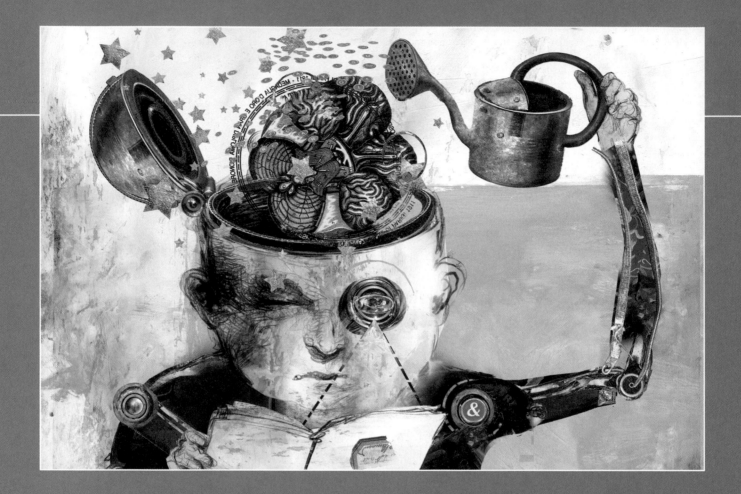

7

Vision
From Eye to Brain

When Seeing Isn't Seeing

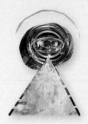

It was cold in the bathroom, so the young woman turned on a small heater before she got in the shower. She didn't know that the heater was malfunctioning, filling the room with deadly, odorless carbon monoxide gas. Her husband found her unconscious on the floor and called for an ambulance to rush her to the emergency room. When she regained consciousness, "D.F." seemed to have gotten off lightly, avoiding what could have been a fatal accident. She could understand the doctors' questions and reply sensibly, move all her limbs, and perceive touch on her skin. But something was wrong with her sight.

D.F. had lost the ability to identify things that she viewed. Even the faces of family members had become unfamiliar. More than a decade later, D.F. still could not recognize commonplace objects, yet she was not entirely blind. If you showed her a flashlight, she could tell you that it was made of shiny aluminum with some red plastic, but she didn't recognize it ("Is it a kitchen utensil?"). Without telling her what it was, if you asked her to pick it up, her hand moved directly to grasp the flashlight exactly as one normally does. Shown a slot in a piece of plastic, D.F. could not tell you whether the slot was oriented vertically, horizontally, or diagonally; but if you handed her a disk and asked her to put it through the slot, she invariably turned the disk so that it went smoothly through (Goodale et al., 1991).

Could D.F. see or not?

Many species rely on vision to find food and mates, avoid predators, and locate shelter. However, the sheer volume of visual information poses a serious problem.

Viewing the surrounding world has been compared to drinking from a waterfall. How does the visual system avoid being overwhelmed by the flood of information entering the eyes? One answer is that visual systems are especially sensitive to detecting *movement*, because moving objects are the most likely to represent the danger of predators or the good fortune of prey or mates. So the visual system often ignores information about stationary objects, which is why we have a harder time seeing them.

Another way to deal with information overload is for each species to evolve visual capabilities that are tailored to that species' particular lifestyle. Most nocturnal species have better night vision than do animals that are active during the day, like us. Most rodent species, such as rats and mice, which live in tunnels and close quarters, have poor vision for distant objects, while daytime hunters like hawks have incredibly keen distance vision. Birds and bees can detect ultraviolet light, allowing them to see patterns in flowers that we cannot. But even within our limits of sight, we humans process a remarkable amount of visual information, which keeps about one-third of our cerebral cortex busy analyzing it.

To see the video
Object Recognition,
go to
3e.mindsmachine.com/av7.1

retina The receptive surface inside the eye that contains photoreceptors and other neurons.

transduction The conversion of one form of energy to another, as converting light into neuronal activity.

cornea The transparent outer layer of the eye, whose curvature is fixed. The cornea bends light rays and is primarily responsible for forming the image on the retina.

refraction The bending of light rays by a change in the density of a medium, such as the cornea and the lens of the eyes.

lens A structure in the eye that helps focus an image on the retina.

ciliary muscle One of the muscles that control the shape of the lens inside the eye, focusing an image on the retina.

accommodation The process by which the ciliary muscles adjust the lens to bring nearby objects into focus.

To view the
Brain Explorer,
go to
3e.mindsmachine.com/av7.2

This chapter is organized according to the stages of visual processing. We'll begin by tracing the path of visual information into the eyes and brain, and then we'll move on to how the visual system analyzes forms. We'll conclude with color perception and the mysterious question of how D.F. can see *where* an object is placed in front of her and describe it in fine detail, yet be unable to say *what* that object is.

PART I
Vision Pathways

THE ROAD AHEAD

In the first part of this chapter you'll learn how light entering the eye affects the firing of neurons and how that visual information reaches the brain. By the end of this section, you should be able to:

1. Describe how a visual scene is projected onto the back of the eyes.
2. Identify the major types of neurons there, which detect and analyze light.
3. Explain how we are able to detect visual images over a very broad range of illumination.
4. Describe the orderly mapping of information from a visual scene projecting into the brain.

The Visual System Extends from the Eye to the Brain

The eye is an elaborate structure with optical functions, capturing light and projecting detailed images of the external world onto the back of the eye. There a layer of neurons, called the **retina**, turns the light into neural signals, in a process called **transduction**. So, good vision requires an accurate optical image focused on the retina. In other words, light from a point on a target object must end up as a point of light—rather than a blur—on the retina.

To produce this sharply focused optical image, the eye has many of the features of a camera, starting with the transparent outer layer of the eye, called the **cornea** (**FIGURE 7.1**). Light travels in a straight line until it encounters a change in the density of the medium, such as when it moves from air into water, which causes light rays to bend. This bending of light rays, called **refraction**, is the basis of such instruments as eyeglasses, telescopes, and microscopes. The curvature of the cornea, which does

FIGURE 7.1 Structures of the Human Eye

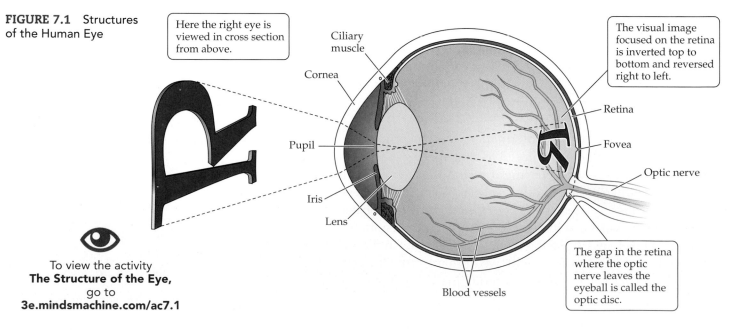

Here the right eye is viewed in cross section from above.

Ciliary muscle

Cornea

Pupil

Iris

Lens

The visual image focused on the retina is inverted top to bottom and reversed right to left.

Retina

Fovea

Optic nerve

Blood vessels

The gap in the retina where the optic nerve leaves the eyeball is called the optic disc.

To view the activity
The Structure of the Eye,
go to
3e.mindsmachine.com/ac7.1

not change shape, refracts light rays and is primarily responsible for focusing on the retina. Light passing through the cornea is further refracted by the **lens**, which changes its shape to fine-tune that image on the retina.

The change in the shape of the lens is controlled by the **ciliary muscles** inside the eye. Contraction of the ciliary muscles alters the focal distance of the eye, causing nearer images to come into focus on the retina; this process is called **accommodation**. As mammals age, their lenses become less elastic and therefore less able to bring nearby objects into focus. Aging humans correct this problem either by holding books and menus farther away from their eyes, or by wearing reading glasses. In young people, the most common vision problem is **myopia** (nearsightedness), which is difficulty seeing distant objects. Myopia develops if the eyeball is too long, causing the cornea and lens to focus images in front of the retina rather than on it (**FIGURE 7.2**). Distance vision can be restored in such cases by lenses that correct refraction of the visual image so that it is on the retina.

If you've ever played around with a magnifying glass, you've probably noticed that if you hold the lens at arm's length, you can see a clearly focused image of a distant scene through the glass but that scene is upside down and reversed. Like a magnifying glass, the biconvex (bulging on both sides) shape of the lens of the eye causes the visual scene that is focused on the retina to be upside down and reversed compared with the real world (see Figure 7.1).

Movement of the eyes is controlled by the **extraocular muscles**, three pairs of muscles that extend from the outside of the eyeball to the bony socket of the eye. Fixating still or moving targets requires delicate control of these muscles to anchor the visual image on the retina. Let's talk about how that sharply focused visual image is processed in the retina.

Visual processing begins in the retina

The first stages of visual information processing occur in the retina, the receptive surface inside the back of the eye. The retina is only 200–300 micrometers thick—not much thicker than the edge of a razor blade—but it contains several types of cells in distinct layers (**FIGURE 7.3A**). Sensory neurons that detect light are called **photoreceptors**. There are two types of photoreceptors in the retina, called **rods** and **cones**, reflecting their respective shapes (**FIGURE 7.3B**). Cones come in several different varieties, which respond differently to light of varying wavelengths, providing us with color vision (as described later in the chapter). Rods respond to visible light of almost any wavelength.

Both rod and cone photoreceptors release neurotransmitter molecules into synapses on the **bipolar cells**, controlling their activity. The bipolar cells, in turn, connect with **ganglion cells**. The axons of the ganglion cells form the **optic nerve**, which carries information to the brain. Two additional types of cells—**horizontal cells** and **amacrine cells**—are especially significant in interactions within the retina. The horizontal cells make contacts among the receptor cells and bipolar cells; the amacrine cells contact both the bipolar cells and the ganglion cells.

Interestingly, the rods, cones, bipolar cells, and horizontal cells generate only graded, local potentials; they do not produce action potentials. Unlike most neurons, these cells affect each other through the *graded* release of neurotransmitters in response to *graded* changes in electrical potentials. The ganglion cells, on the other hand, conduct action potentials in the same way that most other neurons do. From

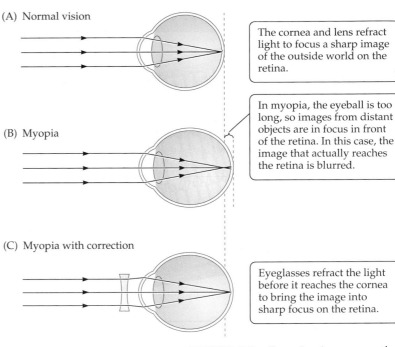

(A) Normal vision

The cornea and lens refract light to focus a sharp image of the outside world on the retina.

(B) Myopia

In myopia, the eyeball is too long, so images from distant objects are in focus in front of the retina. In this case, the image that actually reaches the retina is blurred.

(C) Myopia with correction

Eyeglasses refract the light before it reaches the cornea to bring the image into sharp focus on the retina.

FIGURE 7.2 Focusing Images on the Retina

myopia Nearsightedness; the inability to focus the retinal image of objects that are far away.

extraocular muscle One of the muscles attached to the eyeball that controls its position and movements.

photoreceptor A neural cell in the retina that responds to light.

rod A photoreceptor cell in the retina that is most active at low levels of light.

cone Any of several classes of photoreceptor cells in the retina that are responsible for color vision.

bipolar cell An interneuron in the retina that receives information from rods and cones and passes the information to retinal ganglion cells.

ganglion cell Any of a class of cells in the retina whose axons form the optic nerve.

optic nerve Cranial nerve II; the collection of ganglion cell axons that extends from the retina to the brain.

horizontal cell A specialized retinal cell that contacts both photoreceptors and bipolar cells.

amacrine cell A specialized retinal cell that contacts both bipolar cells and ganglion cells and is especially significant in inhibitory interactions within the retina.

FIGURE 7.5 The Wide Range of Sensitivity to Light Intensity

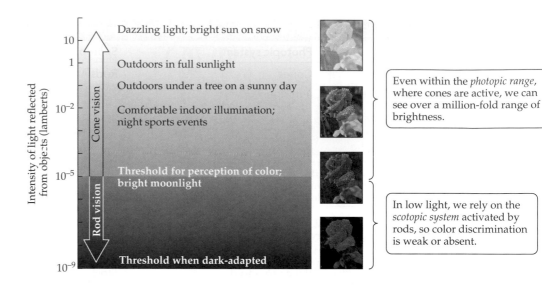

Even within the *photopic range*, where cones are active, we can see over a million-fold range of brightness.

In low light, we rely on the *scotopic system* activated by rods, so color discrimination is weak or absent.

Different mechanisms enable the eyes to work over a wide range of light intensities

Our visual system must respond to stimuli of vastly different intensities: a very bright light is about 10 billion times as intense as the weakest lights we can see (**FIGURE 7.5**). One way the visual system deals with this large range of intensities is by adjusting the size of the **pupil**, which is an opening in the colorful disc called the **iris** (see Figure 7.1). In Chapter 2 we mentioned that dilation (opening) of the pupils is controlled by the sympathetic division of the autonomic system and that constriction is triggered by the parasympathetic division. Because usually both divisions are active, pupil size reflects a balance of influences. Drugs that block acetylcholine transmission in the parasympathetic synapses onto muscles controlling the iris relax them, opening the pupil widely. One drug that has this effect—belladonna—got its name (Italian for "beautiful woman") because it was thought to make a woman more beautiful by giving her the wide-open pupils of an attentive person. Other drugs, such as morphine, constrict the pupils.

In bright light, the pupil contracts quickly to admit only about one-sixteenth as much light as when illumination is dim (**FIGURE 7.6**). Although rapid, the 16-fold difference in light controlled by the pupil doesn't come close to accounting for the *billion*-fold range of visual sensitivity. Another mechanism for handling different light intensities is **range fractionation**, the handling of different intensities by different receptors—some with low thresholds (rods) and others with high thresholds (cones) (see Figure 7.5). But the main reason we can see over such a vast range of light is **photoreceptor adaptation**: each photoreceptor constantly adjusts its sensitivity to match

pupil The opening, formed by the iris, that allows light to enter the eye.

iris The circular structure of the eye that provides an opening to form the pupil.

range fractionation The means by which sensory systems cover a wide range of intensity values, as each sensory receptor cell specializes in just one part of the overall range of intensities.

photoreceptor adaptation The tendency of rods and cones to adjust their light sensitivity to match current levels of illumination.

(A) Bright illumination

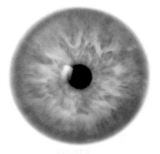

While the size of the pupil can change rapidly, it affects light entry by only about 16-fold. So it cannot possibly account for our ability to see over a billion-fold range of illumination.

(B) Dark

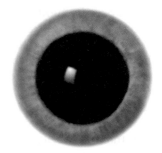

FIGURE 7.6 The Iris Controls the Size of the Pupil Opening

the average level of ambient illumination, over a tremendous range. Thus, the visual system is concerned with *differences*, or changes, in brightness—not with the absolute level of illumination.

At any given time, a photoreceptor operates over a range of intensities of about a hundred-fold; that is, it is completely depolarized by a stimulus about one-tenth the ambient level of illumination, and a light 10 times more intense than the ambient level will completely hyperpolarize it. The receptors constantly shift their whole range of response to work around the prevailing level of illumination. Further adaptation, controlled by neural circuits, occurs in the brain.

Acuity is best in foveal vision

Visual acuity, commonly known as the *sharpness of vision*, is a measure of how much detail we can see. Our visual acuity is especially fine in the center of the visual field and falls off rapidly toward the periphery. That's why when we want to look at something closely, we center our gaze on the object of interest.

The fine structure of the retina explains why our acuity is best in the center of the visual field, called the **fovea** (**FIGURE 7.7A**). Notice how much more densely packed cones are in the fovea, where acuity is highest (**FIGURE 7.7B**), than in other parts of the retina. The fovea has an especially dense concentration of cones, absorbing so much light that the region looks dark in the photo (Figure 7.7A). That is one reason

visual acuity   Sharpness of vision.

fovea   The central portion of the retina, which is packed with the highest density of photoreceptors and is the center of our gaze.

(A) Distributions of rods and cones across the retina

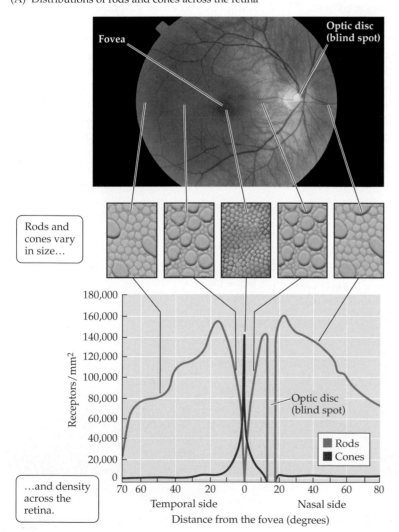

(B) Variation of visual acuity across the retina

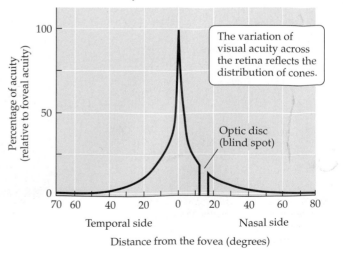

FIGURE 7.7   **Densities of Retinal Receptors and Visual Acuity** (Photo © Paul Parker/SPL/ Science Source. After G. Osterberg, 1935. *Acta. Ophthamol. Suppl.* 13:1.)

visual acuity is so high in this region. People differ in their concentrations of cones (Curcio et al., 1987), and this variation may be related to individual differences in visual acuity. Species differences in visual acuity also reflect the density of cones in the fovea. For example, hawks, whose acuity is much greater than that of humans, have much narrower and more densely packed cones in the fovea than we do. Acuity is reduced in the periphery of the retina in part because both rods and cones are larger there.

The rods show a different distribution from the cones: they are absent in the fovea but more numerous than cones in the periphery of the retina (see Figure 7.7A). This is why, if you want to see a dim star, you do best to search for it a little off to the side of your center of gaze. Not only are rods more sensitive than cones to dim light, but as we mentioned earlier, input from many rods converges on each ganglion cell in the scotopic system, further increasing the system's sensitivity to weak stimuli. But that greater convergence of rods comes at the cost of diminished acuity compared with the fovea. Rods provide high sensitivity with limited acuity; cones provide high acuity with limited sensitivity. Thus, really fine vision requires good lighting.

In addition to the tight packing of cones in the fovea, another reason acuity is greater there than elsewhere on the retina is that in this region light reaches the cones directly, without having to pass through other layers of cells and blood vessels (**FIGURE 7.8**). In the rest of the retina, many light particles hit those upper layers without reaching the photoreceptors. This is why the surface of the retina is depressed at the fovea (see Figure 7.1A), giving the structure its name (*fovea* means "pit" in Latin).

The **optic disc**, to the nasal side of the fovea, is where blood vessels and ganglion cell axons leave the eye (see Figure 7.7A). There are no photoreceptors at the optic disc, so there is a **blind spot** here that we normally do not notice. You can locate your blind spot, and experience firsthand some of its interesting features, with the help of **FIGURE 7.9**. The blind spot is much bigger than we usually appreciate; it is about 10 times larger than the image of a full moon, yet we typically don't even notice it! Again, brain systems "fill in" the missing information so that we perceive an uninterrupted visual scene.

Before we consider how information is processed at different levels of the visual system, we need to describe the pathway from the eye to the cortex, which we'll consider next.

optic disc The region of the retina that is devoid of photoreceptors because ganglion cell axons and blood vessels exit the eyeball there.

blind spot The portion of the visual field from which light falls on the optic disc.

occipital cortex Also called *visual cortex*. The cortex of the occipital lobe of the brain, corresponding to the visual area of the cortex.

optic chiasm The point at which parts of the two optic nerves cross the midline.

FIGURE 7.8 An Unobstructed View

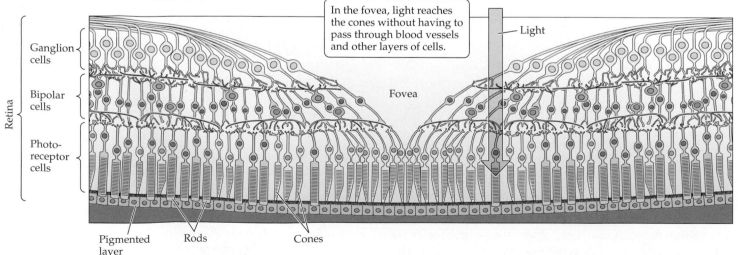

In the fovea, light reaches the cones without having to pass through blood vessels and other layers of cells.

Light

Retina

Ganglion cells

Bipolar cells

Photo-receptor cells

Fovea

Pigmented layer

Rods

Cones

(A)

If you close your left eye and focus on the F, you'll notice that when the book is about 10 inches away, the red dot seems to disappear, as its image falls on the blind spot (see Figure 7.7).

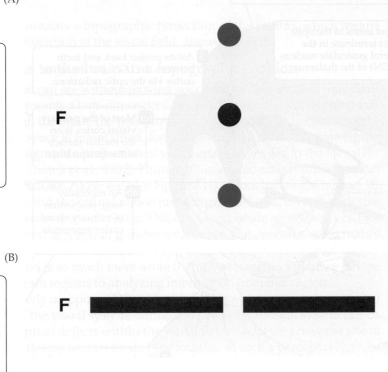

(B)

Here when you focus your right eye on the F and hold the book the right distance away, the red line appears unbroken.

F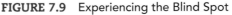

FIGURE 7.9 Experiencing the Blind Spot

HOW'S IT GOING ❓

1. Describe how structures of the eye refract light to focus an image on the retina.
2. How do the photopic and scotopic visual systems vary?
3. How are we able to discriminate differences in light over such a wide range of illumination?
4. Why is our vision so much more acute at the fovea than it is elsewhere?

Neural signals travel from the retina to several brain regions

The ganglion cells in each eye produce action potentials that are conducted along their axons to send visual information to the brain. These axons make up the optic nerve (also known as *cranial nerve II*), which brings visual information into the brain, eventually reaching the **occipital cortex** at the back of the brain.

In vertebrates, some or all of the axons of each optic nerve cross to the opposite cerebral hemisphere. The optic nerves cross the midline at the **optic chiasm** (named for the Greek letter χ [chi] because of its crossover shape). Proportionally more axons cross the midline in prey animals, such as rabbits, that have laterally placed eyes with little overlap in their fields of vision (**FIGURE 7.10**). This arrangement gives a prey animal an especially wide field of view (good for spotting threats) at the cost of poor depth perception (which predators gain by comparing the overlapping visual fields of their front-facing eyes).

FIGURE 7.10 Visual Fields

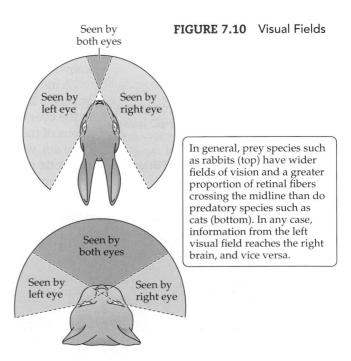

In general, prey species such as rabbits (top) have wider fields of vision and a greater proportion of retinal fibers crossing the midline than do predatory species such as cats (bottom). In any case, information from the left visual field reaches the right brain, and vice versa.

194 CHAPTER 7

required to demonstrate its existence. As with the blind spots we all have, people may not be aware of scotomas that arise.

Within a scotoma, a person cannot *consciously* perceive visual cues, but some visual discrimination in this region may still be possible; this paradoxical phenomenon has been called **blindsight**. People with blindsight say they cannot see, but when asked to *guess* whether a stimulus is present, they're correct more often than could be expected by chance alone, or they may walk down a corridor strewn with objects without running into them (De Gelder et al., 2008).

HOW'S IT GOING ?

1. Describe the path of information from the left visual field to the right side of the brain.
2. Name the structures that carry information from the eye to the brain.
3. Why is the proportion of primary visual cortex devoted to the fovea so large compared with other parts of the retina?

PART II
Visual Analysis

THE ROAD AHEAD

This next section describes how neurons in the retina and brain respond to light that reaches the retina. Reading this section should enable you to:

1. Describe the kinds of light stimuli that best excite or inhibit neurons in the retina, LGN, and striate and extrastriate cortex.
2. Understand why our perception of light and dark is not a simple function of how much light strikes the eye.
3. Explain how simple receptive fields of the retina can be combined to produce more complex receptive fields in V1.
4. Contrast hierarchical models of visual processing with a spatial-frequency model.
5. Identify extrastriate brain regions specialized to detect complex forms and motion.

Neurons at Different Levels of the Visual System Have Very Different Receptive Fields

As we noted in Chapter 5, the **receptive field** of a sensory cell consists of the stimulus region and the features that excite or inhibit the cell. Understanding the receptive fields in the visual system begins with the response of photoreceptors. At rest, both rod and cone photoreceptors steadily release the synaptic neurotransmitter glutamate. Light always hyperpolarizes the photoreceptors, causing them to release *less* glutamate. But the *responses* of the bipolar cells that receive this glutamate differ, depending on the type of glutamate receptor they possess.

One group of bipolar cells consists of **on-center bipolar cells.** Glutamate is *inhibitory* to this type of cell, so light on the on-center bipolar cell's receptive field (which would cause the photoreceptor to release *less* glutamate) would *excite* this bipolar cell (think of taking the brakes off a system) (**FIGURE 7.13A**). The second group consists of **off-center bipolar cells.** Glutamate is *excitatory* to off-center bipolar cells, so shining light on this cell's receptive field (which causes the photoreceptor to release less glutamate) would *inhibit* this bipolar cell. It's called an *off-center bipolar cell* because turning *off* a light in the center of its receptive field excites it (**FIGURE 7.13B**).

Bipolar cells also *release* glutamate, which always depolarizes ganglion cells. Therefore, when light is turned on, on-center bipolar cells depolarize (excite) **on-center**

blindsight The paradoxical phenomenon whereby, within a scotoma, a person cannot *consciously* perceive visual cues but may still be able to make some visual discrimination.

receptive field The stimulus region and features that affect the activity of a cell in a sensory system.

on-center bipolar cell A retinal bipolar cell that is excited by light in the center of its receptive field.

off-center bipolar cell A retinal bipolar cell that is inhibited by light in the center of its receptive field.

on-center ganglion cell A retinal ganglion cell that is activated when light is presented to the center, rather than the periphery, of the cell's receptive field.

(A) On-center receptive fields

(B) Off-center receptive fields

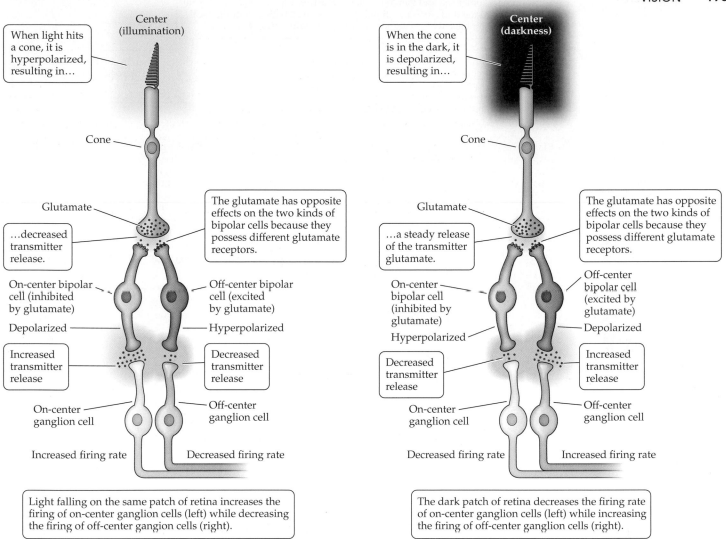

FIGURE 7.13 **Connections of Cones to Bipolar Cells** (After D. Purves et al., 2001. *Neuroscience* [2nd ed.]. Oxford University Press/Sinauer. Sunderland, MA.)

ganglion cells; when light is turned off, off-center bipolar cells depolarize (excite) **off-center ganglion cells** (see Figure 7.13). The stimulated on-center and off-center ganglion cells then fire nerve impulses and report "light" or "dark" to higher visual centers.

Neurons in the retina and the LGN have concentric receptive fields

Recordings from single ganglion cells show that in addition to the on- or off-center portion we've just discussed, their receptive fields also include a ring around that center, which is usually called a *surround* because it surrounds the central patch. Thus the entire receptive field is *concentric*, consisting of a roughly circular central area and the ringlike area surrounding it. Through various retinal connections, the photoreceptors in the central area and those in the ring surrounding it tend to have opposite effects on the next cells in the circuit. Thus, both bipolar cells and ganglion cells have two basic types of retinal receptive fields: **on-center/off-surround** (**FIGURE 7.14A**) and **off-center/on-surround** (**FIGURE 7.14B**). These antagonistic effects of the center and its surround explain why uniform illumination of the visual field has little effect on ganglion cell activity, compared with a well-placed small spot of light on the cell's receptive field. Neurons in the LGN, which are stimulated by retinal ganglion cells, also have these concentric on-center/off-surround or off-center/on-surround receptive fields.

To understand why the effect of light falling on the surround of a firing ganglion cell is opposite to the effect of light falling in the center, we need to understand the

off-center ganglion cell A retinal ganglion cell that is activated when light is presented to the periphery, rather than the center, of the cell's receptive field.

on-center/off-surround Referring to a concentric receptive field in which stimulation of the center excites the cell of interest while stimulation of the surround inhibits it.

off-center/on-surround Referring to a concentric receptive field in which stimulation of the center inhibits the cell of interest while stimulation of the surround excites it.

Each retinal bipolar cell and ganglion cell has a concentric receptive field, with antagonistic center and surround. Bipolar cells respond with changes in local membrane potentials, while ganglion cells respond with action potentials.

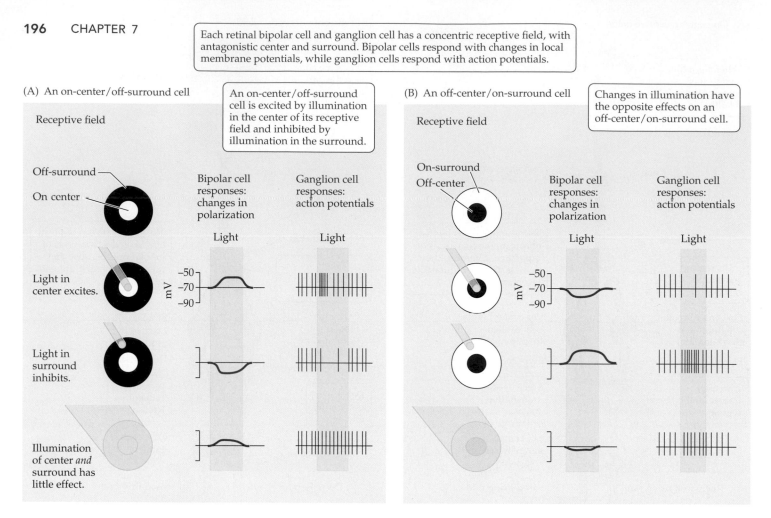

FIGURE 7.14   Receptive Fields of Retinal Cells

To view the animation
Receptive Fields in the Retina,
go to
3e.mindsmachine.com/av7.4

lateral inhibition   The phenomenon by which interconnected neurons inhibit their neighbors, producing contrast at the edges of regions.

concept of **lateral inhibition**, in which sensory receptor cells inhibit the reporting of information from neighboring receptor cells. As illustrated in **FIGURE 7.15**, the bipolar cells that relay information from photoreceptors to ganglion cells also inhibit one another. So when one bipolar cell is active, it inhibits its neighbors.

Because of this lateral inhibition, the ganglion cells stimulated by the right-hand edge of each dark band in **FIGURE 7.16A** are inhibited by the neighboring photoreceptors stimulated by the lighter band next door. Thus, ganglion cells stimulated by the right edge of each bar report receiving less light than they actually do (i.e., that edge looks darker to us). Conversely, the left edge of each bar looks lighter than the rest of the bar.

Again, in **FIGURE 7.16B** two indicated patches, which clearly differ in the brightness we perceive, *reflect the same amount of light*. If you use your pinkie to cover the edge where the two tiles meet, you'll see that the two patches are the same shade of gray. How are such puzzling effects produced? Although the contrast effect in Figure 7.16A is determined, at least in part, by lateral inhibition among adjacent retinal cells, the entire areas indicated in Figure 7.16B, not just the edges, appear different, so the effect must be produced higher in the visual system. One explanation is that we are accustomed to light sources coming from overhead (such as the sun, or a room light), so our brain assumes that the upper patch must actually be darker than the lower patch, because the upper one should be receiving more light than the lower one.

Whether or not that particular explanation is correct, the important point is that our *visual experience is not a simple reporting of the physical properties of light*. Rather, our perception of light versus dark is created by the brain in response to many factors, including surrounding stimuli. For example, if you read this book in bright sunlight, the black ink reflects far more light to your eyes than the blank parts of the page do indoors. Yet, whether you're in sunlight or indoors, you perceive the ink as black and the blank parts as white. Later in the chapter we'll find that our experience of color is also created by the visual system and that it is not a simple reporting of the wavelengths of light.

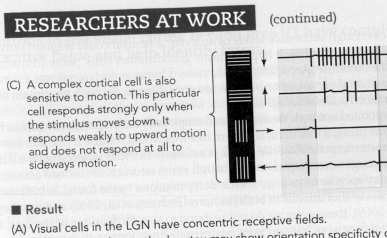

RESEARCHERS AT WORK (continued)

(C) A complex cortical cell is also sensitive to motion. This particular cell responds strongly only when the stimulus moves down. It responds weakly to upward motion and does not respond at all to sideways motion.

■ **Result**

(A) Visual cells in the LGN have concentric receptive fields.

(B) Visual cells in the cerebral cortex may show orientation specificity or respond only to motion, or...

(C) ...they may respond only to motion in a particular direction.

■ **Conclusion**

Neurons at each level of the visual system combine input from neurons at lower levels to make progressively more complex receptive fields. Thus, retinal and LGN neurons respond best to spots of light on the retina, while cortical cells respond best to lines of particular orientation, or lines that move in a particular direction.

Spatial-frequency analysis is unintuitive but efficient

Hubel and Wiesel's theoretical model of visual analysis can be described as hierarchical; that is, more-complex receptive fields are built up from inputs of simpler ones. For example, a simple cortical cell can be thought of as receiving input from a row of LGN cells (**FIGURE 7.18**), and a complex cortical cell can be thought of as receiving input from a row of simple cortical cells.

Other theorists extrapolated from this hierarchical model, suggesting that higher-order circuits of cells could detect any possible form. Thus it was suggested that,

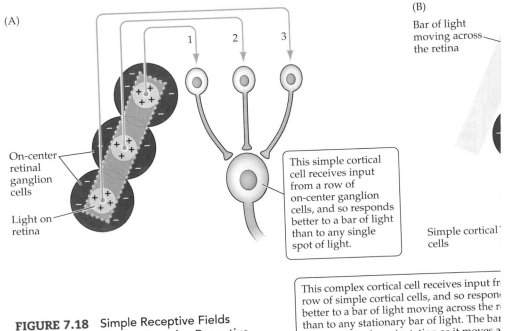

FIGURE 7.18 Simple Receptive Fields Can Combine to Make Complex Receptive Fields (After D. H. Hubel and T. N. Wiesel, 1962. *J. Physiol.* 160: 106.)

(A)

On-center retinal ganglion cells

Light on retina

(B) Bar of light moving across the retina

This simple cortical cell receives input from a row of on-center ganglion cells, and so responds better to a bar of light than to any single spot of light.

Simple cortical cells

This complex cortical cell receives input fr[om] row of simple cortical cells, and so respon[ds] better to a bar of light moving across the r[etina] than to any stationary bar of light. The bar have a particular orientation as it moves a[cross] the retina to best stimulate this neuron.

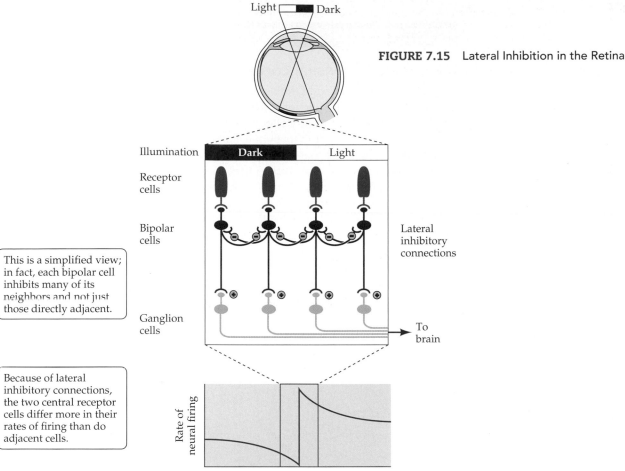

FIGURE 7.15 Lateral Inhibition in the Retina

Light ▪ Dark

Illumination Dark / Light

Receptor cells

Bipolar cells

This is a simplified view; in fact, each bipolar cell inhibits many of its neighbors and not just those directly adjacent.

Ganglion cells

Lateral inhibitory connections

To brain

Because of lateral inhibitory connections, the two central receptor cells differ more in their rates of firing than do adjacent cells.

Rate of neural firing

Position of ganglion cells

HOW'S IT GOING ❓

1. Given that all photoreceptors are hyperpolarized by light, how can the same photoreceptor excite some bipolar cells while inhibiting others?

2. What is a receptive field, and what two kinds of receptive fields are displayed by retinal ganglion cells?

3. Describe lateral inhibition in the retina and how it can sharpen our vision yet make us susceptible to the optical illusion we experience in Figure 7.16A.

(A)

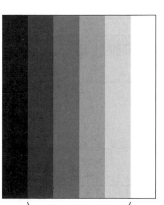

Each strip is uniform, yet they all look lighter on the left edge and darker on the right edge.

(B)

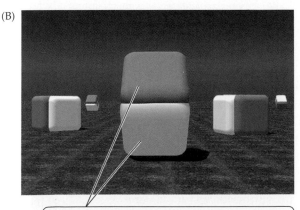

Of the two indicated patches, the upper one looks darker, even though they are in fact the same shade of gray. If you don't believe this, use your finger to cover up the line where they meet. See?

FIGURE 7.16 The Effect of Context on the Perception of Brightness (Part B from D. Purves et al., 1999. *J. Neurosci.* 19: 8543.)

simple cortical cell   Also called *bar detector* or *edge detector*. A cell in the visual cortex that responds best to an edge or a bar that has a particular width, as well as a particular orientation and location in the visual field.

complex cortical cell   A cell in the visual cortex that responds best to a bar of a particular size and orientation anywhere within a particular area of the visual field and that needs movement to make it respond actively.

RESEARCHERS AT WORK

Neurons in the visual cortex have v

Neurons from the LGN send their axons to cells i
but the *spots* of light that are effective stimuli for
also Figure 7.14A) are not very effective for cortic
and Torsten Wiesel reported that visual cortical c
gated stimuli than those that activate LGN cells a

Hubel and Wiesel categorized cortical cells a
that produced maximum responses. So-called **s**
best to an edge or a bar that has a particular wid
and location in the visual field (**FIGURE 7.17B**). T
times called *bar detectors* or *edge detectors*. Li
cortical cells have elongated receptive fields, b
of the stimulus to make them respond actively.
movement in their field is sufficient; others are r
tion in a specific direction (**FIGURE 7.17C**).

FIGURE 7.17   Receptive Fields of Cells at Vario

■ **Hypothesis**
Cells at higher levels of the visual system respon
complex stimuli.

■ **Test**
Compare receptive fields of neurons at each leve
one another.

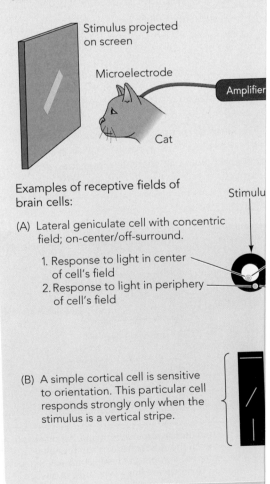

Stimulus projected
on screen

Microelectrode

Amplifier

Cat

Examples of receptive fields of
brain cells:

(A) Lateral geniculate cell with concentric
field; on-center/off-surround.

  1. Response to light in center
    of cell's field
  2. Response to light in periphery
    of cell's field

(B) A simple cortical cell is sensitive
to orientation. This particular cell
responds strongly only when the
stimulus is a vertical stripe.

The four main types of
spectrally opponent cells are:

Each type is excited by
one band of wavelengths
and inhibited by another.

(A) +L/–M

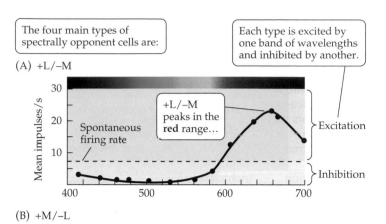

+L/–M
peaks in the
red range…

Spontaneous
firing rate

Excitation

Inhibition

(B) +M/–L

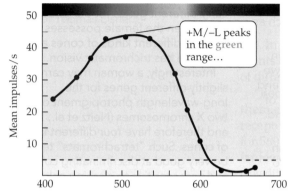

+M/–L peaks
in the green
range…

(C) +(L+M)/–S

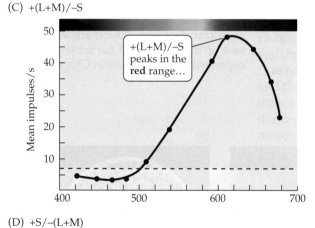

+(L+M)/–S
peaks in the
red range…

(D) +S/–(L+M)

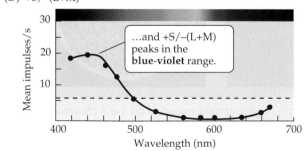

…and +S/–(L+M)
peaks in the
blue-violet range.

Wavelength (nm)

FIGURE 7.28   Responses by the Four Main Types
of Spectrally Opponent Cells in Monkey LGN
(After R. L. De Valois and K. K. De Valois, 1993.
Vision Res. 33: 1053.)

Some retinal ganglion cells and LGN cells show spectral opponency

Monkeys discriminate colors about as well as humans do. Recordings made from monkeys reveal that most ganglion cells and LGN cells are excited and fire in response to some wavelengths and are inhibited by other wavelengths. **FIGURE 7.28A** shows the response of one such LGN cell as a light centered on its receptive field changes from one wavelength to another. Firing is stimulated by wavelengths above 600 nm, where the L cones are most sensitive; it is inhibited at shorter wavelengths, where the L cones are less sensitive than the M cones. A cell exhibiting this response pattern is therefore called a *plus L/minus M cell* (+L/–M). This is an example of a **spectrally opponent cell** (or *color-opponent cell*) because two regions of the spectrum have opposite effects on the cell's rate of firing. Figure 7.28 shows the responses of the four main kinds of spectrally opponent cells.

Each spectrally opponent ganglion cell receives input from two or three different kinds of cones through bipolar cells. The connections from at least one type of cone are excitatory, and those from at least one other type are inhibitory. The spectrally opponent ganglion cells thus record the *difference* in stimulation of different types of cones. For example, a +M/–L cell responds to the difference in the excitation of M and L cones.

The peaks of the sensitivity curves of the M and L cones are not very different (see Figure 7.26). However, whereas the M-minus-L *difference* curve (**FIGURE 7.28B**) shows a clear peak at about 500 nm (in the green part of the spectrum), the L-minus-M difference function (see Figure 7.28A) shows a peak at about 650 nm (in the red part of the spectrum). Thus, +M/–L and +L/–M cells yield distinctly different neural response curves. LGN cells that are excited by the L and M cells but inhibited by S cells—that is, +(L+M)/–S cells—peak in the red range (**FIGURE 7.28C**), while cells excited by S but inhibited by L and M—that is, +S/–(L+M) cells—peak in the blue-violet range (**FIGURE 7.28D**).

Spectrally opponent neurons are the second stage in the system for color perception, but they still cannot be called *color cells*, because (1) they send their outputs into many higher circuits—for detection of form, depth, and movement, as well as hue; and (2) their peak wavelength sensitivities do not correspond precisely to the wavelengths that we see as the principal hues. **FIGURE 7.29** diagrams the presumed inputs to not only the four kinds of spectrally opponent ganglion cells, but also the ganglion cells that detect brightness and darkness. The brightness detectors receive stimulation from both M and L cones (+M/+L); the darkness detectors are inhibited by those same cones (–M/–L).

In the monkey LGN, 70–80% of the cells are spectrally opponent; in the cat, very few spectrally opponent cells are found—only about 1%. This difference explains why monkeys so easily distinguish between colors and it's so difficult to train cats to discriminate even large differences in color.

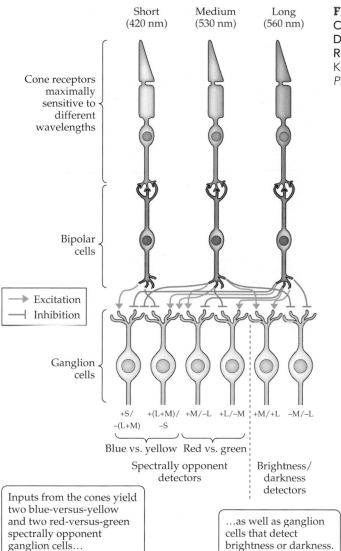

Cone receptors maximally sensitive to different wavelengths

Short (420 nm)   Medium (530 nm)   Long (560 nm)

Bipolar cells

→ Excitation
⊣ Inhibition

Ganglion cells

+S/ −(L+M)   +(L+M)/ −S   +M/−L   +L/−M   +M/+L   −M/−L

Blue vs. yellow   Red vs. green

Spectrally opponent detectors

Brightness/ darkness detectors

Inputs from the cones yield two blue-versus-yellow and two red-versus-green spectrally opponent ganglion cells…

…as well as ganglion cells that detect brightness or darkness.

FIGURE 7.29   A Model of the Connections of Wavelength Discrimination Systems in the Primate Retina   (After R. L. De Valois and K. K. De Valois, 1980. *Annu. Rev. Psychol.* 31: 309.)

Some visual cortical cells and regions appear to be specialized for color perception

In the cortex, spectral information is used for various kinds of information processing. Forms are segregated from their background by differences in color or intensity (or both). The most important role that color plays in our perception is to denote which parts of a complex image belong to one object and which belong to another. Some animals use displays of brightly colored body parts to call attention to themselves, but color can also be used as camouflage.

Some spectrally opponent cortical cells contribute to the perception of color, providing the third stage of the color vision system. These cells are not just responding to the differences between two types of cones, as retinal ganglion cells and LGN cells do. Rather, they are responding to differences in colors that we *perceive*; in other words, they are perceptually opponent: red versus green, blue versus yellow, and black versus white (R. L. De Valois and De Valois, 1993). The spectral responses of these cells correspond to the wavelengths of the principal hues specified by human observers, and their characteristics also help explain other color phenomena.

spectrally opponent cell   Also called *color-opponent cell*. A visual system neuron that has opposite firing responses to different regions of the spectrum.

SIGNS & SYMPTOMS

Correcting "Color Blindness"?

You may have seen one of the poignant videos on YouTube of men putting on special glasses that supposedly let them see many colors for the first time. Take these testimonials with a grain of salt. First, most so-called color-blind men detect blue objects just fine; their difficulty is only in distinguishing red from green. The most common cause of this color deficiency is that the M and L cone photopigments have peak responses that are too close together, caused by a mutation in the gene for one or the other (**FIGURE 7.30A**). That means that red and green light stimulate the two cones equally, so the brain has no basis to know which color the object is. Engineers at EnChroma (www.enchroma.com) were working on color filters for another purpose entirely when they realized they might address this problem. Their filters selectively block wavelengths between those two peaks (**FIGURE 7.30B**). While this reduces the total amount of light reaching the retina, if the remaining light is in the green part of the spectrum, it will stimulate the M cone significantly more than the L cone. Conversely, remaining light in the red portion of the spectrum will stimulate the L cone more than the M cone. Now that the person's M and L cones are getting differential stimulation, they perceive these colors differently. But are they really experiencing red and green the way most people do? Probably not. For example, putting on the glasses does not let color-deficient people read the numbers in figures like that in Box 7.1 (Almutairi et al., 2017). Why, then, do the men in the videos have such emotional reactions upon donning the glasses? Even people with typical color vision see the world differently through these glasses, so the men may interpret this distortion as providing them with new color information. Note that color deficiency sometimes happens because the photopigment for either the M or L cones is missing or totally dysfunctional. These glass filters can't make any difference in color perception in those cases.

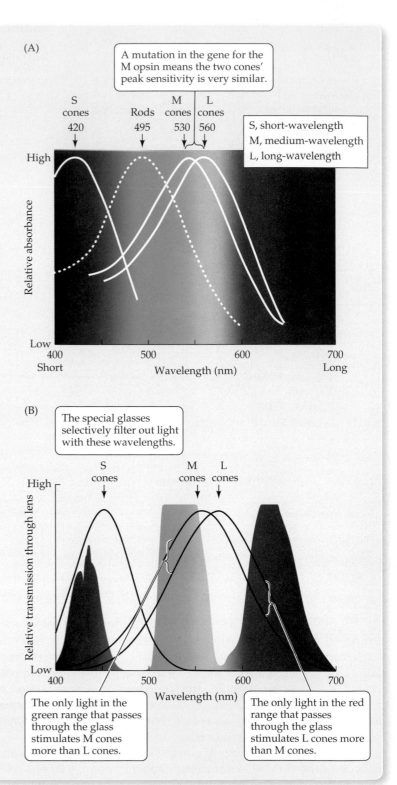

FIGURE 7.30   Filtering Out Wavelengths (Part B after N. Almutairi et al., 2017. *College of Optometry* 21.)

Visual cortical region V4 is particularly rich in color-sensitive cells; each of these cells truly responds best to a particular hue, including the four that Hering postulated (blue, green, yellow, red). V4 cells respond best if the color outside the receptive field is different from the color preferred inside the receptive field (Schein and Desimone, 1990; Zeki et al., 1991).

1. What two main hypotheses were developed to explain our ability to discriminate colors? Which aspects of the visual system appear to match each hypothesis?
2. Describe some examples in which our perception of color is not simply the detection of particular wavelengths of light.
3. Why do we label cones as S cones, M cones, and L cones rather than blue, green, and red cones?
4. Why are men more likely than women to have difficulty distinguishing some colors?
5. Why is it a good idea to make life rafts yellow if they are to be detected on a blue sea?

optic ataxia   Spatial disorientation in which the patient is unable to accurately reach for objects using visual guidance.

PART IV
What versus Where

THE ROAD AHEAD

Vision is so crucial for us primates that we devote lots of brain space to analyzing visual stimuli and work hard to correct vision deficiencies. After reading this final section of the chapter, you should be able to:

1. Identify the major streams of visual processing that deal with what a stimulus is, and where it is.
2. Understand why D.F. can use vision to guide her movements but not to recognize objects.
3. Describe the underlying causes of nearsightedness and how it can be avoided.
4. Understand the role of visual experience in sharpening vision, especially in children.

The Many Cortical Visual Areas Are Organized into Two Major Streams

Mortimer Mishkin and Leslie Ungerleider (1982) proposed that primates have two main visual processing streams, both originating in primary visual cortex: a ventral processing stream responsible for visually *identifying* objects, and a dorsal stream responsible for appreciating the spatial *location* of objects and for visually guiding our movement toward them (**FIGURE 7.31**). They called these processing streams, respectively, the *what* and *where* streams.

PET studies, as well as brain lesions in patients, indicate that the human brain possesses *what* and *where* visual processing streams similar to those that have been found in monkeys (Ungerleider et al., 1998). The two streams are not completely separate, because there are normally many cross connections between them. In the ventral stream, including regions of the occipitotemporal, inferior temporal, and inferior frontal areas, information about faces becomes more specific as one proceeds farther forward. In Chapter 15, we'll discuss a portion of the ventral stream, the fusiform gyrus, that is specialized to identify faces.

Discovery of these separate visual cortical streams helps us understand the case of patient D.F., described at the start of this chapter. Recall that, as a result of carbon monoxide poisoning, D.F. lost the ability to perceive faces and objects but retained the ability to reach and grasp objects under visual control (A. D. Milner et al., 1991). D.F.'s visual ventral (*what*) stream appears to have been devastated, but her dorsal (*where*) stream seems unimpaired. An opposite kind of dissociation had already been reported: damage to the dorsal parietal cortex often results in **optic ataxia**, in which patients have difficulty using vision to reach for and grasp objects, yet some of these patients can still identify objects correctly (Perenin and Vighetto, 1988).

The ventral (*what*) pathway, shown in yellow and red, and the dorsal (*where*) pathway, shown in green and blue, serve different functions.

Dorsal stream: vision for movement, location

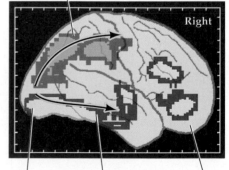

Occipital lobe   Ventral stream: vision for recognition (objects, faces)   Frontal lobe

FIGURE 7.31 Parallel Processing Pathways in the Visual System (Courtesy of Leslie Ungerleider.)

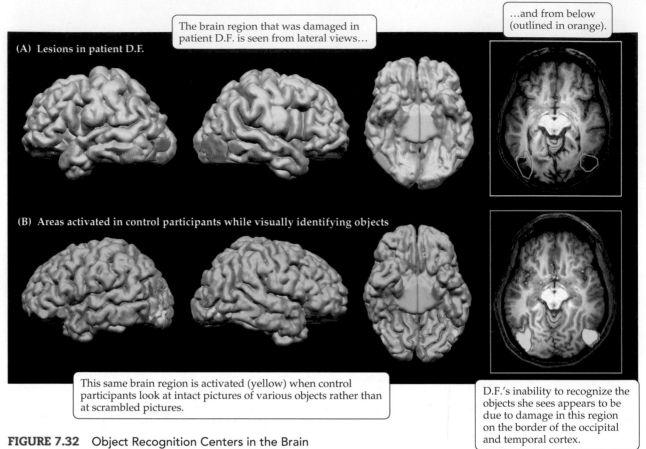

(A) Lesions in patient D.F.

The brain region that was damaged in patient D.F. is seen from lateral views...

...and from below (outlined in orange).

(B) Areas activated in control participants while visually identifying objects

This same brain region is activated (yellow) when control participants look at intact pictures of various objects rather than at scrambled pictures.

D.F.'s inability to recognize the objects she sees appears to be due to damage in this region on the border of the occipital and temporal cortex.

FIGURE 7.32   Object Recognition Centers in the Brain
(From T. W. James et al., 2003. *Brain* 126: 2463.)

High-resolution MRI of D.F.'s brain (**FIGURE 7.32A**) reveals diffuse damage concentrated in the ventrolateral occipital cortex (T. W. James et al., 2003). Throughout the brain there is evidence of atrophy, indicated by shrunken gyri and enlarged sulci. **FIGURE 7.32B** shows the area activated in fMRI recordings when healthy participants viewed pictures of objects; it corresponds to D.F.'s lateral occipital lesion. When D.F. reached for and grasped objects, her fMRI activation in the parietal lobe was similar to that of control participants, indicating that her dorsal stream is largely intact. D.F.'s intact dorsal pathway not only tells her where objects are, but also guides her movements to use these objects properly.

It is still puzzling that one part of D.F. knows exactly how to grasp a pencil held in front of her, yet another part of her—the part that talks to you—has no idea whether the object she's holding is a pencil, a ruler, or a bouquet of flowers. This condition is reminiscent of the cortical damage that causes blindsight, mentioned earlier: people with such damage report being unable to see, but they show evidence that they can. In Chapter 14 we'll learn about other people who can see only one thing at a time, or who can see faces but cannot identify to whom they belong. Imagining what such disjointed visual experience must be like helps us appreciate how effortlessly our brains usually bind together information with our marvelous sense of sight.

Visual Neuroscience Can Be Applied to Alleviate Some Visual Deficiencies

Vision is so important that many investigators have sought ways to prevent its impairment, to improve inadequate vision, and to restore sight to the blind. In the United States, half a million people are blind. Recent medical advances have reduced some causes of blindness but have increased blindness from other causes. For example, medical advances permit people with diabetes to live longer, but because we don't know how to prevent blindness associated with diabetes, there are more people alive today with diabetes-induced blindness. In the discussion that follows, we will first consider ways of avoiding the impairment of vision. Then we will take up ways of improving an impaired visual system.

Impairment of vision often can be prevented or reduced

Studies of the development of vision show that the incidence of myopia (nearsightedness) can be reduced. Myopia develops if the eyeball is too long, causing the eye to focus images in front of the retina rather than on the retina (see Figure 7.2). As a result, distant objects appear blurred. Considerable evidence suggests that the reason some children develop myopia is that certain environmental factors cause the eyeball to grow excessively. Previously it was thought that the modern habit of looking closely at nearby objects (books, computer screens, and so on) might be responsible for myopia, but mounting evidence suggests that indoor lighting may be to blame (Lagrèze and Schaeffel, 2017).

Before civilization, most people spent the bulk of their time outdoors, looking at objects illuminated by sunlight. But with the advent of indoor lighting, we've come to spend a lot of time looking at things with light that, while containing many wavelengths, does not exactly match the composition of sunlight. Several studies found that children with myopia spend less time outdoors than do other children, but that correlation could be caused by genes that favor both myopia and indoor activities, like reading. Indeed, the advent of public schools in various nations is accompanied by increased rates of myopia. However, one of these studies focused on people of Chinese origin who lived in either Singapore, where crowded conditions mean that people spend little time outdoors, or Sydney, Australia. Even though these populations should be genetically similar, 30% of the Chinese children living in Singapore, who averaged only 30 minutes a day outdoors, were myopic, versus only 3% of those living in Sydney, who averaged 2 hours a day outdoors (Rose et al., 2008). What's more, in these populations myopia correlates much more strongly with time spent indoors than with time spent reading.

Of course, too much sunlight can be a bad thing, especially for our skin. So almost all children in Australia wear hats to shield their faces when outdoors, yet they still benefit from being outdoors in terms of avoiding myopia. Likewise, there's no evidence that wearing sunglasses blocks the benefit of light from the sun. The next challenge will be to determine what it is about indoor lighting, as opposed to sunlight, that encourages the eyeball to grow excessively in children, leading to myopia.

Increased exercise can restore function to a previously deprived or neglected eye

The misalignment of the two eyes (*lazy eye*) can lead to a condition called **amblyopia**, in which acuity is poor in one eye, even though the eye and retina are normal. If the two eyes are not aligned properly during the first few years of life, the primary visual cortex of the child tends to suppress the information traveling to the cortex from one eye, and that eye becomes functionally blind. Studies of the development of vision in children and other animals show that most cases of amblyopia are avoidable.

The balance of the eye muscles can be surgically adjusted to bring the two eyes into better alignment. Alternatively, if the weak eye is given regular practice, with the good eye covered, vision can be preserved in both eyes. Attempts to alleviate amblyopia by training alone, however, have produced mixed results. The optimal treatment appears to be a combination of both surgical correction *and* eye patches and visual exercises (Pediatric Eye Disease Investigator Group, 2005).

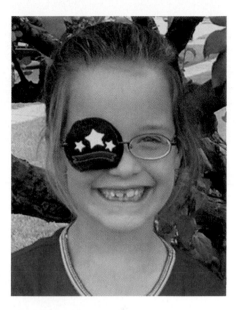

Hey There, You with the Stars over Your Eye As a treatment for amblyopia, this girl is wearing a patch over her "good" eye—the one she has been relying on while ignoring information from her other, "weak" eye. Increased visual experience through the weak eye will strengthen its influence on the cortex. (Courtesy of Patch Pals, www.PatchPals.com.)

amblyopia Reduced visual acuity that is not caused by optical or retinal impairments.

HOW'S IT GOING ❓

1. What are the two main streams of visual processing in the cortex, and what aspects of vision does each stream support?

2. Describe D.F.'s symptoms, and relate them to the brain damage revealed by MRIs.

3. What is the evidence that indoor lighting may cause myopia in children?

Recommended Reading

De Valois, R. L., and De Valois, K. K. (1988). *Spatial Vision.* New York, NY: Oxford University Press.

Gregory, R. L. (2015). *Eye and Brain: The Psychology of Seeing* (5th ed.). Princeton, NJ: Princeton University Press.

Ings, S. (2008). *A Natural History of Seeing: The Art and Science of Vision.* New York, NY: Norton.

Purves, D., and Lotto, R. B. (2011). *Why We See What We Do Redux: A Wholly Empirical Theory of Vision.* Sunderland, MA: Oxford University Press/Sinauer.

Rodieck, R. W. (1998). *The First Steps in Seeing.* Sunderland, MA: Oxford University Press/Sinauer.

Wolfe, J. M., Kluender, K. R., Levi, D. M., Bartoshuk, L. M. et al. (2018). *Sensation & Perception* (5th ed.). Sunderland, MA: Oxford University Press/Sinauer.

7 ■ Visual Summary

3e.mindsmachine.com/vs7

You should be able to relate each summary to the adjacent illustration, including structures and processes. If you go to the website for our text (3e.mindsmachine.com), you can follow links to figures, animations, and activities that will help you consolidate the material.

1 Light is bent, or **refracted**, by the transparent outer layer of the eye, the **cornea**, focusing an image on the **retina** in the back of the eye. We vary the thickness of the **lens** to fine-tune the image. The refracted light forms an image on the retina that is upside down and reversed. Review **Figures 7.1** and **7.2**, **Animation 7.2**, **Activity 7.1**

Dazzling light; bright sun on snow

Outdoors in full sunlight

Outdoors under a tree on a sunny day

Comfortable indoor illumination

Threshold for perception of color

Threshold when dark-adapted

Cone vision / Rod vision

Photopic range / Scotopic range

2 The retina contains two different types of **photoreceptors** to detect light forming the focused image. **Rods** are very sensitive, working even in very low light, and they respond to light of any **wavelength**. Rods drive the **scotopic system**, which can work in dim light. Each of the three different types of **cones** responds better to some wavelengths of light than others, allowing us to detect colors. The cones provide information for the **photopic system**, which requires more light to function. Photoreceptors **adapt** to function across a wide range of light intensities. Review **Figures 7.3–7.6, Table 7.1**

3 The retina consists of layers of neurons, with the photoreceptors in the very back stimulating **bipolar cells**, which stimulate **ganglion cells**. The ganglion cells of the retina project their axons to the brain via the **optic nerve**. **Amacrine cells** and **horizontal cells** communicate across the retina, using processes such as **lateral inhibition** to analyze **brightness**. Review **Figures 7.3, 7.14,** and **7.15**

Cone cell

Rod cell

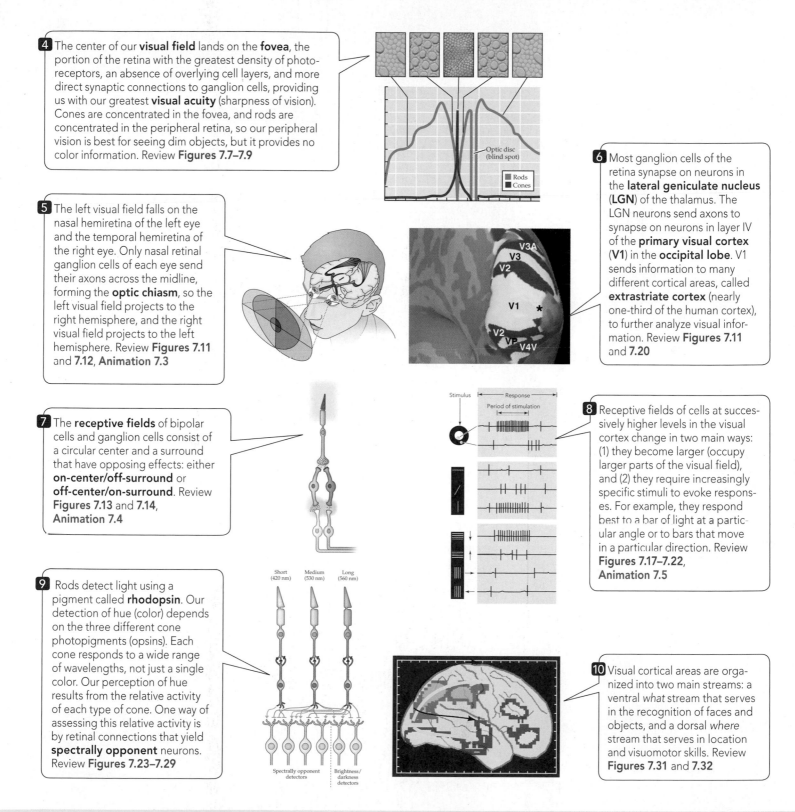

4 The center of our **visual field** lands on the **fovea**, the portion of the retina with the greatest density of photoreceptors, an absence of overlying cell layers, and more direct synaptic connections to ganglion cells, providing us with our greatest **visual acuity** (sharpness of vision). Cones are concentrated in the fovea, and rods are concentrated in the peripheral retina, so our peripheral vision is best for seeing dim objects, but it provides no color information. Review **Figures 7.7–7.9**

5 The left visual field falls on the nasal hemiretina of the left eye and the temporal hemiretina of the right eye. Only nasal retinal ganglion cells of each eye send their axons across the midline, forming the **optic chiasm**, so the left visual field projects to the right hemisphere, and the right visual field projects to the left hemisphere. Review **Figures 7.11** and **7.12**, **Animation 7.3**

6 Most ganglion cells of the retina synapse on neurons in the **lateral geniculate nucleus** (**LGN**) of the thalamus. The LGN neurons send axons to synapse on neurons in layer IV of the **primary visual cortex** (**V1**) in the occipital lobe. V1 sends information to many different cortical areas, called **extrastriate cortex** (nearly one-third of the human cortex), to further analyze visual information. Review **Figures 7.11** and **7.20**

7 The **receptive fields** of bipolar cells and ganglion cells consist of a circular center and a surround that have opposing effects: either **on-center/off-surround** or **off-center/on-surround**. Review **Figures 7.13** and **7.14**, **Animation 7.4**

8 Receptive fields of cells at successively higher levels in the visual cortex change in two main ways: (1) they become larger (occupy larger parts of the visual field), and (2) they require increasingly specific stimuli to evoke responses. For example, they respond best to a bar of light at a particular angle or to bars that move in a particular direction. Review **Figures 7.17–7.22**, **Animation 7.5**

9 Rods detect light using a pigment called **rhodopsin**. Our detection of hue (color) depends on the three different cone photopigments (opsins). Each cone responds to a wide range of wavelengths, not just a single color. Our perception of hue results from the relative activity of each type of cone. One way of assessing this relative activity is by retinal connections that yield **spectrally opponent** neurons. Review **Figures 7.23–7.29**

10 Visual cortical areas are organized into two main streams: a ventral *what* stream that serves in the recognition of faces and objects, and a dorsal *where* stream that serves in location and visuomotor skills. Review **Figures 7.31** and **7.32**

Go to **3e.mindsmachine.com** for study questions, quizzes, flashcards, and other resources.

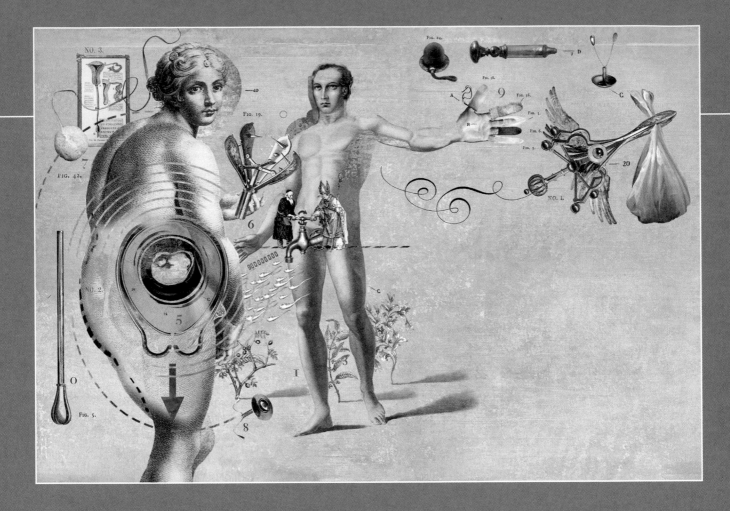

8
Hormones and Sex

Genitals and Gender: What Makes Us Male and Female?

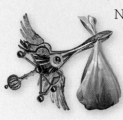

No aspects of human biology are as impressive and humbling as the making of a baby; it is a developmental ballet of staggering complexity and critical timing. Given the countless processes that must unfold perfectly and in precisely the right order, it is a marvel that, in most cases, development proceeds without a hitch. Inevitably, though, there are times when a crucial part of the program is derailed along the way and a baby is born with a heartbreaking deformity.

Such is the case with **cloacal exstrophy**, which affects about one in 400,000 babies, characterized by an incomplete closing of the abdomen that leaves the bladder and intestines exposed. A genetic male with this condition is typically born with normal testes but a very short, split penis or no penis at all. Surgery is required to close up the abdomen, but it isn't really possible to surgically fashion a normal penis, so the parents are faced with a dilemma. Is it better to raise the child as a boy without a penis, despite the emotional costs of the deformity? Or would it be better to assign the child to the female gender, surgically remove the testes and fashion female-looking genitals, and then raise the child as a girl? Which would you choose?

Arguments for each course of action boil down to different opinions about the extent to which our gender is shaped through nurturing and socialization, rather than biological factors. In other words, we need to consider the larger question of why men and women behave differently. Is it because as boys and girls they were treated differently and trained to grow into their gender roles, or do the forces that provide a fetus with testes or ovaries also induce the developing brain to take on a masculine or feminine form?

In this chapter we'll discuss research that informs us about this long-standing question: How do biological and social forces combine to direct development in male-typical and female-typical ways? In Part I we'll learn how hormones can affect the brain to influence behavior. Part II will explain how hormones act on different parts of the brain to influence sexual behavior and parental behavior in particular. Part III will take up the question of how the fetus normally develops into either a male or a female form, not just in terms of the body, but also in terms of the brain and behavior. In animals, prenatal hormones have a tremendous influence on the brain and sexual behaviors. We'll close by reviewing growing evidence that those same prenatal hormones also affect our development into boys or girls, men or women, as well as our sexual orientation.

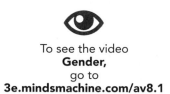

To see the video
Gender,
go to
3e.mindsmachine.com/av8.1

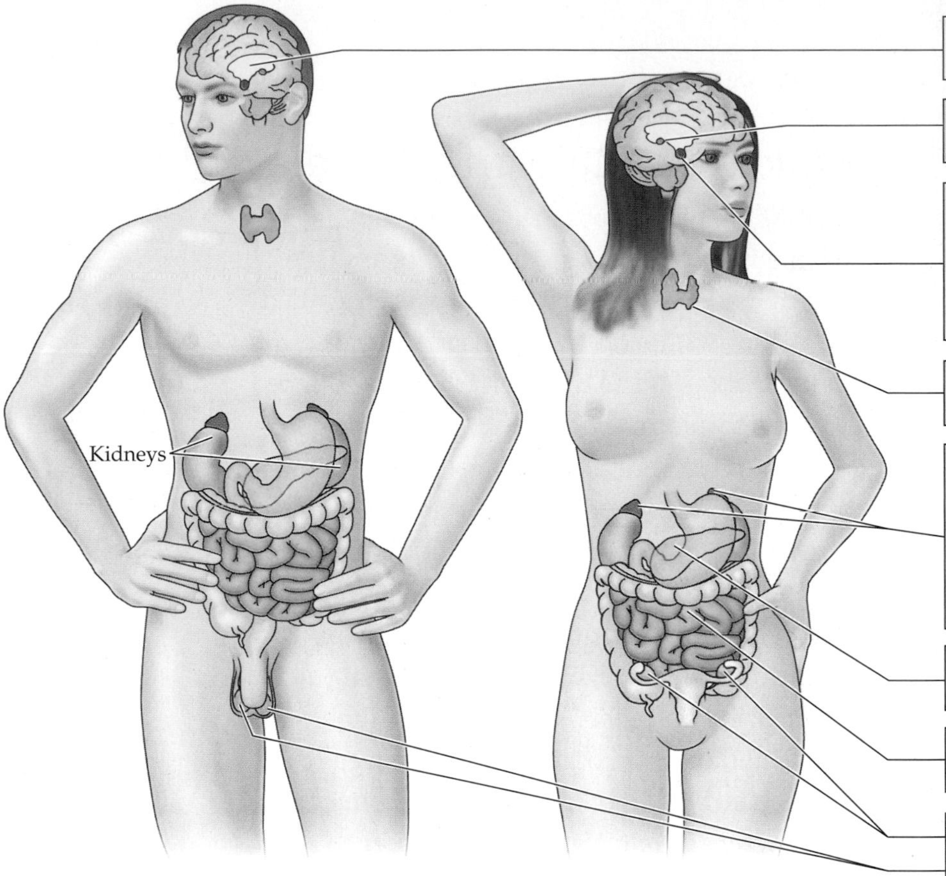

Major endocrine structures	Some main functions regulated by secretion
Hypothalamus	Control of hormone secretions
Pineal gland	Reproductive maturation; body rhythms
Pituitary gland:	
Anterior pituitary	Hormone secretion by thyroid, adrenal cortex, and gonads; growth
Posterior pituitary	Water balance; salt balance
Thyroid	Growth and development; metabolic rate
Adrenal glands:	
Adrenal cortex (outer bark)	Salt and carbohydrate metabolism; inflammatory reactions
Adrenal medulla (inner core)	Emotional arousal (epinephrine)
Pancreas	Sugar metabolism
Gut	Digestion and appetite control
Gonads (testes/ovaries)	Body development; maintenance of reproductive organs in adults

Kidneys

FIGURE 8.1 Major Endocrine Glands and Their Functions

To view the activity
Major Endocrine Glands,
go to
3e.mindsmachine.com/ac8.1

cloacal exstrophy   A rare medical condition in which XY individuals are born completely lacking a penis.

hormone   A chemical, usually secreted by an endocrine gland, that is conveyed by the bloodstream and regulates target organs or tissues.

endocrine gland   A gland that secretes hormones into the bloodstream to act on distant targets.

castration   Removal of the gonads, usually the testes.

PART I
The Endocrine System

THE ROAD AHEAD

The first section of this chapter concerns the way chemical signals, hormones, coordinate action in different parts of the body. After reading this material, you should be able to:

1. Distinguish the different classes of chemical signaling, from neurotransmitters to hormones and pheromones.

2. Contrast the mechanisms of action of peptide hormones versus steroid hormones.

3. Contrast the modes of hormone release from the posterior pituitary versus the anterior pituitary.

4. Explain how the brain regulates circulating levels of hormone.

5. Give examples of the interaction of hormonal and neuronal communication in controlling behavior.

Hormones Act in a Great Variety of Ways throughout the Body

Hormones are chemicals secreted by one group of cells and carried through the bloodstream to other parts of the body, where they act on specific target tissues to produce physiological effects. Most hormones are produced by **endocrine glands** (from the Greek *endon*, "within," and *krinein*, "to secrete"), so called because they release their hormones *within* the body (**FIGURE 8.1**). Endocrine glands are sometimes contrasted with *exocrine glands* (tear glands, salivary glands, sweat glands), which use ducts to secrete fluid *outside* the body.

Our current understanding of hormones developed in stages

Ancient civilizations understood the importance of hormones. In the fourth century BCE, Aristotle described the effects of **castration** (removal of the testes) in chickens and compared them with the effects in eunuchs (castrated men). The first major endocrine experiment, carried out in 1849 by German physician Arnold Berthold (1803–1861), followed up Aristotle's report that when roosters are castrated as juveniles, they fail to develop normal reproductive behavior and secondary sexual characteristics, such as the rooster's comb, in adulthood. Berthold observed, however, that returning one testis back into the body cavity of the young birds allowed them to develop normal male anatomy and behavior. In adulthood, these animals showed the usual male sexual behaviors—mounting hens, fighting, and crowing (**FIGURE 8.2**). Because no nerves had reestablished contact with the transplanted testis, the organ could not be communicating to the brain through nerves. Berthold (1849) concluded that the testes release a chemical into the blood that affects both male behavior and male body structures. Today we know that the testes make and release the hormone testosterone to exert these effects.

Although Berthold didn't know it, experiments like this also illustrate another principle of hormone action. If he had waited until the castrated chicks were adults before returning their testes, Berthold would have seen little effect. The testosterone must be present *early* in life to have such dramatic effects on the body and behavior. We'll return to this point later in this chapter. For now, let's see how hormones fit into the grand scheme of chemical signaling by the body.

FIGURE 8.2   Berthold's (1849) Experiment Demonstrated the Importance of Hormones for Behavior

■ **Question**

Male chicks that are castrated grow up to have small wattles and combs, and they show little interest in mounting hens, fighting, or crowing. What causes these changes—the loss of a nerve connection between the testes and the body, or the loss of a chemical signal released from the testes?

■ **Experiment**

Berthold removed the testes from their normal position but then reimplanted them elsewhere in the abdomen, disconnected from normal innervation.

Group 1	Group 2	Group 3
Left undisturbed, young roosters grow up to have large red wattles and combs, to mount and mate with hens readily, and to fight one another and crow loudly.	Males whose testes were removed during development displayed neither the appearance nor the behavior of normal roosters as adults.	However, if one of the testes was reimplanted into the abdominal cavity immediately after its removal, the rooster developed normal wattles and normal behavior.

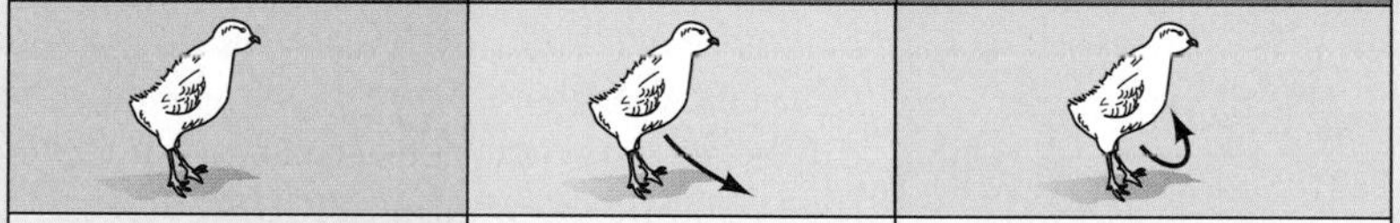

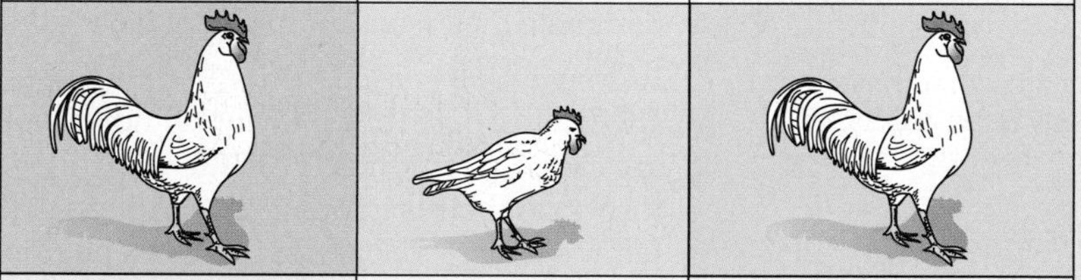

Comb and wattles:	Large	Small	Large
Mount hens?	Yes	No	Yes
Aggressive?	Yes	No	Yes
Crowing?	Normal	Weak	Normal

■ **Outcome**

The animals with the reimplanted testes grew up to look and act like normal males. Berthold reasoned that the testes must have secreted a signal, which today we would call a hormone, that has widespread effects on the body and brain. Today we know that the hormone is testosterone.

(A) Endocrine function

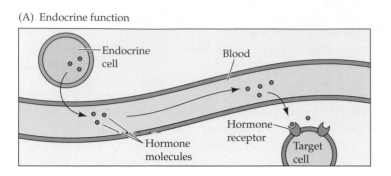

(B) Neural function (synaptic transmission)

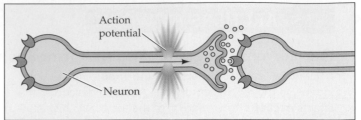

FIGURE 8.3 Chemical Communication Systems

(C) Pheromone function

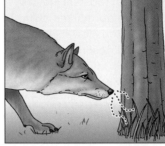

(D) Allomone function

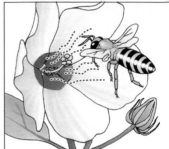

To view the
Brain Explorer,
go to
3e.mindsmachine.com/av8.2

To view the animation
Chemical Communication Systems,
go to
3e.mindsmachine.com/av8.3

endocrine   Referring to glands that release chemicals to the interior of the body. These glands secrete the principal hormones used by the body.

synapse   The cellular location at which information is transmitted from a neuron to another cell.

pheromone   A chemical signal that is released outside the body of an animal and affects other members of the same species.

allomone   A chemical signal that is released outside the body by one species and affects the behavior of other species.

peptide hormone   Also called *protein hormone*. A hormone that consists of a string of amino acids.

amine hormone   Also called *monoamine hormone*. A hormone composed of a single amino acid that has been modified into a related molecule, such as melatonin or epinephrine.

Hormones are one of several types of chemical communication

People had long suspected that special substances circulate to carry messages through the body, but as we discussed above, it wasn't until nineteenth-century scientists started experimenting with hormone-secreting glands that details of chemical communication began to emerge. We can compare hormonal communication with other methods of chemical signaling:

• *Endocrine communication* In **endocrine** communication, our topic for this chapter, the chemical signal is a hormone released into the bloodstream to selectively affect distant target organs (**FIGURE 8.3A**).

• *Synaptic communication* Communication via **synapses** was described in Chapters 3 and 4. In typical synaptic transmission, the released chemical signal diffuses a tiny distance across the synaptic cleft and causes a change in the postsynaptic membrane (**FIGURE 8.3B**).

• *Pheromone communication* Chemicals can be used for communication not only within an individual, but also *between* individuals. **Pheromones** are chemicals that are released outside the body to affect other individuals of the same species (**FIGURE 8.3C**). For example, ants produce pheromones that identify the route to a rich food source (to the annoyance of picnickers). Dogs and wolves urinate on landmarks to designate their territory. In Chapter 6 we discuss pheromones in more detail.

• *Allomone communication* Some chemical signals are released by members of one species to affect the behavior of individuals of *another* species. These substances are called **allomones** (**FIGURE 8.3D**). Flowers exude scented allomones to attract insects and birds in order to distribute pollen. And the bolas spider—nature's femme fatale—releases a moth sex pheromone to lure male moths to their doom (Haynes et al., 2002).

Let's review the basic types of hormones and how they influence cells.

Hormones can be classified by chemical structure

Most hormones fall into one of three categories: peptide hormones, amine hormones, or steroid hormones. Peptides are simply small protein molecules, so, like any other protein, a molecule of **peptide hormone** is made up of a short string of amino acids (**FIGURE 8.4A**). Different peptide hormones consist of different combinations of amino acids. **Amine hormones** are smaller and simpler, consisting of a modified version of

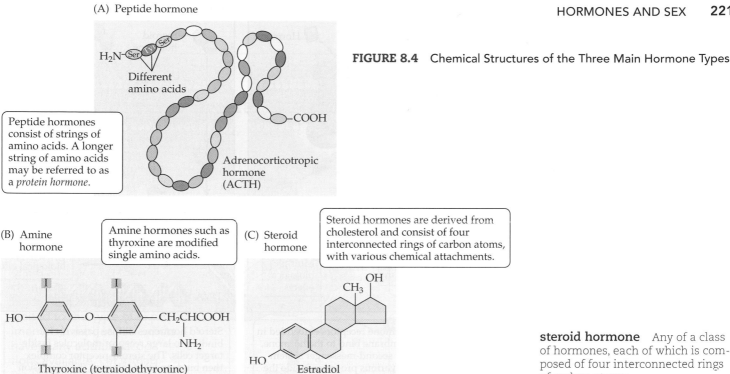

(A) Peptide hormone

H_2N—Ser—Tyr—Ser

Different amino acids

—COOH

Adrenocorticotropic hormone (ACTH)

Peptide hormones consist of strings of amino acids. A longer string of amino acids may be referred to as a *protein hormone*.

FIGURE 8.4   Chemical Structures of the Three Main Hormone Types

(B) Amine hormone

Amine hormones such as thyroxine are modified single amino acids.

HO—⬡—O—⬡—$CH_2CHCOOH$—NH_2
(I, I, I, I attached)

Thyroxine (tetraiodothyronine)

(C) Steroid hormone

Steroid hormones are derived from cholesterol and consist of four interconnected rings of carbon atoms, with various chemical attachments.

CH_3 OH

HO Estradiol

steroid hormone   Any of a class of hormones, each of which is composed of four interconnected rings of carbon atoms.

a single amino acid (hence their alias, *monoamine hormones*) (**FIGURE 8.4B**). The amine hormone melatonin is discussed in **A STEP FURTHER 8.1**, on the website.

Steroid hormones are derived from cholesterol and thus share its structure of four rings of carbon atoms (**FIGURE 8.4C**). Different steroid hormones vary in the number and kinds of atoms attached to the rings. Because steroids dissolve readily in lipids, they can pass through membranes easily (recall from Chapter 2 that cell membranes consist of a lipid bilayer). **TABLE 8.1** gives examples of each class of hormones.

The distinction between peptide or amine hormones and steroid hormones is important because the different types of hormones interact with different types of receptors, as we discuss next.

Hormones Act on a Wide Variety of Cellular Mechanisms

To prepare for later discussions of specific hormonal effects on behavior, let's look briefly at two aspects of hormone activity: first the mechanisms of hormone action, then the types of changes that hormones cause in target cells, including neurons.

Hormones initiate actions by binding to receptor molecules

The three classes of hormones exert their influences on target organs in two different ways. As we'll see next, peptide and amine hormones use one mode of action, while steroid hormones use another.

PEPTIDE AND AMINE HORMONES   Peptide and amine hormones bind to specific receptor proteins *on the surface* of the target cell and activate chemical signals inside the cell that are

TABLE 8.1   ■   Examples of Major Classes of Hormones

Class	Hormone
Peptide hormones	Adrenocorticotropic hormone (ACTH)
	Follicle-stimulating hormone (FSH)
	Luteinizing hormone (LH)
	Thyroid-stimulating hormone (TSH)
	Growth hormone (GH)
	Prolactin
	Insulin
	Glucagon
	Oxytocin
	Vasopressin (arginine vasopressin, AVP; antidiuretic hormone, ADH)
	Releasing hormones, such as:
	Corticotropin-releasing hormone (CRH)
	Gonadotropin-releasing hormone (GnRH)
Amine hormones	Epinephrine (adrenaline)
	Norepinephrine (NE)
	Thyroid hormones (e.g., thyroxine)
	Melatonin
Steroid hormones	Estrogens (e.g., estradiol)
	Progestins (e.g., progesterone)
	Androgens (e.g., testosterone, dihydrotestosterone)
	Glucocorticoids (e.g., cortisol)
	Mineralocorticoids (e.g., aldosterone)

(A)

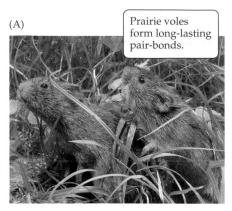

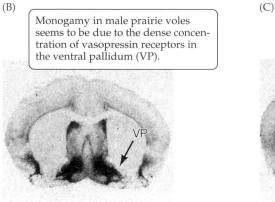

(B)

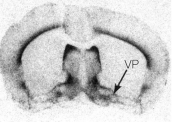

(C)

FIGURE 8.10   Vasopressin and the Monogamous Brain (Part A © Yva Momatiuk and John Eastcott/Minden Pictures; B and C courtesy of Miranda Lim and Larry Young.)

negative feedback   The property by which some of the output of a system feeds back to reduce the effect of input signals.

anterior pituitary   The front division of the pituitary gland. It secretes tropic hormones.

tropic hormone   Any of a class of anterior pituitary hormones that affect the secretion of hormones by other endocrine glands.

To view the animation
The Hypothalamus and Endocrine Function,
go to
3e.mindsmachine.com/av8.5

This is an example of the basic mechanism that regulates all hormone secretion, called **negative feedback**: output of the hormone *feeds back* to inhibit the drive for more of that same hormone (**FIGURE 8.11A**). This negative feedback action of a hormonal system is like that of a thermostat, and just as the thermostat can be set to different temperatures at different times, the set points of a person's endocrine feedback systems can change to meet varying circumstances. We'll discuss negative feedback regulation of other processes in Chapter 9 (see Figure 9.1).

Hormone secretion from the *anterior* pituitary is also regulated by negative feedback, but the mechanism is a bit more complicated, as we'll see next.

Hypothalamic releasing hormones govern the anterior pituitary

The **anterior pituitary** consists of many different endocrine cells, each secreting a different peptide hormone. So, unlike the posterior half of the pituitary, the anterior pituitary actually synthesizes the hormones it releases. The anterior pituitary hormones are called **tropic hormones**. (The *o* in *tropic* is pronounced "oh"; there is

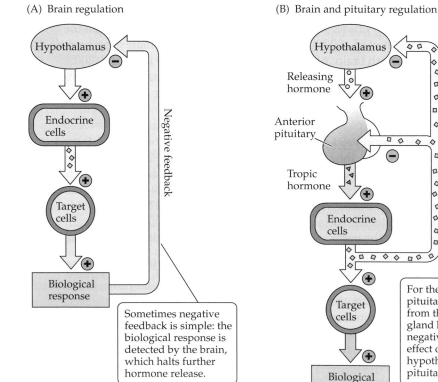

FIGURE 8.11   Endocrine Feedback Loops

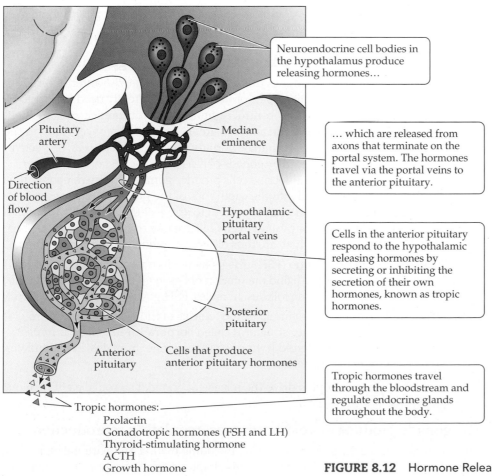

nothing "tropical" about these hormones.) The term *tropic* means "directed toward," and each tropic hormone acts on a different endocrine gland, such as the thyroid or ovaries, as if the tropic hormone were directed toward that gland. Actually, the tropic hormone travels throughout the bloodstream, reaching *all* glands, but only the *target* glands have the appropriate receptors to respond to it. Once the tropic hormone reaches a target gland, it drives the gland to produce its own hormone. For example, one anterior pituitary tropic hormone acts on the thyroid gland to make it secrete thyroid hormones.

To regulate secretions of tropic hormones from the anterior pituitary, the hypothalamus uses another whole set of peptide hormones, called **releasing hormones**. The cells that synthesize the different releasing hormones are neuroendocrine cells residing in various regions of the hypothalamus (**FIGURE 8.11B**). The axons of these neuroendocrine cells converge on the **median eminence**, just above the pituitary stalk. This region contains a profusion of blood vessels that form the **hypothalamic-pituitary portal system**. Here, in response to inputs from the rest of the brain, the axon terminals of the hypothalamic neuroendocrine cells secrete their releasing hormones into the *local* bloodstream (**FIGURE 8.12**). Blood carries the various releasing hormones only a very short distance, into the anterior pituitary. The rate at which releasing hormones arrive at the anterior pituitary controls the rate at which the anterior pituitary cells, in turn, release their tropic hormones into the *general* circulation. These tropic hormones then regulate the activity of major endocrine organs throughout the body. Thus, the brain's releasing hormones affect the anterior pituitary's tropic hormones, which affect the release of hormones from endocrine glands.

releasing hormone   Any of a class of hormones, produced in the hypothalamus, that traverse the hypothalamic-pituitary portal system to control the pituitary's release of tropic hormones.

median eminence   A midline feature on the base of the brain that marks the point at which the pituitary stalk exits the hypothalamus to connect to the pituitary. The median eminence contains one end of the hypothalamic-pituitary portal system.

hypothalamic-pituitary portal system   An elaborate bed of blood vessels leading from the hypothalamus to the anterior pituitary.

Neuroendocrine cell bodies in the hypothalamus produce releasing hormones…

… which are released from axons that terminate on the portal system. The hormones travel via the portal veins to the anterior pituitary.

Cells in the anterior pituitary respond to the hypothalamic releasing hormones by secreting or inhibiting the secretion of their own hormones, known as tropic hormones.

Tropic hormones travel through the bloodstream and regulate endocrine glands throughout the body.

Pituitary artery

Median eminence

Direction of blood flow

Hypothalamic-pituitary portal veins

Posterior pituitary

Anterior pituitary

Cells that produce anterior pituitary hormones

Tropic hormones:
  Prolactin
  Gonadotropic hormones (FSH and LH)
  Thyroid-stimulating hormone
  ACTH
  Growth hormone

FIGURE 8.12   Hormone Release by the Anterior Pituitary

The hypothalamic neuroendocrine cells that synthesize the releasing hormones are themselves subject to two kinds of influences. First, they are directly affected by *circulating messages*, such as other hormones, especially hormones that were secreted in response to tropic hormones (see Figure 8.11B). This hormone sensitivity of the hypothalamic neurons is an important part of the negative feedback we mentioned earlier, because typically the hormones secreted from an endocrine gland feedback to inhibit the secretion of releasing hormones and tropic hormones. Negative feedback in this case goes from the hormone of the endocrine gland to both the hypothalamus and the anterior pituitary.

Second, the hypothalamic neuroendocrine cells that provide releasing hormones also receive *synaptic inputs* (either excitatory or inhibitory) from many other brain regions. As a result, the release of hormones by the anterior pituitary is coordinated with ongoing events, such as time of day, time of the year, safety of the individual, and so on. For example, if a child is living in stressful, abusive conditions, the brain monitors these conditions and reduces the production of releasing hormones that stimulate the anterior pituitary release of **growth hormone** (GH), as we discuss in **A STEP FURTHER 8.3**, on the website.

Thus, the hypothalamic-releasing-hormone system exerts high-level control over endocrine organs throughout the body, translating brain activity into hormonal action. Cutting the pituitary stalk interrupts the portal blood vessels and the flow of releasing hormones, leading to profound atrophy of the pituitary, as well as major hormonal disruptions.

HOW'S IT GOING ?

1. How do hormones and behaviors interact in the milk letdown reflex?
2. How are hormones released from the posterior pituitary?
3. Describe the system regulating hormone release from the anterior pituitary, and explain how that system controls other endocrine glands.

Two anterior pituitary tropic hormones act on the gonads

Driven by various releasing hormones from the hypothalamus, the anterior pituitary gland secretes at least six different tropic hormones. We don't really need to go into all these hormones and the glands they control right now, but you can learn more about them in **A STEP FURTHER 8.4**, on the website. Here we will concentrate on the tropic hormones that affect male and female **gonads** (the *testes* and *ovaries*, respectively), because the hormones produced by gonads play a role in the rest of this chapter.

In the hypothalamus, neuroendocrine cells produce **gonadotropin-releasing hormone** (**GnRH**), which is secreted into the capillaries of the median eminence, traveling via the hypothalamic-pituitary portal system to arrive at the anterior pituitary. In response to this GnRH, anterior pituitary cells release one or both of the tropic hormones that act on the gonads, which are thus collectively known as **gonadotropins**:

1. **Follicle-stimulating hormone** (**FSH**) gets its name from its actions in the ovary, where it stimulates the growth and maturation of egg-containing **follicles** and the secretion of estrogens from the follicles. In males, FSH governs sperm production.
2. **Luteinizing hormone** (**LH**) stimulates the follicles of the ovary to rupture, release their eggs, and form into structures called **corpora lutea** (singular *corpus luteum*) that secrete the sex steroid hormone progesterone. In males, LH stimulates the testes to produce testosterone.

Since both of the gonadotropins drive the release of gonadal steroids, we'll turn our attention to those hormones next.

The gonads produce steroid hormones, regulating reproduction

Almost all aspects of reproductive behavior, including mating and parental behaviors, depend on hormones, as we'll see later in this chapter. Each ovary or testis consists of

---

growth hormone (GH)   Also called *somatotropin* or *somatotropic hormone*. A tropic hormone, secreted by the anterior pituitary, that promotes the growth of cells and tissues.

gonad   Any of the sexual organs (ovaries in females, testes in males) that produce gametes for reproduction.

gonadotropin-releasing hormone (GnRH)   A hypothalamic hormone that controls the release of luteinizing hormone and follicle-stimulating hormone from the pituitary.

gonadotropin   An anterior pituitary tropic hormone that stimulates the cells of the gonads to produce sex steroids and gametes.

follicle-stimulating hormone (FSH)   A gonadotropin, named for its actions on ovarian follicles.

follicle   The structure of the ovary that contains an immature ovum (egg).

luteinizing hormone (LH)   A gonadotropin, named for its stimulatory effects on the ovarian corpora lutea.

corpus luteum   The structure that forms from the collapsed ovarian follicle after ovulation. The corpora lutea are a major source of progesterone.

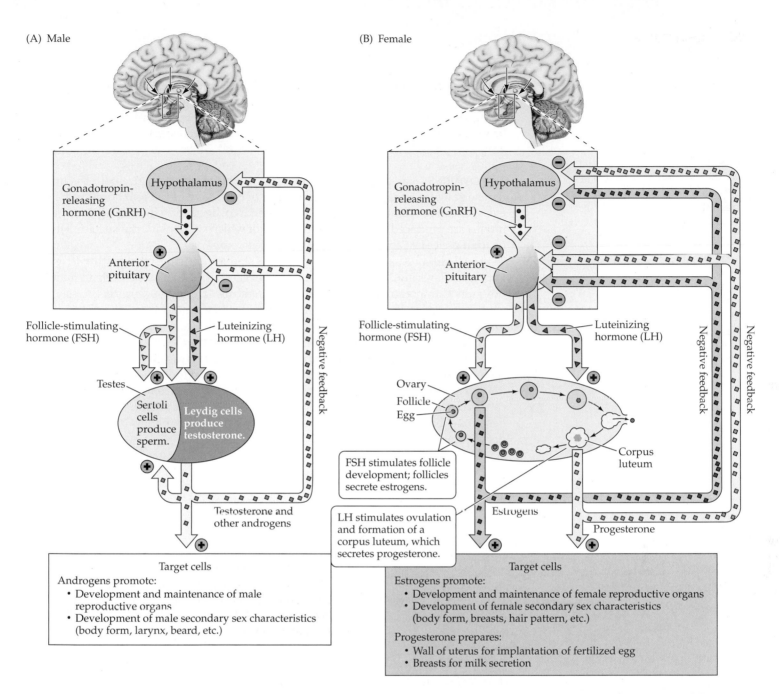

(A) Male

Gonadotropin-releasing hormone (GnRH)

Hypothalamus

⊖

Anterior pituitary

⊕

⊖

Follicle-stimulating hormone (FSH)

Luteinizing hormone (LH)

Negative feedback

Testes

⊕

Sertoli cells produce sperm.

Leydig cells produce testosterone.

⊕

Testosterone and other androgens

⊕

Target cells

Androgens promote:
• Development and maintenance of male reproductive organs
• Development of male secondary sex characteristics (body form, larynx, beard, etc.)

(B) Female

Gonadotropin-releasing hormone (GnRH)

Hypothalamus

⊖

⊖

Anterior pituitary

⊕

⊖

⊖

Follicle-stimulating hormone (FSH)

Luteinizing hormone (LH)

Negative feedback

Negative feedback

Ovary

Follicle

Egg

Corpus luteum

⊕

FSH stimulates follicle development; follicles secrete estrogens.

LH stimulates ovulation and formation of a corpus luteum, which secretes progesterone.

Estrogens

Progesterone

⊕

⊕

Target cells

Estrogens promote:
• Development and maintenance of female reproductive organs
• Development of female secondary sex characteristics (body form, breasts, hair pattern, etc.)

Progesterone prepares:
• Wall of uterus for implantation of fertilized egg
• Breasts for milk secretion

FIGURE 8.13 Regulation of the Gonadal Steroid Hormones

two different subcompartments—one to produce hormones (the sex steroids we mentioned earlier) and another to produce *gametes* (eggs or sperm). The gonadal hormones are critical for triggering both reproductive behavior controlled by the brain, and gamete production.

THE TESTES Within the **testes** (singular *testis*) are Sertoli cells, which produce sperm, and Leydig cells, which produce and secrete the steroid **testosterone**. Testosterone and other male hormones are called **androgens** (from the Greek *andro*, "man," and *gennan*, "to produce").

Testosterone controls a wide range of bodily changes that become visible at puberty, including changes in voice, hair growth, and genital size. In species that breed only in certain seasons of the year, testosterone has especially marked effects on appearance and behavior—for example, the antlers and fighting between males that are displayed by many species of deer. **FIGURE 8.13A** summarizes the regulation of testosterone secretion. As men age, testosterone levels tend to decline. Although elderly men who happen to maintain high levels of circulating testosterone perform better on tests

testes The male gonads, which produce sperm and androgenic steroid hormones.

testosterone A hormone, produced by male gonads, that controls a variety of bodily changes that become visible at puberty. It is one of a class of hormones called *androgens*.

androgen Any of a class of hormones that includes testosterone and similar steroids.

ovaries The female gonads, which produce eggs (ova) for reproduction.

progestin Any of a major class of steroid hormones that are produced by the ovary, including progesterone.

estrogen Any of a class of steroid hormones, including estradiol, produced by female gonads.

estradiol Formally called *17-beta-estradiol*. The primary type of estrogen secreted by the ovary.

progesterone The primary type of progestin secreted by the ovary.

ovulatory cycle The periodic occurrence of ovulation in females.

oral contraceptive A birth control pill, typically consisting of steroid hormones to prevent ovulation.

of memory and attention than do those with low levels (Yaffe et al., 2002), there have been too few studies to tell whether taking supplemental testosterone actually helps aging men (Hua et al., 2016; Snyder et al., 2018). Furthermore, taking supplemental testosterone can sometimes increase aggressive or manic behaviors (Pope et al., 2000), as well as possibly increasing prostate cancer risk.

THE OVARIES The paired female gonads, the **ovaries**, also produce both the mature female gametes—called *ova* (singular *ovum*) or *eggs*—and sex steroid hormones. However, hormone secretion is more complicated in ovaries than in testes. Ovarian hormones are produced in cycles, the duration of which varies with the species. Human ovarian cycles last about 4 weeks; rat cycles last only 4 days.

The ovary produces two major classes of steroid hormones: **progestins** (from the Latin *pro*, "favoring," and *gestare*, "to bear," because these hormones help to maintain pregnancy) and **estrogens** (from the Latin *oestrus*, "frenzy"—*estrus* is the scientific term for the periodic sexual receptivity of females in many species). The most important naturally occurring estrogen is **estradiol** (specifically, 17-beta-estradiol). The primary progestin is **progesterone**.

The **ovulatory cycle** begins when FSH stimulates ovarian follicles to grow and secrete estrogens (**FIGURE 8.13B**). The estrogens induce the hypothalamus and pituitary to release LH, which triggers the release of an egg from a follicle (ovulation) and causes the follicle to develop as a corpus luteum. The corpus luteum then secretes progesterone for a limited time to maintain the uterus for pregnancy. If the female does not become pregnant, the cycle starts over again.

Oral contraceptives contain small doses of synthetic estrogens and/or progestins, which exert a negative feedback effect on the hypothalamus, inhibiting the release of GnRH. The lack of GnRH prevents the release of FSH and LH from the pituitary, and therefore the ovary fails to release an egg for fertilization.

Estrogens may improve aspects of cognitive functioning (Ycaza Herrera and Mather, 2015), although this topic is still debated (Dohanich, 2003; Sherwin, 2009; Korol and Pisani, 2015). Estrogens may also protect the brain from some of the effects of stress and stroke (S. Suzuki et al., 2009; Petrone et al., 2014). For these reasons and others, estrogen replacement therapy has been a popular postmenopausal treatment, but the possibility that these treatments increase the risk of serious diseases like cancer and heart disease (Turgeon et al., 2004; Prentice, 2014) makes the decision of whether to take the hormones difficult for postmenopausal women.

RELATIONS AMONG GONADAL HORMONES All steroid hormones—including androgens, estrogens, and progestins—are based on the chemical structure of cholesterol (see Figure 8.4C). Glands manufacture steroid hormones by using enzymes to modify cholesterol, step by step, into different steroids. For example, ovaries first convert cholesterol into progestins, and then they convert those progestins into androgens, which are then converted into estrogens.

Different organs—and the two sexes—differ in the *relative* amounts of gonadal steroids that they produce. For example, whereas the testes convert only a relatively small proportion of testosterone into estradiol, the ovaries convert most of the testosterone they make into estradiol. What's important to understand is that *no steroid is found exclusively in either males or females.*

Hormonal and neural systems interact to produce integrated responses

The endocrine system and the nervous system work together, each affecting the other, seamlessly integrating various body systems to produce adaptive responses to the environment. So, for example, if our sensory system tells us that a stimulus calls for action—perhaps that faint buzzing sound you're hearing turns out to be coming from a

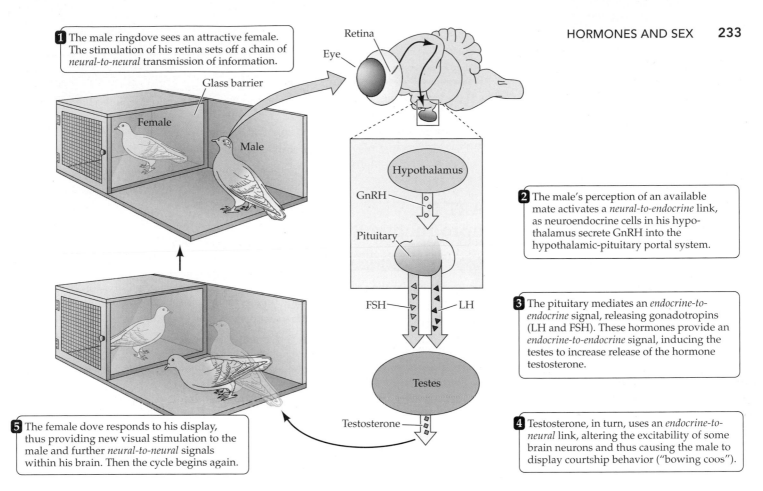

1 The male ringdove sees an attractive female. The stimulation of his retina sets off a chain of *neural-to-neural* transmission of information.

Retina

Eye

Glass barrier

Female

Male

Hypothalamus

GnRH

Pituitary

FSH — LH

Testes

Testosterone

2 The male's perception of an available mate activates a *neural-to-endocrine* link, as neuroendocrine cells in his hypothalamus secrete GnRH into the hypothalamic-pituitary portal system.

3 The pituitary mediates an *endocrine-to-endocrine* signal, releasing gonadotropins (LH and FSH). These hormones provide an *endocrine-to-endocrine* signal, inducing the testes to increase release of the hormone testosterone.

4 Testosterone, in turn, uses an *endocrine-to-neural* link, altering the excitability of some brain neurons and thus causing the male to display courtship behavior ("bowing coos").

5 The female dove responds to his display, thus providing new visual stimulation to the male and further *neural-to-neural* signals within his brain. Then the cycle begins again.

FIGURE 8.14 Four Kinds of Signals between the Nervous System and the Endocrine System

nest of angry wasps—hormones can be released to provide energy to fuel appropriate behaviors (sprinting away, yelling, cursing maybe).

Four kinds of signals are possible between neurons and endocrine cells: neural-to-neural, neural-to-endocrine, endocrine-to-endocrine, and endocrine-to-neural. All four types are illustrated in the courtship behavior of the ringdove. The visual processing that occurs when a male dove sees an attractive female involves neural-to-neural transmission (**FIGURE 8.14**, step 1). The details of the particular visual stimulus—namely, an opportunity to mate—activate a neural-to-endocrine link (step 2), which causes neuroendocrine cells in the male's hypothalamus to secrete GnRH. The GnRH provides an endocrine-to-endocrine signal (step 3), stimulating the pituitary to release gonadotropins, which induce the testes to release more testosterone. Testosterone in turn alters the excitability of neurons in the male's brain through an endocrine-to-neural link (step 4), causing the male to display courtship behavior. The female dove responds to this display (step 5), thus providing new visual stimulation to the male, which triggers another cycle of signaling in him.

The interactions between endocrine activity and behavior are cyclical, as depicted by the circle schema in **FIGURE 8.15**. The levels of circulating hormones can be altered by experience, which in turn can affect future behavior and future experience. For example, men rooting for a sports team will produce more testosterone if their team wins (Bernhardt et al., 1998), which may in turn affect their future behavior and future experience. Physical stresses, pain, and unpleasant emotional situations trigger the release of steroids from the adrenal gland (see Chapter 11).

Conversely, each of these hormonal events will affect the brain, shaping behavior, which will once more affect the person's future hormone production, and so on. It will be important to keep in mind these interactions between hormones and behavior as we consider reproductive behavior in the next section.

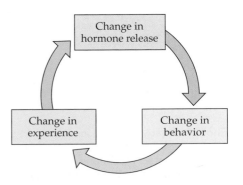

Change in hormone release

Change in behavior

Change in experience

FIGURE 8.15 The Reciprocal Relations between Hormones and Behavior

sexual attraction   The first step in the mating behavior of many animals, in which animals emit stimuli that attract members of the opposite sex.

appetitive behavior   The second stage of mating behavior. It helps establish or maintain sexual interaction.

proceptive   Referring to a state in which a female advertises her readiness to mate through species-typical behaviors.

copulation   Also called *coitus*. The sexual act.

intromission   Insertion of the penis into the vagina during copulation.

vagina   The opening from the outside of the body to the cervix and uterus in females.

ejaculation   The forceful expulsion of semen from the penis.

semen   A mixture of fluid and sperm that is released during ejaculation.

refractory phase   A period following copulation during which an individual does not recommence copulation.

Coolidge effect   The propensity of an animal that appears sexually satisfied with a current partner to resume sexual activity when provided with a new partner.

PART II
Reproductive Behavior

THE ROAD AHEAD

Now we consider the role of hormones in regulating reproductive behavior, including sexual and maternal behavior. Integrating this material should allow you to:

1. Discuss the sequence of mating behaviors in animals and the role of hormones in regulating those behaviors.
2. Outline the brain regions that control sexual behavior in male and female rats.
3. Describe the maternal behaviors of rats and the roles of experience versus hormones in facilitating them.
4. Describe the typical sequence of sexual arousal in women and men, and offer a critical appraisal of whether hormones influence human sexual behavior.

Reproductive Behavior Can Be Divided into Four Stages

Taking a broad view of reproductive behavior, we recognize four distinct stages: (1) sexual attraction, (2) appetitive behavior, (3) copulation, and (4) postcopulatory behavior (**FIGURE 8.16**).

Sexual attraction is the first stage in bringing males and females together. In many species, sexual attraction is closely synchronized with physiological readiness to reproduce. Most male mammals are attracted by particular female odors, which tend to reflect estrogen levels. Because estrogen secretion is associated with the release of eggs, this means female sexual attractiveness peaks alongside fertility. Of course, the female may find a particular male unattractive and refuse to mate with him. Although apparent rape has been described in some nonhuman species (Thornhill and Palmer,

Enough already!   By reducing the refractory phase, when a sexually exhausted male encounters an unfamiliar female, the Coolidge effect permits him to take advantage of a new reproductive opportunity and sire more offspring. (Of course, encountering 24 lovelorn females at once is a situation few males—guinea pig or otherwise—could even dream of.) (© Jane Burton/Minden Pictures.)

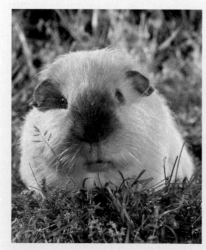

Sooty enjoyed two nights of passion among 24 females.

Guinea pig Don Juan sires 43 offspring in 2 nights

PONTYPRIDD, WALES, 1 DECEMBER 2000

HAVING ESCAPED from captivity at Little Friend's Farm earlier this year, a male guinea pig named Sooty chose to re-enter captivity immediately—in the nearby cage housing 24 females. Two months later he is now the father of 43 offspring.

According to his owner, Carol Feehan, Sooty was missing for two whole days before the staff checked the females' pen. "We did a head count and found 25 guinea pigs," she told the press. "Sooty was fast asleep in the corner.

"He was absolutely shattered. We put him back in his cage and he slept for two days."

2000; Maggioncalda and Sapolsky, 2002), for most species copulation is not possible without the female's active cooperation.

If the animals are mutually attracted, they may progress to the next stage: **appetitive behaviors**—species-specific behaviors that establish, maintain, or promote sexual interaction. A female displaying these behaviors is said to be **proceptive**: she may approach males, remain close to them, or show alternating approach and retreat behaviors. Proceptive female rats typically exhibit "ear wiggling" and a hopping and darting gait to induce a male to mount. Male appetitive behaviors usually consist of staying near the female. In many mammals, the male may sniff around the female's face and vagina. Male birds may engage in elaborate songs or nest-building behaviors, as illustrated for the ringdove in Figure 8.14.

If both animals display appetitive behaviors, they may progress to the third stage of reproduction: **copulation**, also known as *coitus*. In many vertebrates, including all mammals, copulation involves one or more **intromissions**, in which the male inserts his penis into the female's **vagina**, followed by a variable amount of stimulation, usually through pelvic thrusting. When stimulation reaches a threshold level, the male **ejaculates** sperm-bearing **semen** into the female; the length of time required for ejaculation varies greatly between species.

After one bout of copulation, the animals will not mate again for a period of time, which is called the **refractory phase**. The refractory phase varies from minutes to months, depending on the species and circumstances. Many animals will resume mating sooner if they are provided with a new partner—a phenomenon known as the **Coolidge effect** (named after an old joke about U.S. President Calvin Coolidge [Google it]).

The female is often the one to choose whether copulation will take place; when she is willing to copulate, she is said to be **sexually receptive**, in heat, or in **estrus**. In some species, the female may show proceptive behaviors days before she will participate in copulation itself. In most (but not all) species, females are receptive only when mating is likely to produce offspring. Most species are seasonal breeders, with females that are receptive only during the breeding season; some—such as Pacific salmon, octopuses, and cicadas—reproduce only once, at the end of life.

Finally, the fourth stage of reproductive behavior consists of **postcopulatory behaviors**. These behaviors are especially varied, having been strongly shaped by diverse evolutionary pressures related to the different species' mating systems. For example, in some mammals, including dogs and southern grasshopper mice, the male's penis swells so much after ejaculation that he can't remove it from the female for a while. In species like these, where several males may copulate with an ovulating female in quick succession, this phenomenon, called *copulatory lock*, prevents other males from mating, at least for a while (Dewsbury, 1972). Despite wild stories you may have heard or read, humans *never* experience copulatory lock; that urban myth started in 1884 when a physician submitted a fake report as a practical joke (Nation, 1973). For mammals and birds, postcopulatory behavior includes extensive parental behaviors to nurture the offspring, as we describe later in this chapter.

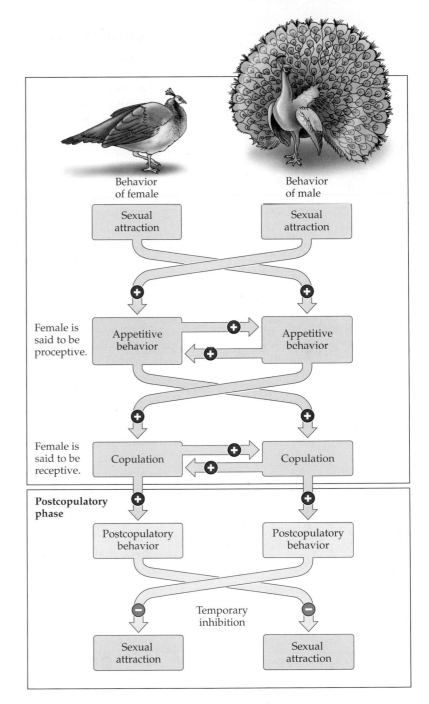

FIGURE 8.16 Stages of Reproductive Behavior (After F. A. Beach, 1976. *Horm. Behav.* 7: 105.)

sexually receptive Referring to the state in which an individual (in mammals, typically the female) is willing to copulate.

estrus The period during which female animals are sexually receptive.

postcopulatory behavior The final stage in mating behavior. Species-specific postcopulatory behaviors include rolling (in the cat) and grooming (in the rat).

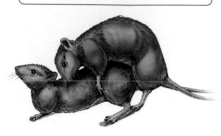

The raised rump and deflected tail of the female (the lordosis posture) make intromission possible in rats.

FIGURE 8.17   Copulation in Rats (After S. A. Barnett, 1975. *The rat: A study in behavior.* University of Chicago Press. Chicago, IL.)

gamete   A sex cell (sperm or ovum) that contains only unpaired chromosomes and therefore has only half of the usual number of chromosomes.

sperm   The gamete produced by males for the fertilization of eggs (ova).

ovum   An egg, the female gamete.

zygote   The fertilized egg.

ovulation   The production and release of an egg (ovum).

lordosis   A female receptive posture in four-legged animals in which the hindquarters are raised and the tail is turned to one side, facilitating intromission by the male.

activational effect   A temporary change in behavior resulting from the availability of a hormone to an adult animal.

Copulation brings gametes together

All mammals, birds, and reptiles employ internal fertilization: the fusion of their **gametes**—**sperm** and **ovum**—within the female's body to form a **zygote**. Most of what we know about the copulatory behavior of mammals comes from studies of lab animals, especially rats. Like most other rodents, rats do not engage in lengthy courtship, nor do the partners tend to remain together after copulation. Rats are attracted to each other largely through odors. Female rats, like humans, are spontaneous ovulators; that is, even when left alone, they **ovulate** (release eggs from the ovary). For a few hours around the time of ovulation, the female rat seeks out a male and displays proceptive behaviors, including vocalizations at frequencies too high for humans to detect but audible to other rats.

These behaviors prompt the male to mount the female from the rear, grasp her flanks with his forelegs, and rhythmically thrust his hips against her rump. If she is receptive, the female adopts a stereotyped posture called **lordosis** (**FIGURE 8.17**), elevating her rump and moving her tail to one side to allow intromission. Once intromission has been achieved, the male rat makes a single deep thrust and then springs back off the female. During the next 6–7 minutes the male and female orchestrate seven to nine such intromissions; then, instead of springing away, the male raises the front half of his body up for a second or two while he ejaculates, then falls backward off the female.

After copulation, the male and female separately engage in grooming their own genitalia, and the male pays little attention to the female for the next 5 minutes or so, until, often in response to the female's proceptive behaviors, the two engage in another bout of intromissions and ejaculation. The cycle may repeat five or six times in one mating session.

Gonadal steroids activate sexual behavior

Hormones play an important role in rat mating behaviors. Testosterone drives the male's interest in copulation: if he is castrated, he will stop ejaculating within a few weeks and will eventually stop mounting receptive females. Although testosterone disappears from the bloodstream within a few hours after castration, the hormone's effects on the nervous system take days or weeks to dissipate. Treating a castrated male with testosterone eventually restores mating behavior; if testosterone treatment is stopped, the mating behavior fades away again. This is an example of a hormone exerting an **activational effect**: the hormone transiently promotes certain behaviors. In normal development, the rise of androgen secretion at puberty activates masculine behavior in males. Estrogens secreted at the beginning of the 4- to 5-day ovulatory cycle facilitate proceptive behavior in female rats, and the subsequent production of progesterone increases proceptive behavior and activates receptivity (**FIGURE 8.18**). An adult female whose ovaries have been removed will show neither proceptive nor receptive behaviors. However, 2 days of estrogen treatment followed by a single injection of progesterone will, about 6 hours later, make the female rat proceptive and receptive for a few hours. Only the correct combination of estrogens and progesterone will fully activate copulatory behaviors in female rats. Because steroids activate sexual behavior, you might wonder if individual differences in hormone levels account for differences in mating vigor, the subject of Researchers at Work, next.

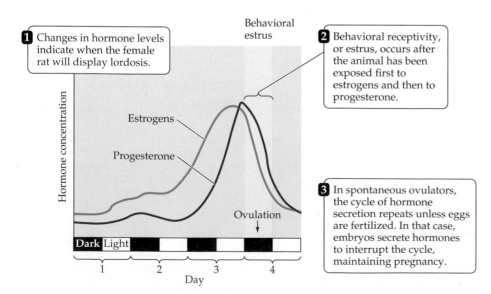

1 Changes in hormone levels indicate when the female rat will display lordosis.

2 Behavioral receptivity, or estrus, occurs after the animal has been exposed first to estrogens and then to progesterone.

3 In spontaneous ovulators, the cycle of hormone secretion repeats unless eggs are fertilized. In that case, embryos secrete hormones to interrupt the cycle, maintaining pregnancy.

Behavioral estrus

Hormone concentration

Estrogens

Progesterone

Ovulation

Dark | Light

1   2   3   4

Day

FIGURE 8.18   The Ovulatory Cycle of Rats

RESEARCHERS AT WORK

Individual differences in mating behavior

Although individual male rats and guinea pigs differ considerably in how eagerly they will mate, blood levels of testosterone clearly are *not* responsible for these differences. For one thing, animals displaying different levels of sexual vigor do not show reliable differences in blood levels of testosterone. Furthermore, when these males are castrated and subsequently all treated with exactly the same dose of testosterone, their precastration differences in sexual activity persist (**FIGURE 8.19**).

FIGURE 8.19   Androgens Permit Male Copulatory Behavior (After J. A. Grunt & W. C. Young, 1953. *J. Comp. Physiol. Psychol.* 46: 138.)

■ Hypothesis

Individual differences in the vigor with which male guinea pigs mate are caused by differences in testosterone secretion.

■ Test

Classify individual males by mating vigor, then castrate and provide them all with the same dose of testosterone.

■ Result

A few weeks after castration, all males stopped mating. But when provided the same dose of testosterone, males returned to their previous levels of mating vigor. Giving a higher dose of testosterone did not eliminate these differences.

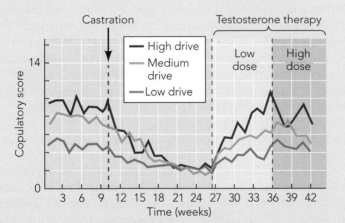

■ Conclusion

Although androgens—especially testosterone—are important for activating normal male sexual function, individual differences in sexual activity are not determined by differences in androgen levels.

   Furthermore, it turns out that a very small amount of testosterone—one-tenth the amount normally produced by the animals—is enough to fully maintain the mating behavior of male rats (Damassa et al., 1977). Thus, since all male rats make more testosterone than is required to maintain their copulatory behavior, some other factor, which we can call drive, must differ across individual males.

Next we'll discuss how steroid hormones affect the brain to activate mating behavior.

1. What are the four stages of reproductive behavior?
2. Describe a typical mating session in laboratory rats.
3. Describe the activational effects of gonadal steroids on mating behaviors in male and female rodents.
4. How do we know whether differences in testosterone secretion are responsible for individual differences in male mating vigor?

The Neural Circuitry of the Brain Regulates Reproductive Behavior

Although most of what we know about the neural circuitry of sexual behavior comes from studies of rats, steroid receptors are found in the same specific brain regions across a wide variety of vertebrate species. Steroid-sensitive regions include the cortex, brainstem nuclei, medial amygdala, hypothalamus, and many others. We'll see that the hypothalamus plays a particularly important role in regulating copulatory behavior.

Estrogen and progesterone act on a lordosis circuit that spans from brain to muscle

Scientists have exploited the steroid sensitivity of the rat lordosis response to develop a map of the neural circuitry that controls this behavior (Pfaff, 1997). Using steroid autoradiography (see Box 8.1), investigators identified hypothalamic nuclei containing many estrogen- and progesterone-sensitive neurons. In particular, the **ventromedial hypothalamus (VMH)** is crucial for lordosis because lesions there abolish the response. Furthermore, tiny quantities of estradiol implanted directly into the brain can induce receptivity in females, but only when the hormone is placed in the VMH (Lisk, 1962).

One action of estrogen treatment is to cause dendrites of VMH neurons to grow and become more complex (Meisel and Luttrell, 1990). Another important action of estrogens is to stimulate the production of progesterone receptors so that the animal will become more responsive to that hormone. Activated progesterone receptors in turn help mediate the lordosis reflex (Mani et al., 2000).

The VMH sends axons to the **periaqueductal gray** region of the midbrain, where again, lesions greatly diminish lordosis. The periaqueductal gray neurons project to other brain regions and the spinal cord. In the spinal cord the sensory information provided by the mounting male will now evoke the motor response of lordosis when the female's estrogen and progesterone levels are right. Thus, the role of the VMH is to monitor steroid hormone concentrations and, at the right time in the ovulatory cycle, activate a neural circuit that allows a lordosis response to a mounting male. **FIGURE 8.20B** schematically represents this neural pathway and its steroid-responsive components.

Androgens act on a neural system for male reproductive behavior

As with the lordosis circuit, mapping the sites of steroid action provided important clues about the neural circuitry controlling male copulatory behavior (**FIGURE 8.20A**). The hypothalamic **medial preoptic area (mPOA)** is chock-full of steroid-sensitive neurons, and lesions of the mPOA abolish male copulatory behavior in a wide variety of vertebrate species (Meisel and Sachs, 1994). Note that lesions of the mPOA do not interfere with males' *motivation* for females; males will still press a bar to gain access to a receptive female (Everitt and Stacey, 1987), but they seem unable to commence mounting. Furthermore, mating can be reinstated in castrated males by small implants of testosterone in the mPOA, but not in other brain regions. Thus, the mPOA seems to provide "higher-order" control of male copulatory behaviors.

ventromedial hypothalamus (VMH)   A hypothalamic region involved in sexual behaviors, eating, and aggression.

periaqueductal gray   A midbrain region involved in pain perception.

medial preoptic area (mPOA) A region of the anterior hypothalamus implicated in the control of many behaviors, including sexual behavior, gonadotropin secretion, and thermoregulation.

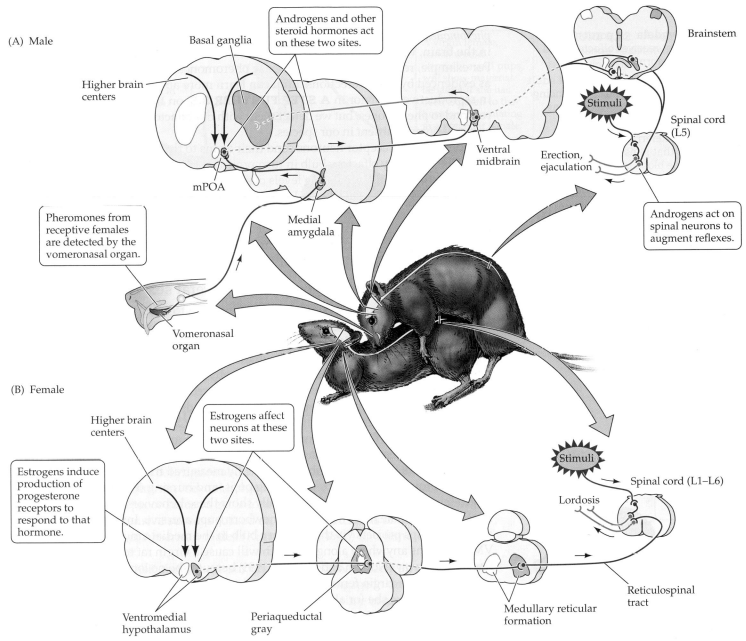

(A) Male

Higher brain centers

Basal ganglia

Androgens and other steroid hormones act on these two sites.

mPOA

Medial amygdala

Ventral midbrain

Brainstem

Stimuli

Spinal cord (L5)

Erection, ejaculation

Androgens act on spinal neurons to augment reflexes.

Pheromones from receptive females are detected by the vomeronasal organ.

Vomeronasal organ

(B) Female

Higher brain centers

Estrogens affect neurons at these two sites.

Estrogens induce production of progesterone receptors to respond to that hormone.

Ventromedial hypothalamus

Periaqueductal gray

Medullary reticular formation

Stimuli

Spinal cord (L1–L6)

Lordosis

Reticulospinal tract

FIGURE 8.20 Neural Circuits for Reproduction in Rodents (After D. W. Pfaff, 1980. *Estrogens and brain function: Neural analysis of a hormone-controlled mammalian reproductive behavior.* Springer-Verlag. New York, NY.)

The mPOA coordinates copulatory behavior by sending axons to the ventral midbrain (which innervates several brain regions to coordinate mounting behaviors) and, via a multisynaptic pathway, to the spinal cord (Hamson and Watson, 2004), which mediates various genital reflexes, such as ejaculation. Brainstem projections of serotonergic fibers to the spinal cord normally hold the penile erection reflex in check (McKenna, 1999). Antidepressant drugs that boost serotonergic activity in the brain—for example, selective serotonin reuptake inhibitors like Prozac (see Chapter 12)—can produce side effects that include difficulty achieving erection, ejaculation, and/or orgasm, probably by enhancing serotonergic inhibition of the spinal cord. (If you're wondering, the drug sildenafil, better known as Viagra, acts directly on tissue in the penis, not in the spinal cord or brain, to promote erection [Boolell et al., 1996].)

We can also learn about male copulatory mechanisms by tracing a sensory system that boosts male arousal in rodents: the vomeronasal system. The **vomeronasal organ**, or **VNO** (see Chapter 9), consists of specialized receptor cells near to, but separate from, the olfactory epithelium. These sensory cells detect chemicals called

vomeronasal organ (VNO)
A collection of specialized receptor cells, near to but separate from the olfactory epithelium, that detects pheromones and sends electrical signals to the accessory olfactory bulb in the brain.

sexual differentiation   The process by which individuals develop either male-like or female-like bodies and behavior.

indifferent gonads   The undifferentiated gonads of the early mammalian fetus, which will eventually develop into either testes or ovaries.

SRY gene   A gene on the Y chromosome that directs the developing gonads to become testes. The name SRY stands for **s**ex-determining **r**egion on the **Y** chromosome.

genital tubercle   In the early fetus, a "bump" between the legs that can develop into either a clitoris or a penis.

wolffian duct   A duct system in the embryo that will develop into male reproductive structures (epididymis, vas deferens, and seminal vesicle) if androgens are present.

müllerian duct   A duct system in the embryo that will develop into female reproductive structures (oviducts, uterus, and upper vagina) in the absence of AMH.

anti-müllerian hormone (AMH)   A peptide hormone secreted by the fetal testes that inhibits müllerian duct development.

dihydrotestosterone (DHT)   The 5-alpha-reduced metabolite of testosterone. DHT is a potent androgen that is principally responsible for the masculinization of the external genitalia in mammals.

5-alpha-reductase   An enzyme that converts testosterone into dihydrotestosterone.

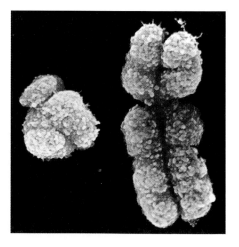

Mammalian Sex Chromosomes   The Y chromosome (*left*) is much shorter than the X (*right*) because it carries far fewer genes. But one of those genes, *SRY*, is critical for masculine development. (© Biophoto Associates/Science Source.)

PART III
Sexual Differentiation and Orientation

THE ROAD AHEAD

Now we take up the question of how developing females and males come to differ. Reading this final section of the chapter should allow you to:

1. Describe the chain of molecular and hormonal events that sculpt the mammalian fetus into a male or female form.
2. Identify several disorders of sexual development that affect that process.
3. Explain the organizational hypothesis of how sex differences in animal behavior arise.
4. Describe the role of hormones in the development of two prominent sexual dimorphisms in neuronal structure.
5. Critically discuss the extent to which prenatal hormones influence sex differences in human behavior, including sexual orientation.

Genetic and Hormonal Mechanisms Guide the Development of Masculine and Feminine Structures

A persistent bias in biomedical science has resulted in males being studied exclusively in most cases, on the assumption that female ovulatory cycles would introduce more variability and that whatever was found in males would hold true for both sexes. However, analysis of the animal literature revealed that in fact there is more variability in males than females (Prendergast et al., 2014), and many biomedical "facts" established in men do not hold for women (Cahill, 2014). For example, heart attacks in women tend to produce symptoms that are very different from those symptoms, derived from observations of men, that were the only ones publicized until recent years. In the USA, the National Institutes of Health (NIH) has now instituted a policy that future research grant applications must either include both sexes or provide a sound rationale for excluding one sex (Sandberg et al., 2015).

Sex chromosomes direct sexual differentiation of the gonads

Sexual differentiation is the process by which individuals develop either male or female bodies and behaviors. In mammals, this process begins before birth and continues into adulthood. In mammals, every egg carries an X chromosome from the mother; fusion with an X- or Y-bearing sperm is the key event in establishing the course of subsequent sexual differentiation of the body. With only occasional exceptions, mammals that receive an X chromosome from the father will become females with an XX sex chromosome complement; those that receive the father's Y chromosome will become XY males. The first major effect of sex chromosomes is on the gonads. Very early in development, each individual has a pair of **indifferent gonads**, glands that vaguely resemble both testes and ovaries. During the first month of gestation in humans, differential genetic instructions determine whether the indifferent gonads begin changing into ovaries or testes.

In mammals, the Y chromosome contains the **SRY gene** (for **s**ex-determining **r**egion on the **Y** chromosome), which is responsible for the development of testes. If an individual has a Y chromosome, the cells of the indifferent gonad begin making the Sry protein, inducing the organ to develop into a testis.

In XX individuals (or XY individuals with a dysfunctional *SRY* gene), no Sry protein is produced, and the indifferent gonad becomes an ovary. This early event of forming either testes or ovaries has a domino effect, setting off a chain of actions that usually results in either a male or a female.

Gonadal hormones direct sexual differentiation of the body

For all mammals, including humans, the gonads secrete hormones to direct sexual differentiation of the body. Fetal ovaries produce very little hormone, but fetal testes produce several hormones. If other embryonic cells are exposed to the testicular hormones, they begin developing masculine characters; if the cells are not exposed to testicular hormones, they develop feminine characters.

We can chart masculine or feminine development by examining the structures that connect the gonads to the outside of the body: these are quite different in adult males and females, but at the embryonic stage all individuals have the precursor tissues of both systems. The early fetus has a **genital tubercle** (a "bump" between the legs) that can form either a clitoris or a penis, as well as two sets of ducts that connect the tubercle to the indifferent gonads: the **wolffian ducts** and the **müllerian ducts** (**FIGURE 8.24A**). In females, the müllerian ducts develop into the oviducts (or *fallopian tubes*), uterus, and inner vagina (**FIGURES 8.24B** and **C** *right*), and only a remnant of the wolffian ducts remains. In males, hormones secreted by the testes orchestrate the converse outcome: each wolffian duct develops into an epididymis, vas deferens, and seminal vesicle (see Figures 8.24B and C *left*), while the müllerian ducts shrink to mere remnants.

The system is masculinized by two testicular secretions: testosterone, which promotes development of the wolffian system; and **anti-müllerian hormone** (**AMH**), which causes regression of the müllerian system. In the absence of testosterone and AMH, the genital tract develops in a feminine pattern, in which the wolffian ducts regress and the müllerian ducts develop into components of the female internal reproductive tract.

Testosterone masculinizes other structures too, acting on exterior tissues to form a scrotum and penis. These effects are aided by the local conversion of testosterone into a more potent androgen, **dihydrotestosterone** (**DHT**), promoted by an enzyme that is found in the genital skin, **5-alpha-reductase**. We'll see later that without the local production of DHT, testosterone alone is able to masculinize the genitalia only partially. If androgens are absent altogether, the genital tissues grow into the female labia and clitoris.

Changes in sexual differentiation processes result in predictable changes in development

Some people have only one sex chromosome: a single X (embryos containing only a single Y chromosome do not survive). This genetic makeup results in **Turner's syndrome**, in which an apparent female has underdeveloped but recognizable ovaries, as you might expect because no *SRY* gene is available. In general, unless the indifferent gonad becomes a testis and begins secreting hormones, immature mammals develop as females in most respects, including women with Turner's syndrome. So the sex chromosomes determine the sex of

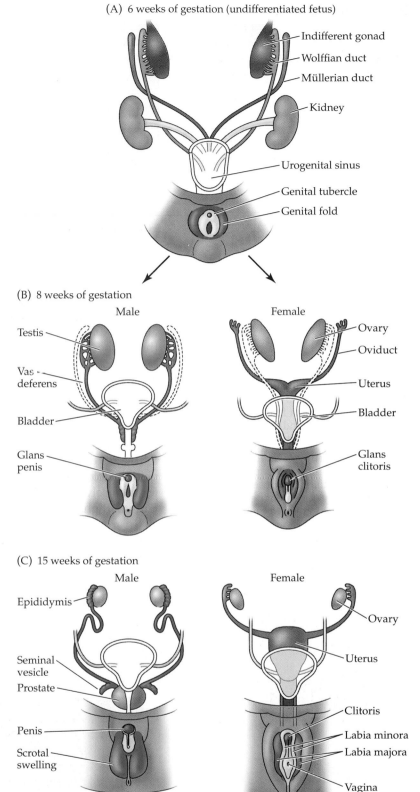

FIGURE 8.24 Sexual Differentiation in Humans

Turner's syndrome A condition, seen in individuals carrying a single X chromosome but no other sex chromosome, in which an apparent female has underdeveloped but recognizable ovaries.

RESEARCHERS AT WORK   (continued)

FIGURE 8.29 Organizational Effects of Testosterone on Rodent Behavior (After C. H. Phoenix et al., 1959. *Endocrinology* 65: 369.)

■ **Hypothesis**

Early in life, androgens organize the brain, and therefore adult behavior, in a masculine fashion.

■ **Test**

Manipulate androgen exposure in genetic male and female rodents early in life, then ask whether hormones in adulthood can elicit male and/or female behaviors.

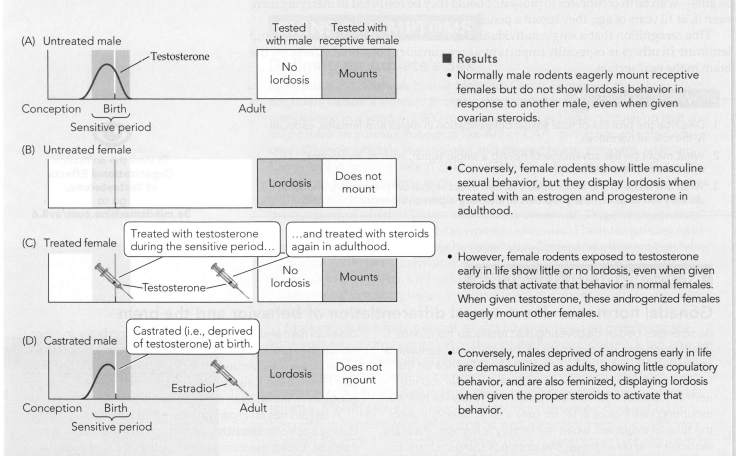

■ **Results**

• Normally male rodents eagerly mount receptive females but do not show lordosis behavior in response to another male, even when given ovarian steroids.

• Conversely, female rodents show little masculine sexual behavior, but they display lordosis when treated with an estrogen and progesterone in adulthood.

• However, female rodents exposed to testosterone early in life show little or no lordosis, even when given steroids that activate that behavior in normal females. When given testosterone, these androgenized females eagerly mount other females.

• Conversely, males deprived of androgens early in life are demasculinized as adults, showing little copulatory behavior, and are also feminized, displaying lordosis when given the proper steroids to activate that behavior.

■ **Conclusion**

When the developing brain is exposed to androgens, the animal's brain is organized in a masculine fashion, so that, as an adult, it is more likely to show malelike behaviors, and less likely to show femalelike behaviors.

Early testicular secretions result in masculine behavior in adulthood

What has come to be called the *organizational hypothesis* provides a unitary explanation for sexual differentiation: that a single steroid signal (androgen) diffuses through all tissues, masculinizing the body, the brain, and behavior (see Figure 8.25). From this point of view the nervous system is just another type of tissue listening for the androgenic signal that will instruct it to organize itself in a masculine fashion. If the nervous system does not detect androgens, it will organize itself in a mostly feminine fashion.

What was demonstrated originally for the lordosis behavior of guinea pigs has been observed in a variety of vertebrate species and for many behaviors. Exposing female rat pups to testosterone either just before birth or during the first 10 days after birth greatly reduces their lordosis responsiveness as adults. This explains the observation that adult male rats show very little lordosis, even when given estrogens and progesterone. However, male rats that are castrated during the first week of life readily display lordosis responses in adulthood if injected with estrogens and progesterone (**FIGURE 8.29D**). In rats, many behaviors conform to the organizational hypothesis: animals exposed to androgens early in life behave like males, whereas animals not exposed to androgens early in life behave like females.

In most cases, full masculine behavior requires androgens both during development (to organize the nervous system to enable the later behavior) and in adulthood (to activate that behavior). Only animals exposed to androgen both in development and in adulthood show fully masculine behavior.

Several regions of the nervous system display prominent sexual dimorphism

The fact that male and female rats behave differently means that their brains must be different in some way, and according to the organizational hypothesis this difference results primarily from androgenic masculinization of the developing brain. The exact form of these neural sex differences can be very subtle; the same basic circuit of neurons will produce very different behavior if the pattern of synapses varies. Sex differences in the number of synapses were identified in the preoptic area (POA) of the hypothalamus (Raisman and Field, 1971). But scientists soon found that there are much more obvious sex differences in the brain, including differences in the number, size, and shape of neurons. Darwin coined a term, **sexual dimorphism**, to describe the condition in which males and females show pronounced sex differences in structure. In all species studied so far, androgens are responsible for the sexual dimorphism seen in the brain: androgens masculinize the brain region, and the absence of androgens leads to a female-typical brain anatomy. We'll discuss two well-studied models.

THE PREOPTIC AREA OF RATS   Roger Gorski et al. (1978) examined the POA of the hypothalamus in rats because of the earlier reports that the number of synapses in this region was different in males and females and because lesions of the POA disrupt ovulatory cycles in female rats and, as we mentioned earlier, reduce copulatory behavior in males. Sure enough, the investigators found a nucleus within the POA that has a much larger volume in males than in females.

This nucleus, dubbed the **sexually dimorphic nucleus of the POA (SDN-POA)**, is much more evident in male rats than in females (**FIGURE 8.30**). The SDN-POA

sexual dimorphism   The condition in which males and females of the same species show pronounced sex differences in appearance.

sexually dimorphic nucleus of the preoptic area (SDN-POA)   A region of the preoptic area that is 5 to 6 times larger in volume in male than in female rats.

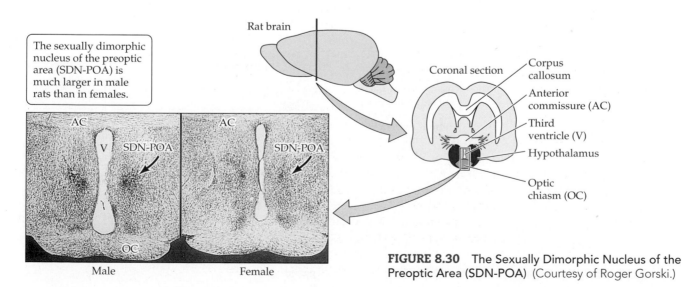

The sexually dimorphic nucleus of the preoptic area (SDN-POA) is much larger in male rats than in females.

Rat brain

Coronal section

Corpus callosum

Anterior commissure (AC)

Third ventricle (V)

Hypothalamus

Optic chiasm (OC)

AC

V   SDN-POA

AC

SDN-POA

Male

Female

FIGURE 8.30   The Sexually Dimorphic Nucleus of the Preoptic Area (SDN-POA) (Courtesy of Roger Gorski.)

conformed beautifully to the organizational hypothesis: males castrated at birth had much smaller SDN-POAs in adulthood, while females androgenized at birth had large, male-like SDN-POAs as adults. Castrating male rats in adulthood, however, did not alter the size of the SDN-POA. Thus, testicular androgens somehow alter the development of the SDN-POA, resulting in a nucleus permanently larger in males than in females (**FIGURE 8.31**).

One quirk of sexual dimorphism in the brains of some lab species, including rodents, is that testosterone reaching the brain is converted into estrogens that act on estrogen receptors, not androgen receptors, to masculinize the SDN-POA and some other brain regions. For example, XY rats that are androgen-insensitive (like the people with AIS discussed earlier) have testes but a feminine exterior. These rats have a masculine SDN-POA because their estrogen receptors are normal. Androgen-insensitive rats also do not display lordosis in response to estrogens and progesterone, because the testosterone that they secreted early in life was converted to an *estrogen* in the brain and masculinized their behavior (Olsen, 1979). Instead, the androgen-insensitive rats show normal male attraction to receptive females, with whom they may attempt to mate, despite the lack of a penis (Hamson et al., 2009). Estrogenic metabolites of testosterone do not seem to play a role in masculinizing the primate brain

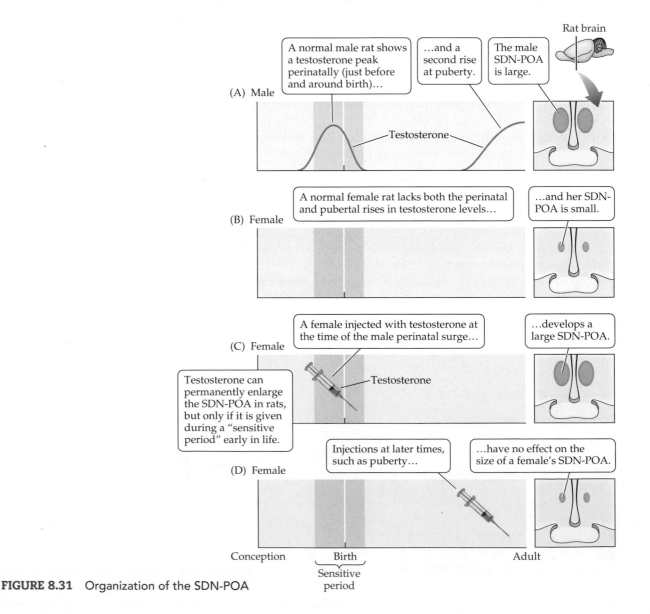

FIGURE 8.31   Organization of the SDN-POA

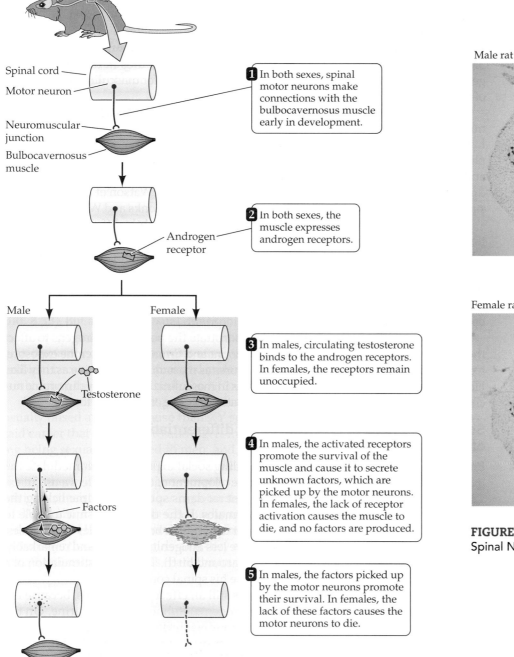

1. In both sexes, spinal motor neurons make connections with the bulbocavernosus muscle early in development.

Spinal cord
Motor neuron
Neuromuscular junction
Bulbocavernosus muscle

2. In both sexes, the muscle expresses androgen receptors.

Androgen receptor

Male | Female

3. In males, circulating testosterone binds to the androgen receptors. In females, the receptors remain unoccupied.

Testosterone

4. In males, the activated receptors promote the survival of the muscle and cause it to secrete unknown factors, which are picked up by the motor neurons. In females, the lack of receptor activation causes the muscle to die, and no factors are produced.

Factors

5. In males, the factors picked up by the motor neurons promote their survival. In females, the lack of these factors causes the motor neurons to die.

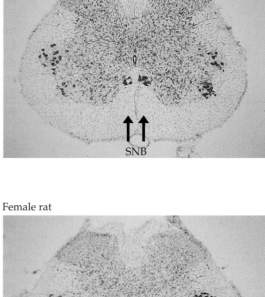

Male rat

SNB

Female rat

FIGURE 8.32 Sexual Differentiation of the Spinal Nucleus of the Bulbocavernosus (SNB)

(Grumbach and Auchus, 1999), so we won't deal with that mechanism any further, but you can learn more about it in **A STEP FURTHER 8.7**, on the website.

THE SPINAL CORD IN MAMMALS In rats, the bulbocavernosus (BC) muscles that surround the base of the penis are innervated by motor neurons in the **spinal nucleus of the bulbocavernosus (SNB)**. Male rats have about 200 SNB cells, but females have far fewer motor neurons in this region of the spinal cord.

On the day before birth, female rats have BC muscles attached to the base of the clitoris that are nearly as large as the BC muscles of males and that are innervated by motor neurons in the SNB region (Rand and Breedlove, 1987). In the days just before and after birth, however, many SNB cells die, especially in females (Nordeen et al., 1985), and the BC muscles of females die (**FIGURE 8.32**).

A single injection of androgens delivered to a newborn female rat permanently spares some SNB motor neurons and their muscles. Castration of newborn males,

spinal nucleus of the bulbocavernosus (SNB) A group of motor neurons in the spinal cord of rats that innervate muscles controlling the penis.

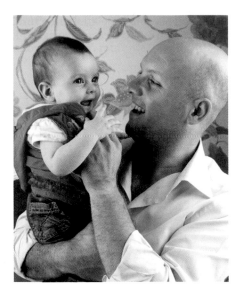

Training Girls to Be Verbal Adults tend to spend more time talking to a baby if they believe the baby is a girl (whether it actually is a girl or not) (Seavey et al., 1975). (Photo © istock.com/Murat Sarica.)

describe themselves as heterosexual, but they are more likely than other women to report being lesbians. Interestingly, as females with CAH grow older, the proportion who report being lesbians increases (Dittmann et al., 1992), suggesting that they start off trying to follow the socially approved role of heterosexual female but then become more comfortable with a gay orientation later in life. Do women with CAH exhibit those behaviors because early androgens partially masculinized their brains? Or did their ambiguous genitalia cause parents and others to treat them differently from infancy?

The *guevedoces* of the Dominican Republic, who are raised as girls but grow a penis at puberty, behave like males as adults, dressing like men and seeking girlfriends. There are two competing explanations for why these people raised as girls later behave as men. First, prenatal testosterone may masculinize their brains; thus, despite being raised as girls, when they reach puberty, their brains lead them to seek out females for mates. This explanation suggests that the social influences of growing up—assigning oneself to a gender and mimicking role models of that gender, as well as gender-specific playing and dressing—are unimportant for later behavior and sexual orientation.

An alternative explanation is that early hormones have no effect—that the local culture simply recognizes and teaches children that some people can start out as girls and change to boys later. If so, then the social influences on gender role development might be completely different in this society from those in ours. Of course, a third option is that both mechanisms contribute to the final outcome.

At the opening of the chapter, we discussed the dilemma of cloacal exstrophy, in which genetic boys are born with functional testes but without penises. Historically in these cases, neonatal sex reassignment has been recommended on the assumption that unambiguously raising these children as girls, and surgically providing them with the appropriate external genitalia, could produce a more satisfactory outcome. In a long-term follow-up of 14 such cases, however, Reiner and Gearhart (2004) found that 8 of these "girls" eventually declared themselves to be boys, even though several were unaware that they had ever been operated on. Although this finding indicates that prenatal exposure to androgens strongly predisposes subsequent male gender identity, 5 of the remaining 6 cases were apparently content with their female identities, suggesting that socialization can also play a strong role. However, almost all of these teenagers, including those who felt comfortable as girls, reported being sexually attracted to girls. These reports are part of a growing body of evidence suggesting that prenatal testosterone does in fact influence sexual orientation in humans, as we'll see next.

What determines a person's sexual orientation?

There are two kinds of developmental influences that could shape human sexual orientation. Sociocultural influences instruct children about how they should behave when they grow up (think of all those charming princes wooing princesses in Disney movies). But, as we discussed in the previous section, differences in fetal exposure to testosterone could also organize developing brains to be attracted to females or males in adulthood. For that great majority of people who are heterosexual, there's no way to distinguish between these two influences, because they both favor the same outcome. Gay people provide a test, because homosexuality (and other sexual minorities) remains stigmatized by various social groups and cultural institutions (Herek and Mc-Lemore, 2013). Is there evidence that early hormones are responsible for causing some people to ignore society's prescription and become gay? If so, then maybe hormones play a role in heterosexual development too.

Homosexual behavior is certainly seen in other species—mountain sheep, swans, gulls, and dolphins, to name a few (Bagemihl, 1999). Interestingly, homosexual behavior is more common among apes and monkeys than in prosimian primates like lemurs and lorises (Vasey, 1995), so perhaps greater complexity of the brain makes homosexual behavior more likely. In the most-studied animal model—sheep—some rams consistently refuse to mount females but prefer to mount other rams. There is

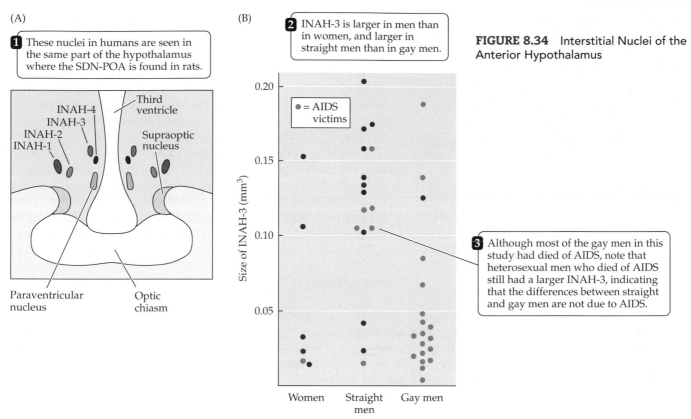

(A)

1 These nuclei in humans are seen in the same part of the hypothalamus where the SDN-POA is found in rats.

INAH-4
INAH-3
INAH-2
INAH-1

Third
ventricle

Supraoptic
nucleus

Paraventricular
nucleus

Optic
chiasm

(B)

2 INAH-3 is larger in men than in women, and larger in straight men than in gay men.

FIGURE 8.34 Interstitial Nuclei of the Anterior Hypothalamus

● = AIDS victims

Size of INAH-3 (mm³)

Women   Straight men   Gay men

3 Although most of the gay men in this study had died of AIDS, note that heterosexual men who died of AIDS still had a larger INAH-3, indicating that the differences between straight and gay men are not due to AIDS.

solid evidence of differences in the POA of "gay" versus "straight" rams (Roselli et al., 2004), apparently organized by testosterone acting on the brain during fetal development (Roselli and Stormshak, 2009).

Simon LeVay (1991) performed postmortem examinations of the POA in humans and found a nucleus (the third interstitial nucleus of the anterior hypothalamus, or INAH-3) (**FIGURE 8.34A**) that is larger in men than in women, and larger in heterosexual men than in gay men (**FIGURE 8.34B**). All but one of the gay men in the study had died of AIDS, but the brain differences could not be due to AIDS pathology, because straight men with AIDS still had a significantly larger INAH-3 than did the gay men (Byne et al., 2001). To the press and the public, this finding sounded like strong evidence that sexual orientation is "built in." It's still possible, however, that early social experience affects the development of INAH-3 to determine later sexual orientation. Furthermore, sexual experiences as an adult could affect INAH-3 structure, so the smaller nucleus in some homosexual men may be the *result* of their gay orientation, rather than the *cause*, as LeVay himself was careful to point out.

In women, purported markers of exposure to androgen as a fetus—sounds emitted from the ears (McFadden and Pasanen, 1998), patterns of eye blinks (Rahman, 2005), and finger length patterns (**FIGURE 8.35**)—all indicate that lesbians, on average, were exposed to slightly more fetal androgen than were heterosexual women. These findings suggest that fetal exposure to androgen

FIGURE 8.35 Bodily Indicators of Prenatal Androgen Note that these are group differences in averages; you cannot reliably determine an *individual's* orientation by examining digit ratios. (After T. J. Williams et al., 2000. *Nature* 404: 455.)

$\frac{2D}{4D}$

The ratio of the length of the index finger divided by the ring finger (2D:4D) is affected by prenatal androgen and indicates that lesbians, on average, were exposed to more prenatal testosterone than were straight women.

2D:4D ratio

0.97
0.96
0.95
0.94

Hetero-
sexual
men

Gay
men

Hetero-
sexual
women

Lesbians

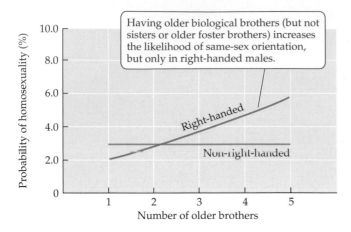

Having older biological brothers (but not sisters or older foster brothers) increases the likelihood of same-sex orientation, but only in right-handed males.

FIGURE 8.36 Older Brothers Increase the Chance That a Boy Will Grow Up Gay (After R. Blanchard et al., 2006. *Horm. Behav.* 49: 405.)

fraternal birth order effect
A phenomenon in human populations, such that the more older biological brothers a boy has, the more likely he is to grow up to be gay.

increases the likelihood that a girl will grow up to be gay. There is always considerable overlap between the two groups, so you cannot use these features to predict whether a particular woman is gay, and clearly fetal androgens cannot account for all lesbians. But if early androgen exposure results in later being attracted to women, maybe the reason most men are attracted to women is because they were exposed to prenatal androgen.

Yet there's little evidence that variation in prenatal androgen can account for gay versus straight men; some markers suggest that gay men were exposed to less prenatal testosterone, and others suggest that they were exposed to *more* prenatal testosterone than were straight men. However, another nonsocial factor influences the probability of homosexuality in men: the more older brothers a boy has, the more likely he is to grow up to be gay (Blanchard et al., 2006). Your first guess might be that this is a social influence of older brothers, but it turns out that older stepbrothers that are raised with the boy have no effect, while biological brothers (sharing the same mother) increase the probability of the boy's being gay *even if they are raised apart* (Bogaert, 2006). Furthermore, this **fraternal birth order effect** is seen in boys who are right-handed, but not in left-handed boys (Blanchard et al., 2006; Bogaert, 2007), providing another indication of differences in early development between gay and straight men (**FIGURE 8.36**). Statistically, the birth order effect is strong enough that about one in every seven gay men in North America—about a million people—is gay because his mother had sons before him (Cantor et al., 2002). One theory is that the immune system of a mother carrying a son is exposed for the first time to proteins from the Y chromosome, so it may produce antibodies that affect development of subsequent sons (Bogaert et al., 2018).

There is good evidence that human sexual orientation is at least partly heritable (Sanders et al., 2017), reinforcing the notion that both biological and social factors have a say. About 50% of variability in human sexual orientation is accounted for by genetic factors, leaving ample room for early social influences. Monozygotic twins, who have exactly the same genes, do not always have the same sexual orientation (J. M. Bailey et al., 1993). A gene or genes in the Xq28 region of the X chromosome increases the chances that a boy will be gay (Hamer et al., 1993); but again the genetic explanation accounts for only some, not all, of the cases. It seems clear that there are several different pathways to sexual orientation.

From a political viewpoint, the controversy—whether sexual orientation is determined before birth or determined by early social influences—is irrelevant. Laws and prejudices against homosexuality are based primarily on religious views that it is a sin that some people "choose." But almost all gay and straight men report that, from the beginning, their interests and romantic attachments matched their adult orientation. So any social influence would have to be acting very early in life and without any conscious awareness (do you remember "choosing" whom to find attractive?). Furthermore, despite extensive efforts, no one has come up with a reliable way to change sexual orientation (Spitzer, 2012). These findings, added to evidence that older brothers and prenatal androgens affect the probability of being gay, have convinced most scientists that we do not choose our sexual orientation.

HOW'S IT GOING ?

1. What does the sexual orientation of people with various syndromes of sexual differentiation suggest about hormonal influences on human sexual orientation?

2. If human sexual orientation were shown definitively to be influenced by prenatal factors such as hormones and the fraternal birth order effect, would you be more or less inclined to accept homosexuality?

Recommended Reading

Colapinto, J. (2000). *As Nature Made Him.* New York, NY: HarperCollins.

Eugenides, J. (2002). *Middlesex: A Novel.* New York, NY: Farrar, Straus, and Giroux.

Komisaruk, B. R., and González-Mariscal, G. (2017). *Behavioral Neuroendocrinology*. Boca Raton, FL: CRC Press.

LeVay, S., Baldwin, J., and Baldwin, J. (2018). *Discovering Human Sexuality* (4th ed.). Sunderland, MA: Oxford University Press/Sinauer.

Nelson, R. J., and Kriegsfeld, L. J. (2016). *An Introduction to Behavioral Endocrinology* (5th ed.). Sunderland, MA: Oxford University Press/Sinauer.

Patisaul, H. B., and Belcher, S. M. (2017). *Endocrine Disruptors, Brain and Behavior.* New York, NY: Oxford University Press.

8 ■ Visual Summary   3e.mindsmachine.com/vs8

You should be able to relate each summary to the adjacent illustration, including structures and processes. If you go to the website for our text (3e.mindsmachine.com), you can follow links to figures, animations, and activities that will help you consolidate the material.

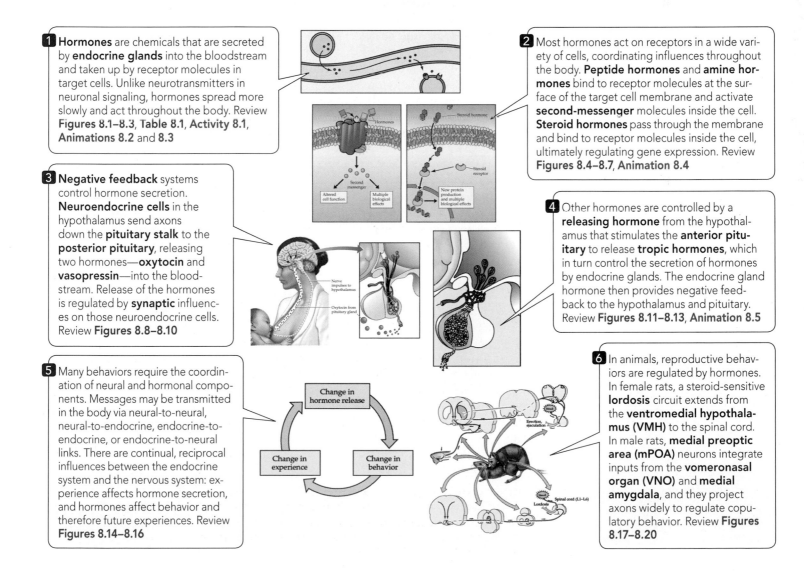

1 **Hormones** are chemicals that are secreted by **endocrine glands** into the bloodstream and taken up by receptor molecules in target cells. Unlike neurotransmitters in neuronal signaling, hormones spread more slowly and act throughout the body. Review **Figures 8.1–8.3, Table 8.1, Activity 8.1, Animations 8.2 and 8.3**

2 Most hormones act on receptors in a wide variety of cells, coordinating influences throughout the body. **Peptide hormones** and **amine hormones** bind to receptor molecules at the surface of the target cell membrane and activate **second-messenger** molecules inside the cell. **Steroid hormones** pass through the membrane and bind to receptor molecules inside the cell, ultimately regulating gene expression. Review **Figures 8.4–8.7, Animation 8.4**

3 **Negative feedback** systems control hormone secretion. **Neuroendocrine cells** in the hypothalamus send axons down the **pituitary stalk** to the **posterior pituitary**, releasing two hormones—**oxytocin** and **vasopressin**—into the bloodstream. Release of the hormones is regulated by **synaptic** influences on those neuroendocrine cells. Review **Figures 8.8–8.10**

4 Other hormones are controlled by a **releasing hormone** from the hypothalamus that stimulates the **anterior pituitary** to release **tropic hormones**, which in turn control the secretion of hormones by endocrine glands. The endocrine gland hormone then provides negative feedback to the hypothalamus and pituitary. Review **Figures 8.11–8.13, Animation 8.5**

5 Many behaviors require the coordination of neural and hormonal components. Messages may be transmitted in the body via neural-to-neural, neural-to-endocrine, endocrine-to-endocrine, or endocrine-to-neural links. There are continual, reciprocal influences between the endocrine system and the nervous system: experience affects hormone secretion, and hormones affect behavior and therefore future experiences. Review **Figures 8.14–8.16**

6 In animals, reproductive behaviors are regulated by hormones. In female rats, a steroid-sensitive **lordosis** circuit extends from the **ventromedial hypothalamus (VMH)** to the spinal cord. In male rats, **medial preoptic area (mPOA)** neurons integrate inputs from the **vomeronasal organ (VNO)** and **medial amygdala**, and they project axons widely to regulate copulatory behavior. Review **Figures 8.17–8.20**

7 In humans, very low levels of **testosterone** are required for either men or women to display a full interest in sex, but additional testosterone has no additional effect. In animals, hormones significantly influence **maternal behavior** by acting on the same brain regions that are important for sexual behavior (mPOA, VMH). Review **Figures 8.18** and **8.21–8.23**

9 In animals, **androgens** also organize the developing brain, masculinizing regions such as the **sexually dimorphic nucleus of the preoptic area (SDN-POA)** and the **spinal nucleus of the bulbocavernosus (SNB)**. There is evidence that prenatal androgens also masculinize the human brain. Review **Figures 8.29–8.32, Animation 8.6**

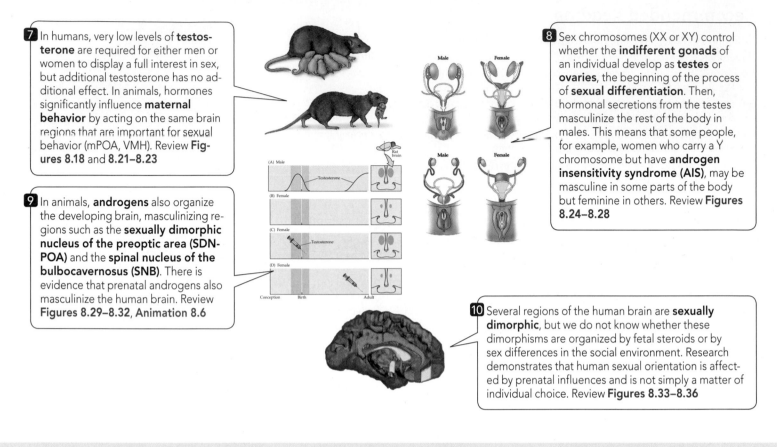

8 Sex chromosomes (XX or XY) control whether the **indifferent gonads** of an individual develop as **testes** or **ovaries**, the beginning of the process of **sexual differentiation**. Then, hormonal secretions from the testes masculinize the rest of the body in males. This means that some people, for example, women who carry a Y chromosome but have **androgen insensitivity syndrome (AIS)**, may be masculine in some parts of the body but feminine in others. Review **Figures 8.24–8.28**

10 Several regions of the human brain are **sexually dimorphic**, but we do not know whether these dimorphisms are organized by fetal steroids or by sex differences in the social environment. Research demonstrates that human sexual orientation is affected by prenatal influences and is not simply a matter of individual choice. Review **Figures 8.33–8.36**

Go to **3e.mindsmachine.com** for study questions, quizzes, flashcards, and other resources.

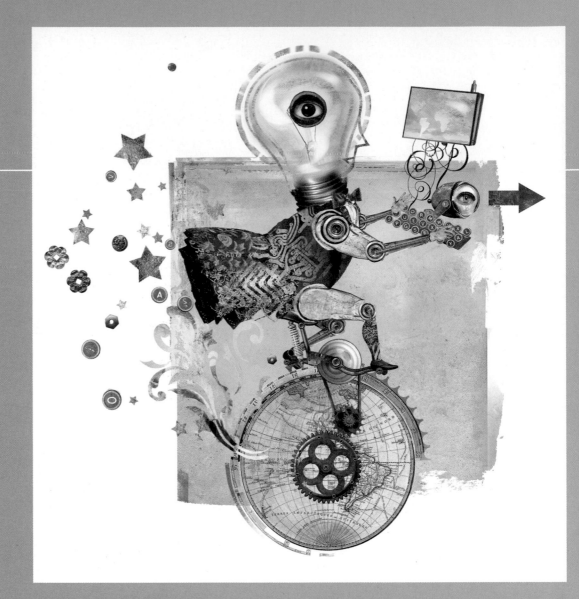

9

Homeostasis
Active Regulation of the Internal Environment

Harsh Reality TV

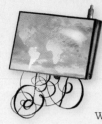

Introduced in 2004, the reality television show *The Biggest Loser* went on to become a huge prime-time hit. The premise of the show was simple enough—the contestant who lost the most weight during the season won—but the effort required from the contestants was immense.

The biggest loser of them all in season 8 (2009) was Danny C. Through a punishing combination of near-starvation dieting and all-day exercise, Danny shed an incredible 239 pounds (108 kilograms), dropping from 430 pounds to a svelte 191 pounds in just 7 months. Other initially obese contestants similarly accomplished exceptional weight loss and delighted in revealing their new, slimmer silhouettes to their friends, families, and viewers.

Recognizing an unusual opportunity, a group of scientists followed Danny and other *Biggest Loser* contestants for 6 years following their weight loss: the longest-term study of its kind ever conducted (Fothergill et al., 2016). The results are discouraging. In the years after his appearance on the show, and despite exceptional ongoing efforts, Danny regained more than 100 pounds of the weight he had lost. In fact, all but one of the 14 contestants who were tracked in the study regained significant weight; some were even heavier after the show than they were before the contest started. The pattern of results confirms a common observation: it is very hard to keep the weight off after dieting. But what could explain the additional discovery that even after 6 long years of hard work, the metabolisms of these contestants still had not adjusted and instead strived to return them to their original obese state?

Millions of years of evolution have endowed our bodies with complex physiological mechanisms, and multiple backup systems, devoted to producing a stable internal environment, monitored and regulated by the brain at every stage. But in the context of modern society, some of these ancient systems are making trouble for us; obesity, for example, is reaching epidemic proportions and placing a severe burden on health care resources. The physiological and behavioral processes governing the internal environment, and their role when things go wrong, are our topic in this chapter.

To see the video
Regaining the Weight,
go to
3e.mindsmachine.com/av9.1

To view the
Brain Explorer,
go to
3e.mindsmachine.com/av9.2

PART I
Principles of Homeostasis

THE ROAD AHEAD

In the first part of the chapter, we use body temperature to explore the general principles of homeostasis. By the end of this section you should be able to:

1. Define homeostasis and allostasis, and their relationship to drive states.
2. Distinguish between endothermy and ectothermy, with examples, and discuss the pros and cons of each system.
3. Describe, with appropriate examples, how the engineering concepts of negative feedback and redundancy apply to homeostatic systems.
4. Discuss some of the ways in which animals use specialized behaviors to maintain a stable internal environment.

Homeostatic Systems Share Several Key Features

The bodies of many animals exhibit some degree of **homeostasis**: a relatively stable, balanced internal environment that is optimized for cellular activities. Variables such as acidity, saltiness, water level, oxygenation, temperature, and energy availability are closely monitored and controlled by elaborate physiological systems. Deviations from optimum states can affect **motivation**, the psychological process that induces or sustains a particular behavior, and the effect can escalate rapidly as the deviation worsens from a minor distraction (like the urge to take a couple of sips if water is handy) to an overwhelmingly powerful need (like the raging thirst of someone lost in the desert).

Because it is a relatively simple system, we'll start by using **thermoregulation** (the regulation of body temperature) to look at some important general concepts of homeostasis: negative feedback, redundancy, behavioral compensation, and the concept of allostasis. These topics will arise again when we talk about fluid balance, appetite, and body weight in the remainder of the chapter.

We mammals are **endotherms**, meaning that we make our own heat *inside* our bodies, using metabolism and muscular activity (and if our muscles aren't making enough heat, we can shiver them to make more). Endothermy gives us clear advantages over **ectotherms** (animals that get their heat mostly from *outside* the body—from the environment) by allowing us to roam more widely. Like endotherms, ectotherms such as lizards and snakes try to regulate their temperature within a range that is optimal for the functioning of their cells, but this means they need to stay near sources of warmth. Furthermore, the evolution of endothermy involved enhanced capacity for oxygen utilization, with the result that the muscles of mammals can work hard for longer periods of time: endothermic hares will always outrun ectothermic tortoises. (For more on the pros and cons of endothermy and ectothermy, see **A STEP FURTHER 9.1**, on the website.) So it's no surprise that we have dedicated systems for creating warmth and regulating our body temperature. The systems that govern body temperature operate according to several general principles common to almost all homeostatic systems.

Negative feedback allows precise control

The homeostatic mechanisms that regulate temperature, body fluids, and metabolism are primarily **negative feedback** systems, where deviation from a desired value, called the **set point**, triggers a compensatory action of the system. Restoring the desired value turns off the response (this is why it is called negative feedback). A simple analogy for this mechanism is a household thermostat (**FIGURE 9.1**): a temperature drop below the set point activates the thermostat, which turns on the heating system. The heat that is produced has a negative feedback effect on the thermostat, so it stops calling for heat. Most heating systems have at least a little bit of tolerance built

homeostasis   The maintenance of a relatively constant internal physiological environment.

motivation   The psychological process that induces or sustains a particular behavior.

thermoregulation   The active process of maintaining a relatively constant internal temperature through behavioral and physiological adjustments.

endotherm   An animal whose body temperature is regulated chiefly by internal metabolic processes.

ectotherm   An animal whose body temperature is regulated by, and whose heat comes mainly from, the environment.

negative feedback   The process whereby a system monitors its own output and reduces its activity when a set point is reached.

set point   The point of reference in a feedback system.

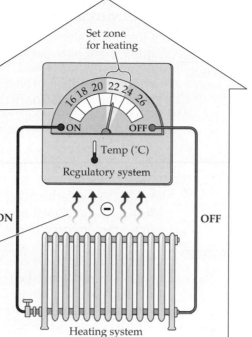

FIGURE 9.1 Negative Feedback

A household thermostat uses negative feedback control. Such systems always include a sensor (a thermometer in this case) to monitor the controlled variable, and a response system (the heating system here) to change the monitored variable.

Set zone for heating

Heat from the heating system provides negative feedback, inhibiting the thermostat from calling for more heat.

To view the animation **Negative Feedback,** go to **3e.mindsmachine.com/av9.3**

in—otherwise the system would be going on and off too frequently—so there is generally a **set zone** rather than a rigid set point.

Just like a thermostat, your set zone for body temperature can be changed under certain circumstances. For example, your body temperature drops at night for much the same reason that people turn down their home thermostats at night: to conserve energy. Or your set zone may be temporarily elevated, producing a fever to help your body fight off an infection. But in either case there are narrow limits. Too hot, and proteins begin to lose their correct shape, link together, and malfunction (this modification of proteins is called *denaturing* or, if it is really hot, *cooking*), with lethal results if critical brain regions are compromised. If we are too cool, chemical reactions of the body occur too slowly; at very low body temperatures, ice crystals may disrupt cellular membranes, killing the cells.

set zone The optimal range of a variable that a feedback system tries to maintain.

Redundancy ensures critical needs are met

Just as engineers equip critical equipment with several backup systems, our bodies tend to have multiple mechanisms for monitoring our stores, conserving remaining supplies, obtaining new resources, and shedding excesses. Loss of function in one part of the system usually can be compensated for by the remaining parts. This redundancy attests to the importance of maintaining our inner environment, but it also complicates the lives of scientists who are trying to figure out exactly how the body normally regulates temperature, water balance, and food intake.

It has long been known that the hypothalamus senses and controls body temperature, but lesion experiments eventually showed that different hypothalamic sites control two separate thermoregulatory systems. Lesions in the preoptic area (POA) of rats impaired the physiological responses to cold, such as shivering and constriction of the blood vessels, but did not interfere with such behaviors as pressing levers to control heating lamps or cooling fans (Satinoff and Rutstein, 1970; Van Zoeren and Stricker, 1977). Lesions in the lateral hypothalamus of rats abolished behavioral regulation of temperature but did not affect the physiological responses (Satinoff and Shan, 1971; Van Zoeren and Stricker, 1977). This is a clear example of homeostatic redundancy: two different systems for regulating the same variable.

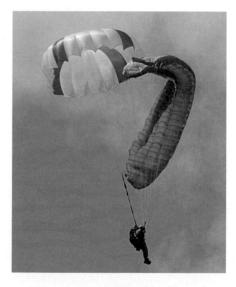

Redundancy Engineers equip critical systems with multiple "fail-safe" redundancies—for example, skydivers generally carry a secondary parachute—so that a backup always protects the critical system (the skydiver, in this example). Multiple redundancy is a feature of many of the body's homeostatic systems, protecting the constant internal environment that is crucial for survival. (© Karen Hadley/Shutterstock.com.)

(A)

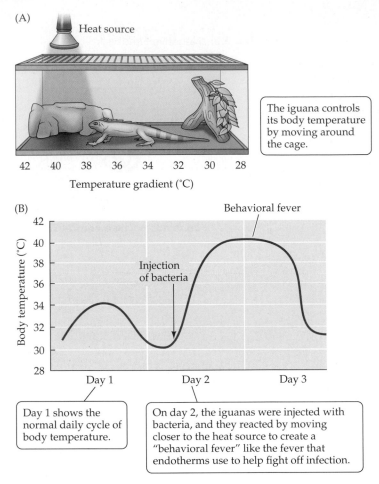

FIGURE 9.2 Behavioral Thermo-regulation in Bacteria-Challenged Iguanas (After M. J. Kluger, 1978. *Amer. Sci.* 66: 38.)

allostasis The varying behavioral and physiological adjustments that an individual makes in order to maintain optimal (rather than unchanging) functioning of a regulated system in the face of changing environmental stressors.

Animals use behavioral compensation to adjust to environmental changes

Organisms also use behavioral measures to help them acquire more heat, water, or food, in order to achieve and maintain homeostasis. In general, both ectotherms and endotherms deploy three kinds of temperature-regulating behavior: (1) behaviors that change *exposure* of the body surface—for example, by huddling or extending limbs; (2) behaviors that change external *insulation*, such as by using clothing or nests; and (3) behaviors that change *surroundings*, by moving into the sun, into the shade, or into a burrow.

Because ectotherms generate little heat through metabolism, behavioral methods of thermoregulation are especially important to them. In the laboratory, iguanas carefully regulate their temperature by moving toward or away from a heat lamp, and when infected by bacteria, they even produce a fever through such behavioral means (**FIGURE 9.2**), which helps them fight off an infection. Endotherms use internal processes to generate a fever when fighting infections, which boosts our immune system response. Unfortunately, sometimes the body goes too far, as a fever above 104°F (40°C) does more harm than good (see **A STEP FURTHER 9.2**, on the website). **FIGURE 9.3** summarizes the basic mammalian thermoregulatory system: receptors in the skin, body core, and hypothalamus detect temperature and transmit that information to three neural regions (spinal cord, brainstem, and hypothalamus). If the body temperature moves outside the set zone, each of these neural regions can initiate physiological and behavioral responses to return it to the set zone.

A wide array of sensors continuously monitors the many internal and external threats to our physiological stability. At any given moment, depending on what's happening in the environment, simultaneous perturbations in multiple regulated systems cause varying degrees of physiological stress. Rather than defending a single set point, many physiological systems must continually shift their responses depending on the nature of the stressors and prior experience—for example, your heart rate and blood pressure are continually shifting to accommodate your current or anticipated activity level—a dynamic process termed **allostasis** (Sterling and Eyer, 1988; McEwen and Wingfield, 2010). Allostatic adjustments are a normal part of dealing with the demands of daily life, but the heavy physiological burden on chronically stressed individuals puts them at risk of pathology due to allostatic overload.

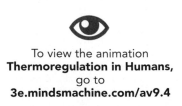

To view the animation **Thermoregulation in Humans,** go to 3e.mindsmachine.com/av9.4

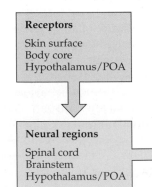

FIGURE 9.3 Basic Elements of Mammalian Thermoregulatory Systems

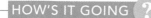

HOW'S IT GOING ?

1. Define homeostasis, and discuss its relation to the psychological concept of motivation. Why do homeostatic systems tend to have a set zone instead of a set point?
2. Distinguish between endotherms and ectotherms, and give a few examples of each.
3. Using examples, define and describe negative feedback as it applies to homeostasis.
4. Many homeostatic systems feature redundancy. What is it and why is it important?
5. Although the concept of homeostasis primarily relates to the physical internal environment, behavior can play an important role too. How?
6. Define allostasis. How does allostasis relate to homeostasis?

PART II
Fluid Regulation

THE ROAD AHEAD

In the next section, we discuss the distribution and movement of water in the body. By the end of this section you should be able to:

1. Describe the compartmentalization of fluids in the body.
2. Briefly define diffusion and osmosis.
3. Describe the semipermeable membrane, and explain its role in the movement of water between compartments.
4. Define and compare osmotic thirst and hypovolemic thirst, and the sensors that monitor each type of fluid loss.
5. Give an overview of physiological responses to thirst, and tell how the brain gauges when to stop drinking.

Water Moves between Two Major Body Compartments

Our homeostatic mechanisms are continually challenged by *obligatory losses*: the unavoidable expenditures of bodily resources that must then be regained from the external environment. Many body functions use up resources. Water (and some salt molecules), for example, are lost when we produce urine to get rid of waste molecules. We even lose water in our breath. Restoring expended water (and food) can take up much of an animal's waking life.

A precise balance of fluids and dissolved salts bathes the cells of the body and enables them to function. The composition of this fluid provides an echo of our evolutionary past. The first living organisms on Earth were single-celled inhabitants of the ancient oceans, and it was in these simple organisms that the fundamental processes of cellular life were established. When multicellular organisms evolved much later and began to exploit opportunities on land and in the air, they had no choice but to bring along with them the watery environment that their cells needed to survive. For this reason, most organisms evolved homeostatic systems that ensure that the composition of their body fluids closely resembles dilute seawater (Bourque, 2008); (**FIGURE 9.4**). Even relatively minor deviation from optimal water and salt balance can be lethal.

FIGURE 9.4 Each Animal Contains a Tiny Sea (After C. W. Bourque, 2008. *Nat. Rev. Neurosci.* 9: 519.)

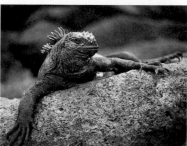

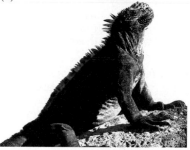

Behavioral Control of Body Temperature
(A) A Galápagos marine iguana, upon emerging from the cold sea, raises its body temperature by hugging a warm rock and lying broadside to the sun. (B) Once its temperature is sufficiently high, the iguana reduces its surface contact with the rock and faces the sun to minimize its exposure. These behaviors control body temperature. (Photographs by Mark R. Rosenzweig.)

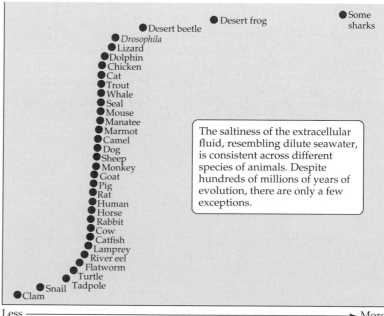

Desert beetle · Desert frog · Some sharks
Drosophila
Lizard
Dolphin
Chicken
Cat
Trout
Whale
Seal
Mouse
Manatee
Marmot
Camel
Dog
Sheep
Monkey
Goat
Pig
Rat
Human
Horse
Rabbit
Cow
Catfish
Lamprey
River eel
Flatworm
Turtle
Snail Tadpole
Clam

The saltiness of the extracellular fluid, resembling dilute seawater, is consistent across different species of animals. Despite hundreds of millions of years of evolution, there are only a few exceptions.

Less ⟶ More
Saltiness of extracellular fluid

intracellular compartment
The fluid space of the body that is contained within cells.

extracellular compartment
The fluid space of the body that exists outside the cells.

diffusion   The passive spread of solute molecules through a solvent until a uniform solute concentration is achieved.

osmosis   The passive movement of a solvent, usually water, through a semipermeable membrane until a uniform concentration of solute (often salt) is achieved on both sides of the membrane.

osmotic pressure   The tendency of a solvent to move across a membrane in order to equalize the concentration of solute on both sides of the membrane.

Scientists typically describe water balance by contrasting the inside versus the outside of our cells. Most of the water in the body is contained within our cells; this water is collectively referred to as the **intracellular compartment**. The fluid that is outside of our cells, called the **extracellular compartment**, is divided between the *interstitial fluid* (the fluid between cells) and *blood plasma* (the protein-rich fluid that carries red and white blood cells). Water is continually moving back and forth between these compartments, in and out of cells.

To understand the forces driving the movement of water, we must understand diffusion and osmosis. In **diffusion**, molecules of a substance, like salt (a *solute*), that are dissolved in a quantity of another substance, such as water (a *solvent*), will passively spread through the solvent because of the random jiggling and movement of the molecules until they are more or less uniformly distributed throughout it. If we divide a container of water with a membrane that is impermeable to water and salt and then put salt in the water on one side, the salt molecules will diffuse only within the water on that side. If instead the membrane impedes salt molecules only a little, then the salt will distribute itself evenly within the water on the initial side but will also—more slowly—invade and distribute itself across the other side. A membrane that is permeable to some molecules but not others is referred to as *selectively permeable* or *semipermeable*. As we saw in Chapter 3, selective permeability of cell membranes is what lets neurons create and transmit electrical potentials.

Osmosis is the movement of water molecules that occurs so as to equalize the concentration of two solutions that are separated by a semipermeable membrane. This is the case we examine in **FIGURE 9.5**, where a semipermeable membrane that permits water to cross, *but not salt*, divides a tank into two sides. Adding extra salt to one side induces water molecules to move into the now-salty side until the concentrations of both solutions equalize. The physical force that pushes or pulls water across the membrane is called **osmotic pressure**.

FIGURE 9.5   Osmosis

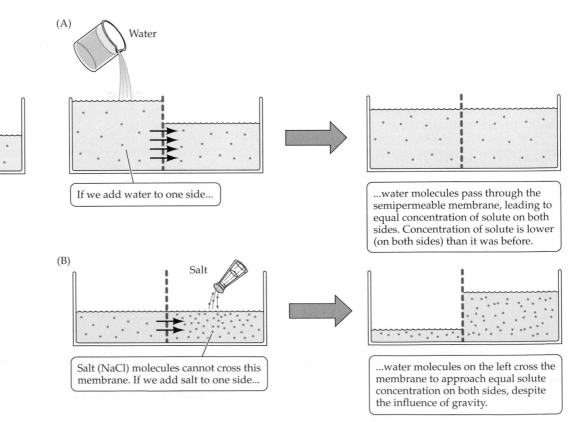

Salt water   Semipermeable membrane

Equal concentration of solute on both sides.

(A)   Water

If we add water to one side...

...water molecules pass through the semipermeable membrane, leading to equal concentration of solute on both sides. Concentration of solute is lower (on both sides) than it was before.

(B)   Salt

Salt (NaCl) molecules cannot cross this membrane. If we add salt to one side...

...water molecules on the left cross the membrane to approach equal solute concentration on both sides, despite the influence of gravity.

Normally the concentration of salt (sodium chloride, or NaCl) in the extracellular fluid of mammals is about 0.9% (which means there's about 0.9 gram of NaCl for every 100 milliliters of water). A solution with this concentration of salt is called *physiological saline* or described as *isotonic*. Because water moves to produce uniform saltiness (see Figure 9.5), cells will lose water if placed in a saltier solution and will gain water in a less salty solution. If excessive, this movement of water will damage or kill the cell. The extracellular fluid serves as a *buffer*, a reservoir of isotonic fluid that provides and accepts water molecules, so cells can maintain proper internal conditions and prevent such damage. The nervous system uses two cues to ensure that the extracellular compartment has about the right amount of water and solute, as we'll see next.

Two Internal Cues Trigger Thirst

The brain contains a dedicated network that carefully monitors the quantity and concentration of the fluid in our bodies, and triggers thirst to stimulate the intake of more water when needed (Zimmerman et al., 2017). Two different signals, combined in varying degrees, can trigger thirst: (1) high extracellular solute concentration (**osmotic thirst**) —a consequence of our extracellular body fluids becoming too salty – and (2) low extracellular volume (**hypovolemic thirst**), resulting from the loss of body fluids (**FIGURE 9.6**). We'll consider each in turn.

Osmotic thirst occurs when the extracellular fluid becomes too salty

Most of the time, we feel thirsty because of the obligatory water losses we mentioned earlier—through respiration, urination, and so on—in which more water is lost than salt. In this case, not only is the *volume* of the extracellular fluid *decreased*, but also the solute *concentration* of the extracellular fluid is *increased*. As a result of the increase in extracellular saltiness, water is pulled out of cells through osmosis.

osmotic thirst A desire to ingest fluids that is stimulated by high concentration of solute (like salt) in the extracellular compartment.

hypovolemic thirst A desire to ingest fluids that is stimulated by a reduction in volume of the extracellular fluid.

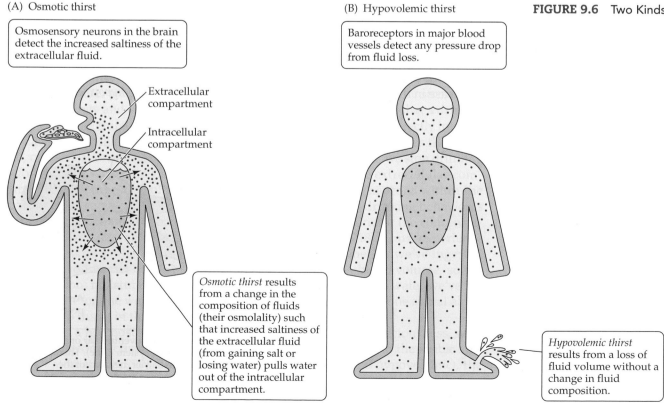

(A) Osmotic thirst

Osmosensory neurons in the brain detect the increased saltiness of the extracellular fluid.

Extracellular compartment

Intracellular compartment

Osmotic thirst results from a change in the composition of fluids (their osmolality) such that increased saltiness of the extracellular fluid (from gaining salt or losing water) pulls water out of the intracellular compartment.

(B) Hypovolemic thirst

Baroreceptors in major blood vessels detect any pressure drop from fluid loss.

Hypovolemic thirst results from a loss of fluid volume without a change in fluid composition.

FIGURE 9.6 Two Kinds of Thirst

that a calorie-reduced diet prompts the body to reduce its basal metabolic rate, which in turn slows the loss of weight (Bray, 1969; C. K. Martin et al., 2007). Along with the other *Biggest Loser* contestants, Danny C., whom we met at the outset of the chapter, has learned the hard way that our brains and bodies vigorously defend our energy balance and body weight, even if we are obese. Due to a dramatic decrease in his basal metabolism following weight loss—a process called *metabolic adaptation*—Danny now needs to consume 800 fewer calories per day than the typical man, just to maintain his current 295 pound body weight. And to make matters worse, this metabolic adaptation is annoyingly persistent; even after 6 long years, the metabolisms of the other contestants also remained very low (**FIGURE 9.11**) as their brains continued to try to regain the lost weight (Fothergill et al., 2016). A major goal for researchers is thus to discover a way to reset the body's set point (or set zone) for energy storage. Mice whose basal metabolic rate has been increased (by an induced increase in the energy used by mitochondria) eat more yet weigh less than normal mice, without increased locomotor activity (Clapham et al., 2000). Perhaps someday a drug will be developed to exert this effect on human mitochondria and produce such wonderful results in humans as well.

In the meantime, the debate about the most effective ways to decrease fat deposition through dieting continues to be immensely popular in the mass media. Although it is counterintuitive, some evidence suggests that diets high in fats and proteins, and correspondingly low in carbohydrates, can help people lose weight and also may increase serum levels of "good" cholesterol while decreasing serum fats (G. D. Foster et al., 2003; Samaha et al., 2003). However, long-term studies will be required to establish the overall safety of low-carbohydrate diets.

The only certain way to lose weight is to decrease the number of calories taken in and/or increase the number of calories spent in physical activity, and for the weight loss to be permanent, these changes in diet and activity must be permanent too. As an added bonus, research with monkeys suggests that long-term restriction of caloric intake can slow the aging process and reduce the prevalence of disease (Colman et al., 2014). And while the effects of caloric restriction on human aging remain to be established, researchers have reported that restricted food intake may have some beneficial effects on cognitive performance in elderly participants, at least over the short term (Witte et al., 2009; Prehn et al., 2017).

FIGURE 9.11 Metabolic Adaptation in the Biggest Losers (After E. Fothergill et al., 2016. *Obesity* 24: 1612.)

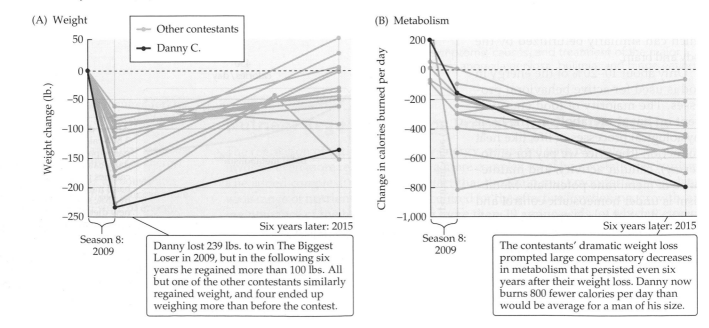

(A) Weight

Danny lost 239 lbs. to win The Biggest Loser in 2009, but in the following six years he regained more than 100 lbs. All but one of the other contestants similarly regained weight, and four ended up weighing more than before the contest.

(B) Metabolism

The contestants' dramatic weight loss prompted large compensatory decreases in metabolism that persisted even six years after their weight loss. Danny now burns 800 fewer calories per day than would be average for a man of his size.

Insulin is essential for obtaining, storing, and using food energy

In addition to converting surplus glucose into glycogen, as we discussed earlier, insulin has another critical function: your body needs insulin to make any use of the circulating glucose. That's because *glucose transporters*—the membrane-spanning proteins that most cells use to import glucose from the blood—need insulin in order to function properly (brain cells are an important exception; they can use glucose without the aid of insulin). The disease **diabetes mellitus** results from a lack of insulin production (in the *type 1*, or *juvenile-onset*, variety of the disease) or from greatly reduced tissue sensitivity to insulin (*type 2*, or *adult-onset*, diabetes, which is often associated with obesity). Although the brain can still make use of glucose from the diet, the rest of the body cannot and is forced to use energy from fatty acids while glucose accumulates in the blood, resulting in gradual severe damage to many tissues.

Insulin release around mealtimes is so important that it is triggered by several different mechanisms at different points in time. First comes the *cephalic phase* of insulin release, triggered by sights, smells, and tastes that we have learned to associate with food (*cephalic* means "of the head"). Then, during the *digestive phase*, food entering the digestive tract prompts an additional release of insulin. We now know that the digestive system contains the same sort of sweet taste receptors as are found on the tongue, and it uses them to help regulate insulin release (Kokrashvili et al., 2009). Finally, during the *absorptive phase*, as digested food is absorbed into the bloodstream, specialized liver cells called **glucodetectors** detect the increase in circulating glucose and signal the pancreas to release still more insulin. Information from the liver's glucodetectors is also conveyed directly to the hypothalamus via the vagus nerve (Powley, 2000), and the brain uses this information about circulating glucose to help control the pancreas and to stimulate feelings of hunger.

Given the crucial role of insulin in mobilizing and distributing food energy, and its fluctuations in association with feeding, it might seem an obvious candidate for signaling the brain to start or stop eating. Lowering an animal's blood insulin level does cause it to become hungry and eat a large meal, and injecting some insulin causes the animal to eat much less. But injecting a larger dose of insulin doesn't produce fully satiated animals; instead, they become hungry again and eat a large meal! The reason for this surprising result is that the high insulin levels direct much of the blood glucose into storage, which means that there is *less* glucose in circulation. The brain learns of this condition, called *hypoglycemia*, directly via glucodetectors, leading to a hunger response. And while it is certainly important, glucose can't be the sole appetite signal either, because people with untreated diabetes have very high levels of circulating glucose yet are constantly hungry. Somehow the brain integrates insulin and glucose levels with other sources of information to decide whether to initiate eating. As we'll

diabetes mellitus A condition, characterized by excessive glucose in the blood and urine and by reduced glucose utilization by body cells, that is caused by the failure of insulin to induce glucose absorption.

glucodetector A specialized type of liver cell that detects and informs the nervous system about levels of circulating glucose.

Not Too Sweet People with type 1 diabetes mellitus must receive insulin in order to utilize glucose. Taking insulin requires careful monitoring of blood glucose and, as shown here, self-administration via (A) daily injections or (B) drug pumps to infuse insulin throughout the day. Until the 1920s, when insulin was discovered as a result of experiments on dogs, this form of diabetes was a dreaded killer of children. (C) In an especially dramatic moment in science, three of the discoverers of insulin—Frederick Banting (right), Charles Best (left), and James Collip (not pictured)—went through a hospital ward full of dying diabetic children, injecting them with the newly purified hormone. By the time the last child had been injected, the first was already waking up from a diabetic coma. The discovery saved millions of lives and garnered a Nobel Prize in 1923. (A © Dmitry Lobanov/Shutterstock; B © istock.com/MarkHatfield. C Library and Archives Canada.)

(A)   (B)   (C)

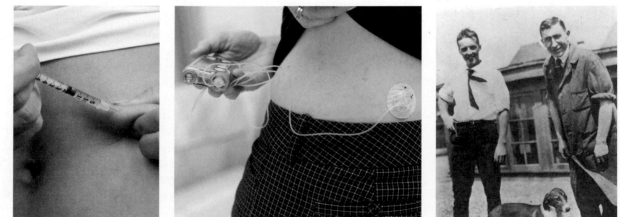

see next, this has become a central theme in research on appetite control—that the brain integrates many different signals rather than relying exclusively on any single signal to trigger hunger.

HOW'S IT GOING ?

1. Provide a review of how glucose is used, stored, and retrieved from storage. Be sure to identify the roles of pancreatic hormones in each step.
2. What is basal metabolism? How is it affected by homeostatic processes, and how does the homeostatic regulation of metabolism frustrate efforts to lose weight?
3. Define the types of diabetes mellitus and discuss their causes. What are some of the ways that insulin release is normally controlled?
4. Discuss the evidence about whether blood levels of insulin and glucose directly control hunger.

The Hypothalamus Coordinates Multiple Systems That Control Hunger

Although no single brain region has exclusive control of appetite, decades of research have confirmed that the hypothalamus is critically important for regulating metabolic rate, food intake, and body weight.

RESEARCHERS AT WORK

Lesion studies showed that the hypothalamus is crucial for appetite

Early researchers made discrete bilateral lesions in the hypothalamus—in either the **ventromedial hypothalamus** (**VMH**) or the **lateral hypothalamus** (**LH**)—of rats (**FIGURE 9.12**). After recovery, VMH-lesioned rats ate to excess and became obese (Hetherington and Ranson, 1940), leading researchers to suggest that the VMH is the *satiety center* of the brain (because the rats didn't show evidence of satiety once the VMH was gone). Rats with LH lesions, conversely, ceased eating and rapidly lost weight, suggesting that the LH acts as a *hunger center* (because rats who lost their LH stopped acting hungry) (Anand and Brobeck, 1951). So, an early model of feeding behavior featured the VMH and LH acting in opposition to control appetite.

It soon became clear that the initial model of appetite was too simple. For one thing, although the VMH was identified as a satiety center, its destruction did not create out-of-control feeding machines. Instead, VMH-lesioned animals exhibited a period of rapid weight gain but then stabilized at a new, higher level. When obese VMH-lesioned animals were forced to either gain or lose weight through dietary manipulation, they returned to their new "normal" weight as soon as they were allowed to eat freely again. So, because VMH-lesioned rats experienced satiety, the VMH cannot be the sole satiety controller.

Similarly, although they initially stopped eating, LH-lesioned rats that were kept alive with a feeding tube soon resumed eating and drinking, and their body weight eventually stabilized at a new, lower level. As with the VMH-lesioned animals, LH-lesioned animals that were later forced to gain weight would swiftly return to their new, lower set point for body weight after they returned to eating at will (see Figure 9.12) (Keesey, 1980). Researchers thus realized that the hypothalamic system controlling feeding must involve multiple

---

ventromedial hypothalamus (VMH) A hypothalamic region involved in eating and sexual behaviors.

lateral hypothalamus (LH) A hypothalamic region involved in the control of appetite and other functions.

(continued)

components that coordinate to establish a set point for metabolic fuels, monitor energy balance in the body, and trigger behavioral responses to meet the established energy goals, with a collective effect on body weight.

FIGURE 9.12   Lesion Studies Revealed That the Hypothalamus Is Involved in Appetite (After R. E. Keesey and P. C. Boyle, 1973. *J. Comp. Physiol. Psychol.* 84: 38. After D. Sclafani et al., 1976. *Physiol. Behav.* 16: 631

■ **Hypothesis**

The hypothalamus contains discrete systems for controlling hunger and satiety.

■ **Test**

Place small lesions in target areas within the hypothalamus.

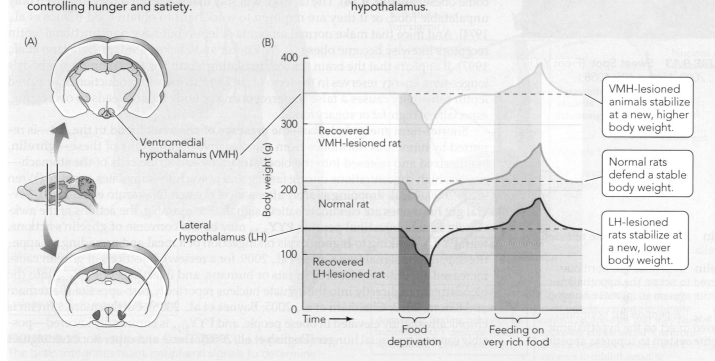

■ **Result**

Animals with lesions of the lateral hypothalamus (LH) decrease their food intake and rapidly lose weight, but they eventually stabilize at a new, lower weight. Following recovery, LH-lesioned animals forced to gain or lose weight return to the new lower weight when allowed to feed freely. Animals with lesions of the ventromedial hypothalamus (VMH) increase their food intake and rapidly gain weight, but they eventually stabilize at a new, higher weight. Following recovery, VMH-lesioned animals forced to gain or lose weight return to their new higher weight when allowed to feed freely.

■ **Conclusion**

The LH and VMH appear to play a role in appetite and body weight control, but because LH- and VMH-lesioned animals eventually show hunger and satiety, these two hypothalamic centers alone cannot constitute the entire appetite control system.

By demonstrating that the hypothalamus contains distinct components of an appetite control network, the early research on hunger and satiety provided a framework for subsequent work. For example, fMRI studies show that elevations in circulating glucose after a period of fasting produce large changes in the activity of the human hypothalamus (**FIGURE 9.13**) (Y. Liu et al., 2000), probably acting via hypothalamic glucodetector neurons that directly monitor blood levels of glucose (Parton et al., 2007).

Hormones from the body drive a hypothalamic appetite controller

A spate of discoveries has sharpened our understanding of the hypothalamic control of appetite. This evidence indicates that a circuit within the **arcuate nucleus** of the

arcuate nucleus   An arc-shaped hypothalamic nucleus implicated in appetite control.

anorexigenic neurons Neurons of the hypothalamic appetite system that inhibit feeding behavior.

paraventricular nucleus (PVN) A nucleus of the hypothalamus involved in the release of peptide hormones and in the control of feeding and other behaviors.

nucleus of the solitary tract (NST) A complicated brainstem nucleus that receives visceral and taste information via several cranial nerves.

cholecystokinin (CCK) A peptide hormone that is released by the gut after ingestion of food that is high in protein and/or fat.

orexin Also called *hypocretin*. A neuropeptide produced in the hypothalamus that is involved in switching between sleep states, in narcolepsy, and in the control of appetite.

endocannabinoid An endogenous ligand of cannabinoid receptors, thus a cannabis analog that is produced by the brain.

orexigenic neurons act to increase appetite and food intake. In contrast, when the balance of arcuate outputs tips toward activation of the **anorexigenic neurons** of the **paraventricular nucleus** (**PVN**), those neurons act to decrease appetite and feeding (Garfield et al., 2015; Krashes et al., 2016) (refer to Figure 9.15B for help in understanding this circuit).

So how do the peripheral hormone signals interact with the arcuate-based appetite controller? As we've discussed, leptin levels (and to a lesser extent, insulin levels) in the blood convey information about the body's longer-term energy reserves, stored in fat cells. Leptin affects both types of arcuate appetite neurons, but in opposite ways. High circulating levels of leptin activate the POMC satiety neurons and simultaneously inhibit the NPY hunger neurons—so in both ways leptin is working to suppress hunger. In contrast to leptin, ghrelin and gut satiety hormones like PYY_{3-36} provide shorter-term hour-to-hour hunger signals from the gut. These peptides act primarily on the appetite-stimulating NPY neurons of the arcuate nucleus. In this model, ghrelin stimulates these cells, leading to a corresponding increase in appetite, while PYY_{3-36} and other gut satiety hormones work in opposition, inhibiting the same cells to *reduce* appetite. Thus, short-term control of appetite seems to reflect a balance between ghrelin and concentrations of PYY_{3-36} and/or other gut satiety hormones in circulation. The net result of all this is a constant balancing act between the appetite-stimulating effects of the NPY system and the appetite-suppressing effects of the POMC system, spread across the hypothalamus.

Other systems also play a role in hunger and satiety

Appetite signals from the hypothalamus converge on the **nucleus of the solitary tract** (**NST**) in the brainstem (see Figure 9.15B). The NST can be viewed as part of a common pathway for feeding behavior, receiving appetite signals from a variety of sources in addition to the hypothalamus. Thus, the sensation of hunger is affected by a wide variety of peripheral sensory inputs, such as oral stimulation and the feeling of stomach distension, transmitted via spinal and cranial nerves. Information about nutrient levels is conveyed directly from the body to the NST via the vagus nerve (Tordoff et al., 1991). For example, the gut peptide **cholecystokinin** (**CCK**), released by the gut after feeding, provides yet another appetite-suppressant signal to the brain directly via the vagus (H. Fink et al., 1998).

In keeping with the concept of multiple redundancy that we discussed earlier in the chapter, a variety of additional signals and brain locations also participate in feeding behavior, either directly or through indirect effects on other processes. The peptide **orexin**, produced by neurons in the lateral hypothalamus, appears to participate in the subsequent control of feeding behavior. Direct injection of orexin into the hypothalamus of rats causes up to a sixfold increase in feeding (Sakurai et al., 1998). And it probably won't surprise you to learn that the brain's reward system is intimately involved with feeding. Activity of a circuit including the amygdala and the dopamine-mediated reward system of the nucleus accumbens (see Chapter 4) is hypothesized to mediate pleasurable aspects of feeding (Ahn and Phillips, 2002; Volkow and Wise, 2005).

The **endocannabinoid** system (see Chapter 4) likewise has a potent effect in appetite and feeding. Endocannabinoids, such as anandamide, are endogenous substances that act much like the active ingredient in cannabis (*Cannabis sativa*) and, like cannabis, can potently stimulate hunger. Acting both in the brain and in the periphery, endocannabinoids might stimulate feeding by affecting the mesolimbic dopamine reward system. However, injection of anandamide into the hypothalamus also stimulates eating (C. D. Chapman et al., 2012), confirming that endocannabinoids act directly on hypothalamic appetite mechanisms, while inhibiting satiety signals from the gut (Di Marzo and Matias, 2005).

Hypothalamic feeding control must be strongly influenced by inputs from higher brain centers, but little is known about these mechanisms. During development, for example, our feeding patterns are increasingly influenced by social factors such as parental and peer group pressures (Birch et al., 2003). Understanding the nature of cortical influences on feeding mechanisms is a major challenge for the future. The list of participants in appetite regulation is long and growing longer, revealing overlapping and complex controls with a high degree of redundancy, as befits a behavioral function of such critical importance to health and survival. With each new discovery, we draw nearer to finally developing safe and effective treatments for obesity and eating disorders, as we discuss next.

HOW'S IT GOING ?

1. Review the early work implicating the LH and VMH in appetite control. Why did researchers abandon the view that the LH and VMH were the sole controllers of appetite and satiety?
2. Sketch or briefly describe the major components of the hypothalamic appetite controller, as currently understood.
3. Describe how the hypothalamic appetite controller functions during hunger, in contrast to just after a meal.
4. What is leptin? Discuss its origins in the body and its effects on feeding behavior.
5. What are some of the gut hormones that may be involved in appetite control, and what are they thought to do?
6. Briefly describe some of the additional (redundant) mechanisms of appetite control that supplement the hypothalamic appetite system. What is the basis of the increased appetite frequently experienced after use of cannabis?

Obesity Is Difficult to Treat

Unfortunately, effective treatments to aid weight loss have been elusive. In our modern world, with its plentiful calories and sedentary lifestyles, the multiple redundant systems for appetite and energy management that evolved in our distant ancestors work all too well in preventing weight loss. Obesity has certainly reached epidemic proportions: a majority of the adults in the United States are overweight as defined by body mass index (BMI) (**TABLE 9.1**)—about two-thirds—and about one in three qualify as obese (**FIGURE 9.16**) (Flegal et al., 2002). Future health care systems will be burdened by obesity-related disease—cardiovascular disease, diabetes,

TABLE 9.1 ■ Body Mass Index (BMI)	
Value	Body weight category
<15	Starvation
15–18.5	Underweight
18.5–25	Ideal weight
25–30	Overweight
30–40	Obese
>40	Morbidly obese

Note:

$$BMI = \frac{weight\,(kg)}{height \times height\,(m \times m)}$$

or

$$BMI = 703\frac{weight\,(lb)}{height \times height\,(in. \times in.)}$$

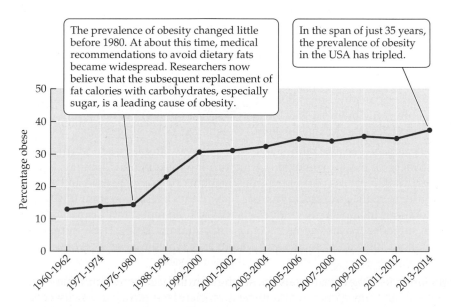

FIGURE 9.16 **An Epidemic of Obesity** (After Fryar et al., 2016. *Natl. Ctr. Hlth. Stat.* July 2016.)

etc.—and parental obesity may program metabolic disadvantages in offspring via **epigenetic transmission** (Ng et al., 2010).

In Lewis Carroll's *Alice's Adventures in Wonderland*, Alice quaffs the contents of a small bottle in order to shrink. The quest for a real-life shrinking potion—but one that makes you thin rather than short—is the subject of intense scientific activity, and several major strategies or targets are emerging:

1. *Appetite control* Hopes are high that drugs designed to reset the hypothalamic appetite controller will be safe and potent obesity treatments. Alteration of leptin levels has not proven to be very effective (Montague et al., 1997). Drugs that directly interfere with endocannabinoid activity, which is normally regulated by leptin in the hypothalamus, effectively produce "anti-munchies"—the reverse of the hunger experienced by cannabis users (Van Gaal et al., 2005; Thornton-Jones et al., 2006). However, significant mood problems (an "anti-high"?) also occur, so the search continues for drugs that can selectively modify the signaling systems in the arcuate appetite controller. Treatments that mimic other signaling hormones are promising, especially those that exploit the shorter-term satiety-signaling peptides from the gut. Simply spraying a PYY_{3-36} solution into the mouths of lab mice is apparently not aversive, yet it powerfully suppresses their appetite (Hurtado et al., 2013). The prescription anti-obesity drug Saxenda (liraglutide) suppresses appetite by mimicking a different gut peptide hormone, called GLP-1 (glucagon-like peptide) (Halford et al., 2010).

2. *Increased metabolism* An alternative approach to treating obesity is to raise the body's metabolic rate and thus expend extra calories in the form of heat. For example, scientists are trying to design drugs that will mimic some of the metabolism-elevating actions of thyroid hormones without producing harmful side effects (Grover et al., 2003). Another promising approach involves inducing fat tissue to start burning stored energy faster than normal (Boström et al., 2012; Kajimura and Saito, 2014).

3. *Inhibition of fat tissue* A third way to treat obesity involves blocking the formation of new fat tissue. For example, in order for fat tissue to grow, it must be able to recruit and develop new blood vessels. Drugs that block this process inhibit weight gain in mice and may have similar anti-obesity benefits in humans (Rupnick et al., 2002; Tam et al., 2009).

4. *Reduced absorption* The anti-obesity medication orlistat (trade name Xenical) works by interfering with the digestion of fat. However, this approach has generally produced only modest weight loss, and it often causes intestinal discomfort.

5. *Reduced reward* A different perspective on treating obesity focuses on the rewarding properties of food. Not only is food delicious, but "comfort foods" also directly reduce circulating stress hormones, thereby providing another reward. Drugs that affect the brain's reward circuitry (see Chapter 4), reducing the rewarding properties of food, may promote weight loss (Volkow and Wise, 2005).

6. *Anti-obesity surgery* Because fat tissue tends to regrow after liposuction (the surgical removal of fat tissue), some people are turning to a different strategy: bariatric surgeries that bypass part of the intestinal tract or stomach, or install a gut liner, in order to reduce the absorptive capacity of the digestive system (**FIGURE 9.17**). Alterations in appetite hormones such as ghrelin reportedly also accompany such surgeries (Baynes et al., 2006; D. E. Cummings, 2006). These surgeries can bring about substantial and lasting weight loss, which may also reverse comorbid conditions like type 2 diabetes and hypertension.

7. *Lifestyle changes* Follow-up research with the *Biggest Loser* contestants has confirmed what many of us already suspected: increased physical activity can help keep the pounds off after dieting. However, the required change may need to be very substantial, and sustained. Compared with the contestants who

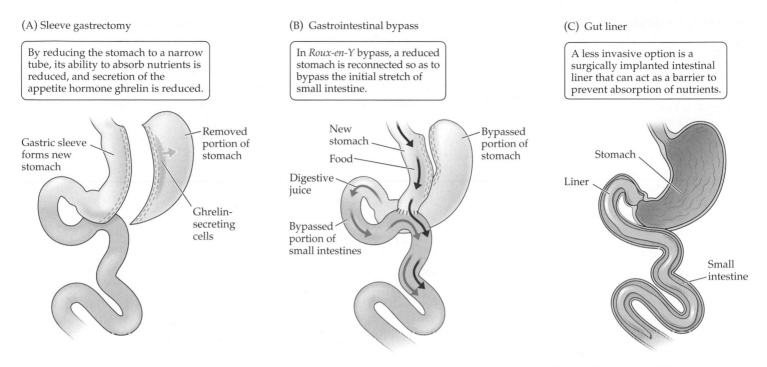

(A) Sleeve gastrectomy

> By reducing the stomach to a narrow tube, its ability to absorb nutrients is reduced, and secretion of the appetite hormone ghrelin is reduced.

Gastric sleeve forms new stomach

Removed portion of stomach

Ghrelin-secreting cells

(B) Gastrointestinal bypass

> In *Roux-en-Y* bypass, a reduced stomach is reconnected so as to bypass the initial stretch of small intestine.

New stomach

Food

Digestive juice

Bypassed portion of small intestines

Bypassed portion of stomach

(C) Gut liner

> A less invasive option is a surgically implanted intestinal liner that can act as a barrier to prevent absorption of nutrients.

Stomach

Liner

Small intestine

FIGURE 9.17 Surgical Options for Obesity

regained all of their former weight, the few who maintained their new lower weight 6 years after the end of the contest had to increase their physical activity level by an average of 160% (Kerns et al., 2017) relative to their pre-contest activity levels. At least in this group, exercise played a significantly greater role than dietary changes.

Eating Disorders Can Be Life-Threatening

Sometimes people shun food, despite having no apparent aversion to it. These people are usually young, become obsessed with their body weight, and become extremely thin—generally by eating very little and sometimes also by vomiting, taking laxatives, overexercising, or drinking large amounts of water to suppress appetite. This condition, which is more common in adolescent and adult women than in men, is called **anorexia nervosa**. The name of the disorder indicates (1) that the afflicted people have no appetite (*anorexia*) and (2) that the disorder originates in the nervous system (*nervosa*).

People who suffer from anorexia nervosa tend to think about food a good deal, and physiological evidence suggests that they respond even *more* than normal people to the presentation of food (Broberg and Bernstein, 1989); for example, food stimuli provoke a large release of insulin, despite cognitive denial of any feelings of hunger. So, in a physiological sense their hunger may be normal or

anorexia nervosa A syndrome in which individuals severely deprive themselves of food.

(A)

(B)

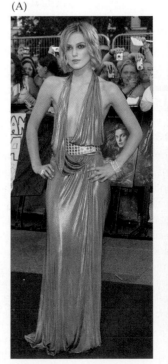

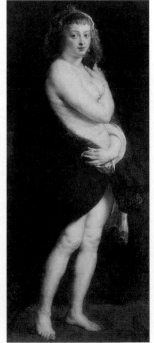

Changing Ideals of Female Beauty Actress Keira Knightley (A) exemplifies modern society's emphasis on thinness as an aspect of beauty, while *Helena Fourment as Aphrodite* (B), which Flemish painter Peter Paul Rubens painted of his wife circa 1630, illustrates the very different fashion of her era. This treatment of the female body as an object, subject to fluctuating cultural norms and whims of fashion, may play a role in the development of eating disorders such as anorexia nervosa and bulimia. (Part A © Fred Duval/FilmMagic/Getty Images; B © Kunsthistorisches Museum, Vienna.)

bulimia Also called *bulimia nervosa*. A syndrome in which individuals periodically gorge themselves, usually with "junk food," and then either vomit or take laxatives to avoid weight gain.

binge eating The rapid intake of large quantities of food, often poor in nutritional value and high in calories.

gut microbiota The microorgansims that normally inhabit the digestive system.

microbiome The collective term for the population of microorganisms that inhabit the body.

enterotype Each individual's personal composition of the gut microbiota.

To see the video
Anorexia,
go to
3e.mindsmachine.com/av9.5

even exaggerated, but this hunger is somehow absent from their conscious perceptions and they refuse to eat. The idea that anorexia nervosa is primarily a nervous system disorder stems from this mismatch between physiology and cognition, as well as from the distorted body image of the people with anorexia (they may consider themselves fat when others see them as emaciated). There may also be abnormalities in the functioning of the dopamine-based reward system that signals pleasurable aspects of eating, persisting even after recovery (Kaye et al., 2009).

Anorexia nervosa is notoriously difficult to treat, because it appears to involve an unfortunate combination of genetic, endocrine, personality, cognitive, and environmental variables. One approach that is successful in some cases is a family-based treatment (sometimes termed *Maudsley therapy* after the hospital where it was introduced) that de-emphasizes the identification of causal factors and instead focuses on intensive, parent-led "refeeding" of the anorexic person (Le Grange, 2005; Kass et al., 2013).

Bulimia (or *bulimia nervosa*, from the Greek *boulimia*, "great hunger") is a related disorder. Like those who suffer from anorexia nervosa, people with bulimia may believe themselves fatter than they are, but they periodically gorge themselves, usually with "junk food," and then either vomit the food or take laxatives to avoid weight gain. Also like sufferers of anorexia nervosa, people with bulimia may be obsessed with food and body weight, but not all of them become emaciated. Both anorexia nervosa and bulimia can be fatal because the person's lack of nutrient reserves damages various organ systems and/or leaves the body unable to battle otherwise mild diseases.

In **binge eating**, people spontaneously gorge themselves with far more food than is required to satisfy hunger, often to the point of illness. Such people are often obese, and the causes of the bingeing are not fully understood. In susceptible people, the strong pleasure associated with food activates opiate and dopaminergic reward mechanisms to such an extent that bingeing resembles drug addiction. Indeed, "binge eating disorder" is now a psychiatric diagnosis in the *Diagnostic and Statistical Manual of Mental Disorders*, 5th edition (*DSM-5*; American Psychiatric Association, 2013).

Despite the epidemic of obesity in our society, or perhaps because of it, our present culture emphasizes that women, especially young women, must be thin to be attractive. This cultural pressure is widely perceived as one of the causes of eating disorders. In earlier times, however, when plump women were considered the most beautiful, some women still fasted severely and may have suffered from anorexia nervosa. The origins of these disorders remain elusive, and to date, the available therapies help only a minority of people with anorexia.

SIGNS & SYMPTOMS

Friends with Benefits

Most people know that the gut is normally inhabited by helpful bacteria, but the extent of that occupation may surprise you. You probably contain in the range of 2.5–5 pounds of gut microbes: trillions of individual organisms belonging to dozens (perhaps hundreds) of different species of bacteria, fungi, and viruses, making up more than half the contents of your large intestine (Guarner and Malagelada, 2003). Put another way, you have more gut microbes than body cells, and they weigh more than your brain. This huge population, known as the **gut microbiota** or, collectively, as the **microbiome**, normally provide a variety of beneficial actions in return for their comfortable lodgings.

Each of us possesses a distinct microbial **enterotype**—a personal combination of different species of microbiota—that researchers increasingly believe to be in extensive two-way communication with your brain via the vagus nerve and chemical signals (Bonaz et al., 2018; Cussotto et al., 2018). Your enterotype reflects the history of your gut, so substantial changes in your diet, or the use of antibiotics to treat infections, can potently alter the composition of the enterotype (David et al., 2014), with uncertain consequences. Preliminary evidence has tentatively linked the microbiome enterotype to such diverse domains as mood, stress, social behavior, and cognitive functioning (Sylvia and Demas, 2018; Tetel et

SIGNS & SYMPTOMS   (continued)

al., 2018) and also various neurological conditions, including autism, schizophrenia, bipolar disorder, and Parkinson's disease (Fung et al., 2017; Tremlett et al., 2017). But one of the areas where an effect of changes in the gut microbiota may be most evident is obesity.

Feeding antibiotics to young mice, even at relatively low doses, changes gut microbiota and circulating hormones, leading to weight gain (I. Cho et al., 2012). Similarly, two studies looking at almost 40,000 babies have found that human infants given antibiotics in their first 6 months were statistically more likely to be overweight at age 7 (Ajslev et al., 2011; Trasande et al., 2013). It remains to be seen how much adult obesity is accounted for by long-lasting changes to our enterotypes, but it is at least possible that early exposure to antibiotics—or even chlorinated drinking water (because the whole point of adding chlorine is to kill bacteria)—is making some of us fat (Cox and Blaser, 2015). What can we do about it?

Scientists hope to turn our new knowledge of the connection between the gut and brain into novel treatments, such as drugs based on metabolites secreted by specific gut bacteria (Suez and Elinav, 2017). Some researchers have also been investigating the possible benefits of a gross-sounding procedure: **fecal transplantation**. Yes, it is just what it sounds like: feces are collected from carefully screened donors, processed to create a liquid suspension, and then passed through a catheter into the colon of the recipient (**FIGURE 9.18**), where the donor's healthy enterotype

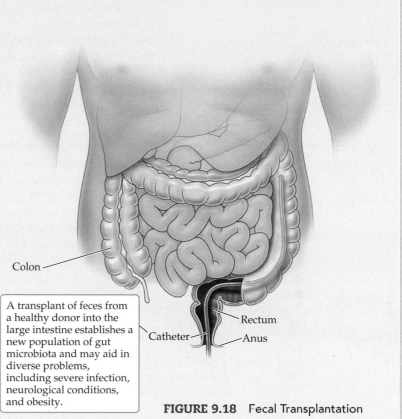

A transplant of feces from a healthy donor into the large intestine establishes a new population of gut microbiota and may aid in diverse problems, including severe infection, neurological conditions, and obesity.

FIGURE 9.18   Fecal Transplantation

establishes itself. Transplantation is an effective treatment for certain dangerous gut infections, and it reportedly improved metabolic function in a sample of obese men (Vrieze et al., 2012), so perhaps our tiny passengers can someday be coaxed to pay their way by supplying benefits like weight loss and better brain health.

HOW'S IT GOING ?

1. What proportion of adults in the United States are overweight or obese? How might homeostasis be part of the problem?
2. If you were designing drugs to combat obesity, what specific parts of the hypothalamic appetite controller might you target? Why?
3. Compare and contrast anorexia nervosa and bulimia. Are people with anorexia interested in food at all? Briefly discuss possible methods of treating anorexia.
4. Drawing on concepts covered in this chapter, discuss the likely contributions of cultural versus biological factors in various eating disorders.
5. Discuss nonpharmacological methods of weight reduction. Is surgery a good option?

fecal transplantation   A medical procedure in which gut microbiota, via fecal matter, are transplanted from a donor to a host.

Recommended Reading

Agras, W. S. (Ed.). (2010). *Oxford Handbook of Eating Disorders*. New York, NY: Oxford University Press.

Blumberg, M. S. (2009). *Body Heat*. Cambridge, MA: Harvard University Press.

Brownell, K. D., and Walsh, B. T. (2017). *Eating Disorders and Obesity* (3rd ed.). New York, NY: Guilford Press.

Daniels, D., and Fluharty, S. J. (2009). Neuroendocrinology of body fluid homeostasis. In D. W. Pfaff, A. P. Arnold, A. M. Etgen, S. E. Fahrbach, and R. T. Rubin (Eds.), *Hormones, Brain and Behavior* (2nd ed.) (pp. 259–288). San Diego, CA: Academic Press.

DeSalle, R., and Perkins, S. L. (2015). *Welcome to the Microbiome: Getting to Know the Trillions of Bacteria and Other Microbes In, On, and Around You*. New Haven, CT: Yale University Press.

Logue, A. W. (2014). *The Psychology of Eating and Drinking* (4th ed.). New York, NY: Routledge.

Lustig, R. H. (2018). *The Hacking of the American Mind: The Science Behind the Corporate Takeover of Our Bodies and Brains*. New York, NY: Avery.

McNab, B. K. (2012). *Extreme Measures: The Ecological Energetics of Birds and Mammals*. Chicago, IL: University of Chicago Press.

Schulkin, J. (Ed.). (2012). *Allostasis, Homeostasis, and the Costs of Physiological Adaptation*. Cambridge, UK: Cambridge University Press.

9 ■ Visual Summary
3e.mindsmachine.com/vs9

You should be able to relate each summary to the adjacent illustration, including structures and processes. If you go to the website for our text (3e.mindsmachine.com), you can follow links to figures, animations, and activities that will help you consolidate the material.

1 Homeostatic systems, such as the processes regulating **thermoregulation** (body temperature), work to maintain a constant internal environment. Like other homeostatic systems, thermoregulation employs negative feedback control: the resulting heat inhibits the system from calling for more. Review **Figure 9.1, Animations 9.2–9.4**

2 Homeostatic systems rely on specialized behaviors to help regulate physiological parameters. For example, most species have specialized behaviors to help warm or cool the body. Review **Figure 9.2**

3 Our cells function properly only when the concentration of salt in the **intracellular compartment** of the body is within a critical range. The **extracellular compartment** is a source of replacement water for osmosis and a buffer between the intracellular compartment and the outside world. Review **Figure 9.5**

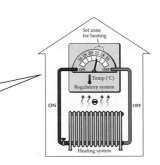

4 Thirst is a powerful motivator, triggered either by **hypovolemic thirst** (decreased volume of the extracellular fluid) or by **osmotic thirst** (increased extracellular saltiness). Because of the importance of solute concentration, we must regulate salt intake in order to regulate water balance effectively. Review **Figure 9.6**

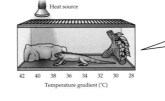

5 Specialized **osmosensory neurons** detect the concentration of extracellular fluid. **Baroreceptors** in the major blood vessels monitor blood pressure and volume. Review **Figure 9.7**

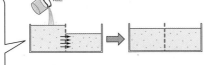

6 Hypovolemic and osmotic thirsts are triggered by different mechanisms and differ in their immediate effects, but both forms of thirst ultimately trigger a complex shared thirst network. Review **Figure 9.8**

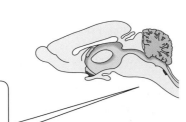

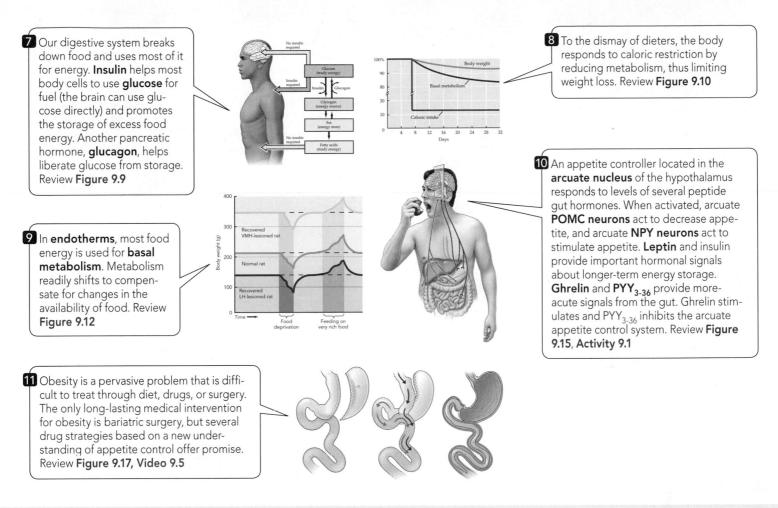

7 Our digestive system breaks down food and uses most of it for energy. **Insulin** helps most body cells to use **glucose** for fuel (the brain can use glucose directly) and promotes the storage of excess food energy. Another pancreatic hormone, **glucagon**, helps liberate glucose from storage. Review **Figure 9.9**

9 In **endotherms**, most food energy is used for **basal metabolism**. Metabolism readily shifts to compensate for changes in the availability of food. Review **Figure 9.12**

11 Obesity is a pervasive problem that is difficult to treat through diet, drugs, or surgery. The only long-lasting medical intervention for obesity is bariatric surgery, but several drug strategies based on a new understanding of appetite control offer promise. Review **Figure 9.17**, **Video 9.5**

8 To the dismay of dieters, the body responds to caloric restriction by reducing metabolism, thus limiting weight loss. Review **Figure 9.10**

10 An appetite controller located in the **arcuate nucleus** of the hypothalamus responds to levels of several peptide gut hormones. When activated, arcuate **POMC neurons** act to decrease appetite, and arcuate **NPY neurons** act to stimulate appetite. **Leptin** and insulin provide important hormonal signals about longer-term energy storage. **Ghrelin** and PYY$_{3-36}$ provide more-acute signals from the gut. Ghrelin stimulates and PYY$_{3-36}$ inhibits the arcuate appetite control system. Review **Figure 9.15**, **Activity 9.1**

Go to **3e.mindsmachine.com** for study questions, quizzes, flashcards, and other resources.

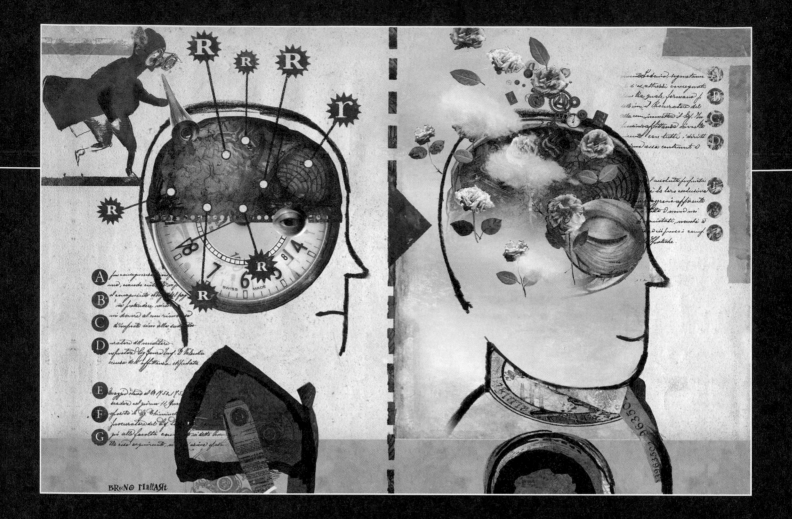

10

Biological Rhythms and Sleep

When Sleep Gets Out of Control

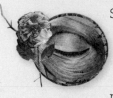

Starting college always brings its share of new experiences and adjustments, but "Barry" knew something was wrong freshman year when he seemed to be sleepy all the time (S. Smith, 1997). Barry napped so often that his friends called him the hibernating bear. Of course, college can be exhausting, and many students seek refuge in long snooze sessions. But one day while Barry was camping with his pals, an even odder thing happened: "I laughed really hard, and I kind of fell on my knees … After that, about every week I'd have two or three episodes where if I'd laugh … my arm would fall down or my muscles in my face would get weak. Or if I was running around playing catch and someone said something, I would get weak in the knees. And there was a time there that my friends kinda used it as a joke. If they're going to throw me the ball and they didn't want me to catch it, they'd tell me a joke and I'd fall down and miss it."

It was as if any big surge in emotion in Barry might trigger a sudden paralysis lasting anywhere from a few seconds to a few minutes, affecting either a body part or his whole body. Sex became something of a challenge because sometimes during foreplay, Barry's body would just collapse. "Luckily, you're probably laying down, so it's not that big a deal. But it just puts a damper on the whole thing."

What was happening to Barry? By the end of this chapter, we'll know a lot more about sleep and what went wrong in Barry's brain to cause these problems.

All living systems show repeating, predictable changes over time. Some rhythms, like brain potentials, are rapid; other rhythms, like annual hibernations, are slow. Daily rhythms, the topic of Part I of this chapter, have an intriguing clocklike regularity and are seen in virtually every physiological measure, including body temperature and hormone secretion. Part II concerns that familiar daily rhythm known as the sleep-waking cycle. By age 60, most humans have spent 20 years asleep (some, alas, on one side or the other of the classroom podium). We'll find that sleep is not a passive state of "nonwaking," but rather the interlocking of several different brain states. We'll conclude with a consideration of sleep disorders, as well as some tips on how to get the sleep you need.

To see the video
Narcolepsy,
go to
3e.mindsmachine.com/av10.1

To view the
Brain Explorer,
go to
3e.mindsmachine.com/av10.2

PART I
Biological Rhythms

THE ROAD AHEAD

The first section of the chapter concerns the evidence that the brain contains a biological clock to synchronize our behavior to the world around us. This material will allow you to:

1. Discuss the evidence that a tiny brain structure imposes a daily rhythm on behavior.
2. Describe the neural pathway by which information about daylight synchronizes that structure.
3. Understand how a molecular clock in brain neurons generates that daily rhythm.
4. Evaluate the evidence that later start times benefit high school students.

Many Animals Show Daily Rhythms in Activity

Biological rhythms are regular fluctuations in any living process. Almost all physiological processes—hormone levels, body temperature, drug sensitivity—change over the course of the day in a repeating pattern. Because such rhythms last about a day, they are called **circadian rhythms** (from the Latin *circa*, "about," and *dies*, "day"). Circadian rhythms are by far the most studied of the biological rhythms, and they will be our major concern in this chapter.

Still, you should know that some biological rhythms are shorter than a day. Such rhythms are referred to as **ultradian** (because they repeat more than once per day; the Latin *ultra* means "beyond"), and they vary from several minutes to hours long. Ultradian rhythms are seen in such behaviors as bouts of activity, feeding, and hormone release.

Biological rhythms that take *more* than a day are called **infradian** rhythms because they repeat less than once per day (the Latin *infra* means "below"). A familiar infradian rhythm is the 28-day human menstrual cycle. Many animal behaviors vary across the year; for example, most animals breed only during a particular season. There's also growing evidence of annual rhythms in the onset of human behavioral disorders, such as depression (see Chapter 12). (By the way, despite the urban myth that cases of depression peak around the holiday season, in fact they peak in the spring.) You might think that breeding seasons in animals would be triggered by changes in temperatures or food availability, but experiments suggest that the duration of light each day is the real trigger: in the laboratory, animals exposed to short days and long nights (mimicking wintertime conditions) reliably change to the nonbreeding condition (**FIGURE 10.1**).

Circadian rhythms are generated by an endogenous clock

Humans and many other primates are *diurnal*—active during the day. But most other mammals, including most rodents, are *nocturnal*—active during dark periods. These circadian activities are extraordinarily precise: the beginning of activity may vary only a few minutes from one day to another. For humans equipped with watches and clocks, this regularity may seem uninteresting, but other animals achieve such remarkable regularity using only a built-in *biological clock*.

A favorite way to study circadian rhythms exploits rodents' love of running wheels. A switch attached to the

biological rhythm   A regular fluctuation in any living process.

circadian rhythm   A pattern of behavioral, biochemical, or physiological fluctuation that has a 24-hour period.

ultradian   Referring to a rhythmic biological event with a period shorter than a day, usually from several minutes to several hours long.

infradian   Referring to a rhythmic biological event with a period longer than a day.

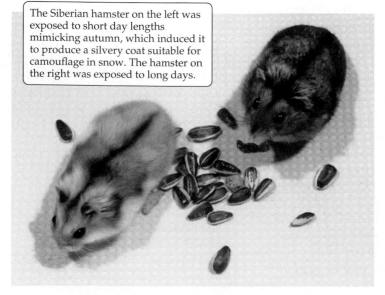

The Siberian hamster on the left was exposed to short day lengths mimicking autumn, which induced it to produce a silvery coat suitable for camouflage in snow. The hamster on the right was exposed to long days.

FIGURE 10.1   A Hamster for All Seasons
(Photo by Carol D. Hegstrom.)

(A)

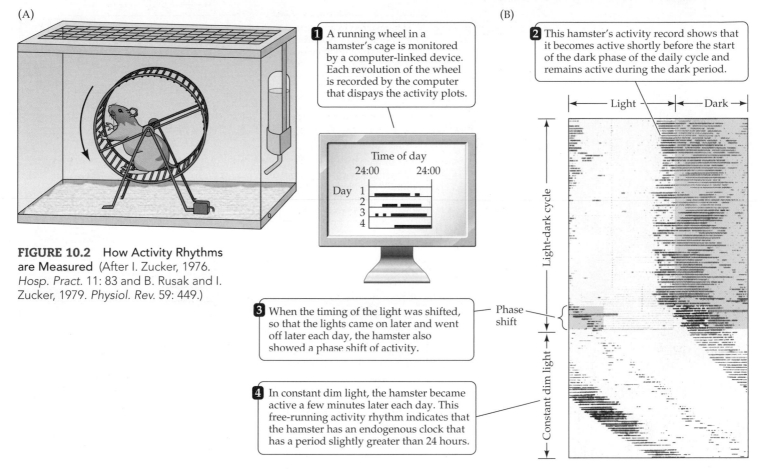

1 A running wheel in a hamster's cage is monitored by a computer-linked device. Each revolution of the wheel is recorded by the computer that dispays the activity plots.

2 This hamster's activity record shows that it becomes active shortly before the start of the dark phase of the daily cycle and remains active during the dark period.

Time of day

24:00   24:00

Day 1
     2
     3
     4

FIGURE 10.2 How Activity Rhythms are Measured (After I. Zucker, 1976. *Hosp. Pract.* 11: 83 and B. Rusak and I. Zucker, 1979. *Physiol. Rev.* 59: 449.)

3 When the timing of the light was shifted, so that the lights came on later and went off later each day, the hamster also showed a phase shift of activity.

Phase shift

4 In constant dim light, the hamster became active a few minutes later each day. This free-running activity rhythm indicates that the hamster has an endogenous clock that has a period slightly greater than 24 hours.

(B)

Light   Dark

Light-dark cycle

Constant dim light

wheel connects to a computer that registers each turn, revealing an activity rhythm as in **FIGURE 10.2A**. A hamster placed in a dimly lit room continues to show a daily rhythm in wheel running despite the absence of day versus night, suggesting that the animal has an internal clock. But even when the light is constantly dim, it is always possible that the animal detects other external cues (e.g., outside noises, temperature, barometric pressure—who knows?) signaling the time of day. Arguing for a biological clock, however, is the fact that in constant light or dark the circadian cycle is not *exactly* 24 hours: activity starts a few minutes later each day, so eventually the normally nocturnal hamster is active while it is daytime outside (**FIGURE 10.2B**, bottom). The animal is said to be **free-running**, maintaining its own personal cycle, which, in the absence of external cues, is a bit more than 24 hours long.

The free-running **period**, the time between two similar points of successive cycles (such as sunset to sunset), differs from one hamster to another. If two hamsters are placed in constant dim light next door to each other, eventually one may be active when the other is asleep—further evidence that they are not detecting some mysterious external cue. Rather, every animal has its own endogenous clock; periods vary from one individual to another.

Normally this internal clock is reset by light. If we expose a free-running nocturnal animal to periods of light and dark, the animal soon synchronizes its wheel running to the beginning of the dark period. The shift of activity produced by a synchronizing stimulus is referred to as a **phase shift** (see Figure 10.2B, middle), and the process of shifting the rhythm is called **entrainment**. Any cue that an animal uses to synchronize its activity with the environment is called a **zeitgeber** (German for "time giver"). Light acts as a powerful zeitgeber, and we can easily manipulate it in the lab. Because light stimuli can entrain circadian rhythms, the endogenous clock must receive input from the visual system, as we'll confirm shortly.

To view the animation **Biological Rhythms,** go to 3e.mindsmachine.com/av10.3

free-running Referring to a rhythm of behavior shown by an animal deprived of external cues about time of day.

period The interval of time between two similar points of successive cycles, such as sunset to sunset.

phase shift A shift in the activity of a biological rhythm, typically provided by a synchronizing environmental stimulus, such as light.

entrainment The process of synchronizing a biological rhythm to an environmental stimulus.

zeitgeber Literally "time giver" (in German). The stimulus (usually the light-dark cycle) that entrains circadian rhythms.

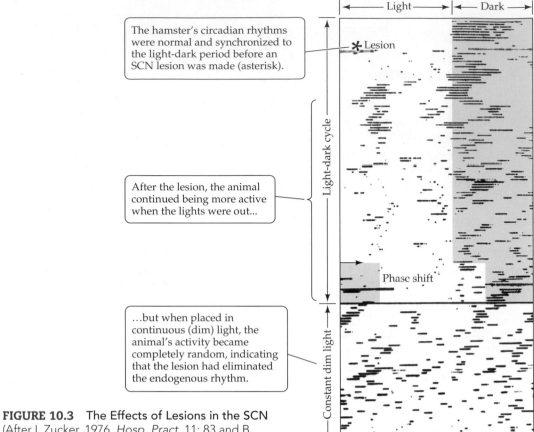

FIGURE 10.3 The Effects of Lesions in the SCN
(After I. Zucker, 1976. *Hosp. Pract.* 11: 83 and B.
Rusak and I. Zucker, 1979. *Physiol. Rev.* 59: 449.

We humans experience a mismatch of internal and external time when we fly
from one time zone to another. Flying three time zones east (say, from California to
New York) means that sunlight arrives 3 hours sooner than our brain expects. The
next morning we'll probably have a hard time waking up at 7:00 AM New York time,
because it's 4:00 AM California time. We need about one day per time zone to entrain
after such travel, and in the meantime we experience jet lag, with symptoms such as
insomnia and daytime fatigue.

The major value of circadian rhythms is obvious: they enable us to *anticipate* an
event, such as sunrise or sunset, and to begin physiological and behavioral preparations *before* that event. Let's talk about how this circadian clock works.

The Hypothalamus Houses a Circadian Clock

Where is the biological clock that drives circadian rhythms, and how does it work?
Early research showed that while removing various endocrine glands had little effect
on the free-running rhythm of rats, large lesions of the hypothalamus interfered with
circadian rhythms (Richter, 1967). It was subsequently discovered that lesions of a tiny
subregion of the hypothalamus—the **suprachiasmatic nucleus** (**SCN**), named for its
location above the optic chiasm—eliminates circadian rhythms of drinking and locomotor behavior (**FIGURE 10.3**) (Stephan and Zucker, 1972) and of hormone secretion
(R. Y. Moore and Eichler, 1972).

The clocklike nature of the SCN is also evident in its metabolic activity. If we take
SCN cells out of the brain and put them in a dish (Earnest et al., 1999; Yamazaki et al.,
2000), their electrical activity continues to show a circadian rhythm for days or weeks.
This striking evidence supports the idea that the SCN contains an endogenous clock.
But even stronger proof that the SCN generates a circadian rhythm comes from trans-
planting the SCN from one animal to another, as we'll see next.

suprachiasmatic nucleus (SCN)
A small region of the hypothalamus
above the optic chiasm that is the location of a circadian clock.

RESEARCHERS AT WORK

Transplants prove that the SCN produces a circadian rhythm

Ralph and Menaker (1988) found a male hamster that exhibited an unusually short free-running activity rhythm in constant conditions. Normally, hamsters free-run at a period slightly longer than 24 hours, but this male showed a free-running period of 22 hours. Half of his offspring also had a shorter circadian rhythm, indicating that he had a genetic mutation affecting the endogenous clock. Grandchildren inheriting two copies of this mutation had an even shorter period: 20 hours. The mutation was named *tau*, after the Greek symbol used by scientists to represent the period (duration) of cyclical processes. These hamsters entrained to a normal 24-hour light-dark cycle just fine; their abnormal endogenous circadian rhythm was revealed only in constant conditions.

Dramatic evidence that the SCN is a master clock was provided by transplant experiments (Ralph et al., 1990), as detailed in **FIGURE 10.4**.

Reciprocal transplants gave comparable results: the endogenous rhythm following the transplant was always that of the *donor* SCN, not the recipient, so the SCN must be driving the circadian rhythms. This remains the only known case of transplanting brain tissue from one individual to another in which the recipient subsequently displayed the donor's behavior!

FIGURE 10.4 Brain Transplants Prove That the SCN Contains a Clock (From M. R. Ralph et al., 1990. *Science* 247: 975.)

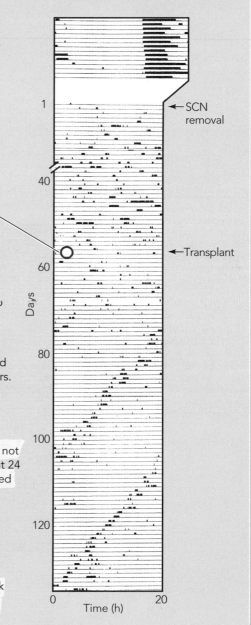

■ **Hypothesis**
The endogenous clock determining an individual hamster's circadian rhythm is in the suprachiasmatic nucleus (SCN).

■ **Test**
The SCN is lesioned in several normal hamsters, rendering them arrhythmic.

Adult hamsters receive SCN transplants from newborn hamsters. This hamster received an SCN from a mutant hamster with a period of about 20 hours.

■ **Alternative Outcomes**
• If the endogenous circadian rhythm is generated outside the SCN, then when the hamster recovers, it should return to its original period of just over 24 hours.
• If the endogenous circadian rhythm is controlled by the SCN, then when the adult hamster recovers, its period should match that of the donor—about 20 hours.

■ **Result**
When the adult hamster recovered, it did not show its original circadian rhythm of about 24 hours, but displayed a rhythm that matched that of its donor, about 20 hours.

■ **Conclusion**
Within the SCN itself there must be a mechanism that can drive a circadian rhythm in activity, and this biological clock is affected by mutation of the gene *tau*.

In mammals, light information from the eyes reaches the SCN directly

Most vertebrates have photoreceptors *outside the eye* that are part of the mechanism of light entrainment (Rusak and Zucker, 1979). For example, the pineal gland of some birds and amphibians is itself sensitive to light (Jamieson and Roberts, 2000) and helps

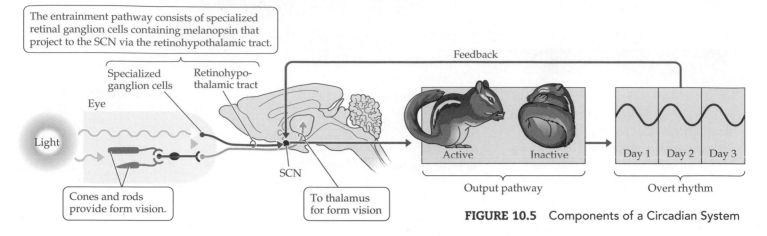

The entrainment pathway consists of specialized retinal ganglion cells containing melanopsin that project to the SCN via the retinohypothalamic tract.

Specialized ganglion cells

Retinohypo-thalamic tract

Eye

Light

Cones and rods provide form vision.

SCN

To thalamus for form vision

Feedback

Active   Inactive

Output pathway

Day 1   Day 2   Day 3

Overt rhythm

FIGURE 10.5   Components of a Circadian System

entrain circadian rhythms to light. Because the skull over the pineal is especially thin in some species, we can think of those species as having a primitive "third eye" in the back of the head. (Some elementary school teachers also seem to have an eye in the back of the head, but this has not been proven to be the pineal gland.) At night, the pineal gland secretes a hormone, **melatonin**, that informs the brain about day length. For more on the nocturnal secretion of melatonin, see **A STEP FURTHER 8.1** (from Chapter 8), on the website.

In mammals, however, cells in the eye tell the SCN when it is light out. Certain retinal ganglion cells send their axons along the **retinohypothalamic pathway**, veering out of the optic chiasm to synapse directly within the SCN. This short pathway carries information about light to the hypothalamus (R. Y. Moore, 2013) to entrain rhythms (**FIGURE 10.5**). Most of the retinal ganglion cells that extend their axons to the SCN do not rely on the traditional photoreceptors—rods and cones—to learn about light. Rather, these retinal ganglion cells themselves contain a special photopigment, called **melanopsin**, that makes them sensitive to light (Do et al., 2009). Transgenic mice that lack rods and cones, and so are blind in every other respect, will still entrain their behavior to light (Freedman et al., 1999) if the specialized melanopsin-containing ganglion cells are present.

Unfortunately, those melanopsin-containing retinal ganglion cells appear to be absent or dysfunctional in most totally blind humans, because people who are blind often show a free-running circadian rhythm, with difficulties getting to sleep at night and staying awake during the day (Sack et al., 1992). Taking melatonin at bedtime, thus mimicking the normal nightly release of the hormone from the pineal gland, helps sighted people to get to sleep (Burgess and Emens, 2018), and it also helps blind people to entrain to daylight (Sack et al., 2000). This result suggests that while humans rely primarily on light stimulation of the retinohypothalamic tract to the SCN in order to entrain to light, our brains have retained enough sensitivity to melatonin that we can use that cue in the absence of information about light.

Deprived of light cues, people free-run just like hamsters (Wever, 1979). Spending weeks in a cave with all cues to external time removed, they display a circadian rhythm of the sleep-waking cycle that slowly shifts from 24 to 25 hours (**FIGURE 10.6**), just as a hamster does (see Figure 10.2). Because the free-running period is greater than 24 hours, some people in these studies are surprised

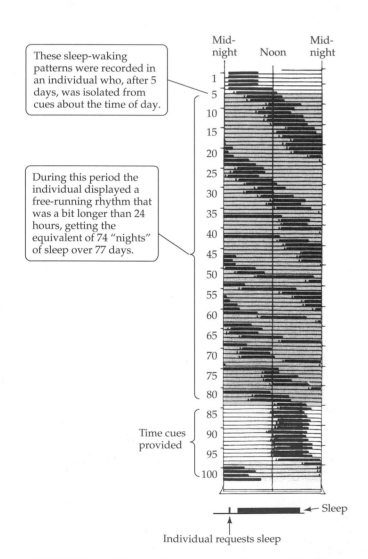

Midnight   Noon   Midnight

These sleep-waking patterns were recorded in an individual who, after 5 days, was isolated from cues about the time of day.

During this period the individual displayed a free-running rhythm that was a bit longer than 24 hours, getting the equivalent of 74 "nights" of sleep over 77 days.

Time cues provided

Sleep

Individual requests sleep

FIGURE 10.6   Humans Free-Run Too (From E. D. Weitzman et al. in J. B. Martin et al., 1981. *Neurosecretion and brain peptides*. Raven Press. New York, NY.)

when they're told that the experiment has ended. They may have experienced only 74 sleep-waking cycles during a 77-day study.

Circadian rhythms have been genetically dissected in flies and mice

Genes that were found to affect circadian rhythms in the fruit fly *Drosophila melanogaster* (Konopka and Benzer, 1971) were later discovered to have differently named but similar-acting counterparts in mammals. This paved the way for understanding the molecular basis of the circadian clock. Neurons in the mammalian SCN make the proteins Clock and Cycle, which bind together to form a dimer (a pair of proteins attached to each other). The Clock/Cycle dimer then binds to the cell's DNA to promote the transcription of other genes, including one called *period* (*per*). The proteins made from these other genes go back to inhibit the action of Clock and Cycle, which started the whole process. Because those inhibitory proteins degrade with time, eventually the inhibition is lifted, starting the whole cycle over again (**FIGURE 10.7**). The entire cycle takes about 24 hours to complete, and it is this 24-hour molecular cycle that drives the 24-hour activity cycle of SCN cells. You can learn more about the molecular basis of the circadian clock in **A STEP FURTHER 10.1**, on the website.

melatonin An amine hormone that is secreted by the pineal gland at night, thereby signaling day length to the brain.

retinohypothalamic pathway The route by which specialized retinal ganglion cells send their axons to the suprachiasmatic nuclei.

melanopsin A photopigment found in those retinal ganglion cells that project to the suprachiasmatic nucleus.

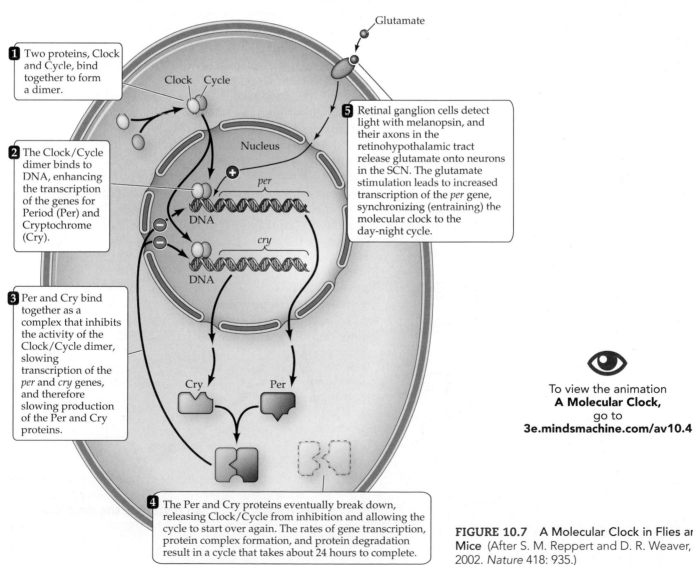

1 Two proteins, Clock and Cycle, bind together to form a dimer.

Clock   Cycle

Glutamate

2 The Clock/Cycle dimer binds to DNA, enhancing the transcription of the genes for Period (Per) and Cryptochrome (Cry).

Nucleus

per

DNA

cry

DNA

5 Retinal ganglion cells detect light with melanopsin, and their axons in the retinohypothalamic tract release glutamate onto neurons in the SCN. The glutamate stimulation leads to increased transcription of the *per* gene, synchronizing (entraining) the molecular clock to the day-night cycle.

3 Per and Cry bind together as a complex that inhibits the activity of the Clock/Cycle dimer, slowing transcription of the *per* and *cry* genes, and therefore slowing production of the Per and Cry proteins.

Cry   Per

4 The Per and Cry proteins eventually break down, releasing Clock/Cycle from inhibition and allowing the cycle to start over again. The rates of gene transcription, protein complex formation, and protein degradation result in a cycle that takes about 24 hours to complete.

To view the animation
A Molecular Clock,
go to
3e.mindsmachine.com/av10.4

FIGURE 10.7 A Molecular Clock in Flies and Mice (After S. M. Reppert and D. R. Weaver, 2002. *Nature* 418: 935.)

FIGURE 10.8 When the Endogenous Clock Goes Kaput (From M. H. Vitaterna et al., 1994. *Science* 29: 719.)

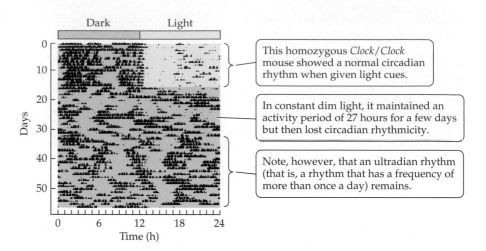

This homozygous *Clock/Clock* mouse showed a normal circadian rhythm when given light cues.

In constant dim light, it maintained an activity period of 27 hours for a few days but then lost circadian rhythmicity.

Note, however, that an ultradian rhythm (that is, a rhythm that has a frequency of more than once a day) remains.

One indication of the importance of the molecular clock in controlling circadian behavior is the effect of differences in the genes involved in the clock. We've already seen that hamsters with a mutation in *tau* have a free-running rhythm that is shorter than normal. Mice in which both copies of the *Clock* gene are disrupted show severe arrhythmicity under constant conditions (**FIGURE 10.8**). People who feel energetic in the morning ("larks") are likely to carry a different version of the *Clock* gene than "night owls" have (Katzenberg et al., 1998). Different versions of other genes in the molecular clock are also associated with being a lark versus an owl in both humans (Blum et al., 2018) and mice (Pfeffer et al., 2015). Human night owls are at greater risk than larks for depression (Foster et al., 2013) and obesity (Roenneberg et al., 2012), perhaps because they are forced to adapt their natural sleep rhythm to fit into an early-bird society.

At puberty, most people shift their circadian rhythm of sleep so that they get up later in the day (**FIGURE 10.9**), basically acting more like night owls. Unfortunately, many school systems require students to come to school *earlier* in the day when they hit adolescence. When high schools shifted their morning start to after 8:30 AM, students showed improved academic performance, including (big surprise!) less sleeping in class, and a reduced incidence of depression (Lo et al., 2018). Plus, the student drivers had 70% fewer car crashes (Wahlstrom et al., 2014)!

Having covered some of the mechanisms that enforce our daily rhythms, we'll spend the rest of the chapter exploring that mysterious circadian behavior called sleep.

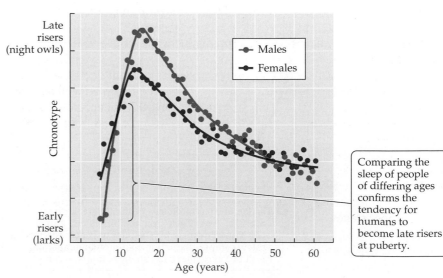

Comparing the sleep of people of differing ages confirms the tendency for humans to become late risers at puberty.

FIGURE 10.9 How I Hate to Get Out of Bed in the Morning! (After T. Roenneberg et al., 2004. *Curr. Biol.* 14: R1038.)

Ultra- hormone
Infra- menstrual cycle

HOW'S IT GOING ❓

1. Give some examples of ultradian and infradian rhythms.
2. What are circadian rhythms, and how can they be studied and manipulated in lab animals?
3. Describe experiments that established which parts of the brain control circadian rhythms.
4. How does information about day and night reach the mammalian brain?
5. Describe in general terms how a molecular process in the brain cycles about every 24 hours.   10.7

PART II
Sleep

THE ROAD AHEAD

The next section concerns our most prominent circadian behavior: sleep. Studying this material should allow you to:

1. Describe the various stages of sleep and how they are distributed across the night.
2. Distinguish the types of mental activity typical of the two major classes of sleep.
3. Describe the changes in sleep as we grow up and grow old.
4. Critically discuss the effects of partial versus total sleep deprivation.
5. Discuss various theories about the function of sleep.
6. Describe four brain systems that influence the sleep-waking cycle.

Human Sleep Exhibits Different Stages

In the 1930s, experimenters found that brain potentials recorded from electrodes on the scalp by **electroencephalography** (**EEG**; see Figure 3.15A) provide a way to define, describe, and classify levels of arousal and states of sleep. In sleep studies, eye movements and muscle tension are monitored in addition to the EEG. Together, these measures led to the groundbreaking discovery that there are two distinct classes of sleep: **rapid-eye-movement (REM) sleep** (Aserinsky and Kleitman, 1953) and **non-REM sleep**.

What are the electrophysiological distinctions that define different sleep states? Let's begin with the pattern of EEG activity in the brain of a fully awake, alert person. It is a mixture of low-amplitude waves with many relatively fast frequencies (greater than 15–20 cycles per second, or hertz [Hz]). This pattern is sometimes referred to as *beta activity* or a **desynchronized EEG** (**FIGURE 10.10A**).

When you relax and close your eyes, a distinctive rhythm appears in the EEG, consisting of a regular oscillation at a frequency of 8–12 Hz, known as the **alpha rhythm**. As drowsiness sets in, the time spent in the alpha rhythm decreases, and the EEG shows waves of smaller amplitude and irregular frequency, as well as sharp waves called **vertex spikes**. This is the beginning of non-REM sleep, called **stage 1 sleep** (**FIGURE 10.10B**), which is accompanied by slowing of the heart rate and relaxation of the muscles; in addition, under the closed eyelids the eyes may roll about slowly. Stage 1 sleep usually lasts several minutes and gives way to **stage 2 sleep** (**FIGURE 10.10C**), which is defined by waves of 12–14 Hz called **sleep spindles** that occur in periodic bursts, and by **K complexes**. If awakened during these first two stages of sleep, many people deny that they have been asleep, even though they failed to respond to signals while in those stages.

Stage 2 sleep leads to (can you guess?) **stage 3 sleep** (**FIGURE 10.10D**), which is defined by the appearance of large-amplitude, *very* slow waves (**delta waves**, about one per second). These waves give stage 3 sleep its other name—*slow wave sleep* (*SWS*). As

electroencephalography (EEG) The recording of gross electrical activity of the brain via large electrodes placed on the scalp.

rapid-eye-movement (REM) sleep Also called *paradoxical sleep*. A stage of sleep characterized by small-amplitude, fast EEG waves, no postural tension, and rapid eye movements. *REM rhymes with "gem."*

non-REM sleep Sleep, divided into stages 1–3, that is defined by the presence of distinctive EEG activity that differs from that seen in REM sleep.

desynchronized EEG Also called *beta activity*. A pattern of EEG activity comprising a mix of many different high frequencies with low amplitude.

alpha rhythm A brain potential of 8–12 Hz that occurs during relaxed wakefulness.

vertex spike A sharp-wave EEG pattern that is seen during stage 1 sleep.

stage 1 sleep The initial stage of non-REM sleep, which is characterized by small-amplitude EEG waves of irregular frequency, slow heart rate, and reduced muscle tension.

stage 2 sleep A stage of sleep that is defined by bursts of EEG waves called *sleep spindles*.

sleep spindle A characteristic 12–14 Hz wave in the EEG of a person said to be in stage 2 sleep.

K complex A sharp, negative EEG potential that is seen in stage 2 sleep.

stage 3 sleep Also called *slow wave sleep* (*SWS*). A stage of non-REM sleep that is defined by the presence of large-amplitude, slow delta waves.

delta wave The slowest type of EEG wave, about 1/sec, characteristic of stage 3 sleep.

FIGURE 10.10 Electrophysiological Correlates of Sleep and Waking (After A. Rechtschaffen and A. Kales, 1968. *A manual of standardized terminology, techniques and scoring system for sleep stages of human subjects.* U.S. NINDB, Neurological Information Network. Bethesda, MD.)

To view the activity
Stages of Sleep,
go to
3e.mindsmachine.com/ac10.1

(A) Waking

An alert, awake human's EEG is desynchronized. This mix of high frequencies with low amplitude is also called *beta activity*.

(B) Stage 1

Alpha rhythms appear during relaxation.

Sharp waves called *vertex spikes* appear during stage 1 sleep.

(C) Stage 2

Brief periods of *sleep spindles* and…

…*K complexes* are characteristic of stage 2 sleep.

(D) Stage 3 SWS

Stage 3 slow-wave sleep is recognized by large, slow *delta waves*.

(E) REM sleep

Despite deep muscle relaxation, the EEG activity in REM sleep resembles that of waking.

200 µV

1 s

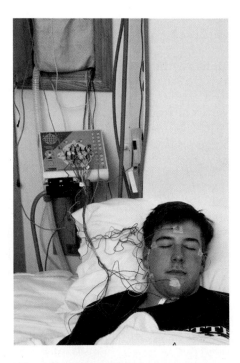

Wired for Sleep Machines measure electrical activity across the various electrodes to monitor EEG, eye movements, and muscle tension across sleep stages. (© Hank Morgan/Science Source.)

the night progresses, the delta waves become even more prominent. (Previously, SWS with delta waves at least half the time was called *stage 4 sleep,* but that distinction is no longer made. Now all sleep with delta waves is called *stage 3* or *SWS.*) The slow waves of electrical potential that give SWS its name represent a widespread synchronization of cortical neuron activity (Poulet and Petersen, 2008) that has been likened to a room of people who are all chanting the same phrase over and over. From a distance, you would be able to hear the rise and fall of the cadence of speech in a slow rhythm. Contrast this with a room full of people all saying something *different.* You would hear only a buzz—the rapid frequencies of many desynchronized speakers. This is like the desynchronized EEG of wakefulness, when many parts of the cortex are communicating different things and fulfilling different functions.

After about an hour, the typical time to progress through the SWS stage, with a brief return to stage 2—something totally different occurs: REM sleep. Quite abruptly, the EEG displays a pattern of small-amplitude, high-frequency activity similar in many ways to the pattern of an awake individual (**FIGURE 10.10E**), except the eyes are darting rapidly about under their lids (the *r*apid *e*ye *m*ovements that give REM sleep its name). Aside from those muscles moving the eyes, all other skeletal muscles not only are relaxed, but show a complete absence of muscle tone, called *atonia.* The active-looking EEG coupled with deeply relaxed muscles is typical of REM sleep. If you see a cat sleeping in the sitting, sphinx position, it cannot be in REM sleep; in REM, it will be sprawled limply on the floor. For the same reason, a student sleeping while sitting upright in class cannot be in REM sleep.

This flaccid muscle state appears, despite intense brain activity, because during REM sleep, brainstem regions are profoundly inhibiting motor neurons. This seeming contradiction—the brain waves look awake, but the muscles are flaccid and

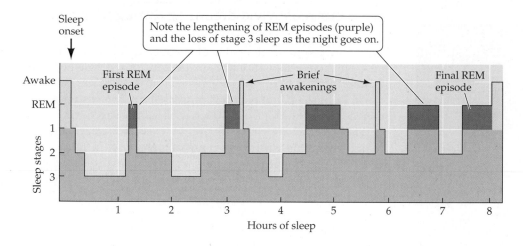

FIGURE 10.11 A Typical Night of Sleep in a Young Adult (After A. Kales and J. Kales, 1970. *JAMA* 213: 2229.)

unresponsive—is what gives REM sleep its other name: *paradoxical sleep*. Unlike SWS, REM sleep is accompanied by irregular breathing and pulse rate, as in wakefulness. It is during REM sleep that we experience vivid dreams, as we'll discuss shortly.

The EEG portrait in Figure 10.10 shows that sleep consists of a complex series of brain states, not just an "inactive" period. The total sleep time of young adults usually ranges from 7 to 8 hours, about half of it in stage 2 sleep. REM sleep accounts for about 20% of total sleep. A typical night of adult human sleep shows repeating cycles approximately 90–110 minutes long, recurring four or five times in a night, reflecting a basic ultradian rest-activity cycle (Kaiser, 2013). These cycles change in a subtle but regular manner through the night. Stage 3 SWS, when we are most deeply asleep and the pituitary releases growth hormone, is more prominent early in the night (**FIGURE 10.11**), and then it tapers off as the night progresses. In contrast, REM sleep is more prominent in the later cycles of sleep. The first REM period is the shortest, while the last REM period, just before waking, may last up to 40 minutes. Brief arousals (yellow bars in Figure 10.11) occasionally occur immediately after a REM period, and the sleeper may shift posture at this time (Amici et al., 2014). **TABLE 10.1** compares the properties of REM and non-REM sleep.

TABLE 10.1 ■ Properties of REM Sleep and Non-REM Sleep

Property	REM sleep	Non-REM sleep
AUTONOMIC ACTIVITIES		
Heart rate	Variable, with high bursts	Slow decline
Respiration	Variable, with high bursts	Slow decline
Brain temperature	Increased	Decreased
Cerebral blood flow	High	Reduced
SKELETAL MUSCULAR SYSTEM		
Postural tension	Eliminated	Progressively reduced
Knee-jerk reflex	Suppressed	Normal
Twitches	Increased	Reduced
Eye movements	Rapid, coordinated	Infrequent, slow, uncoordinated
COGNITIVE STATE		
Dream state	Vivid dreams, well organized	Vague thoughts
HORMONE SECRETION		
Growth hormone secretion	Low	High in SWS
NEURAL FIRING RATES		
Cerebral cortex activity	Increased firing rates	Many cells reduced

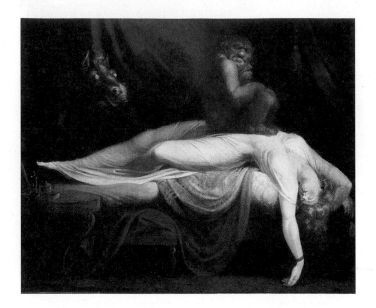

Night Terror This 1781 painting by Henry Fuseli is called *The Nightmare*. It also aptly illustrates night terror, or even sleep paralysis, discussed later in the chapter, as the demon crushes the breath from his victim.

nightmare A long, frightening dream that awakens the sleeper from REM sleep.

night terror A sudden arousal from stage 3 sleep that is marked by intense fear and autonomic activation.

We do our most vivid dreaming during REM sleep

We can record the EEGs of participants to monitor their sleep stages, awaken them at a particular stage (1, 2, 3, or REM), and question them about thoughts or perceptions they were having. Early studies of this sort suggested that dreams happen only during REM sleep, but we now know that dreams also occur in other sleep stages. What is distinctive about dreams during REM sleep is that they are characterized by visual imagery, whereas dreams during non-REM sleep are of a more "thinking" type. REM dreams are apt to include a story that involves odd perceptions and the sense that the dreamer "is there" experiencing sights, sounds, smells, and emotions (McNamara et al., 2010). People awakened from non-REM sleep report thinking about problems rather than seeing themselves in a stage presentation. The dreams of these two states are so different that people can be trained to predict accurately whether a described dream occurred during REM sleep or SWS (Cartwright, 1979).

Almost everyone has terrifying dreams on occasion (Llewellyn and Hobson, 2015). **Nightmares** are defined as long, frightening dreams that awaken the sleeper from REM sleep. They are occasionally confused with **night terror**, which is a sudden arousal from stage 3 SWS marked by intense fear and autonomic activation. In night terror, the sleeper does not recall a vivid dream but may remember a sense of a crushing feeling on the chest, as though being suffocated. Night terrors are common in children during the early part of an evening's sleep.

Many medications, including antidepressants and drugs that control blood pressure, make nightmares more frequent (Pagel and Helfter, 2003), but nightmares are quite prevalent even without such influences. At least 25% of college students report having one or more nightmares per month. Have you had the common one, which Sigmund Freud had, of suddenly remembering that you're supposed to be taking a final exam that is already in progress?

As fascinating as they are, we still do not know what function, if any, is fulfilled by dreams. The *activation-synthesis* theory suggests our experiences in REM sleep are the more or less random results of which neurons happen to get activated (Hobson and Friston, 2012). The brain strings together these disparate activated elements into a more or less coherent story, a narrative. Later we'll discuss evidence that at least some other animals experience dreaming, which suggests that dreaming either fulfills an important function or is an unavoidable consequence of some other function of REM sleep.

FIGURE 10.12 Sleep in Marine Mammals (After L. M. Mukhametov in A. Borbély and J. L. Valatx, 1984. *Experimental brain research: Suppl. 8. Sleep mechanisms*. Springer-Verlag. Berlin, Germany.)

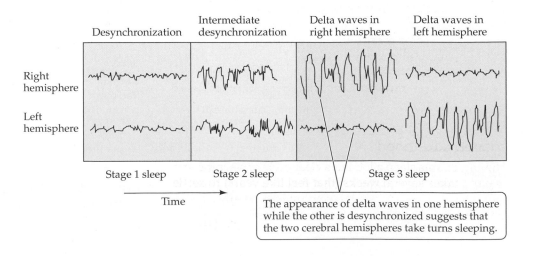

Different species provide clues about the evolution of sleep

With the aid of behavioral and EEG techniques, sleep has been studied in a wide assortment of mammals and, to a lesser extent, in reptiles, birds, and amphibians (Lesku et al., 2009; Hartse, 2011). Nearly all mammalian species that have been investigated thus far, including our most distant mammalian relatives, such as the platypus (Siegel, Manger et al., 1999), display both REM sleep and SWS. Among the other vertebrates, birds display clear signs of both SWS and REM sleep, which indicates that REM sleep was present in an ancestor common to birds and mammals. The recent report of REM sleep in a reptile (Shein-Idelson et al., 2016) suggests that maybe it arose even earlier.

The absence of REM sleep in dolphins is probably a late adaptation that evolved when their land-dwelling ancestors took to the water, because they must come to the surface of the water to breathe. That requirement may be incompatible with the deep relaxation of muscles during REM sleep. Another dolphin adaptation to living in water is that only one side of the dolphin brain engages in SWS at a time (Mukhametov, 1984). It's as if one whole hemisphere is asleep while the other is awake (**FIGURE 10.12**). During these periods of "unilateral sleep," the animals continue to come up to the surface occasionally to breathe. Birds can also display unilateral sleep—one hemisphere sleeping while the other hemisphere watches for predators (Rattenborg, 2006). Unilateral sleep while gliding may also enable birds to fly long distances without stopping; for example, a bar-tailed godwit flew nonstop more than 10,000 miles, from Alaska to Australia, in a week (Gill et al., 2009). You can learn more about comparing patterns of sleep in different species in **A STEP FURTHER 10.2**, on the website.

HOW'S IT GOING ❓

1. What are the different stages of sleep, and what measures define them?
2. What happens to our muscles during the sleep stage characterized by the most vivid dreams?
3. Contrast the mental activity present in REM sleep versus SWS.
4. Describe one way that certain species manage to remain active around the clock and still sleep.

Our Sleep Patterns Change across the Life Span

How much sleep and what kind of sleep we get changes across our lifetime. As infants, we sleep a lot; as we grow, we sleep less and less until we hit adolescence, when once again sleep seems precious. After that, we sleep less and less as we age, sometimes to our disappointment. These changes as we grow up and grow old suggest that the function(s) of sleep are more important during some stages of life than others.

Mammals sleep more during infancy than in adulthood

Human infants sleep a lot, but a clear cycle of sleeping and waking takes several weeks (that feel like years) to settle in (**FIGURE 10.13**). A 24-hour rhythm is generally evident by 16 weeks of age. Infant sleep is characterized by shorter sleep cycles than those of adults, probably reflecting the

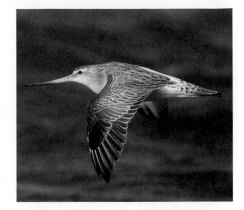

Sleeping on the Go A female bar-tailed godwit flew over 10,000 miles, nonstop, from Alaska to Australia in a week. Were both sides of its brain awake the entire time? (© Robin Chittenden/Alamy Stock Photo.)

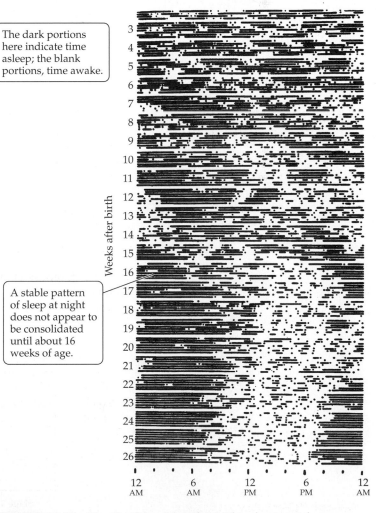

The dark portions here indicate time asleep; the blank portions, time awake.

A stable pattern of sleep at night does not appear to be consolidated until about 16 weeks of age.

Weeks after birth

FIGURE 10.13 **The Trouble with Babies** This classic study may represent an extreme example of a baby slow to entrain to the day-night rhythm. (From N. Kleitman and T. Engelmann, 1953. *J. App. Physiol.* 6: 269.)

FIGURE 10.14 Human Sleep Patterns Change with Age (After H. P. Roffwarg et al., 1966. *Science* 152: 604.)

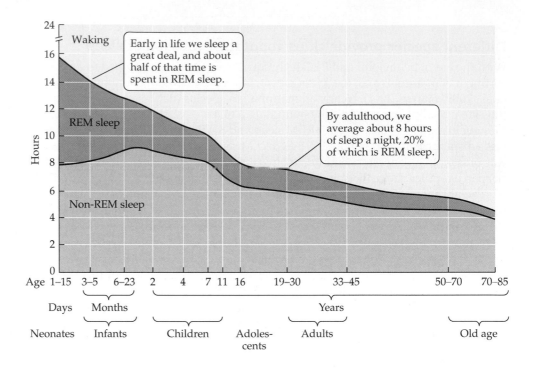

relative immaturity of the brain, since sleep cycles in prematurely born infants are even shorter than in full-term newborns.

Infant mammals also show a large percentage of REM sleep. In humans, for example, half of sleep in the first 2 weeks of life is REM sleep. The prominence of REM sleep is even greater in premature infants. Unlike most adults, human infants can move directly from an awake state to REM sleep. The REM sleep of infants is quite active, accompanied by muscle twitching, smiles, grimaces, and vocalizations. The preponderance of REM sleep early in life (**FIGURE 10.14**) suggests that this state provides stimulation that is essential to maturation of the nervous system. By contrast, killer whales and bottlenose dolphins appear to spend little or no time in REM sleep (or any other sleep stage) for the first month of life (Lyamin et al., 2005), presumably because they have to surface often to breathe. So, either REM sleep does not fill a crucial need in all mammalian infants, or dolphin and whale infants have evolved an alternative way to fill that need.

Most people sleep appreciably less as they age

The character of sleep changes in old age, though more slowly than in early development. **FIGURE 10.15** shows the sleep pattern typical of an elderly person. The total amount of sleep declines, while the number of awakenings increases (compare with Figure 10.11). Lack of sleep, or *insomnia* (which we discuss at the end of this chapter), is a common complaint of the elderly and is associated with a variety of physical and cognitive impairments (Cooke and Ancoli-Israel, 2011).

In humans and other mammals, the most dramatic decline is in stage 3 sleep; 60-year-old people spend only about half as much time in stage 3 as they did at age 20 (Bliwise, 1989). By 90 years of age, stage 3 sleep has disappeared. This decline in stage 3 sleep may be related to diminished cognitive functioning, since an especially marked reduction of stage 3 SWS characterizes the sleep of people who suffer from senile dementia. Growth hormone is secreted primarily during stage 3 SWS (see Table 10.1), so perhaps the loss of growth hormone due to disrupted sleep in the elderly leads to the cognitive deficits. Loss of SWS probably also impairs memory processes (discussed below) in older people and patients with dementia (Westerberg et al., 2012).

Most elderly people fall asleep easily enough, but then they may have a hard time staying asleep, which causes sleep "dissatisfaction." As in so many things, attitude may be important for how you experience sleep loss as you age. Objective measures of sleep suggest that elderly people who complain of poor sleep may actually sleep

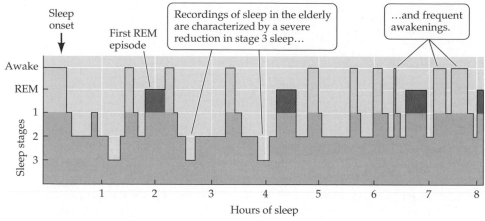

FIGURE 10.15 The Typical Pattern of Sleep in an Elderly Person Compare this recording with the young adult sleep pattern shown in Figure 10.11. (After A. Kales and J. D. Kales, 1974. *New England J. Med.* 290: 487.)

more than those who are satisfied with their sleep (McCrae et al., 2005). Perhaps if, as you grow older, you can regard waking up at 3:00 AM as a "bonus" (a little more time awake before you die), you will be more satisfied with the sleep you get.

Manipulating Sleep Reveals an Underlying Structure

Another persuasive clue that sleep is important is revealed when we go without it. First of all, our mental function is impaired. This is bad news for college students, who rarely get enough sleep, just when they're supposed to be learning how to make their way in the world. In addition, after sleep deprivation we tend to sleep more than we would have, as though catching up on something we need, as we'll see.

Sleep deprivation impairs cognitive functioning but does not cause insanity

Most of us at one time or another have been willing or not-so-willing participants in informal **sleep deprivation** experiments. Thus, most of us are aware of the primary effect of partial or total sleep deprivation: it makes us sleepy. It has other effects as well. Early reports from sleep deprivation studies emphasized a similarity between schizophrenia and "bizarre" behavior provoked by sleep deprivation. A frequent theme in this early work was the functional role of dreams as a "guardian of sanity." But examination of people with schizophrenia does not fit this view. For example, these patients can show sleep-waking cycles similar to those of typical adults, and sleep deprivation does not exacerbate their symptoms.

The behavioral effects of prolonged, total sleep deprivation vary appreciably and may depend on some general personality factors and on age. In studies employing prolonged total deprivation—205 hours (8.5 days!)—a few participants showed occasional episodes of hallucinations. But the most common behavior changes were increases in irritability, difficulty in concentrating, and episodes of disorientation. The sleep-deprived participants' ability to perform tasks was summed up like this: "Performance is like a motor that after much use misfires, runs normally for a while, then falters again" (L. C. Johnson, 1969, p. 216).

You don't need to resort to total sleep deprivation to see effects. Moderate effects of sleep debt can accumulate with successive nights of little sleep. Voluntary experimental participants who got 6 or 4 hours of sleep per night for 2 weeks showed ever-mounting deficits in attention tasks and in speed of reaction, compared with those sleeping 8 hours per night (Van Dongen et al., 2003). Interestingly, the sleep-deprived participants often reported not feeling sleepy, yet they still exhibited behavioral deficits. By the end of the study, the people getting less than 8 hours of sleep per night had cognitive deficits equivalent to those of participants who had been totally sleep-deprived for 3 days!

Finally, it is clear that prolonged, total sleep deprivation in mammals compromises the immune system and leads to death, as we'll see in Signs & Symptoms next.

sleep deprivation The partial or total prevention of sleep.

SIGNS & SYMPTOMS

Total Sleep Deprivation Can Be Fatal

Sustained sleep deprivation in rats causes them to increase their metabolic rate, lose weight, and, within an average of 19 days, die (Everson et al., 1989). Allowing them to sleep prevents their death. After the fatal effect of sleep deprivation had been shown, researchers undertook studies in which they terminated the sleep deprivation before the fatal end point and looked for pathological changes in different organ systems (Rechtschaffen and Bergmann, 1995). No single organ system seems affected in chronically sleep-deprived animals, but early in the deprivation they develop sores on their bodies. These sores mark the beginning of the end; shortly thereafter, blood tests reveal infections from a host of bacteria, which probably enter through the sores (Everson, 1993).

These bacteria are not normally fatal, because the rat's immune system and body defenses keep the bacteria in check, but severely sleep-deprived rats fail to develop a fever in response to these infections. (Fever helps the body fight infection.) In fact, the sleep-deprived animals show a *drop* in body temperature, which probably speeds bacterial infections that in turn cause diffuse organ damage. The decline of these severely sleep-deprived rats is complicated, but it seems clear that getting sleep improves immune system function (Bryant et al., 2004). So perhaps Shakespeare's theory of the function of sleep, "Sleep that knits up the ravell'd sleave of care," isn't so far from the truth. Even fruit flies will die without sleep (P. J. Shaw et al., 2002).

Some unfortunate humans inherit a defect in the gene for the prion protein, which can transmit mad cow disease, and although they sleep normally at the beginning of life, in midlife they simply stop sleeping—with fatal effect. People with this disease, called **fatal familial insomnia**, die 7–24 months after the insomnia begins (Medori et al., 1992; Mastrianni et al., 1999). Autopsy reveals degeneration in the cerebral cortex (**FIGURE 10.16**) and thalamus, which may cause the insomnia (Almer et al., 1999). Like sleep-deprived rats, sleep-deprived humans with this disorder don't have obvious damage to any single organ system, but they suffer from diffuse bacterial infections. Apparently, these patients die because they are chronically sleep-deprived, and these results, combined with research on rats, certainly support the idea that prolonged insomnia is fatal. Given that, it's surprising how long people can do without sleep and apparently be okay, as we'll see next.

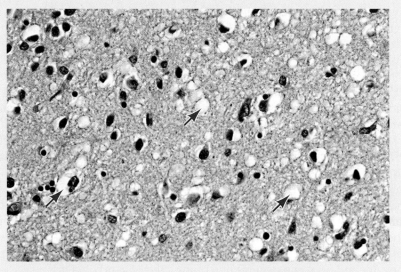

FIGURE 10.16   Fatal Sleeplessness Note the large holes (arrows) that have developed in this section of frontal cortex from a victim of fatal familial insomnia. (Micrograph courtesy of H. Budka.)

fatal familial insomnia   An inherited disease that causes people in middle age to stop sleeping, which after a few months results in death.

sleep recovery   The process of sleeping more than normally after a period of sleep deprivation, as though in compensation.

Sleep recovery may take time

One of the most famous cases of sleep deprivation began as a high school student's science project. Researchers became involved only after Randy Gardner had started his deprivation schedule, which is why we have no data about his sleep before he decided to stay awake for, believe it or not, 11 days! As in other studies, Randy's performance on some tests was impaired, but he could still hold a conversation and was articulate and clear in a press conference at the end of his experiment. In other words, he showed no signs of insanity—he just acted really, really sleepy.

Randy's **sleep recovery** after 11 days of sleep deprivation, depicted in **FIGURE 10.17**, shows the same pattern of sleep recovery as in controlled studies with shorter periods of deprivation. In the first night of sleep recovery, stage 3 sleep shows the

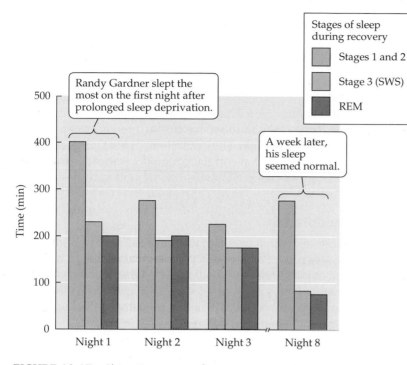

Randy Gardner slept the most on the first night after prolonged sleep deprivation.

A week later, his sleep seemed normal.

Stages of sleep during recovery
- Stages 1 and 2
- Stage 3 (SWS)
- REM

FIGURE 10.17 Sleep Recovery After 11 Days Awake
(After G. Gulevich et al., 1966. *Arch. Gen. Psychiatry* 15: 29.)

Skipping Sleep for Science   As a young man, Randy Gardner decided to see how long he could stay awake as a science fair project. The answer? Just over 11 days. Is that a record for the most demanding science fair project? (© San Diego History Center.)

greatest relative difference from normal. This increase in stage 3 sleep is usually at the expense of stage 2 sleep. However, the added stage 3 sleep during recovery never completely makes up for the deficit accumulated over the deprivation period. In fact, Randy had no more additional stage 3 sleep than do people deprived of sleep for half as long. REM sleep in recovery nights is more "intense" than normal, with a greater number of rapid eye movements per period of time. So you never recover all the sleep time you lost, but you may make up for the loss by having more intense sleep for a few nights. The sooner you get to sleep, the sooner you recover.

The effects of sleep deprivation suggest that sleep plays an important function, or even several functions, that we'll consider next.

HOW'S IT GOING ❓
---

1. Describe how sleep changes as we grow up and grow old.
2. What happens when we are deprived of sleep?
3. Describe the outcome of Randy Gardner's famous self-study.

What Are the Biological Functions of Sleep?

Doesn't it seem like a big waste of time to spend one-third of our lifetime asleep? Most of us have fantasized about how great it would be if we could stay awake and chipper all the time, but we've seen that it's just not possible. What is so important about sleep that we can't seem to live without it? Let's consider the four functions that are most often ascribed to sleep:

1. Energy conservation
2. Niche adaptation
3. Body and brain restoration
4. Memory consolidation

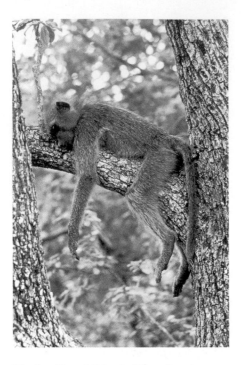

Finding Your Niche in Life Species that can sleep in secure circumstances tend to sleep more than other species. (© Hoberman Collection/Alamy Stock Photo.)

ecological niche The unique assortment of environmental opportunities and challenges to which each organism is adapted.

Sleep conserves energy

We use up less energy when we sleep than when we're awake. For example, SWS is marked by reduced muscular tension, lowered heart rate, reduced blood pressure, reduced body temperature, and slower respiration. This diminished metabolic activity during sleep suggests that one role of sleep is to conserve energy. We can see the importance of this function by considering small animals. Small mammals and birds have very high metabolic rates (see Chapter 9). In general, the smaller the mammal, the higher its metabolic rate and the more time it spends asleep (Siegel, 2005). Larger mammals, like elephants, have low metabolic rates and sleep only a few hours per day (Gravett et al., 2017). That correlation supports the idea that sleep helps conserve energy. But energy savings from sleep seem modest at best (Lesku et al., 2009).

Sleep enforces niche adaptation

Almost all animals are either nocturnal or diurnal. This specialization for either nighttime or daytime activity is part of each species' **ecological niche**, that unique assortment of environmental opportunities and challenges to which each organism is adapted. Thanks to these adaptations, each species is better at gathering food either at night or in the daytime, and it is also better at avoiding predators either during the day or at night. If you're a nocturnal mammal, like a mouse, you are adept at sneaking around in the dark, using your acute senses of hearing and smell to navigate and find food. The rest of the time, during daylight, you should spend holed up somewhere safe to stay away from keen-eyed predators. Sleep debt and the unpleasant feelings of sleepiness have the effect of enforcing the circadian rhythm characteristic of your species. So, one important function of sleep, or of the results of sleep deprivation, is to force the individual to conform to the particular ecological niche for which it is well adapted (Meddis, 1975), and natural selection must have played an important role in its evolution.

Sleep restores the body and brain

If someone asked you why you wanted to go to sleep, you might answer that you "feel worn out." Indeed, one of the proposed functions of sleep is simply the rebuilding or restoration of materials used during waking, such as proteins (Moruzzi, 1972; Pulak and Jensen, 2014). Maybe this is why most growth hormone release happens during slow wave sleep.

We've seen that prolonged and total sleep deprivation—either forced on rats or, in humans, as a result of inherited pathology—interferes with the immune system and leads to death. Even relatively mild deprivation, having sleep shortened or disrupted (e.g., by a nurse taking vital signs every hour), makes people more sensitive to pain the following day (Edwards et al., 2009). A study of over a million Americans found that those sleeping less than 6 hours per night were more likely to die over the next 6 years, although interestingly, people who slept *more than 8* hours per night were also at greater risk (Kripke et al., 2002). People who sleep less than 5 hours per night are more likely to develop diabetes (Gangwisch et al., 2007). Perhaps the most alarming link between sleep and health is the finding that people who work at night and sleep in the daytime are more likely to develop cancer (Erren et al., 2009). So the widespread belief that sleep helps the body ward off illness is well supported by research (S. Cohen et al., 2009; Imeri and Opp, 2009).

There's also evidence that sleep may help "clean out" the brain. Glia control the flow of cerebrospinal fluid through a network of microscopic channels throughout the brain, the glymphatic system we mentioned in Chapter 2, collecting and disposing of toxins that build up. This flow is much faster during sleep than wakefulness (Xie et al., 2013), flushing out brain waste products as we snooze.

Sleep may aid memory consolidation

A peculiar property of dreams is that, unless we describe them to someone or write them down soon after waking, we tend to forget them as though the brain refuses to store anything that we experience during REM sleep. This seems like a good idea—why waste memory storage space on something that never happened? Similarly, and despite ads you might read in the backs of magazines, you cannot learn new material while you're sleeping (Druckman and Bjork, 1994). Putting a speaker under your pillow to recite material for a final exam will not help you, unless you stay awake to listen (J. M. Wood et al., 1992).

Sleep seems important for learning in another way, however. In 1924 an experiment suggested that sleep helps you learn or remember material or events experienced *before* you went to bed (Jenkins and Dallenbach, 1924). Some participants were trained in a verbal learning task at bedtime and tested 8 hours later on rising from sleep; other people were trained early in the day and tested 8 hours later (with no intervening sleep). The results showed better retention when a period of sleep intervened between a learning period and tests of recall. A surge of supporting evidence has shown that sleep helps with memory formation in many domains, not just verbal memory (Ellenbogen et al., 2007; Korman et al., 2007; Cherdieu et al., 2018; Navarro-Lobato and Genzel, 2018).

Despite early assumptions that REM sleep would play a bigger role in learning and memory (Karni et al., 1994; C. Smith, 1995), most research suggested that it is SWS that helps memory consolidation (Plihal and Born, 1999; Nishida and Walker, 2007). In fact, consolidation of a declarative memory task was even better if the person's cortical slow wave oscillations during SWS were boosted by electrically stimulating electrodes over the skull (Marshall et al., 2006). (Don't try this at home.) What's more, one man who had brainstem injuries that seemed to eliminate REM sleep could still learn, and he earned a law school degree (P. Lavie, 1996). So even if REM sleep *aids* learning, clearly it is not absolutely *necessary* for learning (Ackermann and Rasch, 2018).

Don't rule out a role for REM sleep in learning entirely, however, because synapses are being rearranged during that state (W. Li et al., 2017), and some memory consolidation seems dependent on REM (Boyce et al., 2016).

Some humans sleep remarkably little, yet function normally

One challenge to all the theories about the function of sleep is the existence of a few people who seem perfectly healthy, yet sleep hardly at all. These cases are more than just folktales. A Stanford University professor slept only 3–4 hours a night for more than 50 years and lived to be 80 (Dement, 1974). Sleep researcher Ray Meddis (1977) found a cheerful 70-year-old retired nurse who said she had slept little since childhood. She was a busy person who easily filled up her 23 hours of daily wakefulness. During the night, she sat in bed reading or writing, and at about 2:00 AM she fell asleep for an hour or so, after which she readily awakened.

For her first two nights in Meddis's laboratory, she did not sleep at all, because it was all so interesting to her. On the third night, she slept a total of 99 minutes, and her sleep contained both SWS and REM sleep periods. In a later session, her sleep was recorded for 5 days. She didn't sleep the first night, but on subsequent nights she slept an average of 67 minutes. She never complained about not sleeping more, and she did not feel drowsy during either the day or the night. Meddis described several other people who slept only an hour or two per night. Some of these people reported having parents who slept little, so there may be a genetic tendency for little sleep. Whatever the function of sleep is, some people (and elephants) have a way of fulfilling it in just a few hours per night. Why aren't their immune systems compromised? We don't know, but perhaps their immune systems don't need much sleep either. Or perhaps the small amount of sleep they have almost every night is more efficient at doing whatever sleep does. The important point, though, is that no healthy person has ever been found who does not sleep at all.

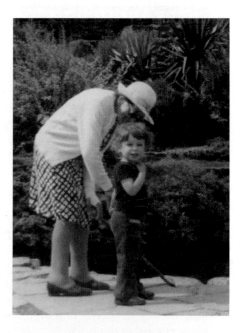

A Nonsleeper   When Ray Meddis brought this 70-year-old nurse into the lab for sleep recording, he confirmed that she slept only about an hour per night. Yet she was a healthy and energetic person. Here she's touring a garden with Meddis's son. (Photo courtesy of Ray Meddis.)

HOW'S IT GOING   **?**

1. Describe the four most prominent theories about the function of sleep and the evidence to support them.
2. What can we conclude about the function of sleep when we consider people who sleep very little?
3. What happens when we stop sleeping altogether?

isolated brain   An experimental preparation in which an animal's brainstem has been separated from the spinal cord by a cut below the medulla.

isolated forebrain   An experimental preparation in which an animal's nervous system has been cut in the upper midbrain, dividing the forebrain from the brainstem.

basal forebrain   A ventral region in the forebrain that has been implicated in sleep.

tuberomammillary nucleus
A region of the basal hypothalamus, near the pituitary stalk, that plays a role in generating slow wave sleep.

general anesthetic   A drug that renders an individual unconscious.

At Least Four Interacting Neural Systems Underlie Sleep

At one time sleep was regarded as a passive state, as though most of the brain simply stopped working while we slept, leaving us unaware of events around us. We now know that sleep is an active state mediated by at least four interacting neural systems:

1. A *forebrain* system that generates SWS
2. A *brainstem* system that activates the sleeping forebrain into wakefulness
3. A *pontine* system that triggers REM sleep
4. A *hypothalamic* system that coordinates the other three brain regions to determine which state we're in

Let's examine each of these systems in some detail.

RESEARCHERS AT WORK

The forebrain generates slow wave sleep

Some of the earliest studies of sleep indicated that a system in the forebrain promotes SWS. These are experiments in which an animal's brain is transected—literally cut into two parts: an upper part and a lower part. The entire brain can be isolated from the body by an incision between the medulla and the spinal cord. This preparation was first studied by the Belgian physiologist Frédéric Bremer (1892–1982), who called it the **isolated brain** (Bremer, 1938).

The EEGs of such animals showed signs of waking alternating with sleep (**FIGURE 10.18A**). During EEG-defined wakeful periods, the pupils were dilated and the eyes followed moving objects. During EEG-defined sleep, the pupils were small, as in normal sleep. REM sleep can also be detected in the isolated brain. These results demonstrated that wakefulness, SWS, and REM sleep are all mediated by *networks within the brain*.

When Bremer made the transection higher along the brainstem—in the midbrain—a very different result was seen. Bremer referred to such a preparation as an **isolated forebrain**, and he found that the EEG from the brain in front of the cut displayed constant SWS (**FIGURE 10.18B**), with no indications of wakefulness or REM sleep. This result demonstrates that the forebrain alone can generate SWS, without contributions from the lower brain regions.

The constant SWS seen in the cortex of the isolated forebrain appears to be generated by the **basal forebrain** in the ventral frontal lobe and anterior hypothalamus (**FIGURE 10.19**, step 1). Electrical stimulation of the basal forebrain can induce SWS activity (Clemente and Sterman, 1967), while lesions there suppress sleep (McGinty and Sterman, 1968). Neurons in this region become active at sleep onset and release gamma-aminobutyric acid (GABA) (Gallopin et al., 2000) to stimulate $GABA_A$ receptors in the nearby **tuberomammillary nucleus** in the posterior hypothalamus. These same $GABA_A$ receptors are stimulated by **general anesthetics**—drugs such as barbiturates and anesthetic gases that render people unconscious during surgery. Thus, general anesthetics produce slow waves in the EEG that resemble those seen in SWS (Franks, 2008).

So the basal forebrain promotes SWS by releasing GABA into the nearby tuberomammillary nucleus, and if left alone, this system would keep the cortex asleep forever. But as we'll see next, the brainstem contains a system that arouses the forebrain from slumber.

RESEARCHERS AT WORK (continued)

FIGURE 10.18   Transecting the Brain at Different Levels

■ Hypothesis

The forebrain contains a neural system promoting SWS.

■ Test

Bremer transected the brain at one of two levels: between the spinal cord and medulla, or between the midbrain and the forebrain. If neural systems in the forebrain generate SWS, then the isolated forebrain should show SWS.

■ Result

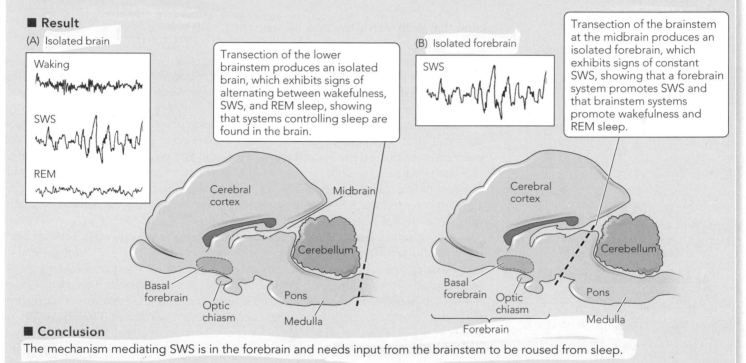

(A) Isolated brain

Waking

SWS

REM

Transection of the lower brainstem produces an isolated brain, which exhibits signs of alternating between wakefulness, SWS, and REM sleep, showing that systems controlling sleep are found in the brain.

Cerebral cortex   Midbrain

Cerebellum

Basal forebrain   Optic chiasm   Pons

Medulla

(B) Isolated forebrain

SWS

Transection of the brainstem at the midbrain produces an isolated forebrain, which exhibits signs of constant SWS, showing that a forebrain system promotes SWS and that brainstem systems promote wakefulness and REM sleep.

Cerebral cortex

Cerebellum

Basal forebrain   Optic chiasm   Pons

Forebrain   Medulla

■ Conclusion

The mechanism mediating SWS is in the forebrain and needs input from the brainstem to be roused from sleep.

The reticular formation wakes up the forebrain

In the late 1940s, scientists found that they could wake sleeping animals by electrically stimulating an extensive region of the brainstem known as the **reticular formation** (**FIGURE 10.19**, step 2) (Moruzzi and Magoun, 1949). The reticular formation is a diffuse group of cells whose axons and dendrites course in many directions, extending from the medulla through the thalamus. Because electrical stimulation anywhere along this region activates the forebrain, the reticular formation is sometimes called the *reticular activating system* of the brainstem. Conversely, lesions of these regions produced persistent sleep in the animals. So the basal forebrain region actively imposes SWS on the brain, and the brainstem reticular formation seems to push the brain from SWS to wakefulness. What system imposes REM sleep?

The pons triggers REM sleep

Several experiments indicated that a region of the pons is important for REM sleep. Lesions of the region just ventral to the **locus coeruleus** abolish REM sleep (**FIGURE 10.19**, step 3) (Friedman and Jones, 1984). Electrical stimulation of the same region, or pharmacological stimulation of this region with cholinergic agonists, can induce or

reticular formation   Also called *reticular activating system.* An extensive region of the brainstem (extending from the medulla through the thalamus) that is involved in arousal.

locus coeruleus   A small nucleus in the brainstem whose neurons produce norepinephrine and modulate large areas of the forebrain.

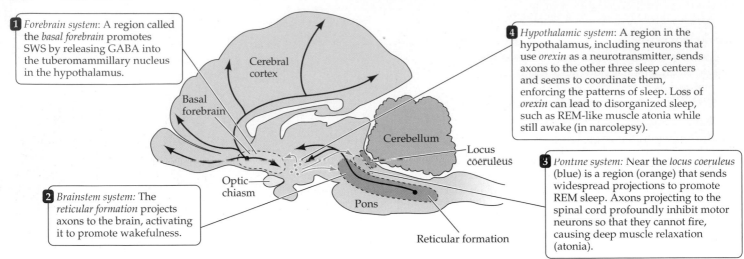

1 *Forebrain system:* A region called the *basal forebrain* promotes SWS by releasing GABA into the tuberomammillary nucleus in the hypothalamus.

4 *Hypothalamic system:* A region in the hypothalamus, including neurons that use *orexin* as a neurotransmitter, sends axons to the other three sleep centers and seems to coordinate them, enforcing the patterns of sleep. Loss of *orexin* can lead to disorganized sleep, such as REM-like muscle atonia while still awake (in narcolepsy).

2 *Brainstem system:* The *reticular formation* projects axons to the brain, activating it to promote wakefulness.

3 *Pontine system:* Near the *locus coeruleus* (blue) is a region (orange) that sends widespread projections to promote REM sleep. Axons projecting to the spinal cord profoundly inhibit motor neurons so that they cannot fire, causing deep muscle relaxation (atonia).

FIGURE 10.19 Brain Mechanisms Underlying Sleep

To view the activity
Sleep Mechanisms,
go to
3e.mindsmachine.com/ac10.2

prolong REM sleep. Finally, some neurons in this region seem to be active only during REM sleep (Siegel, 1994). So the pons has a REM sleep center near the locus coeruleus.

One important job of the pontine REM sleep center is to prevent motor neurons from firing. During REM sleep, the inhibitory transmitters GABA and glycine produce powerful inhibitory postsynaptic potentials (discussed in Chapter 3) in spinal motor neurons, preventing them from reaching threshold and producing an action potential (Kodama et al., 2003). Thus, the dreamer's muscles are not just relaxed, but flaccid. This loss of muscle tone during REM sleep can be abolished by small lesions that damage only a part of the REM center, suggesting that this subregion is what normally disables the motor system during REM.

Cats with such lesions seem to act out their dreams. They enter SWS as they normally would, but when they begin to display the EEG signs of REM sleep, instead of becoming completely limp as normal cats do, these cats stagger to their feet (A. R. Morrison, 1983; A. R. Morrison et al., 1995). Are they awake or in REM sleep? They move their heads as though visually tracking moving objects (that aren't there), bat with their forepaws at nothing, and ignore objects that are present (**FIGURE 10.20**). In addition, the cats' *inner eyelids*, the translucent nictitating membranes, partially cover the eyes. Thus, the cats appear to be in REM sleep, but motor activity is not being inhibited by the brain. These results strongly suggest that animals dream too. What do cats dream of? If their actions while sleeping are any indication, they dream of stalking prey, perhaps a mouse or a ball of yarn.

So far we've described three interacting brain systems controlling sleep: an SWS-promoting region in the forebrain, an arousing reticular formation in the brainstem, and a system in the pons that triggers REM sleep, including paralysis of the body

To see the video
Animal Sleep Activity,
go to
3e.mindsmachine.com/av10.5

(A) This cat received a small lesion near the locus coeruleus that blocked the completely limp muscles (atonia) that normally accompanies REM sleep.

(B) The cat stands up wobbly, "looking" at something we cannot see. These behaviors indicate the cat is dreaming—seeing and interacting with objects that aren't really there.

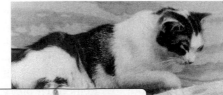

Following a bout of SWS, the cat in REM rises up as though about to pounce, but its eyes are nearly closed and nothing is there.

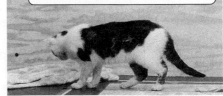

FIGURE 10.20 Acting Out a Dream (From A. R. Morrison et al., 1995. *Behav. Neurosci.* 109: 972.)

during that state. There is a fourth important system, which seems to act as a "co-ordinating center" among these three centers, in the hypothalamus (**FIGURE 10.19**, step 4). To understand how we learned about this fourth system, we need to consider sleep disorders because a rare but fascinating condition taught us about a specific neurotransmitter that is crucial in the control of sleep.

HOW'S IT GOING ❓

1. Describe the four brain systems that control different stages of the sleep-waking cycle, discussing the experiments that revealed each.
2. What receptor systems do anesthetics act upon to render people unconscious?
3. What happens when brainstem systems to inhibit movement during REM sleep are damaged?

PART III
Sleep Disorders

THE ROAD AHEAD

The final part of the chapter concerns disorders of sleep and wakefulness. Studying this material will enable you to:

1. Discuss narcolepsy and how study of this disorder revealed a neural system controlling sleep.
2. Describe several different sleep disorders associated with particular sleep stages or partial arousals.
3. Distinguish between different types of insomnia, and offer advice for good sleep hygiene.

Sleep Disorders Can Be Serious, Even Life-Threatening

For some people, the peace and comfort of regular, uninterrupted sleep is routinely disturbed by the inability to fall asleep, by prolonged sleep, or by unusual awakenings. Other people suffer from attacks where they cannot move, despite remaining conscious. Study of this disruptive disorder, first in dogs and then in people, revealed an important system for coordinating sleep states.

A hypothalamic sleep center was revealed by the study of narcolepsy

You might not consider getting lots of sleep an affliction, but some people are either drowsy all the time or suffer sudden attacks of sleep. At the extreme of such tendencies is **narcolepsy**, an unusual disorder in which the person is afflicted by frequent, intense attacks of sleep that last 5–30 minutes and can occur at any time during usual waking hours. These sleep attacks occur several times a day—usually about every 90 minutes (Dantz et al., 1994).

Most people display SWS for an hour or more before entering REM; individuals who suffer from narcolepsy, however, tend to enter REM in the first few minutes of sleep. People with this disorder exhibit an otherwise normal sleep pattern at night, but they suffer abrupt, overwhelming sleepiness during the day. Some people with narcolepsy also show **cataplexy**, a sudden loss of muscle tone, leading to collapse of the body *without loss of consciousness*. Cataplexy can be triggered by sudden, intense emotional stimuli, including both laughter and anger. Narcolepsy usually manifests itself between the ages of 15 and 25 years and continues throughout life. Remember Barry from the start of this chapter? His narcolepsy symptoms began in his freshman year of college, when he started showing the classic signs of excessive daytime sleepiness and partial cataplexy, like having his legs go limp while running.

narcolepsy A disorder that involves frequent, intense episodes of sleep, which last from 5 to 30 minutes and can occur anytime during the usual waking hours.

cataplexy Sudden loss of muscle tone, leading to collapse of the body without loss of consciousness. Cataplexy is sometimes a component of narcoleptic attacks.

FIGURE 10.21 Canine Narcolepsy (Courtesy of Seiji Nishino.)

To see the video
Narcoleptic Dachshund,
go to
3e.mindsmachine.com/av10.6

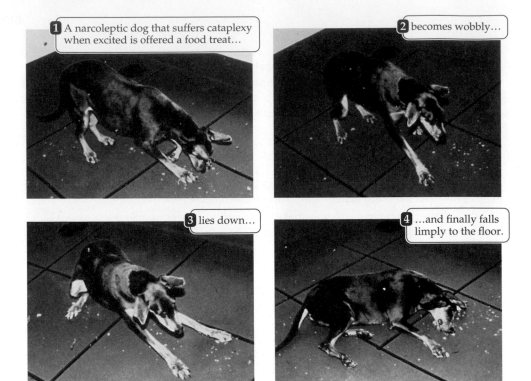

Several strains of dogs exhibit narcolepsy (Aldrich, 1993), complete with sudden collapse and very rapid sleep onset (**FIGURE 10.21**). Just like humans who suffer from narcolepsy, these dogs often show REM signs immediately upon falling asleep. Abrupt collapse in these dogs is suppressed by the same drugs (discussed shortly) that are used to treat human cataplexy.

Finding the mutant gene responsible for narcoleptic dogs revealed a hypothalamic system that is responsible for narcolepsy in people too. This was the gene for a neuropeptide called **orexin** (also known as *hypocretin*; see Chapter 9) (L. Lin et al., 1999). Mice with the *orexin* gene knocked out also display narcolepsy (Chemelli et al., 1999). Genetically normal rats can be made narcoleptic if injected with a toxin that destroys neurons possessing orexin receptors (Gerashchenko et al., 2001). The narcoleptic dogs start losing orexin neurons at about the age when symptoms of narcolepsy appear (Siegel, Nienhuis et al., 1999).

Similarly, humans with narcolepsy have lost about 90% of their orexin neurons (**FIGURE 10.22**) (Thannickal et al., 2000). This degeneration of orexin neurons seems to cause inappropriate activation of the cataplexy pathway that normally happens only during REM sleep. So, orexin normally keeps sleep at bay and prevents the transition from wakefulness directly into REM sleep.

The neurons that produce orexin are found almost exclusively in the hypothalamus. Where do these neurons send their axons to release the orexin? Not so coincidentally, the axons go to each of the three brain centers that we mentioned before: basal forebrain, reticular formation, and locus coeruleus (Sutcliffe and de Lecea, 2002). The orexin neurons also project axons to the hypothalamic tuberomammillary nucleus—the same structure that is inhibited by the basal forebrain to induce SWS. So, it looks as if the hypothalamus contains an orexin-based "switching station" (see Figure 10.19) that switches the brain between states, from wakefulness to non-REM sleep to REM sleep (Saper et al., 2010). This system normally triggers paralysis only during REM, so loss of the system in narcolepsy leads to paralysis while awake (cataplexy).

The traditional treatment for narcolepsy was the use of amphetamines in the daytime. The drug GHB (gamma-hydroxybutyrate, trade name Xyrem) helps some narcoleptics (although there are concerns about potential abuse of this drug [Tuller, 2002]). A newer drug, modafinil (Provigil), is sometimes effective for preventing narcoleptic attacks and has been proposed as an "alertness drug" for people with attention deficit hyperactivity disorder. There is also debate about whether modafinil should be

orexin Also called *hypocretin*. A neuropeptide produced in the hypothalamus that is involved in switching between sleep states, in narcolepsy, and in the control of appetite.

(A) Normal

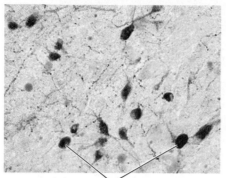

Immunocytochemistry reveals orexin containing neurons in the lateral hypothalamus of a person who did not have narcolepsy.

(B) Narcoleptic

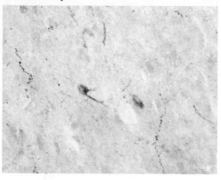

This same region of the brain from someone who suffered from narcolepsy has far fewer orexin neurons.

FIGURE 10.22 Neural Degeneration in Humans with Narcolepsy (Courtesy of Jerome Siegel.)

available to anyone who feels sleepy or needs to stay awake (Pack, 2003), but at least one study found the drug no more effective than caffeine in this regard (Wesensten et al., 2002). Our friend Barry, from the chapter opener, eventually found a combination of mild stimulants that worked for him, and he ultimately earned an MD degree. Now that narcolepsy is known to be caused by a loss of orexin signaling, there is hope of developing synthetic drugs to stimulate orexin receptors, both for the relief of symptoms in narcolepsy and to combat sleepiness in people without narcolepsy.

Many people who do not suffer from narcolepsy nevertheless occasionally experience the cataplexy that accompanies narcolepsy (Fukuda et al., 1998). **Sleep paralysis** is the temporary inability to move or talk either just before dropping off to sleep or, more often, just after waking. In this state people may experience sudden sensory hallucinations (Cheyne, 2002), including the belief that something is crushing their chest. Sleep paralysis never lasts more than a few minutes, so it's best to relax and avoid panic. One hypothesis is that sleep paralysis results when the pontine center (see Figure 10.19, step 3) continues to impose paralysis for a short while after a person awakes from a REM episode.

Some minor dysfunctions are associated with sleep

Some dysfunctions associated with sleep are much more common in children than in adults. Two sleep disorders in children—night terrors (described earlier) and **sleep enuresis** (bed-wetting)—are associated with SWS. Most people grow out of these conditions without intervention, but pharmacological approaches can be used to reduce the amount of stage 3 sleep (as well as REM time) while increasing stage 2 sleep. For sleep enuresis, some doctors prescribe a nasal spray of the hormone vasopressin (see Chapter 9) before bedtime, which decreases urine production.

Somnambulism (sleepwalking) consists of getting out of bed, walking around the room, and appearing awake. Although more common in childhood, it sometimes persists into adulthood. These episodes last a few seconds to minutes, and the person usually does not remember the experience. Because such episodes occur during stage 3 SWS, they are more common in the first half of the night when that stage predominates. Likewise, episodes of "sexsomnia," when adults have sex but afterward have no memory of it (Muza et al., 2016), happen during non-REM sleep, early in the night. Narcolepsy and other sleep disorders (**TABLE 10.2**) have made sleep disorder clinics common in major medical centers.

Some people appear to be acting out their nightmares

While most sleepwalkers are not acting out a dream, there is a disorder where people appear to be acting out a dream. **REM behavior disorder** (RBD) is characterized by organized behavior—such as fighting an imaginary foe, eating a meal, or acting like a wild animal—by a person who appears to be asleep (Schenck and Mahowald, 2002). Sometimes the person remembers a dream that fits well with his behavior (C. Brown,

sleep paralysis A state, during the transition to or from sleep, in which the ability to move or talk is temporarily lost.

sleep enuresis Bed-wetting.

somnambulism Sleepwalking.

REM behavior disorder (RBD) A sleep disorder in which a person physically acts out a dream.

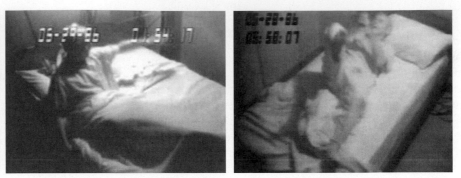

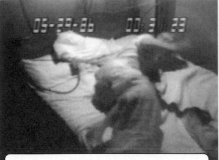

People with RBD seem to be acting out a dream, often of running away from or fighting an unseen foe.

FIGURE 10.23 Battling in Your Dreams (From M. W. Mahowald and C. H. Schenck, 2005. *Nature* 437: 1279.)

To see the video
REM Behavior Disorder,
go to
3e.mindsmachine.com/av10.7

2003), like the gentleman in the low-light video on our website (**FIGURE 10.23**). This disorder usually begins after the age of 50 and is more common in men than in women. Individuals with RBD are reminiscent of the cats with a lesion near the locus coeruleus, mentioned earlier, that were no longer paralyzed during REM and so acted out their dreams. In both cases, they no longer benefit from brainstem inhibition of motor neurons that would normally prevent them from moving. Unfortunately, the onset of RBD is often followed by symptoms of Parkinson's disease and dementia (Abbott and Videnovic, 2014), suggesting that the disorder marks the beginning of widespread neurodegeneration. The breakdown appears to begin in the brainstem region that imposes muscle atonia (see Figure 10.18) (Peever et al., 2014). RBD may be controlled by antianxiety drugs (benzodiazepines like Valium) taken at bedtime.

Insomniacs have trouble falling asleep or staying asleep

Almost all of us have trouble falling asleep on occasion, but many people persistently find it difficult to get as much sleep as they would like. Estimates of the prevalence of insomnia range from 15% to 30% of the adult population (Parkes, 1985). Insomnia is more commonly reported by older people, females, and users of drugs like tobacco, caffeine, and alcohol. It is not a trivial disorder; recall that adults who regularly sleep for short periods show a higher mortality rate than those who regularly sleep 7–8 hours each night (Kripke et al., 2002).

Insomnia seems to be the final common outcome for various conditions. Situational factors such as shift work, time zone changes, and changes in the daily routine

TABLE 10.2 ■ Classification of Sleep Disorders

DISORDERS OF INITIATING AND MAINTAINING SLEEP (INSOMNIA)	DISORDERS OF SLEEP-WAKING SCHEDULE
Ordinary, uncomplicated insomnia	Temporary disruption caused by:
Drug-related insomnia caused by:	Time zone change by airplane flight (jet lag)
Use of stimulants	Shift work, especially night work
Withdrawal of depressants	Persistent disruption (irregular rhythm)
Chronic alcoholism	DYSFUNCTIONS ASSOCIATED WITH SLEEP, SLEEP STAGES, OR PARTIAL AROUSALS
Insomnia associated with psychiatric disorders	Sleepwalking (somnambulism)
Insomnia associated with sleep-induced respiratory impairment (sleep apnea)	Sleep enuresis (bed-wetting)
DISORDERS OF EXCESSIVE DROWSINESS	Night terror
Narcolepsy	Nightmares
Drowsiness associated with psychiatric problems	Sleep-related seizures
Drug-related drowsiness	Teeth grinding
Drowsiness associated with sleep-induced respiratory impairment (sleep apnea)	REM behavior disorder (RBD)

Source: After E. D. Weitzman, 1981. *Annu. Rev. Neurosci.* 4: 381.

(that hard motel bed) can lead to insomnia. Usually these conditions produce transient **sleep-onset insomnia**, a difficulty in falling asleep. Drugs, as well as neurological and psychiatric factors, seem to cause **sleep-maintenance insomnia**, a difficulty in remaining asleep. In this type of insomnia, sleep is punctuated by frequent nighttime arousals.

People with **sleep state misperception** (Lichstein, 2017; Rezaie et al., 2018) *report* that they didn't sleep even when the EEG showed signs of sleep and they failed to respond to stimuli. They are sleeping without knowing it. Sometimes these people, upon learning that they really are sleeping, are more satisfied with the sleep they get.

In some people, respiration becomes unreliable during sleep. Breathing may cease for a minute or so, or it may slow alarmingly; blood levels of oxygen drop markedly. This syndrome, called **sleep apnea**, arises either from the progressive relaxation of muscles of the chest, diaphragm, and throat cavity or from changes in the pacemaker respiratory neurons of the brainstem. In the former instance, relaxation of the throat obstructs the airway—a kind of self-choking. This mode of sleep apnea is common in very obese people, but it also occurs, often undiagnosed, in non-obese people. Sleep apnea is frequently accompanied by loud, interrupted snoring, so loud snorers should consult a physician about the possibility that they suffer from sleep apnea.

Investigators have speculated that **sudden infant death syndrome** (**SIDS**, or *crib death*) arises from sleep apnea as a result of immature systems that normally control respiration. Autopsies of SIDS victims reveal abnormalities in brainstem serotonin systems (Kinney, 2009); interfering with this system in mice renders them unable to regulate respiration effectively (Audero et al., 2008). The incidence of SIDS has been cut almost in half by the Safe to Sleep campaign, which urges parents to place infants on their backs to sleep rather than on their stomachs. Placing the baby face down may lead to suffocation if the baby cannot regulate breathing or arouse properly. Exposure to cigarette smoke also increases the risk of crib death.

Although many drugs affect sleep, there is no perfect sleeping pill

Throughout recorded history, humans have reached for substances to enhance sleep. Ancient Greeks used opium from the juice of the poppy, as well as products of the mandrake plant, to aid sleep (Hartmann, 1978). The preparation of barbituric acid in the mid-nineteenth century started the development of many drugs—*barbiturates*—that were widely used to combat insomnia.

Most modern sleeping pills—including benzodiazepines (see Chapter 4) like triazolam (Halcion), and nonbenzodiazepine sedatives like zolpidem (Ambien) and eszopiclone (Lunesta)—bind to GABA receptors, inhibiting broad regions of the brain. But reliance on sleeping pills poses many problems (Rothschild, 1992). Viewed solely as a way to deal with sleep problems, current drugs fall far short of being a suitable remedy, for several reasons. First, even the newest class of sleeping pills produce little more sleep than placebos (Huedo-Medina et al., 2012). Second, continued use of sleeping pills causes them to lose effectiveness (Walker, 2017), and this declining ability to induce sleep often leads to increased self-prescribed dosages that can be dangerous. Another major drawback is that sleeping pills produce marked changes in the pattern of sleep, both while the drug is being used and for days afterward.

Use of sleeping pills may lead to a persistent "sleep drunkenness," coupled with drowsiness, that impairs waking activity or to memory gaps about daily activity. Police have reported cases of "Ambien drivers," people who have taken a sleeping pill and then got up a few hours later to go for a spin, with sometimes disastrous results, while apparently asleep (Saul, 2006). In other cases, people taking such medicines eat snacks, shop over the internet, or even have sex, with no memory of these events the next day (Dolder and Nelson, 2008).

Everyone should practice good sleep hygiene

Certainly, the treatment for insomnia that has the fewest side effects, and that is very effective for most people, is not to use any drug, but to practice good sleep hygiene. One strategy is to develop a regular routine to exploit the body's circadian clock. The best

sleep-onset insomnia Difficulty in falling asleep.

sleep-maintenance insomnia Difficulty in staying asleep.

sleep state misperception Commonly, a person's perception that he has not been asleep when in fact he has. It typically occurs at the start of a sleep episode.

sleep apnea A sleep disorder in which respiration slows or stops periodically, waking the patient. Excessive daytime sleepiness results from the frequent nocturnal awakening.

sudden infant death syndrome (SIDS) Also called *crib death*. The sudden, unexpected death of an apparently healthy human infant who simply stops breathing, usually during sleep.

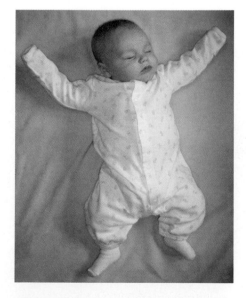

Back to Sleep Placing infants on their backs for sleep reduces the risk of sudden infant death syndrome (SIDS) by half. (Courtesy of Joanne Delphia.)

TABLE 10.3 ■ Some Simple Tips to Promote Sleep Hygiene

Keep your internal clock set with a consistent sleep schedule (get up at the same time each day).

Seek sunlight in the daytime, avoid lights at night.

Turn your bedroom into a sleep-inducing environment.

Avoid caffeine, alcohol, and nicotine before bedtime.

Establish a soothing presleep routine.

Only go to sleep when you're truly tired.

If you're going to nap, do it early in the day.

Lighten up on evening meals.

Balance fluid intake to avoid night trips to the bathroom.

Avoid using computer screens before bedtime.

Don't exercise late in the day.

Source: Healthy Sleep, http://healthysleep.med.harvard.edu/healthy/getting/overcoming/tips

advice for insomniacs is to use an alarm clock to wake up faithfully at the same time each day (weekends included) and then simply go to bed *once they feel sleepy* (Webb, 1992). They should also avoid daytime naps and having caffeine at night. Going through a bedtime routine in a quiet, dark environment can also help to condition sleep onset. Melanopsin, the retinal photopigment that tells the SCN about light and dark, is especially sensitive to bluish light (Gooley et al., 2010), such as the light that comes from LCD screens. So avoiding the use of smart phones and laptops at bedtime (or at least dimming their light) can thus improve sleep (Bedrosian et al., 2013). These steps will let you get the sleep you need (**TABLE 10.3**), and sleeping pills will not (no matter what the millions of dollars in annual pharmaceutical advertising might say).

Unfortunately, many college students adopt schedules that virtually guarantee they won't get enough sleep. Waking up early on Monday and Wednesday to attend one class, sleeping a bit later on Tuesday and Thursday, and then sleeping a *lot* later on weekends disrupts your circadian sleep cycle, making it hard to fall asleep when you should on the nights before an early class. It's unpopular advice, but if you want enough sleep, get up at the same time *every* day, not just the days you have that early class, and go to bed about the same time each night. True, you'll miss out on some late night activities with your friends, but you'll get to feel so self-righteous being awake and working while they are sleeping in. Plus you'll stay awake in lectures (we hope).

HOW'S IT GOING ❓

1. What is narcolepsy, and what brain system seem to be responsible for this disorder?
2. During what stage of sleep does sleepwalking tend to happen? During what time of night?
3. What are the different types of insomnia, and why are sleeping pills an imperfect long-term solution?
4. Describe REM behavior disorder.

Recommended Reading

Aserinsky, E., and Kleitman, N. (1955). "Regularly Occurring Periods of Eye Motility, and Concomitant Phenomena, during Sleep." *Science*, 118, pp. 273–274.

Dunlap, J. C., Loros, J. J., and DeCoursey, P. J. (2004). *Chronobiology: Biological Timekeeping*. Sunderland, MA: Oxford University Press/Sinauer.

Kryger, M. K., Roth, T., and Dement, W. C. (Eds.). (2016). *Principles and Practice of Sleep Medicine* (6th ed.). Philadelphia, PA: Saunders/Elsevier.

Max, D. T. (2007). *The Family That Couldn't Sleep: A Medical Mystery*. New York, NY: Random House.

Mendelson, W. B. (2017). *The Science of Sleep: What It Is, How It Works, and Why It Matters*. Chicago, IL: University of Chicago Press.

Walker, M. (2017). *Why We Sleep: Unlocking the Power of Sleep and Dreams*. New York, NY: Scribner.

You should be able to relate each summary to the adjacent illustration, including structures and processes. If you go to the website for our text (**3e.mindsmachine.com**), you can follow links to figures, animations, and activities that will help you consolidate the material.

1 Animals show **circadian rhythms** of activity that can be **entrained** by light. These rhythms synchronize behavior to changes in the environment. In constant dim light, animals **free-run**, displaying a period of about 24 hours. Review **Figures 10.2** and **10.6**, **Animations 10.2** and **10.3**

2 Lesions of the **suprachiasmatic nucleus (SCN)** abolish activity rhythms in constant conditions. Transplanting the SCN from one animal into another results in a free-running rhythm of the donor, demonstrating that the SCN contains a clock that can drive circadian activity. Several proteins (including Clock and Cycle) interact, increasing and decreasing in a cyclic fashion that takes about 24 hours. This molecular clock, pooled from many SCN neurons, drives circadian rhythms. Review **Figures 10.3–10.8**, **Animation 10.4**

3 Almost all mammals show two sleep states: **rapid-eye-movement (REM)** sleep and **non-REM sleep**. Human non-REM sleep has three distinct stages—**stages 1, 2, 3**—defined by **electroencephalography (EEG)** criteria, including **sleep spindles** and large, slow **delta waves** in stage 3. Review **Figure 10.10**, **Table 10.1**, **Activity 10.1**

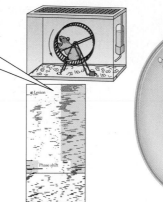
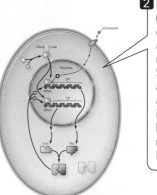

4 REM sleep is characterized by rapid, low-amplitude EEG waves (almost like an EEG while awake) but also by profound muscle relaxation because motor neurons are inhibited. People awakened from REM frequently report vivid dreams, while people awakened from SWS report ideas or thinking. Review **Table 10.1**

5 Sleep stages cycle through the night, with stage 3 SWS prominent early, while REM predominates later. Infants sleep a lot, with lots of REM, but as we grow up we sleep less, with less REM. Elderly people sleep even less, and stage 3 sleep eventually disappears. Review **Figures 10.11–10.15**

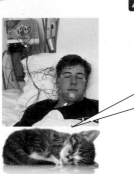

6 Four proposed functions of sleep are energy conservation, **ecological niche** adaptation, body and brain restoration, and memory consolidation. A few people sleep only an hour per night, suggesting that they accomplish the function(s) of sleep very efficiently, but all healthy people sleep.

7 **Sleep deprivation** leads to impairments in vigilance and reaction times. It also incurs sleep debt, although the lost SWS and REM may be partially restored in subsequent nights. Prolonged sleep deprivation compromises the immune system and leads to death. Review **Figure 10.16**

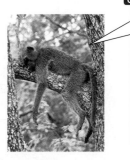

8 Four brain systems control sleep and waking. The **basal forebrain** promotes SWS, the brainstem **reticular formation** promotes arousal, a pontine system triggers REM sleep, and hypothalamic neurons releasing **orexin** regulate these three centers. Review **Figures 10.18–10.20**, **Activity 10.2**, **Video 10.5**

9 **Narcolepsy** is characterized by sudden, uncontrollable periods of sleep, which may be accompanied by **cataplexy**, paralysis while remaining conscious. Disruption of orexin signaling causes narcolepsy. Review **Figures 10.21** and **10.22**, **Video 10.6**

10 Sleep disorders fall into four categories: **sleep-onset** and **sleep-maintenance insomnia**; excessive drowsiness (e.g., narcolepsy); disruption of the sleep-waking schedule; and dysfunctions associated with sleep, sleep stages, or partial arousals (e.g., **somnambulism, RBD**). No pill guarantees a normal night's sleep. Review **Figure 10.23**, **Table 10.2**, **Video 10.7**

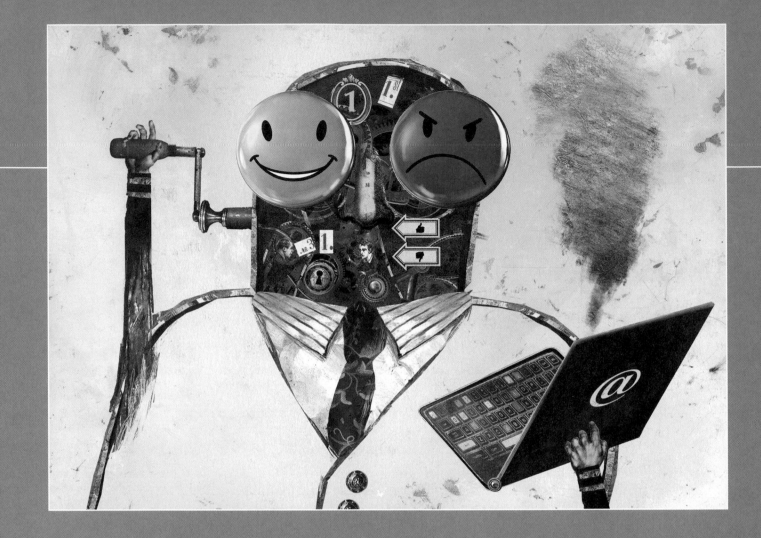

11
Emotions, Aggression, and Stress

The Hazards of Fearlessness

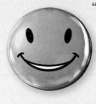

"Fear has its use, but cowardice has none," wrote the Mahatma Gandhi. But wouldn't it be great to never feel fear at all? When we say that heroes are "fearless," what we really mean is that they manage to function effectively despite the fear they experience, not that they never feel afraid. However, there are people who literally do not experience fear. One such woman, known as S.M. in the scientific literature, lost her ability to feel fear in late childhood because of a genetic disorder so rare, fewer than 300 cases have been reported (Feinstein et al., 2011).

In Chapter 8 we saw how the absence of an unpleasant experience, pain, can be hazardous to your health. S.M. similarly shows us the survival value of fear. Not only is she unafraid of snakes or spiders, but she once walked right up to a knife-wielding robber and basically dared him to stab her. He was so disquieted by her strange response that he ran away! Another time she was nearly killed in an act of domestic violence. While her behavioral responses and self-report appear typical for other emotions, S.M. shows very little of the physiological response, organized by the sympathetic nervous system, that the rest of us experience in frightening situations. Similarly, S.M. produces almost no startle response to a sudden, loud noise (Aschwanden, 2013).

S.M. is not deliberately reckless; she has learned to follow simple safety rules like looking both ways before crossing the street. But there are other consequences of S.M.'s fearlessness that you might not predict. When talking to someone, she tends to get much closer than other people do, sometimes just a foot away (Kennedy et al., 2009), suggesting she has a distorted sense of personal space. When strangers talk to her in public, like the mugger she encountered, she tends to stroll right up to them. S.M. also fails to perceive risk in more mundane social situations, so she's an easy target for internet scams. Although she's very outgoing and might fondly address a waiter she's only met once before, she has few long-term friendships, perhaps because she speaks without fear. Maybe being fearless isn't all it's cracked up to be.

What happened to S.M. to make her this way, and is there really nothing she is afraid of?

The sound of unexpected footsteps in the eerie quiet of the night brings fear to many of us. But the sound of music we enjoy and the voice of someone we love summon feelings of comfort or happiness. For some of us, feelings and emotions can become vastly exaggerated; fears, for example, may become paralyzing attacks of anxiety, or even panic. No story about human behavior is complete without considering these powerful feelings.

To see the video
The Case of S.M.,
go to
3e.mindsmachine.com/av11.1

emotion A subjective mental state that is usually accompanied by distinctive behaviors as well as involuntary physiological changes.

sympathetic nervous system The part of the autonomic nervous system that acts as the fight-or-flight system, generally preparing the body for action.

parasympathetic nervous system The part of the autonomic nervous system that generally prepares the body to relax and recuperate.

To view the
Brain Explorer,
go to
3e.mindsmachine.com/av11.2

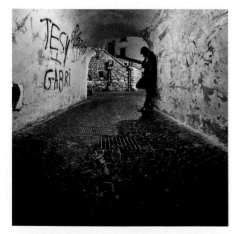

Fear and Loathing Can Save You
Strong emotions, like fear in unfamiliar and threatening circumstances, are evolved adaptations that swiftly activate behavioral and physiological responses appropriate to the situation. (© istock.com/zodebala.)

Our chapter begins with emotions, the bodily responses and brain mechanisms underlying happiness and joy, fear and loathing. We'll discuss both the development of emotions in individuals and how emotions evolved to help guide our reactions to the world around us. Part I's examination of brain mechanisms related to emotional states emphasizes fear and aggression because both are important for survival and they are readily studied in animals. That discussion will lead us to Part II, where we consider aggression. Part III rounds out our discussion by turning to the neural origins of stress and its impact on health.

PART I
Emotional Processing

THE ROAD AHEAD

In the first part of the chapter we survey the behavioral neuroscience of emotion. We'll start by looking at theoretical accounts of the perception of emotions, and then we'll discuss the display of emotion via facial expressions, before turning to neural mechanisms of emotion. After reading this section you should be able to:

1. Describe and compare the dominant accounts of emotion, considering the integration of autonomic responses with the perception of specific emotions.
2. Review the evidence for a core set of emotions as well as their role in guiding preprogrammed responses to environmental challenges.
3. Discuss the role of facial expressions of emotion and the ways in which cultural differences influence facial displays.
4. Sketch and describe the major brain mechanisms involved in emotional behaviors, noting the behavioral manifestations of activity in the major pathways.
5. Describe the process of fear conditioning, the neural mechanisms responsible for fear reactions, and the role of this system in pathological states.

Broad Theories of Emotion Emphasize Bodily Responses

The topic of emotions is complicated by the fact that we apply the word emotion to several different things. Emotion is a private, subjective feeling that we may have without anyone else being aware of it. But the word emotional is also used to describe many behaviors that people show, such as fearful facial expressions, frantic arm movements, or angry shouting. Furthermore, during strong emotion we often experience physiological changes, such as a rapidly beating heart, shortness of breath, or excessive sweating. To encompass all three of these aspects, we will define **emotion** as a subjective mental state that is usually accompanied by distinctive behaviors as well as involuntary physiological changes.

In many emotional states the heart races, the hands and face become warm, the palms sweat, and the stomach feels queasy. Common expressions capture this emotional-physical association: "my hair stood on end," "a sinking feeling in my stomach." These sensations are the result of activation of the autonomic nervous system—either the **sympathetic nervous system** (the "fight-or-flight" system that generally activates the body for action) or the **parasympathetic nervous system** (which generally prepares the body to relax and recuperate) (see Figure 2.9).

Several theories have tried to explain the close ties between the subjective feelings of emotions and the activity of the autonomic nervous system. Folk wisdom suggests that the autonomic reactions are caused by the emotion—"I was so angry, my hands were shaking"—as though the anger produces the shaking (**FIGURE 11.1A**). Yet research indicates that the relationship between emotion and physiological arousal is more subtle.

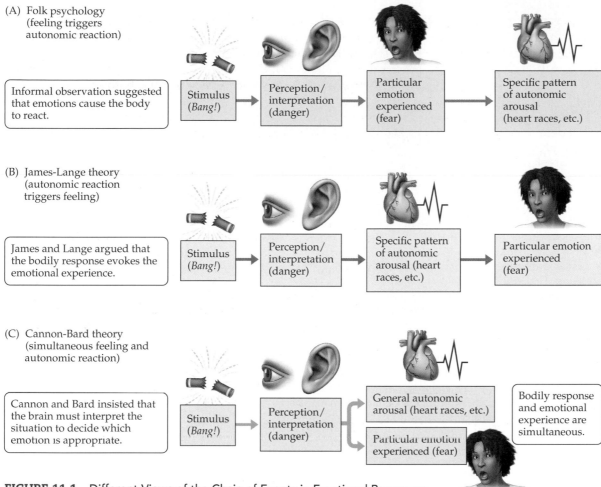

(A) Folk psychology (feeling triggers autonomic reaction)

Informal observation suggested that emotions cause the body to react.

Stimulus (*Bang!*) → Perception/interpretation (danger) → Particular emotion experienced (fear) → Specific pattern of autonomic arousal (heart races, etc.)

(B) James-Lange theory (autonomic reaction triggers feeling)

James and Lange argued that the bodily response evokes the emotional experience.

Stimulus (*Bang!*) → Perception/interpretation (danger) → Specific pattern of autonomic arousal (heart races, etc.) → Particular emotion experienced (fear)

(C) Cannon-Bard theory (simultaneous feeling and autonomic reaction)

Cannon and Bard insisted that the brain must interpret the situation to decide which emotion is appropriate.

Stimulus (*Bang!*) → Perception/interpretation (danger) → General autonomic arousal (heart races, etc.) / Particular emotion experienced (fear) → Bodily response and emotional experience are simultaneous.

FIGURE 11.1 Different Views of the Chain of Events in Emotional Responses

Do emotions cause bodily changes, or vice versa?

William James (1842–1910) and Carl Lange (1834–1900) turned the folk notion on its head, suggesting that the emotions we experience are caused by the bodily changes. From this perspective, we experience fear because we perceive the activity that dangerous conditions trigger in our body (**FIGURE 11.1B**). Different emotions thus feel different because they are generated by different constellations of physiological responses.

The James-Lange theory inspired many attempts to link specific emotions to specific bodily responses. These attempts mostly failed because it turns out that there is no distinctive autonomic pattern for each emotion. Fear, surprise, and anger, for example, tend to be accompanied by sympathetic activation, while parasympathetic activation tends to accompany both joy and sadness.

In addition, the physiological reactions are rather slow, as physiologists Walter Cannon (1871–1945) and Philip Bard (1898–1977) pointed out (Cannon, 1929). In Cannon and Bard's view, it is the brain's job to decide which particular emotion is an appropriate response to the stimuli. According to this model, the cerebral cortex simultaneously decides on the appropriate emotional experience (fear, surprise, joy) and activates the autonomic nervous system to appropriately prepare the body, using either the parasympathetic system to help the body rest, or the sympathetic system to ready the body for action (**FIGURE 11.1C**). It is because the sympathetic system is activated by any threatening situation that so-called lie detectors are very poor at distinguishing liars from truthful people who are anxious (**BOX 11.1**).

BOX 11.1
Lie Detector?

One of the most controversial attempts to apply biomedical science in legal settings is the so-called lie detector test. In this procedure, properly called a **polygraph** test (from the Greek polys, "many," and graphein, "to write"), multiple physiological measures are recorded in an attempt to detect lying during a carefully structured interview. The test is based on the assumption that people have emotional responses when lying because they fear detection and/or feel guilty about lying. Emotions are usually accompanied by bodily responses that are difficult to control, such as changes in respiratory rate, heart rate, blood pressure, and skin conductance (a measure of sweating). In polygraph recordings like the one in **FIGURE A**, each wiggly line, or trace, provides a measurement of one of these physiological variables. Taken together, the measurements are assumed to track the physiological arousal, over time, of the person being tested. When a person lies in response to a direct question (arrows), momentary changes in several of the measured variables may occur.

People who administer polygraph examinations for a living claim that polygraphs are accurate in 85–95% of tests, but the estimate from impartial research is an overall accuracy of about 65% (Nietzel, 2000; Gougler et al., 2011). Even if the higher figure were correct, the fact that these tests are widely used would mean that thousands of truthful people could be branded as liars and fired, disciplined, or not hired. On the other hand, many criminals and spies have been able to pass the tests without detection (Wollan, 2015). For example, longtime CIA agent Aldrich Ames, who was sentenced in 1995 to life in prison for espionage, successfully passed polygraph tests after becoming a spy; former operators have even offered how-to guides to beating polygraph tests (www.polygraph.com). In the wake of the terrorist attacks of

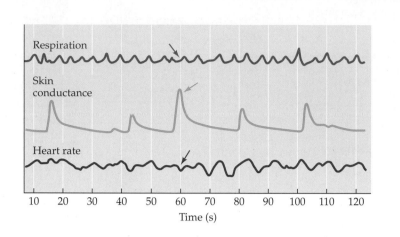

(A) **Are You Lying?** The polygraph measures signs of arousal.

2001, a federally appointed panel of scientists noted that even if polygraphs were correct 80% of the time (which is much higher than impartial research suggests), then giving the test to a group of 10,000 people that included 10 spies would condemn 1,600 innocent people—and let 2 spies go free (National Academy of Sciences, 2003)!

Some scientists believe that modern neuroscience may provide new methods of lie detection someday. Conscious lying may trigger unusual activation of executive control mechanisms of the prefrontal cortex (**FIGURE B**) (Abe et al., 2007). Fear results in activation of the amygdala (as we'll discuss later in this chapter) that, in the case of deception, also might be visible with fMRI (see Chapter 2). Functional MRI

shows that the anterior cingulate cortex (another region associated with executive control) becomes more active when study participants are lying (Langleben et al., 2002). Although such initial results from brain-imaging studies of deception are intriguing, much more work will be required to establish that brain imaging can detect lies with enough reliability to be useful in making important decisions about individual people. And of course, even if they are validated, such lie detectors will be more costly and less widely available than polygraphs.

polygraph Popularly but inaccurately referred to as a *lie detector*. A device that measures several bodily responses, such as heart rate and blood pressure.

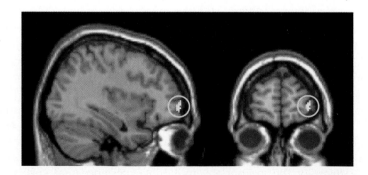

(B) **Your Cheatin' Brain** PET images reveal selective activation (relative to a control scan) of prefrontal cortex in a study participant engaged in lying. (From N. Abe et al., 2007. *J. Cogn. Neurosci.* 19: 287, courtesy of Nobuhito Abe.)

Stanley Schachter proposed a cognitive interpretation of stimuli and visceral states

Like Cannon and Bard, Stanley Schachter (1975) emphasized cognitive mechanisms in emotion. Under Schachter's model, however, emotional labels (e.g., anger, fear, joy) are attributed to relatively nonspecific feelings of physiological arousal. Which emotion we experience depends on cognitive systems that assess the context—our current social, physical, and psychological situation.

In a famous test of this idea, participants were injected with epinephrine (adrenaline) and told either that there would be no effect or that their hearts would race (Schachter and Singer, 1962).

Participants who were warned of the reaction reported no emotional experience, but some participants who were not forewarned experienced emotions when their bodies responded to the drug.

However, which emotion was experienced could be affected by whether a confederate in the room acted angry or happy. The unsuspecting participants injected with epinephrine were much more likely to report feeling angry when in the presence of an "angry" confederate, and more likely to report feeling elated when with a "happy" confederate (**FIGURE 11.2A**).

FIGURE 11.2 The Classic Schachter and Singer Experiment

■ **Hypothesis**
Circumstances provoke autonomic arousal; we then attribute arousal to a particular emotion on the basis of context.

■ **Test**
Activate the sympathetic nervous system with an injection of epinephrine to see whether the participants, uninformed about the drug's effects, experience one particular emotion as they fill out some forms. To test the hypothesis that our emotional experience is determined by cognitive processes, expose the participants to a confederate who acts either angry or happy while filling out the forms.

(A)

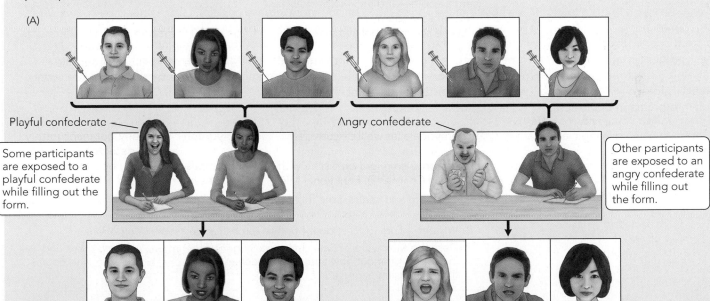

Playful confederate — Angry confederate

Some participants are exposed to a playful confederate while filling out the form.

Other participants are exposed to an angry confederate while filling out the form.

These participants were more likely to report feeling elated.

These participants were more likely to report feeling angry and frustrated.

■ **Result**
Participants who were warned that the injection might affect heart rate reported no emotional reaction. Participants who were not warned about the sympathetic arousal reported more intense emotional reactions than those who were given a control injection. However, among the participants who were not warned about the effects of the injection, *which* emotion they experienced (angry or happy) tended to match that of the confederate.

(Continued)

RESEARCHERS AT WORK (continued)

■ **Conclusion**

While autonomic responses can *intensify* our emotional experience, they cannot explain why we have different emotional experiences in different situations. Rather, our cognitive analysis of the environment affects which emotion we experience.

(B) Schachter's cognitive theory

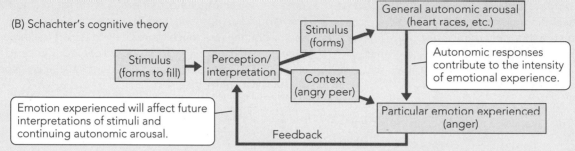

These findings contradict the James-Lange prediction that feelings of anger or elation should each be associated with a unique profile of autonomic reactions. Schachter and Singer concluded that the participants experienced their epinephrine-induced physiological arousal as whichever emotion seemed appropriate, based on their cognitive assessment of the situation: "My heart's really pounding; I'm so angry!" or "My heart's really pounding; I'm so elated!" depending on the environment. Thus, they said, our emotional states are the results of interaction between physiological arousal and cognitive interpretation of that arousal. This cognitive theory of emotions emphasizes that our interpretation of the context, including social factors

such as other people's emotions, determines which emotion we'll experience. The cognitive theory also suggests that our emotional experience at one time may affect how we interpret later events (**FIGURE 11.2B**).

Another interesting outcome of the experiment is that the participants receiving epinephrine reported experiencing more intense emotions than other participants who were given saline, as would be predicted by the James-Lange theory. The autonomic responses do not specify which emotion is being experienced, but our awareness of the body's autonomic responses intensifies our experience of emotion (G. W. Hohmann, 1966).

HOW'S IT GOING ?

1. Compare and contrast the folk psychology view of bodily responses to emotions with the James-Lange theory.
2. What two findings cast doubt on the James-Lange theory of emotions?
3. Describe the results of Schachter and Singer's experiment. What do these findings suggest about how autonomic reactions, emotional experience, and cognitive processing are related?

Is There a Core Set of Emotions?

Just as the colors of the spectrum combine into subtle hues, researchers think there may be a core set of basic emotions underlying the more varied and delicate nuances of our world of feelings. In his book The Expression of the Emotions in Man and Animals (1872), Charles Darwin presented evidence that certain expressions of emotions are universal among people of all regions of the world. Furthermore, Darwin argued that some nonhuman animals show some comparable expressions, suggesting that aspects of emotional expression may have originated in a common ancestor. He noted that nonhuman primates have the same facial muscles that humans have, and a century later, Redican (1982) noted distinct facial expressions in nonhuman primates that appeared to signal emotional states; for example, chimpanzees show a play face, which

(A)

(B)

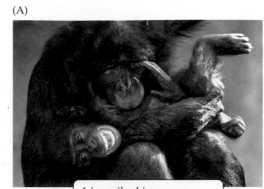

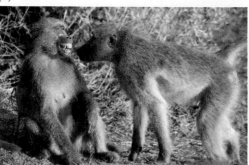

A juvenile chimpanzee shows a play face while being tickled. He also makes a guttural laughing sound.

The female chacma baboon on the left bares her teeth, grinning to signal submission to a dominant animal. In humans, teeth baring has gained a different, friendlier meaning.

FIGURE 11.3 Facial Expression of Emotions in Nonhuman Primates (*Left* © blickwinkel/Alamy Stock Photo; *right* © Nic van Oudtshoorn/Alamy Stock Photo.)

may be homologous to the human laugh (**FIGURE 11.3**). This connection may even extend beyond primates: for example, tickling and playing with rats can elicit ultrasonic vocalizations that may be analogous to laughter. Expression of positive emotions of this sort may facilitate social contact and learning in a variety of species (Panksepp, 2007; Burgdorf et al., 2008).

So, why did emotions and their expression evolve, and how do they help individuals survive and reproduce? Most of us have experienced the frightening nighttime perception of being stalked by a predator—real or imagined, human or nonhuman. Through natural selection, a program for dealing with this situation evolved: we call that program fear. The emotion of fear shifts our perception, attention, cognition, and action to focus on avoiding danger and seeking safety, while preparing us physiologically for fighting or fleeing. Other activities, such as seeking food, sleep, or mates, are suppressed. In the face of an imminent threat to survival, it is better to be afraid, thereby activating a recipe for action that was developed and tested over the ages, than to ad-lib something new.

Viewed in this way, emotions can be seen as evolved preprogramming that helps us deal quickly and effectively with a wide variety of situations. As another example, feelings of disgust for body fluids may help us avoid exposure to germs (Curtis et al., 2004), so it may be wise to recognize disgust in others. Our unfortunate tendency to make snap judgments about other people, based on their appearance and facial expressions, may be an overgeneralization of mechanisms that evolved to help us recognize signs of threat or danger from others (Todorov et al., 2008).

One formulation (Plutchik, 1994) proposes there are eight basic emotions, grouped in four pairs of opposites—joy/sadness, affection/disgust, anger/fear, and expectation/surprise—with all other emotions arising from combinations of this basic array (**FIGURE 11.4**). But researchers do not yet agree about the number of basic emotions (six, seven, eight?). While there may be no way to determine once and for all the number of basic emotions, one clue comes from examining the number of different kinds of facial expressions that we produce and can recognize in others.

FIGURE 11.4 One Classification of Basic Emotions (After R. Plutchik, 1994. *The psychology and biology of emotion.* HarperCollins. New York, NY.)

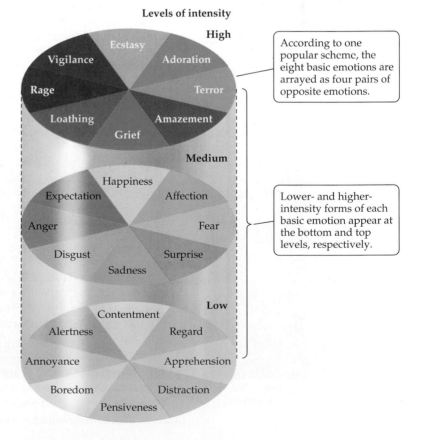

Levels of intensity

High

Medium

Low

According to one popular scheme, the eight basic emotions are arrayed as four pairs of opposite emotions.

Lower- and higher-intensity forms of each basic emotion appear at the bottom and top levels, respectively.

According to Paul Ekman and colleagues, the basic emotional facial expressions shown here are displayed in all cultures.

Anger 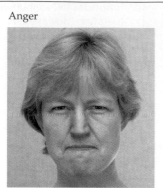 Sadness 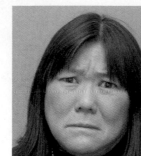 Happiness 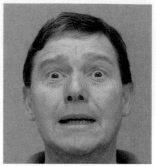 Fear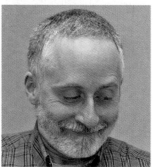

Disgust 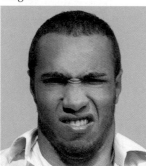 Surprise 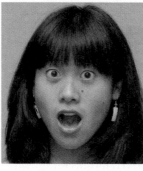 Contempt 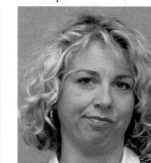 Embarrassment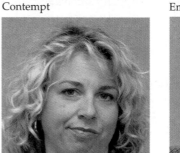

FIGURE 11.5 The Eight Universal Facial Expressions of Emotion ("Happiness" photo © istock.com/ UberImages; "Disgust" photo © Volodymyr Melnyk/Alamy Stock Photo; others © Sinauer Associates.)

Facial expressions have complex functions in communication

How many different emotions can be detected in facial expressions? According to Paul Ekman and collaborators, there are distinctive expressions for anger, sadness, happiness, fear, disgust, surprise, contempt, and embarrassment (**FIGURE 11.5**) (Keltner and Ekman, 2000). Facial expressions of these emotions are interpreted similarly across many cultures without explicit training. (In case you're keeping track, whereas Plutchik included

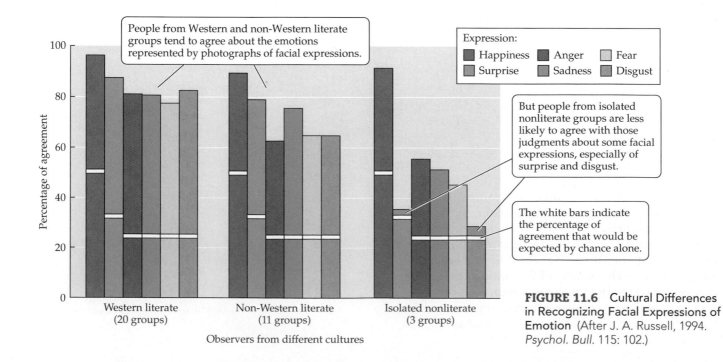

FIGURE 11.6 Cultural Differences in Recognizing Facial Expressions of Emotion (After J. A. Russell, 1994. *Psychol. Bull.* 115: 102.)

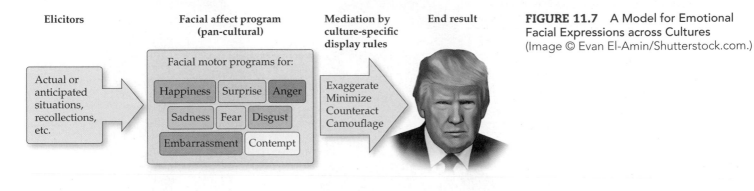

Elicitors   Facial affect program (pan-cultural)   Mediation by culture-specific display rules   End result

Actual or anticipated situations, recollections, etc.

Facial motor programs for:
Happiness | Surprise | Anger
Sadness | Fear | Disgust
Embarrassment | Contempt

Exaggerate
Minimize
Counteract
Camouflage

FIGURE 11.7   A Model for Emotional Facial Expressions across Cultures (Image © Evan El-Amin/Shutterstock.com.)

affection and expectation in his eight basic emotions, Keltner and Ekman include, instead, facial expressions of contempt and embarrassment. The other six emotions—anger, sadness, happiness, fear, disgust, and surprise—are recognized in both schemes.)

Cross-cultural similarity is also noted in the production of expressions specific to particular emotions. For example, people in a preliterate New Guinea society show emotional facial expressions like those of people in industrialized societies. However, facial expressions are not unfailingly universal. Although some degree of agreement is generally evident across cultures, researchers have repeatedly found isolated groups whose identifications of the emotions from facial expressions did not fully agree with those of Westerners, such as those for surprise and disgust (**FIGURE 11.6**), suggesting that different cultures have adopted different ways to express some of the emotions (Russell 1994; Crivelli et al., 2016).

These subtle cultural differences suggest that cultures prescribe rules for facial expression and that they control and enforce those rules by cultural conditioning. Everyone agrees that cultures affect the facial display of emotion; the remaining controversy is over the extent of that cultural influence (**FIGURE 11.7**).

Facial expressions are mediated by muscles, cranial nerves, and CNS pathways

The human face is a complicated object, a network of small muscles that are carefully controlled by the nervous system. We use subsets of those muscles to produce nuanced facial expressions, from grimace to grin, alongside less subtle facial behaviors, like eating and speaking. Facial muscles can be divided into two categories:

1. *Superficial facial muscles* mostly attach only between different points of facial skin (**FIGURE 11.8**), so when they contract, they change the shape of the mouth, eyes, or nose or maybe create a dimple.

2. *Deep facial muscles* attach to bone and produce larger-scale movements, like chewing.

These facial muscles are innervated by two cranial nerves: (1) the facial nerve (VII), which innervates the superficial muscles of facial expression; and (2) the motor branch of the trigeminal nerve (V), which innervates muscles that move the jaw (see Figure 2.7). The activity of the cranial nerves is governed by the face area of motor cortex: a disproportionately large brain region in humans (see Figure 5.10), probably reflecting the importance of emotional expression in our species.

FIGURE 11.8   Superficial Facial Muscles and Their Neural Control

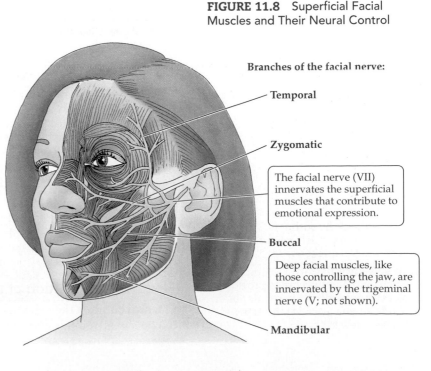

Branches of the facial nerve:

Temporal

Zygomatic

The facial nerve (VII) innervates the superficial muscles that contribute to emotional expression.

Buccal

Deep facial muscles, like those controlling the jaw, are innervated by the trigeminal nerve (V; not shown).

Mandibular

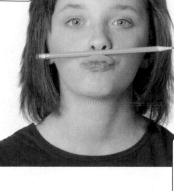

Several studies indicate that when people are manipulated into mimicking facial expressions of sadness...

...or happiness, their emotional mood is actually affected.

So putting on a happy, cheerful expression may actually help you to feel better.

FIGURE 11.9 Facial Feedback Hypothesis (*Left* photo © Richard Green/Commercial/Alamy; *right* photo courtesy of Jennifer Basil-Whitaker.)

Lending support to the James-Lange notion that sensations from our body inform us about our emotions, the **facial feedback hypothesis** suggests that sensory feedback from our facial expressions can affect our mood. In the best tests of this idea, people are given a task, such as holding a pencil either under their nose or between their teeth (**FIGURE 11.9**), that effectively has them take on a sad or happy face, respectively. The participants are then probed to see how happy or sad they feel, or how funny they find a cartoon. People who have been simulating a smile reportedly experience more positive feelings than the folks who have been simulating a frown (Davis et al., 2009). There is controversy about the strength and reliability of this finding (Wagenmakers et al., 2016), but if it turns out to be true that forcing yourself to smile may actually help you feel happier, then the old song that tells us to "just put on a happy face" may be sound advice. People who can't put on a convincing happy face, because they've received Botox injections that paralyzed their facial muscles to reduce wrinkles, reportedly experience emotions less intensely after the treatment than before (Davis et al., 2010). Being forced to display false emotional expressions in stressful situations, however, may have negative consequences for well-being and job happiness (Hülsheger and Schewe, 2011).

HOW'S IT GOING ?

1. List some examples of particular facial expressions that are associated with particular emotions.
2. What is the evidence that emotions, and the facial expressions that accompany them, evolved by natural selection?
3. What evidence suggests that facial expressions of emotional state are inherited rather than taught by culture?
4. Describe the facial feedback hypothesis of emotion, and give an example of an experiment supporting this hypothesis.

Do Distinct Brain Circuits Mediate Different Emotions?

The question of whether different emotions have their own distinct neural mechanisms has been studied using either brain lesions or electrical stimulation. The evidence confirms not only that some brain regions do specialize in emotions, but also that the same regions may be involved in multiple emotions.

Electrical stimulation of the brain can produce emotional effects

One way to study the neuroanatomy of emotion is to electrically stimulate brain sites in conscious animals and then observe the effects on behavior. Classic work in the

facial feedback hypothesis The idea that sensory feedback from our facial expressions can affect our mood.

brain self-stimulation The process in which animals will work to provide electrical stimulation to particular brain sites, presumably because the experience is very rewarding.

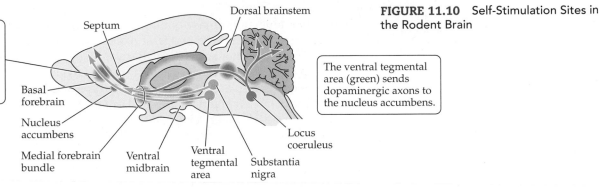

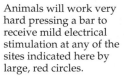

Animals will work very hard pressing a bar to receive mild electrical stimulation at any of the sites indicated here by large, red circles.

The ventral tegmental area (green) sends dopaminergic axons to the nucleus accumbens.

FIGURE 11.10   Self-Stimulation Sites in the Rodent Brain

1950s produced an intriguing finding: rats will enthusiastically press a lever in order to give themselves brief electrical stimulation in a brain region called the septum (**FIGURE 11.10**) (Olds and Milner, 1954). This phenomenon, called **brain self-stimulation**, can also happen in humans. Patients receiving electrical stimulation in the septum feel a sense of pleasure or warmth, or sometimes sexual excitement (Heath, 1972).

A rush of experimentation soon mapped brain sites that support self-stimulation responses. Almost all of these sites are subcortical and are especially concentrated in a large axon tract that ascends from the midbrain through the hypothalamus: the **medial forebrain bundle**. An important destination for the axons of the median forebrain bundle is the **nucleus accumbens**, a major component of the brain's reward circuitry (see Figure 11.10 and Chapter 4). The release of dopamine into the nucleus accumbens appears to produce very pleasurable feelings.

One theory is that the electrical stimulation taps into dopaminergic circuits that are normally activated by behaviors that produce pleasurable feelings, such as feeding or sexual activity (White and Milner, 1992). As we discussed in Chapter 4, researchers have proposed that drugs of abuse are addictive because they activate these same neural circuits with an artificial intensity (R. C. Pierce and Kumaresan, 2006).

Brain lesions also affect emotions

Early in the twentieth century, dogs in which the cortex had been removed were found to respond to routine handling with sudden intense **decorticate rage**—snarling, biting, and so on—sometimes referred to as *sham rage* because it seemed undirected. Clearly, then, emotional behaviors of this type must be organized at a subcortical level, with the cerebral cortex normally inhibiting rage responses. On the basis of studies such as these, combined with observations from brain autopsies of people with emotional disorders, James Papez (1937) proposed a subcortical circuit of emotion. Papez (whose name rhymes with "capes") noted associations between emotional changes and specific sites of brain damage. These interconnected regions, now known as the **limbic system** (MacLean, 1949), include the mammillary bodies of the hypothalamus, the anterior thalamus, the cingulate cortex, the hippocampus, the amygdala, and the fornix. The arrows in **FIGURE 11.11** schematically depict the interconnections of this circuit.

Early support for the limbic model of emotion came from studies of monkeys after removal of their temporal lobes (Klüver and Bucy, 1938). The animals' behavior changed dramatically following surgery; the highlight of this behavioral

medial forebrain bundle
A collection of axons traveling in the midline region of the forebrain.

nucleus accumbens   A region of the forebrain that receives dopaminergic innervation from the ventral tegmental area, often associated with reward and pleasurable sensations.

decorticate rage   Also called *sham rage*. Sudden intense rage characterized by actions (such as snarling and biting in dogs) that lack clear direction.

limbic system   A loosely defined, widespread group of brain nuclei that innervate each other to form a network. These nuclei are implicated in emotions.

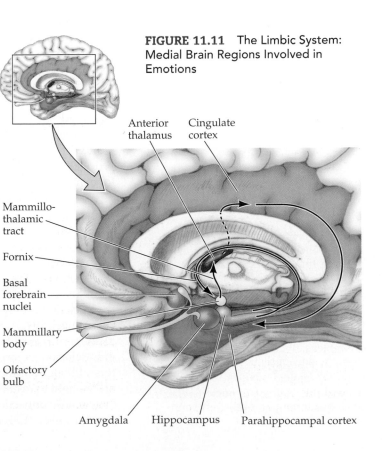

FIGURE 11.11   The Limbic System: Medial Brain Regions Involved in Emotions

Anterior thalamus
Cingulate cortex
Mammillo-thalamic tract
Fornix
Basal forebrain nuclei
Mammillary body
Olfactory bulb
Amygdala
Hippocampus
Parahippocampal cortex

change was an extraordinary taming effect known as the **Klüver-Bucy syndrome**. Animals that had been wild and fearful of humans before surgery became tame and showed neither fear nor aggression afterward. They also showed strong oral tendencies, eating a variety of objects, including rocks. Frequent and often inappropriate sexual behavior was also observed. Because this type of behavior is also seen in monkeys in which only the left and right amygdalas have been destroyed—without damaging any adjacent tissue (Emery et al., 2001)—it appears that the amygdala is a key structure in the behavioral changes in Klüver-Bucy syndrome, especially the loss of fear.

The amygdala is crucial for emotional learning

There is nothing subtle about fear, and fear-provoking situations elicit similar behaviors from individuals of many different species. For example, it is very easy to reliably elicit fear by using classical conditioning, in which the person or animal is presented with a stimulus such as light or sound that is paired with a brief aversive stimulus such as mild electric shock (**FIGURE 11.12A**). After several such pairings, the sound or light by itself effectively elicits behaviors associated with fear, such as freezing in position, and autonomic signs like rapid heart rate and heavy breathing.

Studies of such **fear conditioning** allowed researchers to develop a map of the neural circuitry of emotional learning, which revealed the **amygdala** to be a key structure (**FIGURE 11.12B**). Located at the anterior medial portion of each temporal lobe, the amygdala is composed of about a dozen different nuclei, each with a distinctive set of connections. Lesioning just the central nucleus of the amygdala in rats prevents blood pressure increases and freezing behavior in response to a conditioned fear stimulus. Subsequent research has confirmed that the amygdala is crucial not only for aversive conditioning but also appetitive learning: conditioned positive emotional reactions to attractive stimuli, such as to sex-related stimuli, or other pleasurable signals. In both cases, the amygdala is thought to help form associations between emotional responses and specific memories of stimuli that are stored elsewhere in the brain (Paton et al., 2006; Janak and Tye, 2015).

On its way to the amygdala, sensory information about emotion-provoking stimuli reaches a fork in the road at the level of the thalamus (recall from Chapter 2 that the thalamus acts like a switchboard, directing sensory information to specific brain regions). A direct projection from the thalamus to the amygdala, nicknamed the "low road" for emotional responses in the original fear-conditioning studies (LeDoux, 1996), bypasses conscious processing and allows for immediate emotional reactions to stimuli (de Gelder et al., 2012; Celeghin et al., 2015). An alternate "high road" pathway routes the incoming information through sensory cortex, allowing for processing that, while slower, is conscious, fine-grained, and integrated with higher-level cognitive processes (**FIGURE 11.12C**). You can learn more details about the amygdala circuitry for fear and other emotions in **A STEP FURTHER 11.1**, on the website.

Data from rats and mice about the role of the amygdala in fear mesh well with observations of humans. For example, when people are shown visual stimuli associated with pain or fear, blood flow to the amygdala increases (LaBar et al., 1998), even if the person is not consciously aware of the stimuli (Pegna et al., 2005). Likewise, in people viewing fearful faces, electrophysiological responses occur much more quickly in the amygdala than in visual cortex, reflecting the privileged "low road" access of the fear-inducing stimulus (Méndez-Bértolo et al., 2016). People who suffer from temporal lobe seizures that include the amygdala commonly report that intense fear precedes the start of a seizure (Engel, 1992), and electrical stimulation of temporal lobe sites during brain surgery likewise may elicit feelings of fear (Bancaud et al., 1994). In a rare condition called Capgras delusion, people believe that their significant others have been replaced by impostors; although it is more typically a psychiatric symptom, some cases of Capgras delusion are thought to result from brain damage that robs the afflicted person of the privileged "low road" connection between visual stimuli (like faces) and the emotions they would normally elicit (Ellis and Lewis, 2001). The neural mechanisms of fear conditioning are

Klüver-Bucy syndrome A condition, brought about by bilateral amygdala damage, that is characterized by dramatic emotional changes including reduction in fear and anxiety.

fear conditioning A form of classical conditioning in which a previously neutral stimulus is repeatedly paired with an unpleasant stimulus, like foot shock, until the previously neutral stimulus alone elicits the responses seen in fear.

amygdala A group of nuclei in the medial anterior part of the temporal lobe.

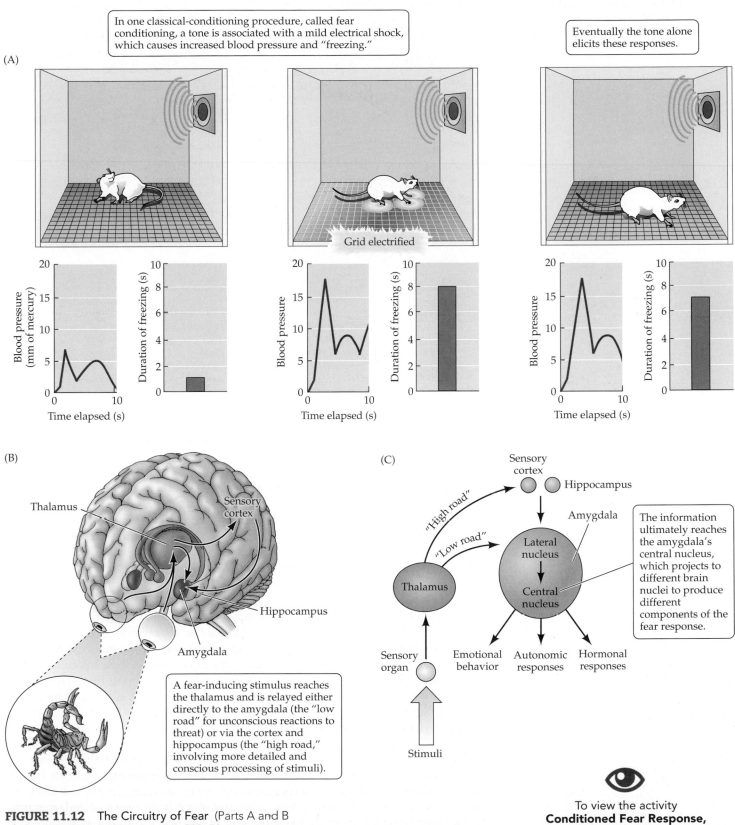

(A)

In one classical-conditioning procedure, called fear conditioning, a tone is associated with a mild electrical shock, which causes increased blood pressure and "freezing."

Eventually the tone alone elicits these responses.

Grid electrified

(B)

Thalamus

Sensory cortex

Hippocampus

Amygdala

A fear-inducing stimulus reaches the thalamus and is relayed either directly to the amygdala (the "low road" for unconscious reactions to threat) or via the cortex and hippocampus (the "high road," involving more detailed and conscious processing of stimuli).

(C)

Sensory cortex

Hippocampus

Amygdala

"High road"

"Low road"

Lateral nucleus

Thalamus

Central nucleus

The information ultimately reaches the amygdala's central nucleus, which projects to different brain nuclei to produce different components of the fear response.

Sensory organ

Emotional behavior

Autonomic responses

Hormonal responses

Stimuli

FIGURE 11.12 **The Circuitry of Fear** (Parts A and B after J. E. LeDoux, 1994. *Sci. Am.* 270: 50, image courtesy of Ian Worpole; C after J. E. LeDoux, 1996. *The emotional brain: The mysterious underpinnings of emotional life.* Simon & Schuster. London, England.)

To view the activity
Conditioned Fear Response,
go to
3e.mindsmachine.com/ac11.1

FIGURE 11.13 The Woman Who Was Never Afraid (After J. S. Feinstein et al., 2011. *Curr. Biol.* 21: 34.)

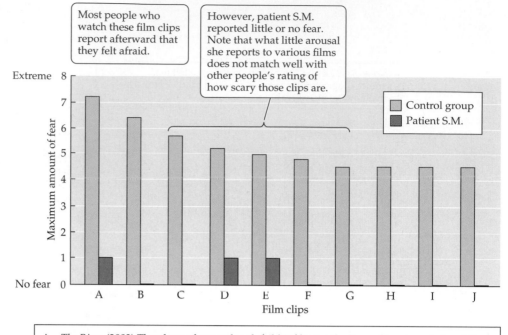

A – *The Ring* (2002) The ghost of a murdered child infiltrates the lives of her soon-to-be victims.
B – *Blair Witch Project* (1999) Campers are attacked by an unknown apparition during the middle of the night.
C – *CSI* (2009) A man struggles to survive after being buried alive.
D – *The English Patient* (1996) A man is tortured by the Germans during World War II.
E – *Se7en* (1995) A mutilated man awakes from the dead.
F – *Cry Freedom* (1987) Armed trespassers attack a woman who is home alone during the night.
G – *Arachnophobia* (1990) A large poisonous spider attacks a girl in the shower.
H – *Halloween* (1978) A woman is being chased by a murderer.
I – *The Shining* (1980) A young boy hears voices in the hallway of a haunted hotel.
J – *The Silence of the Lambs* (1991) A female FBI agent tries to capture a twisted serial killer who is hiding in a dark basement.

also thought to play a central role in post-traumatic stress disorder (PTSD; see Chapter 12), in which memories of horrible events repeatedly intrude into consciousness, reawakening all the autonomic and psychological symptoms of fear.

But perhaps the most compelling evidence that the amygdala is important for fear in our species comes from people like patient S.M., the woman we met at the start of the chapter, who is literally fearless. The fearlessness that she and other people suffering from the disorder display seems almost certainly due to the loss of the amygdala. Her very rare genetic disorder causes the accumulation of calcium deposits in the amygdala, starting in late childhood, which eventually destroys the nuclei in both cerebral hemispheres. When S.M. is shown movie clips that other people find frightening, S.M. reports being unmoved (**FIGURE 11.13**). S.M. is also very poor at recognizing the facial expressions of fear in other people, but she recognizes other emotional expressions—a pattern seen in other people with damaged amygdalas (Adolphs et al., 2005). Interestingly, when S.M. was asked to breathe air with a high concentration of carbon dioxide, she soon felt a panicky fear, flailing her hands about (Feinstein et al., 2013). This result suggests that some other brain system mediates the fear of internal threats, such as a lack of oxygen.

Different emotions activate different regions of the human brain

Several forebrain areas have been consistently implicated in various emotions. Bartels and Zeki (2000) recruited volunteers who professed to be "truly, deeply, and madly in love." Each participant furnished four color photographs: one photo of their romantic partner, and three photos of friends of the same gender as the loved partner and were similar in age and length of friendship. Functional-MRI brain scans were made while each participant was shown counterbalanced sequences of the four photographs. Brain activity elicited by viewing the loved person was compared with that elicited by

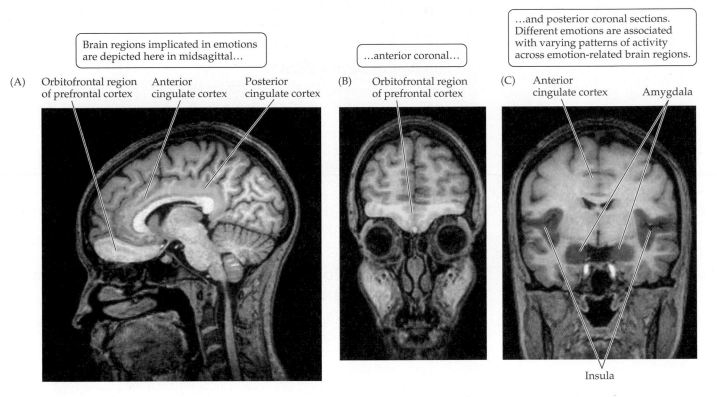

Brain regions implicated in emotions are depicted here in midsagittal...

...anterior coronal...

...and posterior coronal sections. Different emotions are associated with varying patterns of activity across emotion-related brain regions.

(A) Orbitofrontal region of prefrontal cortex   Anterior cingulate cortex   Posterior cingulate cortex

(B) Orbitofrontal region of prefrontal cortex

(C) Anterior cingulate cortex   Amygdala

Insula

FIGURE 11.14   The Emotional Brain (From R. J. Dolan, 2002. *Science* 298: 1191.)

viewing friends. Love, compared with friendship, involved increased activity in the insula and anterior cingulate cortex, and reduced activity in the posterior cingulate and prefrontal cortices (**FIGURE 11.14**). Given its role in fear, you won't be surprised to learn that the amygdala also showed reduced activity when people were contemplating their romantic partners.

Another study compared brain activation during four different kinds of emotion, and again the insula, cingulate cortex, and prefrontal cortex were among the regions implicated. These studies indicate that there is no simple, one-to-one relation between a specific emotion and changed activity of a brain region. There is no "happy center" or "sad center." Instead, each emotion involves differential patterns of activation across a network of brain regions associated with emotion, as you can see in **A STEP FURTHER 11.2**, on the website. For example, activity of the cingulate cortex is altered in sadness, happiness, and anger, and the left somatosensory cortex is deactivated in both anger and fear. Although different emotions are associated with different patterns of activation, there is a good deal of overlap among patterns for different emotions (A. R. Damasio et al., 2000).

In Part II of this chapter we'll focus on the darker side of human emotional experience—aggression—before we address stress and the toll these negative experiences take on our health.

HOW'S IT GOING ?

1. Describe brain self-stimulation and what this phenomenon suggests about emotional experience.
2. What is the limbic system, and what happens when portions of this system are damaged, such as in Klüver-Bucy syndrome?
3. Describe fear conditioning and the evidence that the amygdala plays a role in this process.
4. What evidence suggests that the amygdala mediates fear in humans?

PART II
Aggression

THE ROAD AHEAD

The second part of the chapter is concerned with the neural and hormonal bases of violence and other aggressive behaviors. By the end of this section you should be able to:

1. Define and distinguish between multiple forms of aggression.
2. Summarize research on the role of testosterone in aggression, contrasting between humans and nonhuman animals.
3. Identify the key neural systems implicated in aggression and the environmental stimuli that activate these systems.
4. Discuss the biopsychological origins of violent behavior in humans, and speculate about targets for reducing violent behavior.

Neural Circuitry, Hormones, and Synaptic Transmitters Mediate Violence and Aggression

Violence, assaults, and homicide exact a high price in modern society, and physical assault is not the only form of aggression. Verbal and symbolic aggression—name calling, horn honking, angry glares—also take their toll. We can define **aggression** as behavior that is intended to cause pain or harm (whether physical or emotional) to others, either individually or in groups. We will focus primarily on physical aggression between individuals, excluding the aggression of predators toward their prey, which is better viewed as feeding behavior (Glickman, 1977).

Intermale aggression (aggression between males of the same species) is observed in most vertebrates. The relevance to humans is reflected in the fact that males are 5 times as likely as females to be arrested on charges of murder in the United States. Whatever we may think about aggression, it seems clear that in many species aggressive behavior in males is adaptive for gaining access to food and mates. In the wild, groups of male chimpanzees sometimes band together to kill a rival male (Wilson et al., 2014), increasing the attackers' chances of mating in the future. Further, aggressive behavior between boys, in contrast to that between girls, is evident early, in the form of vigorous and destructive play behavior (J. Archer, 2006). These and similar observations suggest that the hormone that prepares males for reproduction—testosterone—also plays a role in their aggressive behavior.

Androgens seem to increase aggression

At sexual maturity, as the testes begin secreting the steroid hormone **testosterone**, intermale aggression markedly increases in many species (Svare, 2013). In seasonally breeding animals as diverse as birds and primates, intermale aggression waxes and wanes in concert with seasonal changes in levels of testosterone (Wingfield et al., 1987; Munley et al., 2018). Conversely, castrating males to remove the source of testosterone usually reduces aggressive behavior profoundly. Treating castrated males with testosterone restores fighting behavior (**FIGURE 11.15**).

The relationship between testosterone and aggression in humans is more complicated (for a review, see Geniole and Carré, 2018). Treating adult volunteers with extra testosterone does not increase their aggression (O'Connor et al., 2004). Similarly, young men going through puberty experience a sudden large increase in circulating testosterone, yet they do not show a correlated increase in aggressive behavior (J. Archer, 2006). Nevertheless, some human studies report a positive correlation between testosterone levels and the magnitude of hostility, as measured by behavior rating scales (Dabbs and Morris, 1990). Nonaggressive tendencies in males are associated with satisfaction in family functioning and with lower levels of serum

aggression Behavior that is intended to cause pain or harm to others.

intermale aggression Aggression between males of the same species.

testosterone A hormone, produced by male gonads, that controls a variety of bodily changes that become visible at puberty; one of a class of hormones called androgens.

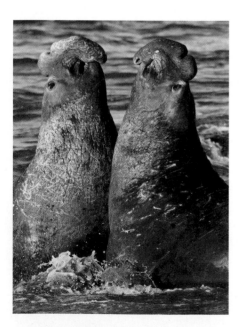

Nature, Red in Tooth and Flipper Fighting male elephant seals draw blood. In most mammalian species, males must compete with one another, often in the form of physical aggression, for the chance to mate with females. (© David Osborn/Alamy.)

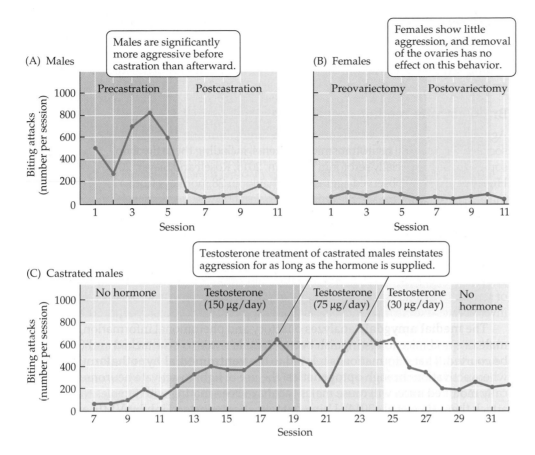

FIGURE 11.15 The Effects of Androgens on the Aggressive Behavior of Mice (After G. C. Wagner et al., 1980. *Aggress. Behav.* 6: 1.)

testosterone (Julian and McKenry, 1979). Among female convicts, testosterone concentrations are highest in women convicted of unprovoked violence and lowest among women convicted of defensive violent crimes (Dabbs et al., 1988; Dabbs and Hargrove, 1997).

At least two variables confound the correlations between testosterone and aggression. First is the observation that experience can affect testosterone levels. In mice and monkeys, the loser in aggressive encounters shows reduced androgen levels (Lloyd, 1971; I. S. Bernstein and Gordon, 1974), so measured levels of testosterone sometimes may be a result, rather than a cause, of behavior. In men, testosterone levels rise in the winners and fall in the losers after competitions ranging from wrestling to chess (van Anders and Watson, 2006). Male sports fans even show a vicarious competition effect in response to simply watching "their" team win or lose a sporting event (Bernhardt, 1997), and during the 2008 U.S. presidential election, men who voted for John McCain experienced a sharp drop in circulating testosterone, compared with backers of Obama, who won (Stanton et al., 2009).

These observations suggest that a second confounding variable between testosterone and aggression is dominance (Mazur and Booth, 1998). According to this model, testosterone levels should be associated with behaviors that confer or protect the individual's social status (and thus reproductive fitness). This type of aggression is said to be proactive—part of an offense strategy to improve the individual's standing in comparison to others or achieve a desired social outcome—in contrast to reactive aggression that often takes the form of a defense against an external threat (Wrangham, 2018). These behaviors may sometimes, but not always, involve overt proactive aggression.

Despite the lack of a close relationship between aggression and androgens, people have tried to modify the behavior of male criminals by manipulating sex hormones, through surgical castration or "chemical" castration with drugs that block androgen

FIGURE 11.17 Physiological Reactions to Stress

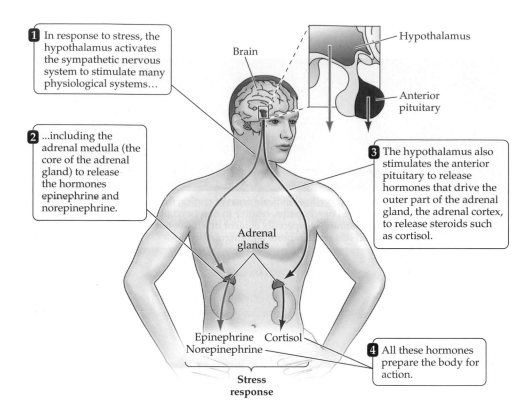

1 In response to stress, the hypothalamus activates the sympathetic nervous system to stimulate many physiological systems…

Brain

Hypothalamus

Anterior pituitary

2 …including the adrenal medulla (the core of the adrenal gland) to release the hormones epinephrine and norepinephrine.

3 The hypothalamus also stimulates the anterior pituitary to release hormones that drive the outer part of the adrenal gland, the adrenal cortex, to release steroids such as cortisol.

Adrenal glands

Epinephrine   Cortisol
Norepinephrine

4 All these hormones prepare the body for action.

Stress response

stress Any circumstance that upsets homeostatic balance.

adrenal medulla The inner core of the adrenal gland.

epinephrine Also called *adrenaline*. A compound that acts both as a hormone (secreted by the adrenal medulla under the control of the sympathetic nervous system) and as a synaptic transmitter.

norepinephrine Also called *noradrenaline*. A neurotransmitter produced and released by sympathetic postganglionic neurons to accelerate organ activity.

adrenal cortex The steroid-secreting outer rind of the adrenal gland.

adrenal steroid hormone A steroid hormone that is secreted by the adrenal cortex.

cortisol A glucocorticoid stress hormone of the adrenal cortex.

research, broadly defined stress as "the rate of all the wear and tear caused by life" (Selye, 1956). Nowadays, researchers try to sharpen their focus by treating **stress** as a multidimensional concept that encompasses stressful stimuli, the stress-processing system (including cognitive assessment of the stimuli), and responses to stress. While many different parts of the body respond to stress, it's clear that the brain carefully monitors and controls those responses (McEwen et al., 2015).

The stress response progresses in stages

Selye called the initial response to stress the alarm reaction. As one part of the alarm reaction, the hypothalamus activates the sympathetic nervous system to ready the body for action; this is the fight-or-flight system we mentioned at the start of the chapter. The sympathetic system stimulates the core of the adrenal gland, which is called the **adrenal medulla**, to release the hormones **epinephrine** (also known as adrenaline) and **norepinephrine** (or noradrenaline). These hormones act on many parts of the body to boost heart rate, breathing, and other physiological processes that prepare the body for action. As another part of the alarm reaction, the hypothalamus stimulates the anterior pituitary to release a hormone that drives the outer layer of the adrenal gland, the **adrenal cortex**, to release **adrenal steroid hormones** such as **cortisol** (**FIGURE 11.17**). These hormones act more slowly than epinephrine, but they also ready the body for action, including releasing body stores of energy. Glucocorticoid receptors—the receptors that respond to cortisol—are found in many locations in the brain, where they are thought to mediate the formation of memories associated with stress and fear (de Quervain et al., 2017).

Hormonal responses to stress were studied in a group of young recruits in the Norwegian military both before and during scary parachute training (Ursin et al., 1978). On each jump day, the anterior pituitary released enhanced levels of hormones, and both the sympathetic and parasympathetic systems were activated (**FIGURE 11.18A**). Initially, cortisol levels were elevated in the blood before each jump, but with more and more successful jumps over successive days, the pituitary-adrenal response soon declined. Epinephrine and norepinephrine were also elevated before the first jumps, but eventually they returned to normal before jumps. Testosterone showed the reverse pattern, falling far below control levels on the first day of training but returning to normal with subsequent jumps (**FIGURE 11.18B**). Once the soldiers mastered the jumps, they no longer showed increased hormonal responses, having adapted to the activity.

(A) Response systems affected in jump situation

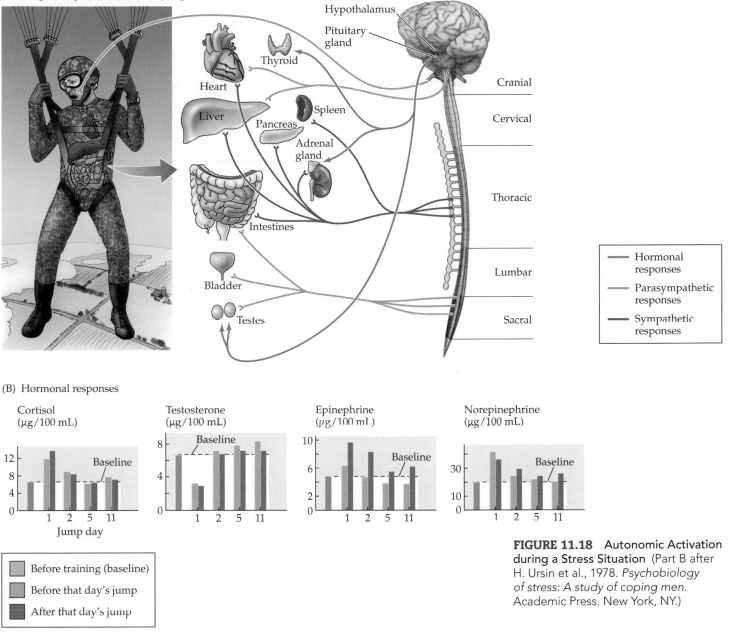

(B) Hormonal responses

FIGURE 11.18 Autonomic Activation during a Stress Situation (Part B after H. Ursin et al., 1978. *Psychobiology of stress: A study of coping men.* Academic Press. New York, NY.)

Less-dramatic real-life situations also evoke clear endocrine responses (Frankenhaeuser, 1978). For example, riding in a commuter train provokes the release of epinephrine; the longer the ride and the more crowded the train, the greater the hormonal response (**FIGURE 11.19A**). Factory work likewise leads to the release of epinephrine; the shorter the work cycle—that is, the more frequently the person has to repeat the same operations—the higher the levels of epinephrine. The stress of a PhD oral exam leads to a dramatic increase in both epinephrine and norepinephrine (**FIGURE 11.19B**). These sorts of social stressors can have enduring medical costs: for example, young people with asthma who experience stress due to peer rejection or a negative emotional climate at home have a more responsive adrenal system, more severe asthma symptoms, and impaired expression of anti-inflammatory genes (Murphy et al., 2015; Farrell et al., 2018).

There are individual differences in the stress response

Why do individuals differ in their responses to stress (Infurna and Luthar, 2016)? One hypothesis focuses on early experience. Rat pups clearly find it stressful to have

FIGURE 11.19 Hormonal Changes in Humans in Response to Social Stresses (Part A after U. Lundberg, 1976. *J. Human Stress* 2: 26; B after M. Frankenhaeuser, 1978. *Nebr. Symp. Motiv.* 26: 123.)

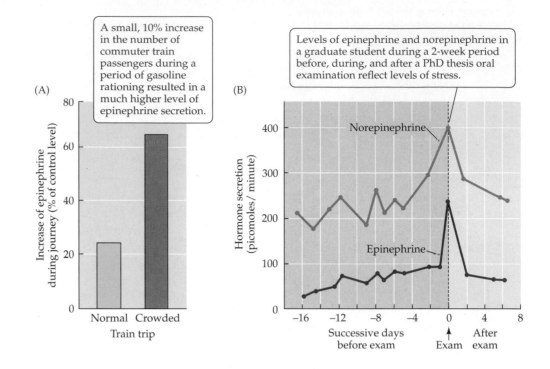

(A)

A small, 10% increase in the number of commuter train passengers during a period of gasoline rationing resulted in a much higher level of epinephrine secretion.

Increase of epinephrine during journey (% of control level)

Normal   Crowded
Train trip

(B)

Levels of epinephrine and norepinephrine in a graduate student during a 2-week period before, during, and after a PhD thesis oral examination reflect levels of stress.

Norepinephrine

Epinephrine

Hormone secretion (picomoles / minute)

Successive days before exam   Exam   After exam

a human pick them up and handle them. Yet rats that have been briefly handled as pups are less susceptible to adult stress than are rats that have been left alone as pups (S. Levine et al., 1967). For example, the previously handled rats secrete lower adrenal steroid amounts in response to a wide variety of adult stressors. Researchers termed this effect **stress immunization** because a little stress early in life seemed to make the animals more resilient to later stress.

Follow-up research showed that there was more to the story. The pups did not benefit because they were stressed; they benefited because their mothers comforted them after the stress. When pups are returned to their mother after a separation, she spends considerable time licking and grooming them. And she will lick the pups much longer if they were handled by humans during the separation. Michael Meaney and colleagues suggest that this gentle tactile stimulation from Mom is crucial for the stress immunization effect. They found that, even among undisturbed litters, the offspring of mother rats that exhibited more licking and grooming behavior were more resilient in their responses to adult stress than other rats were (D. Liu et al., 1997). So the "immunizing" benefit of early stressful experience happens only if the pups are promptly comforted after each stressful event.

If the pups are deprived of their mother for long periods, receiving very little of her attention, then as adults they exhibit a greater stress response, have difficulty learning mazes, and show reduced neurogenesis in the hippocampus (Mirescu et al., 2004). Maternal deprivation exerts this negative effect on adult stress responses by causing long-lasting changes in the expression of adrenal steroid receptors in the brain. This change is termed **epigenetic regulation** because it represents a change in the expression of the gene, rather than a change in the encoding region of the gene (see Figure 13.32).

Dramatic evidence for the same phenomenon has been seen in humans. For example, examination of the brains of suicide victims revealed the same epigenetic change in expression of the adrenal steroid receptor, but only in those victims who had a history of being abused or neglected as children (McGowan et al., 2009). The implication is that the early abuse epigenetically modified expression of the gene, making the person less able to handle stress and thus more likely to become depressed and commit suicide. Suicide victims who had no history of early neglect did

stress immunization The concept that mild stress early in life makes an individual better able to handle stress later in life. The benefits seem to be due to effective comforting after stressful events, not the stressful events themselves.

epigenetic regulation Changes in gene expression that are due to environmental effects rather than to changes in the nucleotide sequence of the gene.

not show the epigenetic change, so their depression may have been a response to other influences.

Early life stress also affects adult health. For example, the children of women who were pregnant during the Dutch famine in World War II were later found to have a greater risk of schizophrenia, depression, and type 2 diabetes as adults (Roseboom et al., 2011). In general, adverse childhood experiences have an enduring effect on multiple aspects of health in later life, including neural and cognitive development, emotional regulation, and measures of lifetime achievement (Felitti et al., 1998; Cameron et al., 2017).

Stress and emotions affect our health

The field of **psychosomatic medicine** studies the distinctive psychological, behavioral, and social factors that influence individual susceptibility or resistance to diverse illnesses. The related field called **health psychology** (or behavioral medicine) emphasizes the role of social factors in the cause, progression, and consequences of health and illness (Ogden, 2012). For example, an active area of research is concerned with the association between heart disease and behavioral and social factors such as hostility, depression, loneliness, and stress at home and at work (Matthews, 2005; Rozanski, 2014).

The field of **psychoneuroimmunology** studies how the immune system—with its collection of cells that recognize and attack intruders—interacts with other organs, especially those of the hormonal systems and nervous system (Ader, 2001). Studies of both human and nonhuman subjects clearly show psychological and neurological influences on the immune system. For example, people with happy social lives are less likely to develop a cold when exposed to the virus (S. Cohen et al., 2006). People exposed to a cold virus have more severe symptoms if they are experiencing conflict with others. But individuals who feel they have more social support, and who receive more hugs from others, are protected from that effect of conflict (S. Cohen et al., 2015). Likewise, people who tend to feel positive emotions will also produce more antibodies in response to a flu vaccination (Rosenkranz et al., 2003), which should help them fight off sickness. These interactions go both ways: the brain influences responses of the immune system, and immune cells and their products affect brain activities, as **FIGURE 11.20** shows. You can learn details of how the immune system, endocrine system, and nervous system communicate with one another in **A STEP FURTHER 11.3**, on the website.

As an example, stressful exam periods usually suppress the immune system (Glaser et al., 1986). Importantly, the student's perception of the stress of the academic program is a predictor of immune system suppression: those who perceive the program as stressful show the most suppression. One experiment considered the effects of university examinations on wound healing in dental students (Marucha et al., 1998). Two small wounds were placed on the roof of the mouth of 11 dental students (sounds like revenge, doesn't it?). The first wound was timed during summer vacation; the second was inflicted 3 days before the first major examination of the term. Two independent daily measures showed that no student healed as rapidly during the exam period, when healing took 40% longer. One measure of immunological response declined 68% during the exam period. The experimenters concluded that even something as transient, predictable, and relatively benign as final exams (do students agree with this description?) can have significant consequences for wound healing.

Why does chronic stress suppress the immune system?

Although brief stress doesn't impair immune function, and may even enhance it (Dhabhar, 2018), longer-lasting stress has a pronounced suppressive effect on the immune system. We discussed earlier how in response to stress, the brain causes adrenal steroid hormones such as cortisol to be released from the adrenal cortex. In chronic stress,

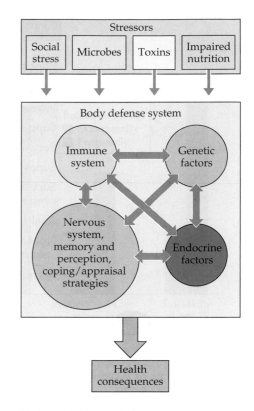

FIGURE 11.20 Factors That Interact during the Development and Progression of Disease

psychosomatic medicine A field of study that emphasizes the role of psychological factors in disease.

health psychology Also called *behavioral medicine*. A field of study that focuses on psychological influences on health-related processes.

psychoneuroimmunology The study of the immune system and its interaction with the nervous system and behavior.

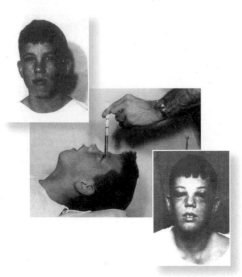

Changed for Life   Twelve-year-old Howard Dully before, during, and after his transorbital lobotomy. The swelling around his eyes eventually went away, but Howard would spend the next four decades in various mental institutions. (From H. Dully and C. Fleming, 2007. *My Lobotomy*. New York, NY: Crown. Courtesy of Howard Dully.)

To view the
Brain Explorer,
go to
3e.mindsmachine.com/av12.2

PART I
Schizophrenia

THE ROAD AHEAD

We begin by considering schizophrenia, a severe disorder occurring in about 1% of the population, no matter where you go in the world. Learning this material should allow you to:

1. Know the most common symptoms of schizophrenia.
2. Understand the strong influence of both genes and the environment on the chances of developing schizophrenia.
3. Describe several of the structural brain differences of people with schizophrenia versus controls.
4. Discuss the several classes of antipsychotic drugs and their mechanisms of action.

The Toll of Psychiatric Disorders Is Huge

Currently in its fifth edition, the American Psychiatric Association's *Diagnostic and Statistical Manual of Mental Disorders,* generally called the *DSM-5*, provides a standardized system for diagnosing and classifying the major psychiatric illnesses according to current knowledge (APA, 2013). Worldwide, between 15% and 50% of the population report psychiatric symptoms at some point in life, with North Americans positioned at the top end of this range (Kessler et al., 2007). About 19% of the adult population of the United States experiences psychiatric symptoms in the course of a year (Substance Abuse and Mental Health Services Administration, 2013), and of this number more than 4% (equating to almost 10 million people) are so ill that they are unable to carry out major life activities, like working or living independently. As shown in **FIGURE 12.1**, these rates are higher for females than for males, primarily because females are more likely to be depressed. (On the other hand, drug dependency and alcoholism, which are not reflected in Figure 12.1, are much more frequent in males.) Note also the high rates that are evident in 18- to 25-year-olds because certain psychiatric disorders—for example,

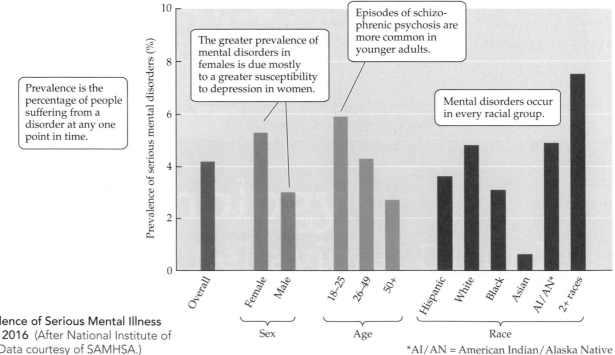

Prevalence is the percentage of people suffering from a disorder at any one point in time.

The greater prevalence of mental disorders in females is due mostly to a greater susceptibility to depression in women.

Episodes of schizophrenic psychosis are more common in younger adults.

Mental disorders occur in every racial group.

FIGURE 12.1   **Prevalence of Serious Mental Illness among U.S. Adults in 2016** (After National Institute of Mental Health, 2017. Data courtesy of SAMHSA.)

*AI/AN = American Indian/Alaska Native

schizophrenia—tend to appear in adolescence and young adulthood. Clearly, mental disorders exact an enormous toll on our lives.

The seeds for a biological perspective in psychiatry were sown at the start of the twentieth century. At that time, almost a quarter of the patients in mental hospitals suffered from so-called paralytic dementia, featuring sudden onset of **delusions** (false beliefs strongly held in spite of contrary evidence), grandiosity (boastful self-importance), euphoria, poor judgment, impulsive behavior, disordered thought, and physiological signs like abnormal pupillary constriction (Argyll-Robertson, 1869). The disorder was originally believed to be caused by "weak character," but analyses of the brains and behavior of the afflicted revealed that their illness had a physiological cause: syphilis. With the advent of antibiotics to cure syphilis, paralytic dementia has virtually disappeared. This finding opened the door to biological explanations for other mental illnesses.

Schizophrenia Is a Major Neurobiological Challenge in Psychiatry

Throughout the world and across the centuries, some people have been recognized as unusual because they hear voices that others don't, feel intensely frightened, sense persecution from unseen enemies, and generally act strangely (Bark, 2002; Heinrichs, 2003). For many, this disordered state—now known as **schizophrenia**—lasts a lifetime. For others, it appears and disappears unpredictably. Schizophrenia is also a public health problem because all too many of the people who suffer from it become homeless.

Schizophrenia is characterized by an unusual array of symptoms

The term *schizophrenia* (from the Greek *schizein*, "to split," and *phren*, "mind") was introduced early in the twentieth century to convey the idea that various functions of the mind—like memory, perception, and thinking—were split from each other (Bleuler, 1950, originally published in 1911). This poetic but vague description of schizophrenia was subsequently replaced with a more objective definition (K. Schneider, 1959) focusing on "first-rank symptoms," which include (1) auditory hallucinations, (2) highly personalized delusions, and (3) changes in affect (emotion). By the 1980s it became clear that many schizophrenia symptoms could be viewed as belonging to two general groups: positive and negative (Crow, 1980). **Positive symptoms** are abnormal behavioral states that have been *gained*; examples include hallucinations, delusions, and excited motor behavior. **Negative symptoms** are abnormalities resulting from the *loss* of normal functions—for example, slow and impoverished thought and speech, emotional and social withdrawal, or blunted affect.

Researchers now recognize that schizophrenia is a complex syndrome in which individuals exhibit varying degrees of distinct but correlated categories of symptoms. The contemporary view of the symptoms of schizophrenia retains the distinction between positive symptoms (psychosis) and negative symptoms (emotional and motivational impairments) but recognizes an additional dimension: cognitive impairment (**TABLE 12.1**). The fact that the various categories of symptoms respond differently to drug treatments suggests that multiple neural mechanisms are involved in the disorder.

Schizophrenia has a heritable component

For many years, genetic studies of schizophrenia were controversial because some early researchers failed to understand that genes need not act in an all-or-none fashion. For any genotype there is often a large range of alternative outcomes determined by both developmental and environmental factors, as we'll see.

FAMILY STUDIES If schizophrenia can be inherited, relatives of people with schizophrenia should show a higher incidence (number of new cases during a period of time) than is found in the general population. In addition, the risk of schizophrenia among

delusion A false belief that is strongly held in spite of contrary evidence.

schizophrenia A severe psychopathological disorder characterized by negative symptoms such as emotional withdrawal and flat affect, by positive symptoms such as hallucinations and delusions, and by cognitive symptoms such as poor attention span.

positive symptom In psychiatry, an abnormal behavioral state. Examples include hallucinations, delusions, and excited motor behavior.

negative symptom In psychiatry, an abnormality that reflects insufficient functioning. Examples include emotional and social withdrawal, and blunted affect.

TABLE 12.1 ■ Symptoms of Schizophrenia	
Symptom dimension	**Symptom category**
POSITIVE SYMPTOMS Refers to symptoms that are present but should not be	PSYCHOSIS Hallucinations Delusions Disorganized thought and speech Bizarre behaviors
NEGATIVE SYMPTOMS Refers to characteristics of the individual that are absent but should be present	EMOTIONAL DYSREGULATION Lack of emotional expression Reduced facial expression (flat affect) Inability to experience pleasure in everyday activities (anhedonia) IMPAIRED MOTIVATION Reduced conversation (alogia) Diminished ability to begin or sustain activities Social withdrawal
COGNITIVE SYMPTOMS Refers to problems with processing and acting on external information	NEUROCOGNITIVE IMPAIRMENT Memory problems Poor attention span Difficulty making plans Reduced decision-making capacity Poor social cognition Abnormal movement patterns

relatives should increase with the closeness of the relationship, because closer relatives share a greater number of genes. Indeed, parents and siblings of people with schizophrenia have a higher risk of becoming schizophrenic than do individuals in the general population (**FIGURE 12.2**). However, the mode of inheritance of schizophrenia is not simple; that is, it does not involve a single recessive or dominant gene (Hyman, 2018). Rather, multiple genes play a role.

ADOPTION STUDIES   It is easy to find fault with family studies. They confuse hereditary and environmental factors because members of a family share both. But what about children who are not raised with their biological parents? In fact, studies of adopted people confirm a strong genetic factor in schizophrenia. The biological parents of adoptees who suffer from schizophrenia are far more likely to have suffered from this disorder than are the adopting parents (Kety et al., 1994).

TWIN STUDIES   In twins, nature provides researchers with an excellent opportunity for a genetic experiment. In identical (or *monozygotic*) twins, who derive from a single fertilized egg and thus share the same set of genes, if one of the twins develops schizophrenia, the other twin has a roughly fifty-fifty chance of also developing the disorder. But in fraternal (or *dizygotic*) twin pairs, who come from two fertilized eggs and thus share about 50% of their genes, just like any pair of siblings, this **concordance** (sharing of a characteristic) drops to about 17% (see Figure 12.2) (Cardno and Gottesman, 2000). The higher concordance in the

concordance   Sharing of a characteristic by both individuals of a pair of twins.

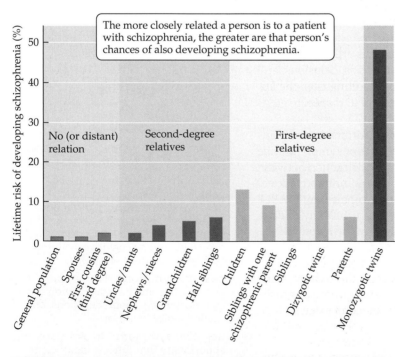

FIGURE 12.2   **The Heritability of Schizophrenia** (After I. I. Gottesman, 1991. *Schizophrenia genesis: The origins of madness.* Freeman. New York, NY.)

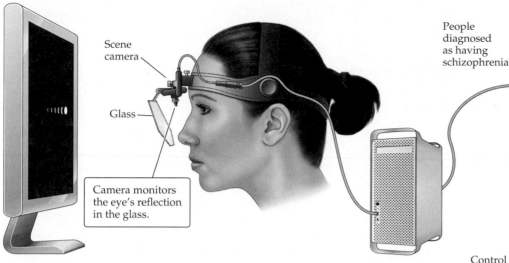
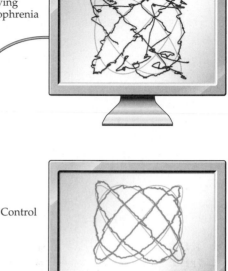

Scene camera

Glass

Camera monitors the eye's reflection in the glass.

People diagnosed as having schizophrenia

Smooth pursuit of moving cursor

Control

FIGURE 12.3 Eye Tracking in People with Schizophrenia versus Controls (After P. J. Benson et al., 2012. *Biol. Psychiatry* 72: 716. Courtesy of Dr. Philip Benson.)

genetically identical twins is thus strong evidence of a genetic factor. Yet even with identical twins, the concordance rate for schizophrenia is only about 50% (some estimates are higher [Hilker et al., 2018], some lower [Joseph, 2013b]), so genes alone cannot fully explain whether a person will develop schizophrenia. Presumably, other factors, especially environmental influences, account for the 50% of identical twin pairs that are discordant (only one twin develops the disorder). Often, the twin who goes on to develop schizophrenia has an abnormal developmental history, such as lower birth weight, more physiological distress in early life, and behavior that seems more submissive, tearful, and sensitive than that of the unaffected twin (Torrey et al., 1994). Subtle neurological signs, such as impaired motor coordination and difficulty with smooth movements of the eyes to follow a moving target (**FIGURE 12.3**), are also common (Avila et al., 2006). In short, the twin studies show that schizophrenia has both environmental and genetic origins.

INDIVIDUAL GENES It has been difficult to identify any single gene that causes schizophrenia to develop or increases susceptibility (Hyman, 2018). In fact, genetic analyses suggest that over 100 genes influencing the likelihood of schizophrenia are scattered across many different human chromosomes (Birnbaum and Weinberger, 2017; Foley et al., 2017). Nonetheless, a few genes have been identified that appear to be abnormal in a small proportion of schizophrenia cases, including genes that are known to participate in synaptic plasticity (Kennedy et al., 2003; Mei and Xiong, 2008). In one large Scottish family, several members who had schizophrenia also carried a mutant, disabled version of a gene, which was therefore named *disrupted in schizophrenia 1* (*DISC1*). We'll discuss *DISC1* further a little later in the chapter.

An interesting *epigenetic* factor (see Chapter 13) in schizophrenia is paternal age: children fathered by older men have a greater risk of developing schizophrenia (de Kluiver et al., 2017). It is thought that, because they are the product of more cell divisions than the sperm of younger men, the sperm of older men have had more opportunity to accumulate mutations caused by errors in copying the chromosomes; these mutations may contribute to the development of schizophrenia in some cases.

Taken together, the studies make it clear that certain genes can indeed increase the risk of developing schizophrenia but that the environment also matters. As we'll see next, a big factor in whether a person will develop schizophrenia is stress.

RESEARCHERS AT WORK

Stress increases the risk of schizophrenia

We've established that there is genetic influence on schizophrenia but also that genes alone cannot account for the disorder. What environmental factors contribute to the probability of developing schizophrenia? Research suggests that a variety of stressful events significantly increase the risk. For example, schizophrenia usually appears during a time in life that many people find stressful—the transition from childhood to adulthood, when people deal with physical, emotional, and lifestyle changes (e.g., going away to college).

Another risk factor seen in multiple studies is the stress of city living. As **FIGURE 12.4** shows, people living in a medium-sized city are about 1½ times more likely to develop schizophrenia than are people living in the country. What's more, the earlier in life a person begins living in the city, the greater the risk. People living in a *big* city are even more likely to develop the disorder (Pedersen and Mortensen, 2001). Conversely, children who move from the city to the country have a *reduced* risk of developing schizophrenia (Van Os et al., 2010). We don't know what it is about living in a city that makes schizophrenia more likely. Pollutants, greater exposure to minor diseases, crowded conditions, tense social interactions—all of these could be considered stressful.

FIGURE 12.4   City Living Increases the Risk of Schizophrenia (After C. B. Pedersen and P. B. Mortensen, 2001. *Arch. Gen. Psychiatry* 58: 1039.)

■ **Hypothesis**
Stress increases the risk of schizophrenia.

■ **Test**
Find a data set that lets you compare people from a relatively homogeneous culture and genetic background, such as Denmark. Assuming that city living is more stressful than living in the country, determine whether populations living in a big city, in other (smaller) cities, or in the country differ in the proportion of people diagnosed with schizophrenia.

■ **Result**

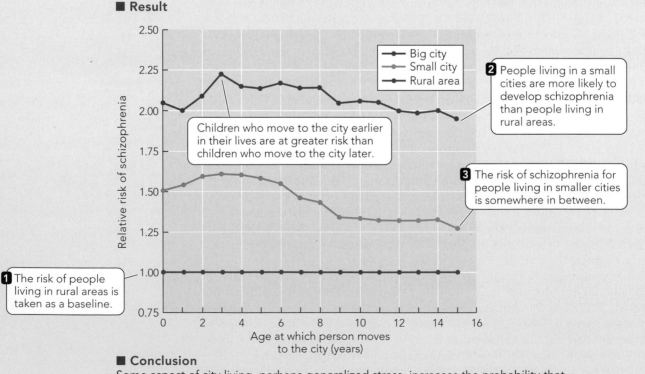

■ **Conclusion**
Some aspect of city living, perhaps generalized stress, increases the probability that a person will develop schizophrenia.

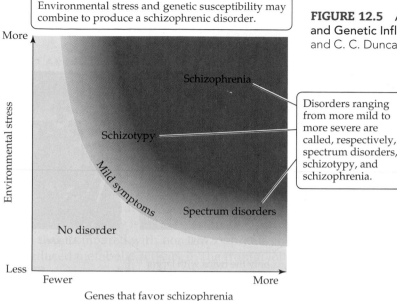

Environmental stress and genetic susceptibility may combine to produce a schizophrenic disorder.

FIGURE 12.5 A Model of the Interaction between Stress and Genetic Influences in Schizophrenia (After A. F. Mirsky and C. C. Duncan, 1986. *Annu. Rev. Psychol.* 37: 291.)

Disorders ranging from more mild to more severe are called, respectively, spectrum disorders, schizotypy, and schizophrenia.

An integrative model of schizophrenia emphasizes the interaction of factors

Prenatal stress, such as infection during pregnancy, increases the likelihood that the baby will develop schizophrenia later in life (P. H. Patterson, 2007; A. S. Brown, 2011). Likewise, if the mother and baby have incompatible blood types, or the mother becomes diabetic during pregnancy, or if there is a low birth weight for some reason, the baby is more likely to develop schizophrenia (King et al., 2010). Birth complications that deprive the baby of oxygen also increase the probability of schizophrenia (Clarke et al., 2011).

These findings suggest that relatively minor stress during development can make the difference in whether schizophrenia develops. It is fascinating, and frightening, to think that events in the womb or early childhood can affect the outcome 16 or 20 years later, when the schizophrenia appears.

Thus the evidence indicates that schizophrenia results from a complex interaction of genetic factors and stress. Each life stage has its own specific features that increase vulnerability to schizophrenia: infections before birth, complications at delivery, urban living in childhood and adulthood (Powell, 2010). From this perspective, the emergence of schizophrenia and related disorders depends on whether a genetically susceptible person is subjected to environmental stressors (**FIGURE 12.5**). The hope is that through the development of sensitive diagnostic approaches that combine brain imaging with genetic and behavioral measures, we will be able to accurately identify and understand the at-risk child early in life, when interventions to reduce stress might prevent schizophrenia later in life.

Once the interaction of genetic susceptibility and stress results in schizophrenia, the condition affects not only the person's behavior but also the physical state of the brain, as we'll see next.

The brains of some people with schizophrenia show structural and functional changes

Because the symptoms of schizophrenia can be so marked and persistent, investigators hypothesized early on that the brains of people with this illness would show distinctive and measurable structural abnormalities. Later, CT and MRI scans confirmed this idea, revealing significant, consistent anatomical differences in the brains of many people with schizophrenia (Trimble, 1991). Interestingly, these scans also confirm the idea that genes alone cannot account for whether a person will develop schizophrenia.

SIGNS & SYMPTOMS

Mixed Feelings about SSRIs

At their introduction, selective serotonin reuptake inhibitors (SSRIs) represented a major revolution in depression treatment. Heavily marketed to the public and to health professionals, SSRIs soon became one of the most widely prescribed medications, propelling an incredible 400% increase in antidepressant prescriptions by 2008. In fact, for 18- to 44-year-olds, antidepressants are prescribed more than any other drug; more than one in ten adult Americans is currently using antidepressant medication (Pratt et al., 2011). Needless to say, the development and sales of antidepressants have provided a huge windfall for the pharmaceuticals industry.

Now that SSRIs have been with us for more than 20 years, researchers have turned to retrospective analyses to reevaluate the efficacy of SSRIs. In part, these large-scale **meta-analyses** (analyses that combine the results of many previously published studies) have been prompted by the concern that for various reasons—public appetite, profit motives, the tendency of journals to publish only positive findings—studies that failed to find effects of SSRIs may historically have been underreported. The results of these meta-analyses have been mixed, but they at least give us cause to take a sober second look at SSRI usage.

As illustrated in **FIGURE 12.14**, one influential large-scale review concluded that only a minority of depressed people, the 13% constituting the most severe cases, responded significantly better to SSRIs than to placebos (Fournier et al., 2010). Furthermore, only about half of the people getting the drug are completely "cured," and about 20% show no improvement at all. And while there are reservations about the efficacy of SSRIs for children or teenagers (Bower, 2006), millions of American children have been given prescriptions for SSRIs despite a reported increased risk of suicide in these age groups (Olfson et al., 2006).

However, other large meta-analytic studies, also based on multiple clinical trials, find evidence of clear beneficial effects of SSRIs relative to placebos for people of all ages and with all levels of severity of depression (Gibbons et al., 2012). These authors argue that the apparent relationship of severity and SSRI efficacy is a statistical artifact of the methodology employed in order to combine studies in a meta-analysis.

This controversy seems likely to rage on for a while. In the meantime, a prudent course of action is to deploy cognitive behavioral therapy as a first-rank treatment in moderate cases, supplemented with antidepressant medication in more severe or nonresponsive cases.

FIGURE 12.14 When Are Antidepressants More Effective Than Placebos? (After J. C. Fournier et al., 2010. *JAMA* 303: 47.)

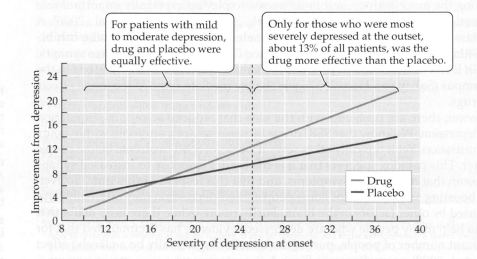

meta-analysis A type of quantitative review of a field of research, in which the results of multiple previous studies are combined in order to identify overall patterns that are consistent across studies.

A newer class of antidepressants comprises the serotonin-norepinephrine reuptake inhibitors (SNRIs) like Cymbalta (duloxetine) and Effexor (venlafaxine) (Hillhouse and Porter, 2015). Several other medications for depression are currently under study. For example, compounds being investigated as potential antidepressants include the glutamate receptor antagonist ketamine (see Chapter 4), which relieves depression almost instantly (E. E. Lee et al., 2015), in contrast to SSRIs and SNRIs, which typically must be taken several weeks before elevating mood.

Despite the popularity of SSRIs for treating depression, treatment with **cognitive behavioral therapy** (**CBT**), a type of psychotherapy aimed at correcting negative thinking and improving interpersonal relationships, is about as effective as SSRI treatment (Butler et al., 2006). Furthermore, the rate of relapse is lower for CBT than for SSRI treatment (DeRubeis et al., 2008). Interestingly, CBT and SSRI treatment *together* are more effective in combating depression than either one is alone (Schramm et al., 2008). Typically, CBT helps the client to recognize self-defeating modes of thinking and encourages breaking out of a cycle of self-fulfilling depression (**FIGURE 12.15**) and has proven effective in avoiding suicide (Mewton and Andrews, 2016).

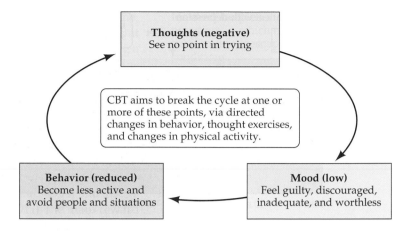

FIGURE 12.15 Depression's Endless Treadmill

An unusual treatment for depression involves a pacemaker that periodically applies mild electrical stimulation to the vagus nerve (cranial nerve X; see Chapter 2). This treatment is offered in cases where drugs or ECT have been ineffective, but it remains to be established whether vagal stimulation is a long-term solution (Grimm and Bajbouj, 2010; Blumberger et al., 2015). For extremely difficult cases of depression, researchers have turned again to psychosurgery—but nothing that resembles the ravages suffered by Howard Dully. In **deep brain stimulation** (**DBS**) surgery, delicate electrodes are surgically implanted in the cingulate cortex or other brain sites (Kringelbach et al., 2007). The effectiveness of DBS or vagal nerve stimulation for depression is difficult to evaluate, because most studies have no placebo control (R. Robinson, 2009). In the few placebo-controlled studies, where the patient was unaware of whether electrical stimulation was provided, the treatment appeared to be less effective than it seemed in initial, uncontrolled reports (Kisely et al., 2018; Widge et al., 2018), suggesting that the promising early results of DBS and vagal stimulation may have been due to placebo effects.

Why do more females than males suffer from depression?

Studies all over the world show that more women than men suffer from major depression. In the United States, women are twice as likely as men to suffer major depression (CDC, 2010; Altemus et al., 2014). Some researchers suggest that the apparent sex difference reflects different patterns of help-seeking behavior by males and females—that women are willing to use health facilities, while men see that as a sign of weakness. But sex differences in the incidence of depression also are evident in door-to-door surveys (Robins and Regier, 1991), which would appear to rule out the simple explanation that women seek treatment more often than men do.

Some researchers have emphasized gender differences in endocrine physiology. The appearance of clinical depression often is related to events in the female reproductive cycle—for example, before menstruation, during use of contraceptive pills, following childbirth, and during menopause. Although there is little relation between circulating levels of individual hormones and measures of depression, the phenomenon of **postpartum depression**, a bout of depression immediately preceding and/or following childbirth, suggests that some combination of hormones can precipitate depression. About one out of every seven pregnant women will show symptoms of depression (Dietz et al., 2007). Because postpartum depression may affect the mother's

cognitive behavioral therapy (CBT) Psychotherapy aimed at correcting negative thinking and consciously changing behaviors as a way of changing feelings.

deep brain stimulation (DBS) Mild electrical stimulation through an electrode that is surgically implanted deep in the brain.

postpartum depression A bout of depression that afflicts a woman either immediately before or after giving birth.

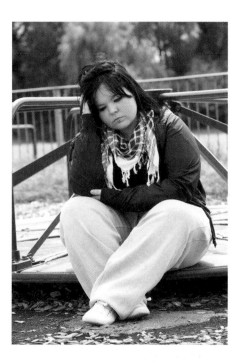

Depression For reasons that are not understood, women are more likely than men to suffer from depression. (© MBI/Alamy Stock Photo.)

RESEARCHERS AT WORK

The entirely accidental discovery of lithium therapy

The effect of lithium on bipolar disorder was discovered purely by accident when it was intended as an inert control in an experiment focusing on the urea in lithium urate (**FIGURE 12.17**), so the mechanism of action is not understood. Lithium has wide-ranging effects on the brain. Because lithium has a narrow range of safe doses (see Chapter 4), care must be taken to avoid toxic side effects of an overdose. Nevertheless, well-managed lithium treatment produces marked relief for many people with bipolar disorder and even has been reported to increase the volume of gray matter in their brains (G. J. Moore et al., 2000).

FIGURE 12.17   Surprisingly Calm Guinea Pigs (After J. F. Cade, 1949. *Med. J. Aust.* 2: 349.)

■ **Question**
Do people with bipolar disorder suffer from having too much urea in circulation?

■ **Hypothesis**
Injecting urea into guinea pigs will make them manic.

■ **Test**
Cade (1949) found that he could dissolve higher concentrations of urea into solution if he used a urea-lithium combination, lithium urate, rather than urea alone. Other guinea pigs got injections of lithium alone as a control group.

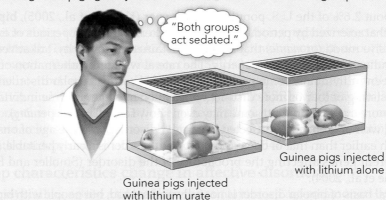

"Both groups act sedated."

Guinea pigs injected with lithium urate

Guinea pigs injected with lithium alone

■ **Results**
Instead of the lithium urate making the guinea pigs manic, it calmed them. But in another surprise, the control injections of lithium alone were just as effective for calming the animals (Howland, 2007). Intrigued, Cade took some lithium himself and, upon finding it harmless, tried giving it to patients with bipolar disorder. Almost all of the patients showed a remarkable recovery, and many who had been institutionalized for years could finally return home.

■ **Conclusion**
Lithium alone calms guinea pigs and relieves symptoms of bipolar disorder in humans. Note that this conclusion has nothing to do with the original question. This experiment demonstrates the importance of having a good control group. If Cade had not injected some guinea pigs with lithium alone, he might have wrongly concluded that urea has a calming effect.

The fact that the manic phases blocked by lithium are so exhilarating may be the reason that some people with bipolar disorder stop taking the medication. Unfortunately, doing so means that the depressive episodes return as well. As in depression, transcranial magnetic stimulation may provide a nonpharmacological treatment alternative in difficult cases of bipolar disorder (Michael and Erfurth, 2004). Furthermore, mounting evidence suggests that some forms of CBT for mild cases of bipolar disorder can be as effective as drug treatments (Hollon et al., 2002) and perhaps can be beneficially combined with other forms of treatment.

HOW'S IT GOING ?

1. What are the symptoms of depression, and how does depression differ from simple sadness?
2. What treatments for depression arose in the twentieth century, and which treatment is used most often today?
3. Summarize the evidence for and against the use of SSRIs in depression. Why is the use of SSRIs controversial?
4. What is bipolar disorder, and how does it compare with depression and with schizophrenia? How is it treated?

PART III
Anxiety Disorders

THE ROAD AHEAD

We conclude the chapter by considering anxiety disorders, among the most common of psychiatric conditions. The material will permit you to:

1. Describe the symptoms of several anxiety disorders.
2. Name the various medications used to treat anxiety disorders and their mechanisms of action.
3. Discuss the data indicating whether some people are initially more vulnerable to post-traumatic stress disorder (PTSD).
4. Describe the several treatments for obsessive-compulsive disorder (OCD), including controversial trials of brain surgery and stimulation.

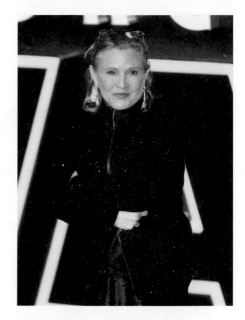

A Disturbance in the Force   Actress Carrie Fisher (1956–2016), who played Princess Leia/Leia Organa in five *Star Wars* movies, wrote about her struggles with bipolar disorder. (© Cpuk/Alamy Stock Photo.)

There Are Several Types of Anxiety Disorders

All of us have at times felt apprehensive and fearful. But some people experience this state with an intensity that is overwhelming and includes irrational fears; a sense of terror; body sensations such as dizziness, difficulty breathing, trembling, and shaking; and a feeling of loss of control. Anxiety can be lethal: men with panic disorder are more likely than others to die from cardiovascular disease or suicide (Coryell et al., 1986).

The *DSM-5* distinguishes several major types of **anxiety disorders**: *Phobic disorders* are intense, irrational fears that become centered on a specific object, activity, or situation that the person feels compelled to avoid. Another type of anxiety disorder is *panic disorder*, characterized by recurrent transient attacks of intense fearfulness. In *generalized anxiety disorder*, persistent, excessive anxiety and worry are experienced for months. There is a strong genetic contribution to each of these disorders (Shih et al., 2004; Oler et al., 2010) and distinctive underlying neurobiological predispositions to the development of anxiety disorders (Shackman et al., 2013).

Some people who suffer from recurrent panic attacks have temporal lobe abnormalities, especially in the left hemisphere (Vythilingam et al., 2000; Van Tol et al., 2010). Given the special role of the amygdala in mediating fear (see Chapter 11), changes may be particularly evident in the amygdala and associated circuitry within the temporal lobes (Rauch et al., 2003).

Drug treatments provide clues to the mechanisms of anxiety

Throughout history, people have consumed all sorts of substances in the hopes of controlling anxiety. The list includes alcohol, bromides, scopolamine, opiates, and

anxiety disorder   Any of a class of psychological disorders that includes recurrent panic states and generalized persistent anxiety disorder.

This PET scan of benzodiazepine receptors shows their wide distribution in the brain, especially the cortex. Highest concentrations are in red; lowest concentrations are in blue.

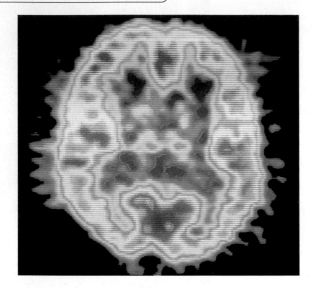

FIGURE 12.18 The Distribution of Benzodiazepine Receptors in the Human Brain (Courtesy of Goran Sedvall.)

barbiturates. In the 1950s the tranquilizing drug meprobamate (Miltown) was introduced, and it became an instant best seller, ushering in the modern age of anxiety pharmacotherapy. Soon researchers discovered a new class of drugs called **benzodiazepines**, which quickly replaced Miltown as the favored drugs for treating anxiety. One type of benzodiazepine—diazepam (trade name Valium)—is one of the most prescribed drugs in history. Other commonly prescribed benzodiazepines include Xanax, Halcion, and Ativan. Such drugs that combat anxiety are termed **anxiolytics** ("anxiety-dissolving"), although they also may have anticonvulsant and sleep-inducing properties. The anxiolytic drugs are also discussed in Chapter 4.

Anxiolytic benzodiazepines interact with binding sites that are part of GABA receptors, especially the $GABA_A$ receptors, where they act as noncompetitive agonists. Recall from Chapter 4 that GABA is the most common inhibitory transmitter in the brain. When GABA is released from a presynaptic terminal and activates postsynaptic receptors, it hyperpolarizes the target neuron and therefore inhibits it from firing. Benzodiazepines alone have little effect on the $GABA_A$ receptor, but when benzodiazepines are present, GABA produces a markedly enhanced hyperpolarization. In other words, benzodiazepines boost GABA-mediated postsynaptic inhibition, reducing the excitability of postsynaptic neurons.

Interestingly, the brain probably makes its own anxiety-relieving substances that interact with the benzodiazepine-binding site on the GABA receptor; the neurosteroid allopregnanolone is a prime candidate for this function. Drugs developed to act at this site are effective anxiolytics in both rats and humans (Rupprecht et al., 2009). As you can see in **FIGURE 12.18**, benzodiazepine/$GABA_A$ receptors are widely distributed throughout the brain, especially in the cerebral cortex and some subcortical areas, such as the hippocampus and the amygdala.

Although the benzodiazepines remain an important category of anxiolytics, especially for acute attacks, other anxiety-relieving drugs have been developed that lack the abuse potential of the benzodiazepines. A notable example is the drug buspirone (Buspar), an agonist at serotonin 5-HT_{1A} receptors that can provide relief from anxiety. This effect is consistent with functional-imaging research that reveals an abnormal density of 5-HT_{1A} receptors in the brains of people with anxiety disorders (Neumeister et al., 2004). SSRI antidepressants, such as paroxetine (Paxil) and fluoxetine (Prozac), which increase the stimulation of serotonin receptors, are also sometimes effective treatments for anxiety disorders.

In Post-Traumatic Stress Disorder, Horrible Memories Won't Go Away

Some people experience especially awful moments in life that seem indelible, resulting in vivid impressions that persist the rest of their lives. The kind of event that seems particularly likely to produce subsequent stress disorders is intense and is usually associated with witnessing abusive violence and/or death. Examples include the sudden loss of a close friend, rape, torture, kidnapping, or profound social dislocation, such as in forced migration. In these cases, memories of horrible events intrude into consciousness and produce the same intense visceral arousal—the fear and trembling and general autonomic activation—that the original event caused. These traumatic memories are easily reawakened by stressful circumstances and even by harmless stimuli that somehow prompt recollection of the original event. An ever watchful and fearful stance becomes the portrait of individuals afflicted with what is called **post-traumatic stress disorder** (**PTSD**), formerly called *combat fatigue, war neurosis,* or *shell shock.* Although related in

benzodiazepine Any of a class of antianxiety drugs that are noncompetitive agonists of $GABA_A$ receptors in the central nervous system. One example is diazepam (Valium).

anxiolytic A substance that is used to reduce anxiety. Examples include alcohol, opiates, barbiturates, and the benzodiazepines.

post-traumatic stress disorder (**PTSD**) A disorder in which memories of an unpleasant episode repeatedly plague the victim.

some ways to anxiety disorders, post-traumatic stress disorder is now recognized in the *DSM-5* as a separate entity.

Analysis of a random sample of Vietnam War veterans has indicated that 19% had PTSD at some point after service. This was the rate for *all* Vietnam veterans; when the researchers focused more specifically on veterans exposed to intense war zone stressors, more than 35% developed PTSD at some point, and most of them were still suffering from the disorder *decades* later (Dohrenwend et al., 2006). More recently, it has been found that Gulf War veterans likewise suffer from high rates of PTSD (Institute of Medicine, 2010).

Genetic factors affect vulnerability to PTSD, as indicated in twin studies of Vietnam War veterans who had seen combat, which showed that monozygotic twins were more similar than dizygotic twins. People who display combat-related PTSD show (1) memory changes such as amnesia for some war experiences, (2) flashbacks, and (3) deficits in short-term memory. These memory disturbances suggest involvement of the hippocampus (see Chapter 13), and indeed the volume of the right hippocampus is smaller in combat veterans with PTSD than in those without it, with no differences in other brain regions (Bremner et al., 1995). It was once widely assumed that stressful episodes caused the hippocampus to shrink, but some veterans suffering PTSD had left their monozygotic twins at home, and it turns out that the nonstressed twins without PTSD also tended to have a smaller hippocampus (Gilbertson et al., 2002). So some inherited characteristic that's associated with having a small hippocampus, and perhaps a reduced rate of adult neurogenesis (Snyder et al., 2011; Kheirbek et al., 2012), may increase susceptibility to developing PTSD if the person is exposed to stress. In Gulf War veterans with more severe PTSD, marked hippocampal size difference is associated with markers of inflammatory processes (O'Donovan et al., 2015), which can strongly contribute to neural degeneration and decreased neurogenesis.

A comprehensive psychobiological model of the development of PTSD draws connections from PTSD's memory disturbances to the neural mechanisms of fear conditioning, behavioral sensitization, and extinction (Charney et al., 1993). Work in animals has revealed that **fear conditioning**—memory for a stimulus that the animal has learned to associate with a negative event—is very persistent and involves the amygdala and brainstem pathways that are part of a circuit of startle response behavior (see Chapter 11). The persistence of memory and fear in PTSD may depend on the failure of mechanisms to *forget*. There is also a hormonal link, because PTSD sufferers exhibit a paradoxical long-term *reduction* in cortisol (stress hormone) levels (Yehuda, 2002), perhaps due to persistent increases in *sensitivity* to cortisol. If, as a result, they feel the effect of stress hormones more strongly than other people do, that greater effect might repeatedly retrigger the fear response, making it harder for them to forget stressful events (**FIGURE 12.19**). In Chapter 13 we will discuss research-based methods that have been proposed to help people forget traumatic life events by having them recall the event while under the influence of a drug that dampens the stress response.

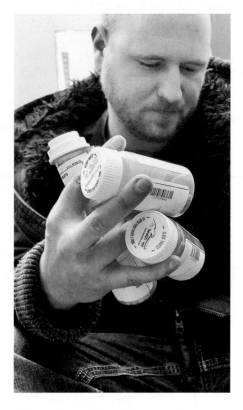

Delayed Reaction   Many combat veterans suffer from PTSD for years afterward. (© ZUMA Press Inc./Alamy Stock Photo.)

fear conditioning   A form of classical conditioning in which fear comes to be associated with previously neutral stimuli.

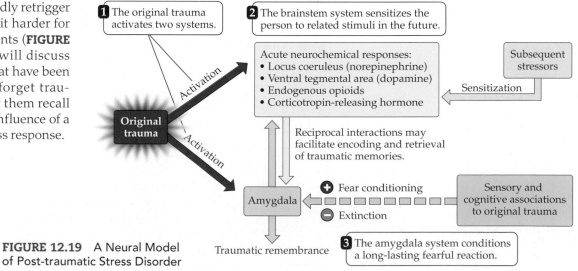

FIGURE 12.19   A Neural Model of Post-traumatic Stress Disorder

In Obsessive-Compulsive Disorder, Thoughts and Acts Keep Repeating

Most of us aspire to be neat and clean, especially when we discover a thick layer of dust under the furniture or perhaps realize we've created yet another tottering pile of papers and bills. And of course, having certain small rituals in our lives—making coffee a certain way in the morning, wishing everyone good night before going to bed—can be a comfort amid the chaos of daily life. But when do orderliness and routine cross the line into pathology? People with **obsessive-compulsive disorder** (OCD) lead lives riddled with repetitive rituals and persistent thoughts that they feel powerless to control or stop, despite recognizing that the behaviors are abnormal. In people with OCD, routine acts that we all engage in, such as checking whether the door is locked when we leave our home, become *compulsions*, acts that are repeated over and over. Recurrent thoughts, or *obsessions*, such as fears of germs or other potential harms in the world, invade the consciousness. These symptoms progressively isolate a person from ordinary social engagement with the world. For many people with OCD, hours each day are consumed by compulsive acts such as repetitive hand washing. **TABLE 12.4** summarizes some of the symptoms of OCD.

Determining the number of people afflicted with OCD is difficult, especially because people with this disorder tend to hide their symptoms (Rapoport, 1989). It is estimated that nearly 1% of adults in the United States will suffer from "severe" OCD in any given year (Kessler et al., 2005). In many cases, the initial symptoms of this disorder appear in childhood; the peak age group for onset of OCD, however, is 25–44

obsessive-compulsive disorder (OCD)   An anxiety disorder in which the affected individual experiences recurrent unwanted thoughts and engages in repetitive behaviors without reason or the ability to stop.

TABLE 12.4 ■ Symptoms of Obsessive-Compulsive Disorder

Symptoms (most to least common by type)

OBSESSIONS (thoughts)
Dirt, germs, or environmental toxins
Something terrible happening (e.g., fire, death or illness of self or loved one)
Symmetry, order, or exactness
Religious obsessions
Body wastes or secretions (urine, stool, saliva, etc.)
Lucky or unlucky numbers
Forbidden, aggressive, or perverse sexual thoughts, images, or impulses
Fear of harming self or others
Household items
Intrusive nonsense sounds, words, or music

COMPULSIONS (acts)
Performing excessive or ritualized hand washing, showering, bathing, tooth brushing, or grooming
Repeating rituals (e.g., going in or out of a door, getting up from or sitting down on a chair)
Checking (doors, locks, stove, appliances, emergency brake on car, paper route, homework, etc.)
Engaging in miscellaneous rituals (such as writing, moving, speaking)
Decontaminating
Touching
Counting
Ordering or arranging
Preventing harm to self or others
Hoarding or collecting
Cleaning household or inanimate objects

Source: After S. E. Swedo et al., 1989. Arch. Gen. Psychiatry 46: 335.

years. People with OCD display increased metabolic rates in the orbitofrontal cortex, cingulate cortex, and caudate nuclei (Chamberlain et al., 2008).

Happily, OCD responds to treatment in most cases. OCD shows excellent response to cognitive behavioral therapy (Öst et al., 2016; Abramowitz et al., 2018) and also to several drugs. What do effective OCD drugs—like fluoxetine (Prozac), fluvoxamine (Luvox), and clomipramine (Anafranil)—tend to have in common? They share the ability to inhibit the reuptake of serotonin at serotonergic synapses, thereby increasing the synaptic availability of serotonin. This observation suggests that the dysfunction of serotonergic neurotransmission plays a central role in OCD. Recall that we already discussed SSRIs like Prozac that inhibit the reuptake of serotonin when we discussed treatments for depression. How can the same drug help two disorders that seem so different? For one thing, depression often accompanies OCD, so the two disorders may be related. Furthermore, functional brain imaging suggests that the same SSRI drugs alter the activity of the orbitofrontal prefrontal cortex in people with OCD (Saxena et al., 2001) while affecting primarily ventrolateral prefrontal cortex in people with depression.

There is a heritable genetic component to OCD; as with schizophrenia and depression, several genes may contribute to susceptibility to this disorder (Pauls et al., 2014), including genes related to serotonin signaling (Sinopoli et al., 2017). There is also evidence that OCD can be triggered by infections (Orlovska et al., 2017). Upon observing that numerous children exhibiting OCD symptoms had recently been treated for strep throat, Dale et al. (2005) found that many children with OCD are producing antibodies to brain proteins. Perhaps, in mounting an immune response to the streptococcal bacteria, these children also make antibodies that attack their own brains. The genetic link may be that some people are more likely than others to produce antibodies to the brain proteins.

In recent years, deep brain stimulation (DBS) has been tried for many psychiatric disorders that do not respond to medication, and OCD is no exception. But again there are few participants and many of the studies have no control condition (when no stimulation is provided to the electrode), so it is difficult to assess whether the DBS is effective (Naesström et al., 2016). Psychosurgery may be a treatment of last resort. Unlike lobotomies, these surgeries target much smaller regions. In one study, about one-third of severely disabled patients with OCD who underwent cingulotomy (making lesions that interrupt pathways in the cingulate cortex) (**FIGURE 12.20**) benefited (Shah et al., 2008; Pepper et al., 2015). Even here it is difficult to rule out a placebo effect of the cingulotomy, as you cannot ethically ask some people to undergo sham neurosurgery, opening up their skull to then *not* make a lesion, to provide a control group. Frontal lobotomy, which causes much more extensive damage to the brain, is virtually never performed today. So we can be pretty confident that no one else will suffer the fate of Howard Dully, lobotomized for being a teenager.

Many researchers also believe that OCD and another disease involving repetitive behaviors, Tourette's syndrome, are part of a spectrum of related disorders (Olson, 2004). OCD and Tourette's are often comorbid (occurring together), and both disorders involve abnormalities of the basal ganglia. However, drug therapy in Tourette's syndrome has typically focused on modifying the actions of dopamine rather than of serotonin (**BOX 12.2**).

FIGURE 12.20 Neurosurgery to Treat Obsessive-Compulsive Disorder (From Martuza et al., 1990, courtesy of Robert L. Martuza.)

These MRIs show the brain of a person who underwent a cingulotomy—the disruption of cingulate cortex connections—in an attempt to treat OCD.

(A) Horizontal view
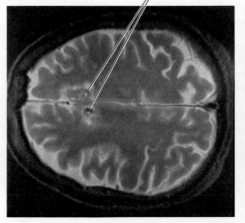

(B) Sagittal view
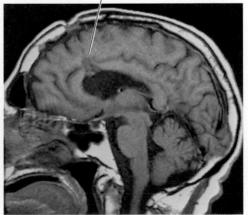

BOX 12.2
Tics, Twitches, and Snorts:
The Unusual Character of Tourette's Syndrome

Their faces twitch in an insistent way, and every now and then, out of nowhere, they blurt out an odd sound. At times they fling their arms, kick their legs, or make violent shoulder movements. People with **Tourette's syndrome** are also supersensitive to tactile, auditory, and visual stimuli (J. H. Cox et al., 2018). Many people with Tourette's report that an urge to emit verbal or phonic tics builds up and that giving in to the urge brings relief. Although popular media often portray people with Tourette's as shouting out insults and profanities (a symptom called *coprolalia*), verbal tics of that sort are rare.

Tourette's syndrome begins early in life; the mean age of diagnosis is 6–7 years (De Groot et al., 1995), and the syndrome is 3–4 times more common in males than in females. **FIGURE A** draws a portrait of the chronology of symptoms. Often people with Tourette's also exhibit attention deficit hyperactivity disorder (ADHD) or OCD (Eapen et al., 2016). Children with Tourette's display a thinning of primary somatosensory and motor cortex representing facial, oral, and laryngeal structures (Sowell et al., 2008), suggesting that the tics mediated by these regions may be underinhibited by cortex.

Family studies indicate that genetics plays an important role in this disorder. Among discordant monozygotic twin pairs, the twin with Tourette's has a greater density of dopamine D_2 receptors in the caudate nucleus of the basal ganglia than the unaffected twin has (Wolf et al., 1996). This observation suggests that differences in the dopaminergic system (Mogwitz et al., 2013), especially in the basal ganglia (Maia and Conceição, 2018), may be important (D_2 receptor binding in an affected individual is illustrated in **FIGURE B**). The contemporary view is that Tourette's syndrome is mediated in a complex manner by many genes rather than just one (Hallett, 2015; Qi et al., 2017).

Treatment with haloperidol, a dopamine D_2 receptor antagonist that is better known as a first-generation antipsychotic drug (see Figure 12.10), significantly reduces tic frequency and is a primary treatment for Tourette's syndrome. Unfortunately, this treatment can have unpleasant side effects (as noted in Box 12.1), but some people with Tourette's also respond well to the second-generation antipsychotics, which may bring fewer side effects. Behavior modification techniques aimed at reducing the frequency of symptoms, especially tics, help some people learn how to replace their obvious tics with behaviors that are more subtle and socially acceptable (McGuire et al., 2015).

DBS, which we mentioned in the text, may also benefit people with Tourette's. In this case, battery-powered stimulating electrodes are aimed bilaterally at targets within the thalamus, in regions associated with the control of movement. Activation of the electrodes can bring dramatic and almost immediate relief from symptoms (Porta et al., 2009; Baldermann et al., 2016). (Figure B from S. S. Wolf et al., 1996. *Science* 273: 1225. Courtesy of Steven Wolf.)

(A) The chronology of Tourette's symptoms

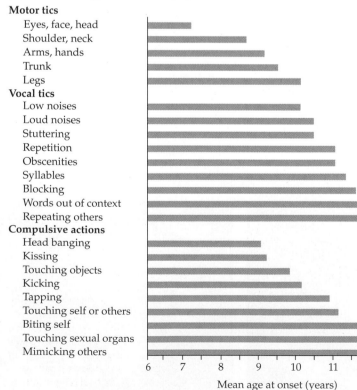

Mean age at onset (years)

(B) D_2 receptor binding in Tourette's syndrome

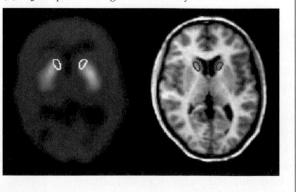

HOW'S IT GOING ?

1. What are the main types of anxiety disorders?
2. What class of drugs is the most common anxiolytic, and what effect do these drugs have on transmitter systems?
3. Describe PTSD and the hypothesis that the disorder is a special case of fear conditioning.
4. What is OCD, and what treatments are available to combat it?

Tourette's syndrome A disorder involving heightened sensitivity to sensory stimuli that may be accompanied by verbal or physical tics.

To view the activity
Concept Matching: Psychopathology,
go to
3e.mindsmachine.com/ac12.1

Recommended Reading

Charney, D. S., Nestler, E. J., Sklar, P., and Buxbaum, J. D. (Eds.). (2018). *Charney & Nestler's Neurobiology of Mental Illness* (5th ed.). New York, NY: Oxford University Press.

Hersen, M., Beidel, D. C., and McCarthy, G. (2014). *Adult Psychopathology and Diagnosis* (7th ed.). New York, NY: Wiley.

Huettel, S. A., Song, A. W., and McCarthy, G. (2014). *Functional Magnetic Resonance Imaging* (3rd ed.). Sunderland, MA: Oxford University Press/Sinauer.

Martino, D., and Leckman, J. F. (Eds.). (2013). *Tourette Syndrome.* Oxford, UK: Oxford University Press.

Meyer, J. S., and Quenzer, L. F. (2018). *Psychopharmacology: Drugs, the Brain, and Behavior* (3rd ed.). Sunderland, MA: Oxford University Press/Sinauer.

Solomon, A. (2001). *The Noonday Demon: An Atlas of Depression.* New York, NY: Scribner.

Steketee, G. (Ed.). (2011). *The Oxford Handbook of Obsessive Compulsive and Spectrum Disorders.* New York, NY: Oxford University Press.

12 ■ Visual Summary   3e.mindsmachine.com/vs12

You should be able to relate each summary to the adjacent illustration, including structures and processes.
If you go to the website for our text (**3e.mindsmachine.com**), you can follow links to figures,
animations, and activities that will help you consolidate the material.

1 Population studies find that psychiatric disorders are prevalent in modern society. Studies of families, twins, and adoptees demonstrate a strong role of genetic factors in **schizophrenia**. Rather than a single gene determining whether a person will develop schizophrenia, several genes contribute to the risk. Review **Figures 12.1** and **12.2**, **Table 12.1**, **Animation 12.2**

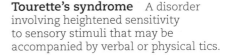

2 Structural changes in the brains of people with schizophrenia—including enlarged ventricles—may arise from early developmental problems. The emergence of schizophrenia depends on the interaction of genes that make a person vulnerable to environmental stressors. Review **Figures 12.3–12.8**

3 The frontal lobes are less active in people with schizophrenia than in people without it. Biochemical theories of schizophrenia emphasize the importance of the dopamine, glutamate, and serotonin receptors. **First-generation antipsychotics** block dopamine D_2 receptors, while **second-generation antipsychotics** block serotonin 5-HT_{2A} receptors in addition to acting on dopamine receptors. Review **Figures 12.9–12.12**, **Box 12.1**, **Video 12.3**

4 **Depression** also has a strong genetic factor. Serotonin has been implicated in this disorder. In general, females are more likely than males to suffer from depression. People suffering from depression show increased activity in the frontal cortex and the amygdala, as well as disrupted sleep patterns. Review **Figures 12.13–12.16**

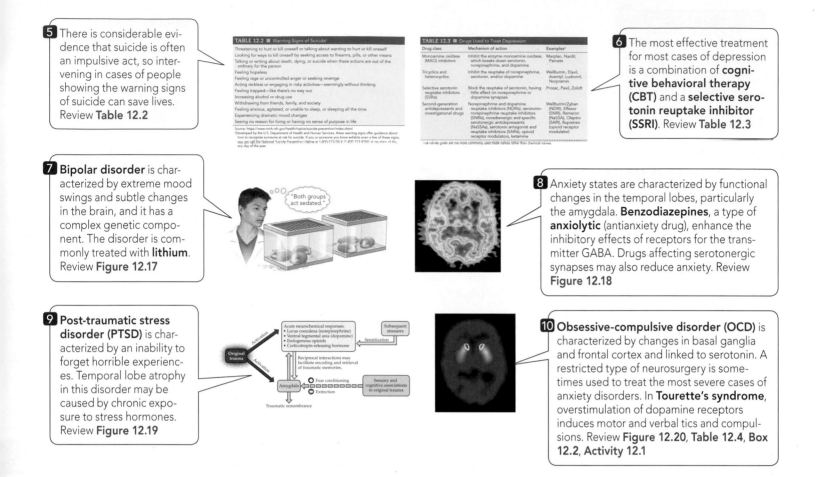

5 There is considerable evidence that suicide is often an impulsive act, so intervening in cases of people showing the warning signs of suicide can save lives. Review **Table 12.2**

6 The most effective treatment for most cases of depression is a combination of **cognitive behavioral therapy (CBT)** and a **selective serotonin reuptake inhibitor (SSRI)**. Review **Table 12.3**

7 **Bipolar disorder** is characterized by extreme mood swings and subtle changes in the brain, and it has a complex genetic component. The disorder is commonly treated with **lithium**. Review **Figure 12.17**

"Both groups act sedated."

8 Anxiety states are characterized by functional changes in the temporal lobes, particularly the amygdala. **Benzodiazepines**, a type of **anxiolytic** (antianxiety drug), enhance the inhibitory effects of receptors for the transmitter GABA. Drugs affecting serotonergic synapses may also reduce anxiety. Review **Figure 12.18**

9 **Post-traumatic stress disorder (PTSD)** is characterized by an inability to forget horrible experiences. Temporal lobe atrophy in this disorder may be caused by chronic exposure to stress hormones. Review **Figure 12.19**

10 **Obsessive-compulsive disorder (OCD)** is characterized by changes in basal ganglia and frontal cortex and linked to serotonin. A restricted type of neurosurgery is sometimes used to treat the most severe cases of anxiety disorders. In **Tourette's syndrome**, overstimulation of dopamine receptors induces motor and verbal tics and compulsions. Review **Figure 12.20**, **Table 12.4**, **Box 12.2**, **Activity 12.1**

Go to **3e.mindsmachine.com** for study questions, quizzes, flashcards, and other resources.

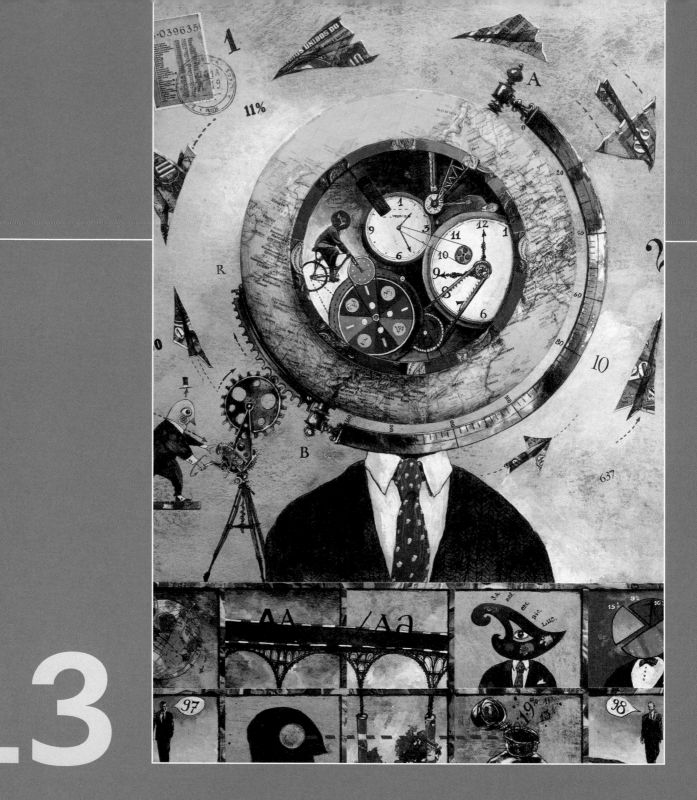

13

Memory, Learning, and Development

Trapped in the Eternal Now

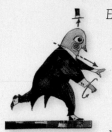

Every day is alone in itself, whatever enjoyment I've had, and whatever sorrow I've had…. Right now, I'm wondering, have I done or said anything amiss? You see, at this moment everything looks clear to me, but what happened just before? That's what worries me. It's like waking from a dream. I just don't remember.

—Henry Molaison (B. Milner, 1970, p. 37)

Known as "Patient H.M." in a classic series of research articles, Henry Molaison was probably the most famous research participant in the history of neuroscience. Henry started to suffer seizures during adolescence, and by his late twenties, his epilepsy was out of control. Because tests showed that Henry's seizures began in both temporal lobes, a neurosurgeon removed most of the anterior temporal lobes in 1953.

Henry's surgery relieved his epilepsy, but that relief came at a terrible, unforeseen price: He couldn't seem to form new memories (Scoville and Milner, 1957). For more than 50 years after the surgery, until his death in 2008, Henry could retain any new fact only briefly; as soon as he was distracted, the newly acquired information vanished. He didn't know his age or the current date. For a while, he carried a note reminding himself that his father had died and his mother was in a retirement home. Henry knew that something was wrong with him, because he had no memories from the years since his surgery, or even memories from earlier the same day, as the quote above indicates.

Henry's inability to form new memories meant that he couldn't have a lasting relationship with anybody new. No matter what experiences he might share with someone he met, Henry would have to start the acquaintance anew the following day, because he would have no recollection of ever meeting the person before. In some ways, this dreadful loss of memory ended Henry's journey as a human being—he could no longer grow in his experience of historical events, his friendships, or even a sense of his own life story.

What happened to Henry, and what does his experience teach us about learning and memory?

All the distinctively human aspects of our behavior are learned: the languages we speak, how we dress, the foods we eat and how we eat them, our skills, and the ways we reach our goals. So much of our own individuality depends on learning and memory. We begin this chapter with a discussion of memory because research in the twentieth century revealed that there are fundamentally different types of memory. In Part II we delve into what we know about how learning alters the structure of the brain, which differs for different types of memory. Part III takes up the fascinating story of brain development and the stupendous rate at which our brains grow, allowing us to learn and remember the masses of information that make us into unique human beings.

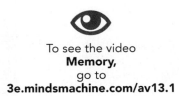

To see the video
Memory,
go to
3e.mindsmachine.com/av13.1

To view the
Brain Explorer,
go to
3e.mindsmachine.com/av13.2

PART I
Types of Learning and Memory

THE ROAD AHEAD

We begin our discussion about learning and memory by examining how they fail. Studying this material should allow you to:

1. Understand the two kinds of amnesia and the two fundamentally different categories of memory.
2. Review the evidence that a particular brain circuit is crucial for forming some types of memory.
3. Understand the two subtypes of declarative memories, which we can describe to other people.
4. List the stages of memory formation and the vulnerability for losing information at each stage.
5. Describe a model of how we encode, consolidate, and retrieve memories.

There Are Several Kinds of Learning and Memory

The terms **learning**, the process of acquiring new information, and **memory**, the ability to store and retrieve that information, are so often paired that it sometimes seems as if one necessarily implies the other. We cannot be sure that learning has occurred unless a memory can be elicited later. Many kinds of brain damage, caused by disease or accident, impair both learning and memory. We'll start by looking at some brain damage cases that revealed different classes of learning and memory.

For Patient H.M., the present vanished into oblivion

Amnesia (Greek for "forgetfulness") is a severe impairment of memory, usually as a result of accident or disease. Loss of memories that formed prior to an event (such as surgery or trauma)—called **retrograde amnesia** (from the Latin *retro*, "backward," and *gradi*, "to go")—is not uncommon. After

(A)

Hippocampus is Latin for "sea horse," and you can see how the brain structure resembles that animal.

Hippocampus

Temporal lobe

Mammillary body

Cerebellum

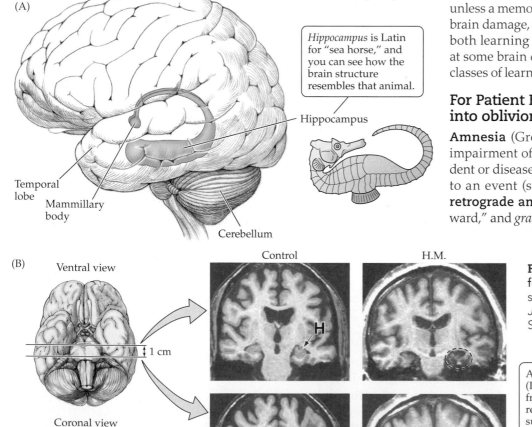

(B)

Ventral view

Coronal view

1 cm

Control   H.M.

H

H

Cer

FIGURE 13.1   Brain Regions Crucial for Forming New Memories (Brain scans from S. Corkin et al., 1997. *J. Neurosci.*, 17, 3964. Courtesy of Suzanne Corkin.)

As a young man, Henry Molaison (Patient H.M.) had the hippocampus (H) from both hemispheres surgically removed, with disastrous results. The surgeons did not remove the cerebellum (Cer), but the loss of hippocampal inputs caused it to shrink as he aged.

an accident that damages the brain, people often have retrograde amnesia regarding events that happened a few hours or days before the accident, or even a year before. Despite dramatic depictions you may see on TV, it is unlikely that longer-term (or "complete") retrograde memory loss has ever occurred.

Patient H.M.—Henry Molaison, whom we met at the start of the chapter—suffered from a far more unusual symptom. In Henry's case, most old memories remained intact, but he had difficulty recollecting any events that took place *after* his surgery. What's more, he was unable to retain any new material for more than a brief period. The inability to form new memories after an event is called **anterograde amnesia** (the Latin *antero* means "forward").

Over the very short term, Henry's memory was normal. If given a series of six or seven digits, he could immediately repeat the list without error. But when he was given a list of words to study and then tested on them after being distracted by another task, he could not repeat the list or even recall that there *was* a list. So Henry's case provided clear evidence that *short-term memory* differs from *long-term memory*—a distinction, long recognized by psychologists on behavioral grounds (W. James, 1890), that we will discuss in more depth later in this chapter.

Henry's surgery removed the amygdala, most of the hippocampus, and surrounding cortex from both temporal lobes (**FIGURE 13.1**). The memory deficit seemed to be caused by loss of the *medial temporal lobe*, including the **hippocampus**, because people who had only the lateral temporal cortex removed had no memory impairment. Despite his obvious memory problems, Henry showed noticeable improvement over days of practice on a mirror-tracing task (**FIGURE 13.2A**) (B. Milner, 1965). Each day, when asked if he remembered the test, Henry said no, yet his performance was better than at the start of the first day (**FIGURE 13.2B**). So, was Henry's memory loss limited to tasks that relied on verbal processing? Not quite. For example, people with amnesia like Henry's can learn the skill of *reading* mirror-reversed text (**FIGURE 13.3**), which is a verbal task.

learning   The process of acquiring new and relatively enduring information, behavior patterns, or abilities, characterized by modifications of behavior as a result of practice, study, or experience.

memory   1. The ability to learn and neurally encode information, consolidate the information for longer-term storage, and retrieve or reactivate the consolidated information at a later time. 2. The specific information that is stored in the brain.

amnesia   Severe impairment of memory.

retrograde amnesia   Difficulty in retrieving memories formed before the onset of amnesia.

Patient H.M.   The late Henry Molaison, a man who was unable to encode new declarative memories because of surgical removal of medial temporal lobe structures.

anterograde amnesia   Difficulty in forming new memories beginning with the onset of a disorder.

hippocampus   A medial temporal lobe structure that is important for learning and memory.

(A)

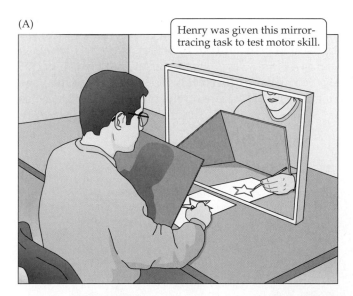

Henry was given this mirror-tracing task to test motor skill.

FIGURE 13.2 Henry's Performance on a Mirror-Tracing Task (After B. Milner, 1965 in P. M. Milner and S. E. Glickman (Eds.), *Cognitive processes and the brain; an enduring problem in psychology* (pp. 97-111). Van Nostrand. USA.)

(B)

Although Henry never recognized the task, his performance progressively improved over successive days, demonstrating a type of long-term memory.

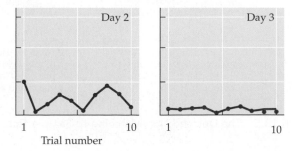

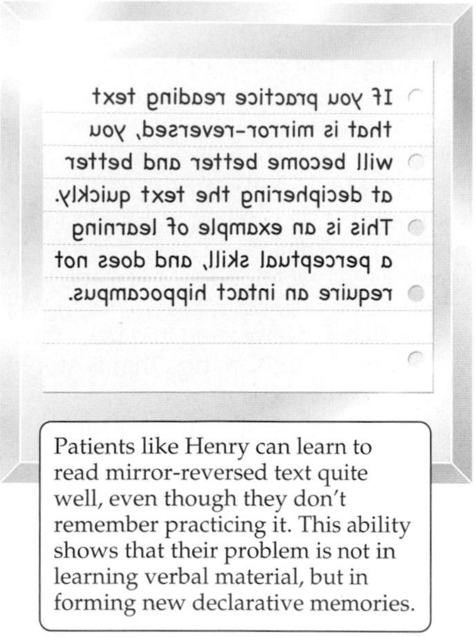

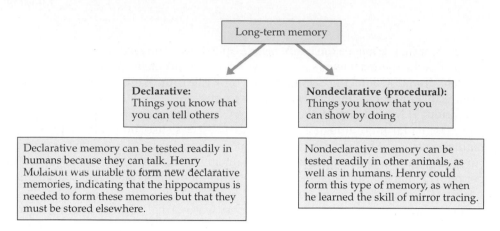

FIGURE 13.4 Two Main Kinds of Memory: Declarative and Nondeclarative

Patients like Henry can learn to read mirror-reversed text quite well, even though they don't remember practicing it. This ability shows that their problem is not in learning verbal material, but in forming new declarative memories.

FIGURE 13.3 Reading Mirror-Reversed Text

declarative memory A memory that can be stated or described.

nondeclarative memory Also called *procedural memory*. A memory that is shown by performance rather than by conscious recollection.

delayed non-matching-to-sample task A test in which the individual must respond to the unfamiliar stimulus in a pair of stimuli.

The important distinction in Henry's deficit is not between motor and verbal performances, but rather between two general categories of memory:

1. **Declarative memory** is what we usually think of as memory: facts and information acquired through learning. It is memory we are aware of accessing, which we can *declare* to others. This is the type of memory that was so profoundly impaired by Henry's surgery. Tests of declarative memory take the form of requests for specific information that was learned previously. It is the type of memory we use to answer "what" questions—and thus is difficult to test in animals.

2. **Nondeclarative memory**, or *procedural memory*—that is, memory about perceptual or motor procedures—is shown by *performance* rather than by conscious recollection. Examples of procedural memory include learning the mirror-tracing task, at which Henry excelled, and the skill of mirror reading or riding a bike (**FIGURE 13.4**). It is the type of memory we use for "how" problems and is often (but not always) nonverbal.

A clever way to measure declarative memory in monkeys and other animals is the **delayed non-matching-to-sample task** (**FIGURE 13.5**), a test of *object recognition* that requires monkeys to declare what they remember by identifying which of two objects was *not* seen previously (Spiegler and Mishkin, 1981). Monkeys with damage to the medial temporal lobe, similar to H.M., are severely impaired on this task, as we'll see next.

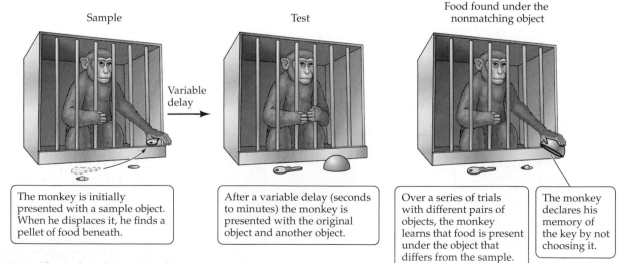

FIGURE 13.5 The Delayed Non-Matching-to-Sample Task

Which brain structures are important for declarative memory?

To determine which parts of the temporal lobe are crucial for declarative memory, researchers selectively removed specific parts of the medial temporal lobes of monkeys to confirm that the amygdala—one of the structures removed in Henry's surgery—is *not* crucial for performance on tests of declarative memory. However, removal of the adjacent hippocampus significantly impaired performance on these tests and, as shown in **FIGURE 13.6**, the deficit was even more pronounced when the hippocampal damage was paired with lesions of nearby cortical regions that communicate with the hippocampus: entorhinal, parahippocampal, and

perirhinal cortices (Zola-Morgan et al., 1994). Humans similarly show larger impairments when both the hippocampus and medial temporal cortex are damaged (Zola-Morgan and Squire, 1986; Rempel-Clower et al., 1996). So Henry's symptoms were probably caused by loss of the medial temporal lobe on both sides of the brain.

The experiments with monkeys, together with Henry's case, indicate that we need at least one intact medial temporal lobe (including the hippocampus) in order to make new declarative memories.

FIGURE 13.6 Memory Performance after Medial Temporal Lobe Lesions (Part A after L. R. Squire and S. Zola-Morgan, 1991. *Science* 253: 1380; B after S. Zola-Morgan, et al., 1994. *Hippocampus* 4: 482.)

■ **Hypothesis**
Particular portions of the medial temporal lobe are required for the formation of new declarative memories.

■ **Test**
Selectively remove different portions of the temporal lobe from both sides of the brain, and test for declarative memories using the delayed non-matching-to-sample task (see Figure 13.5).

■ **Result**

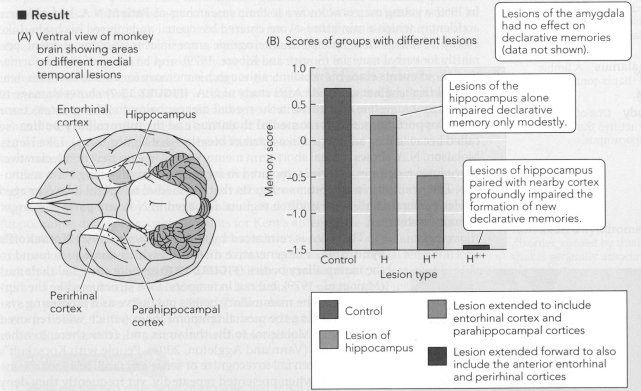

(A) Ventral view of monkey brain showing areas of different medial temporal lesions

Entorhinal cortex
Hippocampus
Perirhinal cortex
Parahippocampal cortex

(B) Scores of groups with different lesions

Memory score

Control H H⁺ H⁺⁺
Lesion type

Lesions of the amygdala had no effect on declarative memories (data not shown).

Lesions of the hippocampus alone impaired declarative memory only modestly.

Lesions of hippocampus paired with nearby cortex profoundly impaired the formation of new declarative memories.

Control
Lesion of hippocampus
Lesion extended to include entorhinal cortex and parahippocampal cortices
Lesion extended forward to also include the anterior entorhinal and perirhinal cortices

■ **Conclusion**
The severe disruption of new declarative memories in Henry Molaison and patients like him is due to damage to both the hippocampus itself and to nearby cortex. But these regions aren't the only brain structures needed for new declarative memories, as we'll see next.

To view the activity
The "Tower of Hanoi" Problem,
go to
3e.mindsmachine.com/ac13.1

skill learning The process of learning to perform a challenging task simply by repeating it over and over.

basal ganglia A group of forebrain nuclei, including the caudate nucleus, globus pallidus, and putamen, found deep within the cerebral hemispheres. They are crucial for skill learning.

priming Also called *repetition priming*. The phenomenon by which exposure to a stimulus facilitates subsequent responses to the same or a similar stimulus.

associative learning A type of learning in which an association is formed between two stimuli or between a stimulus and a response. It includes both classical and instrumental conditioning.

classical conditioning Also called *Pavlovian conditioning*. A type of associative learning in which an originally neutral stimulus acquires the power to elicit a conditioned response when presented alone.

cerebellum A structure located at the back of the brain, dorsal to the pons, that is involved in the central regulation of movement and in some forms of learning.

Different Forms of Nondeclarative Memory Involve Different Brain Regions

So far, we've seen that there are two different kinds of declarative memory: semantic and episodic. Likewise, there are several different types of nondeclarative memory, and we'll see that different brain regions are involved in these different forms.

Different types of nondeclarative memory serve varying functions

Skill learning is the process of learning how to perform a challenging task simply by repeating it over and over. Improving at the mirror-tracing task performed by Henry Molaison (see Figure 13.2) or learning to read mirror-reversed text (see Figure 13.3) are examples of skill learning. So too is the acquisition of everyday skills like learning to ride a bike or to juggle (well, okay, maybe juggling isn't an "everyday" skill, but you get the idea).

Imaging studies have investigated learning and memory for different kinds of skills, including *sensorimotor skills* (e.g., mirror tracing), *perceptual skills* (e.g., reading mirror-reversed text), and *cognitive skills* (tasks involving planning and problem solving, common in puzzles like the Tower of Hanoi problem, which you can play in Activity 13.2, on the website). All three kinds of skill learning are impaired in people with damage to the **basal ganglia** (see Figure 2.14A). Damage to other brain regions, especially the motor cortex and cerebellum, also affects aspects of some skills. Neuroimaging studies confirm that the basal ganglia, cerebellum, and motor cortex are important for sensorimotor skill learning (Makino et al., 2016; Spampinato and Celnik, 2018).

Priming (or *repetition priming*) is a change in the way you process a stimulus, usually a word or a picture, because you've seen it, or something similar, previously. For example, if a person is shown the word *stamp* in a list and later is asked to complete the word stem *STA-*, then she is more likely to reply "stamp" than, say, "start." Priming does not require declarative memory of the stimulus—Henry Molaison and other people with amnesia have shown priming for words they don't remember having seen. In contrast with skill learning, priming is not impaired by damage to the basal ganglia. In functional-imaging studies, perceptual priming (priming based on the visual *form* of words) is related to reduced activity in bilateral occipitotemporal cortex (Schacter et al., 2007), while conceptual priming (priming based on word *meaning*) is associated with reduced activation of the left frontal cortex (Buckner and Koutstaal, 1998). So priming appears to be at least partly a function of the cortex.

Other types of nondeclarative memories include learning that involves relations between events—for example, between two or more stimuli, between a stimulus and

FIGURE 13.9 Pavlovian (Classical) Conditioning

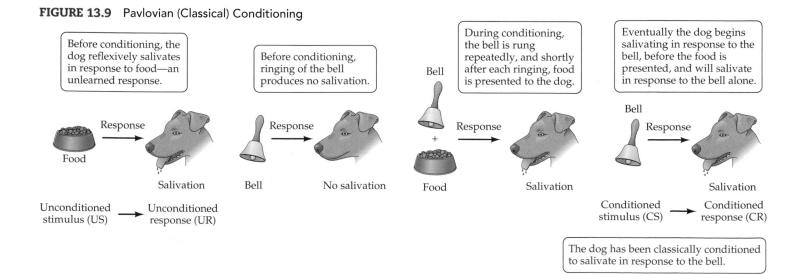

a response, or between a response and its consequence—and is called **associative learning**. In the best-studied form, **classical conditioning**, an initially neutral stimulus comes to predict an event. In famous experiments, Ivan Pavlov (1849–1936) found that a dog would learn to salivate when presented with an auditory or visual stimulus if the stimulus came to predict the presentation of food. So, repeatedly ringing a bell before putting meat powder in a dog's mouth will eventually cause the dog to start salivating when it hears the bell alone. In this case the meat powder in the mouth is called the *unconditioned stimulus* (*US*), which already evokes an *unconditioned response* (*UR*; salivation in this example). The sound of the bell is called the *conditioned stimulus* (*CS*), and the learned response to the CS alone (salivation in response to the bell) is called the *conditioned response* (*CR*) (**FIGURE 13.9**). By the way, several sources on the web smugly declare that Pavlov never actually used a bell for a CS, but there's plenty of evidence that he did (Thomas, 1994; Tully, 2003). Some web "myths" are themselves myths!

Experimental evidence in lab animals shows that circuits in the **cerebellum** are crucial for simple eye-blink conditioning, in which a tone or other stimulus is associated with eye blinking in response to a puff of air. A PET study in humans confirmed this idea by showing a progressive increase in activity in the cerebellum during eye-blink conditioning (Logan and Grafton, 1995). People with hippocampal lesions can acquire the conditioned eye-blink response, but people with damage to the cerebellum on one side can acquire a conditioned eye-blink response *only on the side where the cerebellum is intact* (Papka et al., 1994).

In **instrumental conditioning** (also called *operant conditioning*), an association is formed between the animal's behavior and the consequence(s) of that behavior. An example of an apparatus designed to study instrumental conditioning is called the *Skinner box*, named for its originator, B. F. Skinner (**FIGURE 13.10**). In a common setup, the animal learns that performing a certain action (e.g., pressing a bar) is followed by a reward (such as a food pellet). Research in animals has not pinpointed the brain regions that are crucial for instrumental conditioning, perhaps because this behavior taps so many different aspects of behavior.

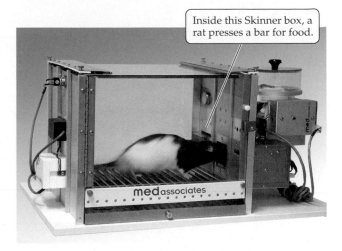

Inside this Skinner box, a rat presses a bar for food.

FIGURE 13.10   A Skinner Box (Courtesy of Med Associates.)

instrumental conditioning Also called *operant conditioning*. A form of associative learning in which the likelihood that an act (instrumental response) will be performed depends on the consequences (reinforcing stimuli) that follow it.

cognitive map   A mental representation of the relative spatial organization of objects and information.

place cell   A neuron in the hippocampus that selectively fires when the animal is in a particular location.

Animal research confirms the various brain regions involved in different attributes of memory

The caricature of the white-coated scientist watching rats run in mazes, a staple of cartoonists to this day, has its origins in the intensive memory research of the early twentieth century. The early work indicated that rats and other animals don't just learn a series of turns but instead form a **cognitive map** (an understanding of the relative spatial organization of objects and information) in order to solve a maze (Tolman, 1949). Animals apparently learn at least some of these details of their spatial environment simply by moving through it (Tolman and Honzik, 1930).

We now know that, in parallel with its role in other types of declarative memory, the hippocampus is crucial for spatial learning. The rat hippocampus contains many neurons that selectively encode spatial location (O'Keefe and Burgess, 2005; Moser et al., 2017). These **place cells** become active when the animal is in—or moving toward—a particular location (**FIGURE 13.11**). If the animal is moved to a new environment, place cell activity indicates that the hippocampus remaps to the new locations

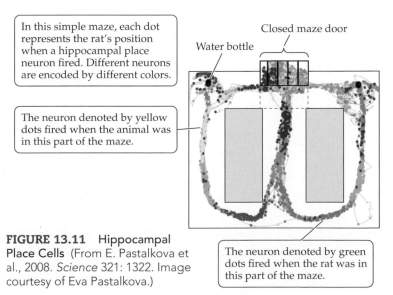

In this simple maze, each dot represents the rat's position when a hippocampal place neuron fired. Different neurons are encoded by different colors.

Closed maze door

Water bottle

The neuron denoted by yellow dots fired when the animal was in this part of the maze.

FIGURE 13.11   Hippocampal Place Cells (From E. Pastalkova et al., 2008. *Science* 321: 1322. Image courtesy of Eva Pastalkova.)

The neuron denoted by green dots fired when the rat was in this part of the maze.

FIGURE 13.12 Subtypes of Declarative and Nondeclarative Memory

To view the activity
Learning and Memory,
go to
3e.mindsmachine.com/ac13.2

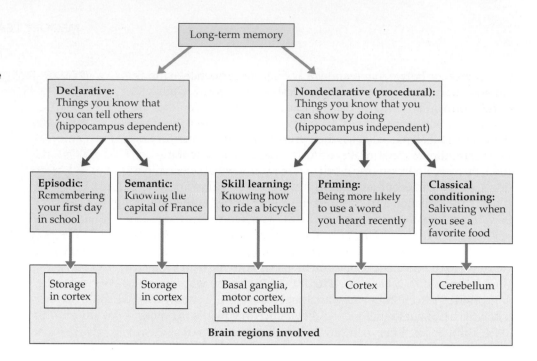

(Moita et al., 2004). Some rat hippocampal neurons act like "grid cells," likened to a latitude and longitude in a maze, which have been recorded in people too (J. Jacobs et al., 2013). The Nobel Prize in Physiology or Medicine for 2014 was awarded to John O'Keefe and the wife-and-husband team of May-Britt and Edvard Moser for their work on understanding hippocampal cells.

Bird species that hide food in many locations have a larger hippocampus than other birds have (Krebs et al., 1989), indicating that natural selection favors enlargement of the hippocampus to enhance spatial learning, as we discuss in **A STEP FURTHER 13.1**, on the website.

Brain regions involved in learning and memory: A summary

FIGURE 13.12 updates and summarizes the classification of long-term memory that we've been discussing. Several major conclusions should be apparent by now, especially (1) that many regions of the brain are involved in learning and memory; (2) that different forms of memory rely on at least partly different brain mechanisms, which may include several different regions of the brain; and (3) that the same brain structure can be a part of the circuitry for several different forms of learning. Next we'll discuss the stages by which memories, of any sort, can be preserved for a lifetime.

HOW'S IT GOING ?

1. Name three different types of nondeclarative memory, giving an example of each. What different parts of the brain have been implicated in each type?
2. What is a cognitive map?
3. What are hippocampal place cells, and why do they suggest a role for the hippocampus in spatial learning?

Successive Processes Capture, Store, and Retrieve Information in the Brain

The span of time over which a piece of information is retained in the brain varies. There are at least three different stages of memory. The briefest memories are called **sensory buffers** (for visual stimuli, they are sometimes called *iconic memories*); an example is the fleeting impression of a glimpsed scene that vanishes from memory seconds later. These brief memories are thought to be residual activity in sensory neurons.

sensory buffer A very brief type of memory that stores the sensory impression of a scene. In vision, it is sometimes called *iconic memory.*

Somewhat longer than sensory buffers are **short-term memories** (**STMs**). If someone tells you a website name and you keep it in mind (perhaps through rehearsal) just until you type it into your browser, you are using STM. In the absence of rehearsal, STMs last only about 30 seconds (J. Brown, 1958; L. R. Peterson and Peterson, 1959). With rehearsal, you may be able to retain an STM until you turn to a new task a few minutes later, but when the STM is gone, it's gone for good. Eventually, some memories become really long-lasting—the address of your childhood home, how to ride a bike, your first crush—and are called **long-term memories** (**LTMs**). A related concept is *working memory*, which refers to the ability to actively manipulate information in your STM, perhaps retrieving information from LTM, to solve a problem or otherwise make use of the information (Aben et al., 2012). We will consider working memory to be a subset of STM where information can be analyzed and manipulated by some "executive" part of our mind.

As shown in **FIGURE 13.13**, the memory system consists of at least three processes: (1) **encoding** of raw information from sensory channels into STM, (2) **consolidation** of the volatile STM into more-durable LTM, and (3) eventual **retrieval** of the stored information from LTM for use in working memory. A problem at any stage can cause us to lose information. Although not depicted in the figure, this model suggests that the flow of information into and out of working memory is supervised by another part of the mind, an *executive function*, which we will discuss in more detail in Chapter 14.

Not all memories are created equal. We all know from firsthand experience that emotion can powerfully affect our memory for past events. For example, an emotionally arousing story is remembered significantly better than a closely matched but emotionally neutral story (Reisberg and Heuer, 1995). But if people are treated with propranolol (a beta-adrenergic antagonist, or beta-blocker, that blocks the effects of epinephrine), this emotional enhancement of memory vanishes. It's not that treated volunteers perceive the story as being any less emotional; in fact, they rate the emotional content of the stories just the same as untreated people do. Instead, the drug seems to directly interfere with the ability of adrenal stress hormones to act on the brain to enhance memory (Cahill et al., 1994). **BOX 13.1** delves further into this topic.

short-term memory (STM)   A form of memory that usually lasts only seconds, or as long as rehearsal continues. Working memory can be considered a portion of STM where information can be manipulated.

long-term memory (LTM)   An enduring form of memory that lasts days, weeks, months, or years. LTM has a very large capacity.

encoding   The first process in the memory system, in which the information entering sensory channels is passed into short-term memory.

consolidation   The second process in the memory system, in which information in short-term memory is transferred to long-term memory.

retrieval   The third process of the memory system, in which a stored memory is used by an organism.

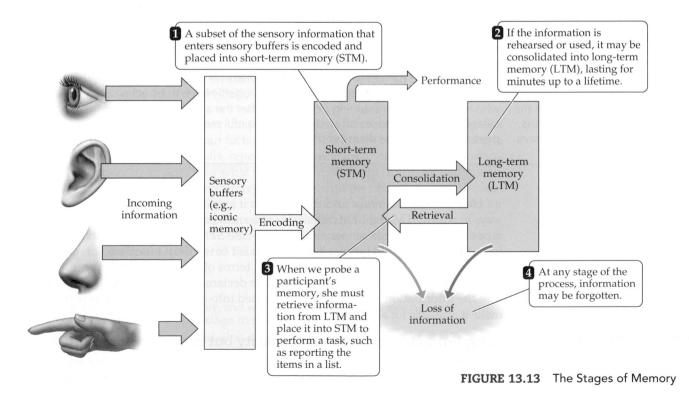

FIGURE 13.13   The Stages of Memory

PART II
Neural Mechanisms of Memory

THE ROAD AHEAD

In this next part of the chapter, we will look at some of the ways in which new learning involves changes in the strength of existing synapses, and we'll look at the biochemical signals that may produce those changes. Reading this material should enable you to:

1. List the possible ways in which changes in neural function and structure could encode memories.
2. Review evidence that exposure to an enriched environment can affect brain structure and affect future behavior.
3. Describe how a circuit involving the cerebellum mediates certain types of conditioning.
4. Explain the properties of a particular type of glutamate receptor that support long-term changes in synaptic strength.
5. Critically evaluate the possibility that such long-term changes in synaptic strength play a role in memory.

Memory Storage Requires Physical Changes in the Brain

In introducing the term *synapse*, Charles Sherrington (1897) speculated that synaptic alterations might be the basis of learning. Sherrington's speculation anticipated what remains one of the most intensive efforts in all of neuroscience, since most theories of learning focus on **neuroplasticity** (or *neural plasticity*), changes in the structure and function of synapses.

Plastic changes at synapses can be physiological or structural

Synaptic changes that may store information can be measured physiologically. The changes can be presynaptic, postsynaptic, or both. They can include changes in the amount of neurotransmitter released and/or changes in the number or sensitivity of the postsynaptic receptors, resulting in larger (or smaller) postsynaptic potentials. Inhibiting inactivation of the transmitter (by altering reuptake or enzymatic degradation) can produce a similar effect (**FIGURE 13.14A**). Synaptic activity can also be influenced by inputs from other neurons, causing extra depolarization or hyperpolarization of the axon terminals and therefore changes in the amount of neurotransmitter released (**FIGURE 13.14B**).

Long-term memories may require changes in the nervous system so substantial that they can be directly observed (with the aid of a microscope, of course). After all, structural changes resulting from use are apparent in other parts of the body, as when exercise tones and shapes muscle. In a similar way, new synapses can form (or old synapses may die back) as a result of use (**FIGURE 13.14C**).

Training can also lead to the reorganization of synaptic connections. For example, it can cause a more active pathway to take over sites formerly occupied by a less active competitor (**FIGURE 13.14D**).

Varied experiences and learning cause the brain to change and grow

The remarkable plasticity of the brain is not all that difficult to demonstrate. Simply living in a complex environment, with its many opportunities for new learning, produces pronounced biochemical and anatomical changes in the brains of rats (Renner and Rosenzweig, 1987).

In standard studies of environmental enrichment, rats are randomly assigned to one of three housing conditions:

neuroplasticity Also called *neural plasticity*. The ability of the nervous system to change in response to experience or the environment.

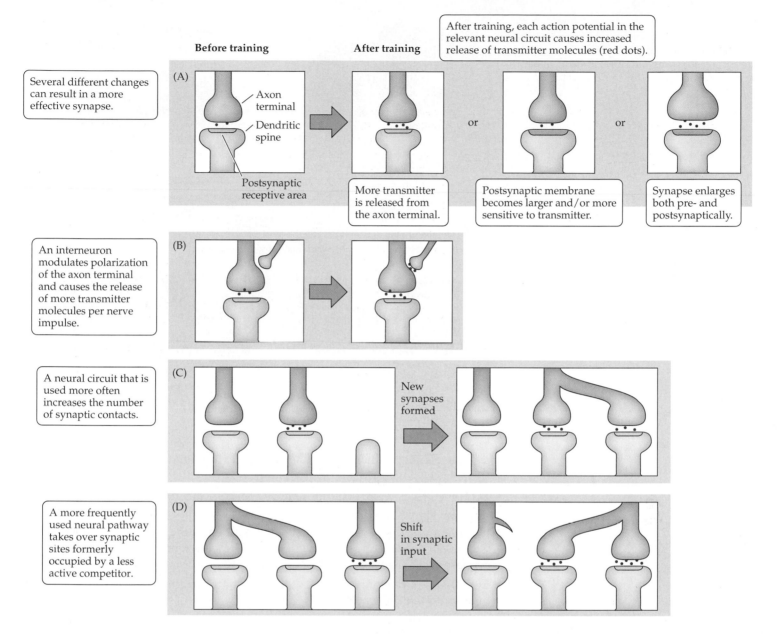

Before training   After training   After training, each action potential in the relevant neural circuit causes increased release of transmitter molecules (red dots).

Several different changes can result in a more effective synapse.

(A)   Axon terminal
Dendritic spine
Postsynaptic receptive area

More transmitter is released from the axon terminal.

Postsynaptic membrane becomes larger and/or more sensitive to transmitter.

Synapse enlarges both pre- and postsynaptically.

An interneuron modulates polarization of the axon terminal and causes the release of more transmitter molecules per nerve impulse.

(B)

A neural circuit that is used more often increases the number of synaptic contacts.

(C)   New synapses formed

A more frequently used neural pathway takes over synaptic sites formerly occupied by a less active competitor.

(D)   Shift in synaptic input

FIGURE 13.14 Synaptic Changes That May Store Memories

1. **Impoverished condition (IC)** Animals are housed individually in standard lab cages (**FIGURE 13.15A**).
2. **Standard condition (SC)** Animals are housed in small groups in standard lab cages (**FIGURE 13.15B**). This is the typical environment for laboratory animals.
3. **Enriched condition (EC)** Animals are housed in large social groups in special cages containing various toys and other interesting features (**FIGURE 13.15C**). This condition provides enhanced opportunities for learning perceptual and motor skills, social learning, and so on.

In dozens of studies over several decades, a variety of changes in the brain were linked to environmental enrichment. For example, compared with IC animals:

- EC animals have a heavier, thicker cortex, especially in somatosensory and visual cortical areas (M. C. Diamond, 1967).

impoverished condition (IC) Also called *isolated condition.* An environment for laboratory rodents in which each animal is housed singly in a small cage without complex stimuli.

standard condition (SC) The usual environment for laboratory rodents, with a few animals in a cage and adequate food and water, but no complex stimulation.

enriched condition (EC) Also called *complex environment.* An environment for laboratory rodents in which animals are group-housed with a wide variety of stimulus objects.

(A) Impoverished condition (IC)   (B) Standard condition (SC)

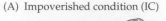

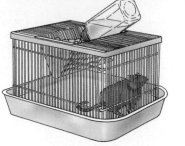

FIGURE 13.15 Experimental Environments to Test the Effects of Enrichment on Learning and Brain Measures (After M. R. Rosenzweig et al., 1972. *Sci. Am.* 226: 22.)

(C) Enriched condition (EC)

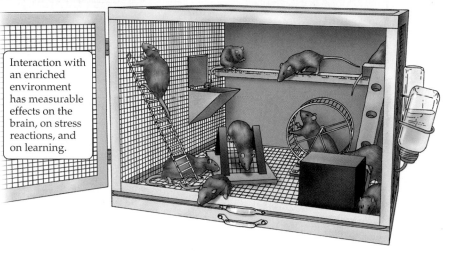

Interaction with an enriched environment has measurable effects on the brain, on stress reactions, and on learning.

- EC animals show enhanced cholinergic activity throughout the cortex (Rosenzweig et al., 1961).

- EC animals have more dendritic branches on cortical neurons, and many more dendritic spines on those branches (**FIGURE 13.16**) (Greenough, 1976).

- EC animals have *larger* cortical synapses (M. C. Diamond et al., 1975), consistent with the storage of long-term memory in cortical areas through changes in synapses and circuits.

- EC animals have more neurons in the hippocampus because newly generated neurons (a topic of Part III of this chapter) live longer (Kempermann et al., 1997).

- EC animals show enhanced recovery from brain damage (Will et al., 2004).

These cerebral effects of experience, which were surprising when first reported for rats in the early 1960s, are now seen to occur widely in the animal kingdom—from flies to philosophers (Mohammed, 2001; Chan et al., 2018). But how can we study the physiology of learning when the mammalian cortex has many billions of neurons, organized in vast networks, and upwards of a billion synapses per cubic centimeter (Merchán-Pérez et al., 2009)? Researchers made progress by studying simple learning circuits, in various species, uncovering basic cellular principles of memory formation that may generalize to neurons throughout the brain.

Invertebrate nervous systems show synaptic plasticity

As we've discussed, neuroplasticity and the ability to learn are ancient adaptations found throughout the animal kingdom. At the neuronal level, even species that are only remotely related likely share the same basic cellular processes for information storage. Indeed, one fruitful research strategy has been to focus on memory mechanisms in the very simple nervous systems of certain invertebrates. Invertebrate nervous systems have relatively few neurons (on the order of hundreds to tens of thousands). Because these neurons are arranged identically in different individuals, it is

(A)

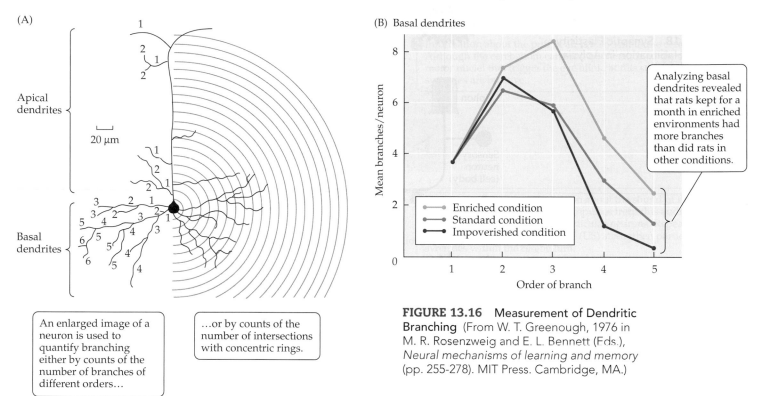

Apical dendrites

20 μm

Basal dendrites

An enlarged image of a neuron is used to quantify branching either by counts of the number of branches of different orders…

…or by counts of the number of intersections with concentric rings.

(B) Basal dendrites

Mean branches/neuron

Order of branch

Enriched condition
Standard condition
Impoverished condition

Analyzing basal dendrites revealed that rats kept for a month in enriched environments had more branches than did rats in other conditions.

FIGURE 13.16 Measurement of Dendritic Branching (From W. T. Greenough, 1976 in M. R. Rosenzweig and E. L. Bennett (Eds.), *Neural mechanisms of learning and memory* (pp. 255-278). MIT Press. Cambridge, MA.)

possible to construct detailed neural circuit diagrams for particular behaviors and study the same few identified neurons in multiple individuals.

Even in these "simple" organisms, the search for memory mechanisms began with the simplest types of learning. Earlier we discussed one of the most basic forms of learning—associative learning about two stimuli, such as the case of a dog learning to associate the sound of a bell with food. Even simpler than associative learning are the types of learning that involve only one stimulus, called *nonassociative learning*. Perhaps the simplest form of nonassociative learning is **habituation**—a decrease in response to a stimulus as it is repeated. To be true habituation, the decreased response cannot be due to failure of the sensory system to detect the stimulus or due to an inability of the motor system to respond. Sitting in a café, you may stop noticing the door chime when someone enters. Your ears still detect the chime, and your body is perfectly capable of looking up to see what happened, but you've habituated to the sound.

Scientists uncovered how the sea slug *Aplysia* learns to habituate to a stimulus (Kandel, 2009). If you squirt water at the slug's siphon—a tube through which it draws water—the animal protectively retracts its delicate gill (**FIGURE 13.17**). But with repeated stimulation the animal retracts the gill less and less, as it learns that the stimulation represents no danger to the gill. Eric Kandel and associates demonstrated that this short-term habituation is caused by changes in the synapse between the sensory cell that detects the squirt of water and the motor neuron that retracts the gill. As less and less transmitter is released at this synapse, the gill withdrawal in response to the stimulation slowly fades (**FIGURE 13.18A**) (M. Klein et al., 1980).

The number and size of synapses can also vary with training in *Aplysia*. For example, if a slug is tested in the habituation paradigm over a series of days, each successive day the animal habituates faster than it did the day before. This phenomenon represents long-term habituation (as opposed to the short-term habituation that we just described), and in this case there is a reduction in the number of synapses between the sensory cell and the motor neuron (**FIGURE 13.18B**) (C. H. Bailey and Chen, 1983).

habituation A form of nonassociative learning in which an organism becomes less responsive following repeated presentations of a stimulus.

In *Aplysia's* usual posture, the siphon is extended and the gill is spread out on the back, with only the tip of the siphon visible.

Siphon

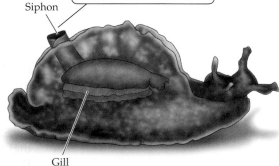

Gill

FIGURE 13.17 The Sea Slug *Aplysia* (After E. R. Kandel, 1976. *Cellular basis of behavior.* Freeman. San Francisco.)

Hebbian synapse A synapse that is strengthened when it successfully drives the postsynaptic cell.

tetanus An intense volley of action potentials.

long-term potentiation (LTP) A stable and enduring increase in the effectiveness of synapses following repeated strong stimulation.

Synaptic Plasticity Can Be Measured in Simple Hippocampal Circuits

Modern ideas about synaptic plasticity have their origins in the theories of Donald Hebb, who proposed that when a presynaptic and a postsynaptic neuron were repeatedly activated together, the synaptic connection between them would become stronger and more stable (the phrase "Cells that fire together wire together" captures the basic idea). These **Hebbian synapses** could then act together to store memory traces (Hebb, 1949).

This idea was eventually confirmed in the 1970s when researchers discovered an impressive form of neuroplasticity in the hippocampus, which appeared to confirm Hebb's theories about synaptic changes (Bliss and Lømo, 1973; Schwartzkroin and Wester, 1975). In experiments like theirs, electrodes are placed within the hippocampus, positioned so that the researchers can stimulate a group of *presynaptic* axons and immediately record the electrical response of a group of *postsynaptic* neurons. Normal, low-level activation of the presynaptic cells produces stable and predictable excitatory postsynaptic potentials (EPSPs) (see Chapter 3), as expected. But when a brief high-frequency burst of electrical stimuli, called a **tetanus**, is applied to the presynaptic neurons, causing them to produce a high rate of action potentials that drive the postsynaptic cell to fire repeatedly, the response of the postsynaptic neurons changes. Now the postsynaptic cells produce much larger EPSPs; in other words, the synapses appear to have become stronger, more effective. This stable and long-lasting enhancement of synaptic transmission, termed **long-term potentiation** (**LTP**; *potentiation* means "strengthening"), is illustrated in **FIGURE 13.20**.

We now know that LTP can be generated in conscious and freely behaving animals, in anesthetized animals, and in tissue slices and that LTP is evident in a variety of invertebrate and vertebrate species. LTP can also last for weeks or more (Bliss and Gardner-Medwin, 1973). So, at least superficially, LTP appears to have the hallmarks of a cellular mechanism of memory: a long-lasting change in synaptic strength. This hint at a cellular origin prompted research into the molecular and physiological mechanisms underlying LTP.

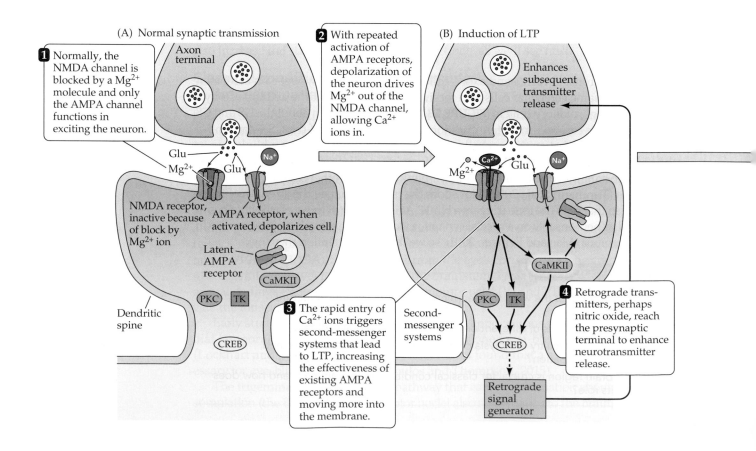

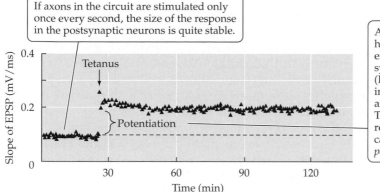

If axons in the circuit are stimulated only once every second, the size of the response in the postsynaptic neurons is quite stable.

Tetanus

Potentiation

After a brief tetanus, however, the excitatory post-synaptic potential (EPSP) response increases markedly and remains high. This greater responsiveness is called *long-term potentiation (LTP)*.

FIGURE 13.20 Long-Term Potentiation Occurs in the Hippocampus

NMDA receptors and AMPA receptors collaborate in LTP

The region called the *hippocampal formation* consists of two interlocking C-shaped structures: the hippocampus itself and the **dentate gyrus**. At least three different pathways in the hippocampal formation display LTP, and it is seen in other brain regions too (Malenka and Bear, 2004). The most studied form of LTP occurs at synapses that use the excitatory neurotransmitter **glutamate**, and it is critically dependent on a glutamate receptor subtype called the **NMDA receptor** (after its selective ligand, *N-m*ethyl-*D-a*spartate). Treatment with drugs that selectively block NMDA receptors completely prevents new LTP in this region, but it does not affect synaptic changes that have already been established. As you might expect, these postsynaptic NMDA receptors—working in conjunction with other glutamate receptors called **AMPA receptors**—have some unique characteristics, which are responsible for LTP.

During normal, low-level activity, the release of glutamate at the synapse activates only the AMPA receptors. The NMDA receptors cannot respond to the glutamate, because magnesium ions (Mg^{2+}) block the NMDA receptor's calcium ion (Ca^{2+}) channel (**FIGURE 13.21A**); thus, few Ca^{2+} ions can enter the neuron. The situation changes, however, if larger quantities of glutamate are released—say, in response to a barrage of action potentials caused by a tetanus. That stronger stimulation of the AMPA receptors

dentate gyrus A strip of gray matter in the hippocampal formation.

glutamate An amino acid transmitter; the most common excitatory transmitter.

NMDA receptor A glutamate receptor that also binds the glutamate agonist NMDA (*N-m*ethyl-*D-a*spartate) and that is both ligand-gated and voltage-sensitive.

AMPA receptor A fast-acting ionotropic glutamate receptor that also binds the glutamate agonist AMPA.

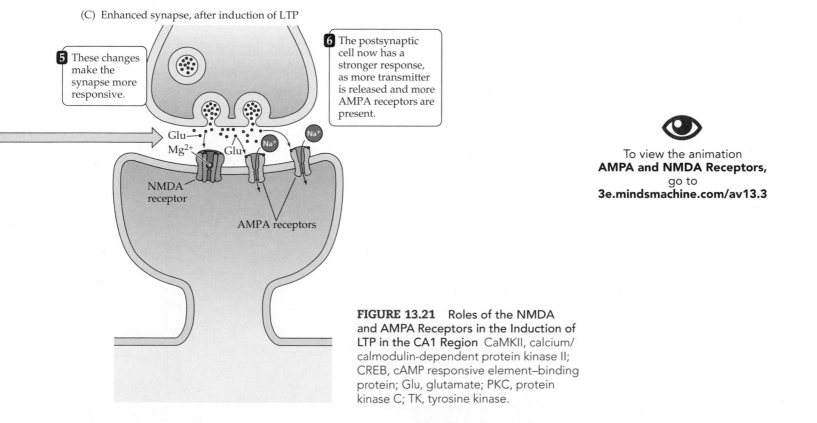

(C) Enhanced synapse, after induction of LTP

5 These changes make the synapse more responsive.

6 The postsynaptic cell now has a stronger response, as more transmitter is released and more AMPA receptors are present.

Glu
Mg^{2+} Glu   Na+   Na+

NMDA receptor

AMPA receptors

To view the animation **AMPA and NMDA Receptors,** go to **3e.mindsmachine.com/av13.3**

FIGURE 13.21 Roles of the NMDA and AMPA Receptors in the Induction of LTP in the CA1 Region CaMKII, calcium/calmodulin-dependent protein kinase II; CREB, cAMP responsive element–binding protein; Glu, glutamate; PKC, protein kinase C; TK, tyrosine kinase.

depolarizes the postsynaptic membrane so much that the Mg^{2+} plug is repulsed from the NMDA receptor's channel (**FIGURE 13.21B**). Now the NMDA receptors are also able to respond to glutamate, admitting large amounts of Ca^{2+} into the postsynaptic neuron. Thus, NMDA receptors are fully active only when "gated" by a combination of strong depolarization (via AMPA receptors) and the ligand (glutamate).

The large influx of Ca^{2+} at NMDA receptors activates a variety of intracellular enzymes that affect AMPA receptors in several important ways (**FIGURE 13.21C**) (Lisman et al., 2002; Kessels and Malinow, 2009). First, the enzymes cause existing nearby AMPA receptors to move to the active synapse (T. Takahashi et al., 2003), and they modify the AMPA receptors to increase their conductance of Na^+ and K^+ ions (Sanderson et al., 2008). In addition, more AMPA receptors are produced and inserted into the postsynaptic membrane. Thus, after the tetanus there are more AMPA receptors, and those receptors are more effective, so the synaptic response to glutamate is strengthened (see Figure 13.21B).

There are *presynaptic* changes in LTP too. When the postsynaptic cell is strongly stimulated and its NMDA receptors become active and admit Ca^{2+}, an intracellular process causes the postsynaptic cell to release a **retrograde transmitter**—often a diffusible gas—that travels back across the synapse and alters the functioning of the presynaptic neuron (see Figure 13.21B). The retrograde transmitter induces the presynaptic terminal to release more glutamate than previously, thereby strengthening the synapse some more. So, LTP involves active changes on both sides of the synapse.

So far, we've talked about how activity can make existing Hebbian synapses stronger. However, evidence suggests that the same mechanisms can affect whether new synapses are formed and old synapses retracted. In these systems it appears that when several presynaptic neurons fire at the same time, they "gang up" on the postsynaptic cell, depolarizing it enough that the NMDA receptors are activated to strengthen those connections. Conversely, any presynaptic neurons that tend to fire *out* of synchrony with the other inputs are not likely to depolarize the postsynaptic neurons enough to activate NMDA receptors. Eventually, the strengthened inputs seem to sprout new, additional connections, while the weakened synapses fade away (**FIGURE 13.22**).

retrograde transmitter   A neurotransmitter that is released by the postsynaptic neuron, diffuses back across the synapse, and alters the functioning of the presynaptic neuron.

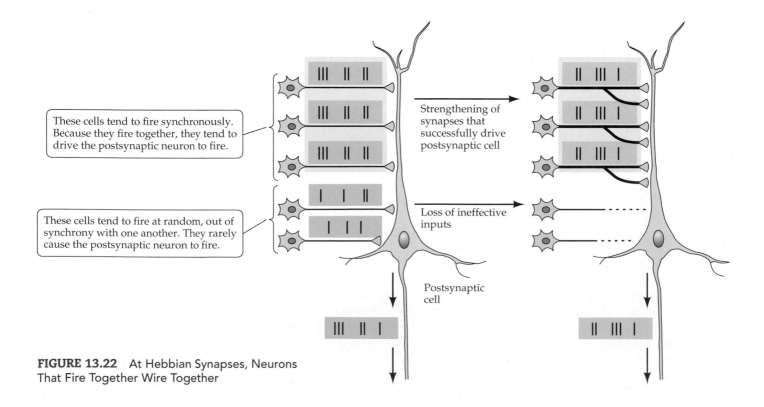

These cells tend to fire synchronously. Because they fire together, they tend to drive the postsynaptic neuron to fire.

These cells tend to fire at random, out of synchrony with one another. They rarely cause the postsynaptic neuron to fire.

Strengthening of synapses that successfully drive postsynaptic cell

Loss of ineffective inputs

Postsynaptic cell

FIGURE 13.22   At Hebbian Synapses, Neurons That Fire Together Wire Together

Many scientists are excited about LTP because this momentary burst of neural activity, the tetanus, can change synaptic strength for a long time. It's easy to imagine how another momentary burst of neural activity, in this case triggered by a learning experience, could change synaptic strength, and that change in synaptic strength might be a memory trace. But is this just a case of an overactive imagination, or is LTP truly involved in learning?

Is LTP a mechanism of memory formation?

Even the simplest learning involves circuits of multiple neurons and many synapses, and more-complex declarative and procedural memory traces must involve vast networks of neurons, so we are unlikely to conclude that LTP is the *only* mechanism of learning. However, evidence from several research perspectives implicates LTP in at least some forms of memory:

1. *Correlational observations* The time course of LTP bears strong similarity to the time course of memory formation (Lynch et al., 1991; Staubli, 1995).

2. *Somatic intervention experiments* In general, pharmacological treatments that interfere with LTP also tend to impair learning. So, for example, NMDA receptor blockade interferes with performance in the Morris water maze (a test of spatial memory) and other types of memory tests (R. G. Morris et al., 1989). Knockout mice that lack functional NMDA receptors only in the CA1 region of the hippocampus appear normal in many respects, but their hippocampi are incapable of LTP and their declarative memory is impaired (Rampon et al., 2000). On the other hand, mice engineered to *overexpress* NMDA receptors in the hippocampus have enhanced LTP and better-than-normal long-term memory (Y. P. Tang et al., 2001). (For the full story of these mice, see **A STEP FURTHER 13.2**, on the website.)

3. *Behavioral intervention experiments* In principle, the most convincing evidence for a link between LTP and learning would be "behavioral LTP": a demonstration that training an animal in a memory task induces LTP somewhere in the brain. Such research is difficult because of uncertainty about exactly where to put the recording electrodes in order to detect any induced LTP. Nevertheless, several examples of successful behavioral LTP have been reported (McKernan and Shinnick-Gallagher, 1997; Rogan et al., 1997; Whitlock et al., 2006).

To see the video
Morris Water Maze,
go to
3e.mindsmachine.com/av13.4

Taken together, these findings support the idea that LTP is a kind of synaptic plasticity that underlies (or is very similar to) certain forms of learning and memory.

Thus it seems that the cause of Henry Molaison's tragic amnesia may have been the loss of medial temporal lobe structures like the hippocampus, which normally use LTP to consolidate short-term memories into long-term memories somewhere in the brain, probably the cortex. It's strange to think that microscopic changes in synapses in a particular brain region could be so crucial for living a full human life. Eventually Henry seemed to stop being shocked when he saw his reflection, and he learned he was no longer in his mid twenties. But it's not clear whether he understood, for long, that his parents had passed away. As a final act of generosity to a field of science that he helped launch, Henry arranged to donate his brain for further study after he died. Through webcasting technology, the dissection of Henry's brain was viewed live by thousands of people (see https://www.thebrainobservatory.org/project-hm), and a series of more than 2,000 brain sections are available.

To the end, although Henry could remember so little of his entire adult life, he was courteous and concerned about other people. Henry remembered the surgeon he had met several times before his operation: "He did medical research on people…. What he learned about me helped others too, and I'm glad about that" (Corkin, 2002, p. 158). Henry never knew how famous he was or how much his dreadful condition taught us about learning and memory; despite being deprived of one of the most important characteristics of a human being, he held fast to his humanity.

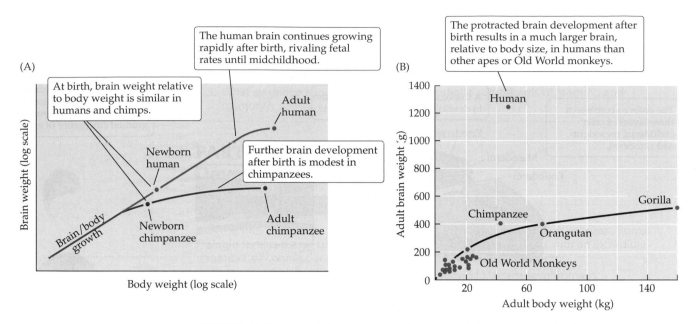

FIGURE 13.24 Fetal-like Rapid Development of the Brain outside the Womb (After B. Bogin, 1997. *Yearb. Phys. Anthropol.* 40: 63.)

Development of the Nervous System Can Be Divided into Six Distinct Stages

From a cellular viewpoint it is useful to consider brain development as a sequence of six distinct stages, most of which occur during prenatal life:

1. *Neurogenesis*, the mitotic division of nonneuronal cells to produce neurons
2. *Cell migration*, the massive movements of nerve cells or their precursors to establish distinct nerve cell populations (nuclei in the CNS, layers of the cerebral cortex, and so on)
3. *Cell differentiation*, the refining of cells into distinctive types of neurons or glial cells
4. *Synaptogenesis*, the establishment of synaptic connections as axons and dendrites grow
5. *Neuronal cell death*, the selective death of many nerve cells
6. *Synapse rearrangement*, the loss of some synapses and the development of others, to refine synaptic connections

The six stages proceed at different rates and times in different parts of the nervous system. Some of the stages may overlap even within a region. In the discussion that follows, we will take up each stage in succession.

Cell proliferation produces cells that become neurons or glia

The production of neurons is called **neurogenesis**. Neurons themselves do not divide, but the cells that will give rise to neurons begin as a single layer of cells along the inner surface of the neural tube. These cells divide in a process called **mitosis**, which takes place within the **ventricular zone** inside the neural tube (**FIGURE 13.25A**). Eventually, some cells leave the ventricular zone and begin transforming into either neurons or glial cells. As the nervous system grows, **cell migration** follows, as the cells move over relatively long distances to fill out the brain (**FIGURE 13.25B**).

To view the animation
Stages of Neuronal Development,
go to
3e.mindsmachine.com/av13.5

neurogenesis The mitotic division of nonneuronal cells to produce neurons.

mitosis The process of division of somatic cells that involves duplication of DNA.

ventricular zone Also called *ependymal layer*. A region lining the cerebral ventricles that displays mitosis, providing neurons early in development and glial cells throughout life.

cell migration The movement of cells from site of origin to final location.

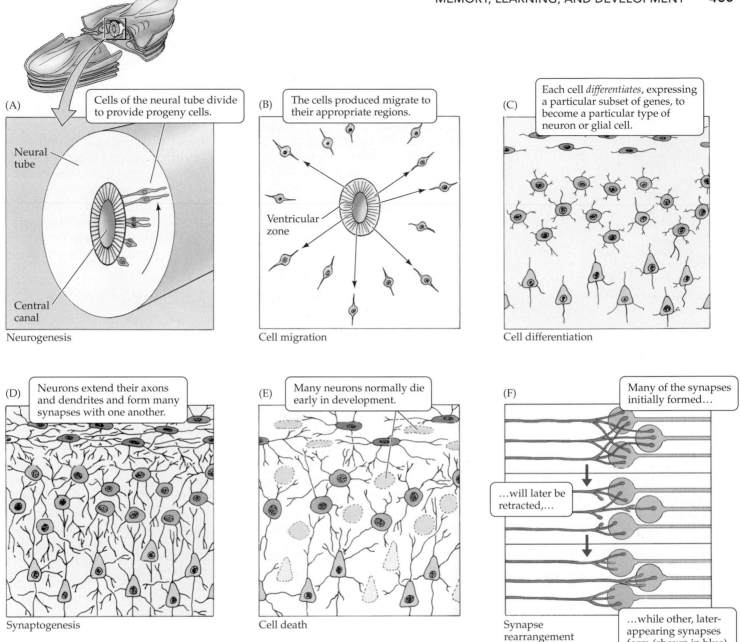

(A) Cells of the neural tube divide to provide progeny cells.

Neural tube

Central canal

Neurogenesis

(B) The cells produced migrate to their appropriate regions.

Ventricular zone

Cell migration

(C) Each cell *differentiates*, expressing a particular subset of genes, to become a particular type of neuron or glial cell.

Cell differentiation

(D) Neurons extend their axons and dendrites and form many synapses with one another.

Synaptogenesis

(E) Many neurons normally die early in development.

Cell death

(F) Many of the synapses initially formed…

…will later be retracted,…

…while other, later-appearing synapses form (shown in blue).

Synapse rearrangement

FIGURE 13.25 The Six Stages of Neural Development

Newly arrived cells in the brain bear no more resemblance to mature nerve cells than they do to the cells of other organs. Once the cells reach their destinations, however, **gene expression** begins, that is, the cells begin to use, or express, particular genes. This means that each type of cell makes use of a particular subset of genes to make the particular proteins that type needs. This process of **cell differentiation** enables cells to acquire the distinctive appearance and functions of neurons characteristic of their particular regions (**FIGURE 13.25C**). Once they take on the characteristics of neurons, they begin making synaptic connections with one another, in the process of **synaptogenesis** (**FIGURE 13.25D**).

The particular fate of a differentiating cell depends on where in the brain the cell happens to be and what the cell's neighbors are doing. Cells in the developing brain are constantly sending chemical signals to one another, each shaping the development of the other. This is the hallmark of vertebrate development: cells sort themselves out via **cell-cell interactions**, taking on fates that are appropriate in the

gene expression The process by which a cell makes an mRNA transcript of a particular gene.

cell differentiation The developmental stage in which cells acquire distinctive characteristics, such as those of neurons, as a result of expressing particular genes.

synaptogenesis The establishment of synaptic connections as axons and dendrites grow.

cell-cell interaction The general process during development in which one cell affects the differentiation of other, usually neighboring, cells.

To see the video
**Migration of a Neuron along
a Radial Glial Cell,**
go to
3e.mindsmachine.com/av13.6

stem cell   A cell that is undifferentiated and therefore can take on the fate of any cell that a donor organism can produce.

adult neurogenesis   The creation of new neurons in the brain of an adult.

context of what neighboring cells are doing. When the negotiations are all over, if things go properly, a new person is formed with all the types of cells in the brain that they need to live.

This system of cell-cell interactions determining how brain cells develop has an important consequence: If cells that have not yet differentiated extensively can be obtained and placed in a particular brain region, they can differentiate in an appropriate way and become properly integrated. Such undifferentiated cells, called **stem cells**, are present throughout embryonic tissues, so they can be gathered from umbilical cord blood, miscarried embryos, or unused embryos produced during in vitro fertilization. It may even be possible someday to take cells from adult tissue and, by treating them with various factors in a dish, transform them into stem cells (Dulak et al., 2015). It is hoped that placing stem cells in areas of brain degeneration, such as loss of myelin in multiple sclerosis or loss of dopaminergic neurons in Parkinson's disease (see Chapters 5 and 15), might reverse such degeneration as the implanted cells differentiate to fill in for the missing components (Wang et al., 2018).

In the adult brain, newly born neurons aid learning

At birth, mammals have already produced most of the neurons they will ever have. The postnatal increase of human brain weight (see Figure 13.24) is due primarily to growth in the size of neurons, branching of dendrites, elaboration of synapses, increase in myelin, and addition of glial cells. But research in the last decade or so has shown that we are also capable of **adult neurogenesis**, the generation of new neurons in adulthood, especially in the dentate gyrus of the hippocampal formation (**FIGURE 13.26**) (Anacker et al., 2018; Boldrini et al., 2018). By one estimate, 700 new neurons are produced every day in the adult human hippocampus (Spalding et al., 2013).

Indeed, although the new neurons acquired in adulthood represent just a tiny minority of the total, there's reason to think they are important. In experimental animals, the birth and/or survival of new neurons is enhanced by factors like exercise, environmental enrichment, and training (Waddell and Shors, 2008; Opendak and Gould, 2015). Neurogenesis appears to enhance various forms of hippocampus-dependent learning, such as spatial memory and fear conditioning, in some (but not all) studies (Saxe et al., 2006; Winocur et al., 2006; Kee et al., 2007). Mice with a genetic manipulation that turns off neurogenesis in the brains of adults showed a marked impairment in spatial learning with little effect on other behaviors (C. L. Zhang et al., 2008).

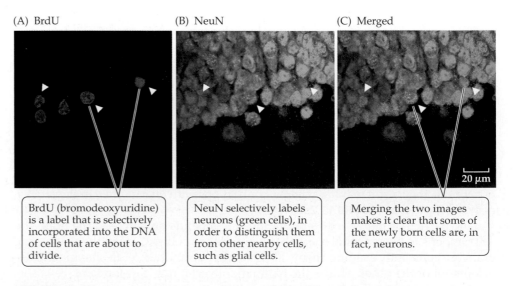

(A) BrdU

(B) NeuN

(C) Merged

BrdU (bromodeoxyuridine) is a label that is selectively incorporated into the DNA of cells that are about to divide.

NeuN selectively labels neurons (green cells), in order to distinguish them from other nearby cells, such as glial cells.

Merging the two images makes it clear that some of the newly born cells are, in fact, neurons.

20 µm

FIGURE 13.26   **Neurogenesis in the Dentate Gyrus** (From E. Bruel-Jungerman et al., 2006. *J. Neurosci.* 26: 5888.)

So by studying this chapter, you may be giving your brain a few more neurons to use on exam day! Physical exercise also boosts neurogenesis in rats—an effect that can be blocked by stressors such as social isolation (Stranahan et al., 2006)—so invest in exercise and a network of friends too.

The death of many neurons is a normal part of development

As strange as it may seem, cell death is a crucial phase of brain development (**FIGURE 13.25E**). This developmental stage is not unique to the nervous system. Naturally occurring **cell death**, also called *apoptosis* (from the Greek *apo*, "away from," and *ptosis*, "act of falling"), is evident as a kind of sculpting process in the emergence of other tissues in both animals and plants.

The number of neurons that die during early development is quite large. In some regions of the brain and spinal cord, *most* of the young nerve cells die during prenatal development. In 1958, Viktor Hamburger (1900–2001) first described naturally occurring neuronal cell death in chicks, in which nearly half the originally produced spinal motor neurons die before the chick hatches. A similar loss of spinal motor neurons was later reported in developing humans (**FIGURE 13.27**) (Forger and Breedlove, 1987).

These cells are not dying because of a defect. Rather, these cells die as a consequence of complex interactions with surrounding cells, so they are actively "committing suicide." Your chromosomes carry *death genes*—genes that are expressed only when a cell undergoes apoptosis (Peter et al., 1997). Genetically interfering with death genes in fetal mice causes them to grow brains that are too large to fit in the skull (Depaepe et al., 2005), so we can see how vital it is that some cells die.

Neurons compete for connections to target structures (other nerve cells or end organs, such as muscle). Cells that make adequate synapses remain; those without a place to form synaptic connections die. Apparently the cells compete not just for synaptic sites, but for a chemical that the target structure makes and releases. Neurons that receive enough of the chemical survive; those that do not, die. Such target-derived chemicals are called **neurotrophic factors** (or simply *trophic factors*) because they act as if they "feed" the neurons to help them survive (in Greek, *trophe* means "nourishment") (**FIGURE 13.28**).

An explosion of synapse formation is followed by synapse rearrangement

Before birth and after, neurons in the human cortex grow ever longer and more elaborate dendrites, each jammed with synapses. As we noted earlier, this massive increase

cell death   Also called *apoptosis*. The developmental process during which "surplus" cells die.

neurotrophic factor   Also called simply *trophic factor*. A target-derived chemical that acts as if it "feeds" certain neurons to help them survive.

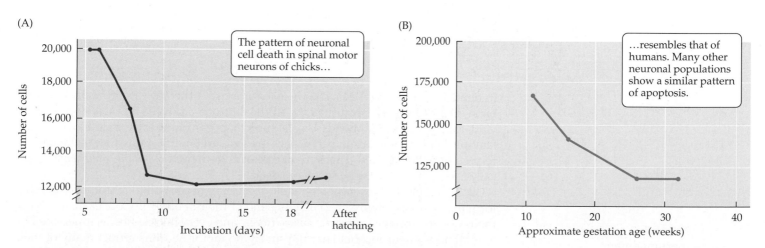

FIGURE 13.27   Many Neurons Die during Normal Early Development (Part A after V. Hamburger, 1975. *J. Comp. Neurol.* 160: 535; B after N. G. Forger and S. M. Breedlove, 1987. *J. Comp. Neurol.* 264: 118.)

FIGURE 13.28 A Model for the Action of Neurotrophic Factors

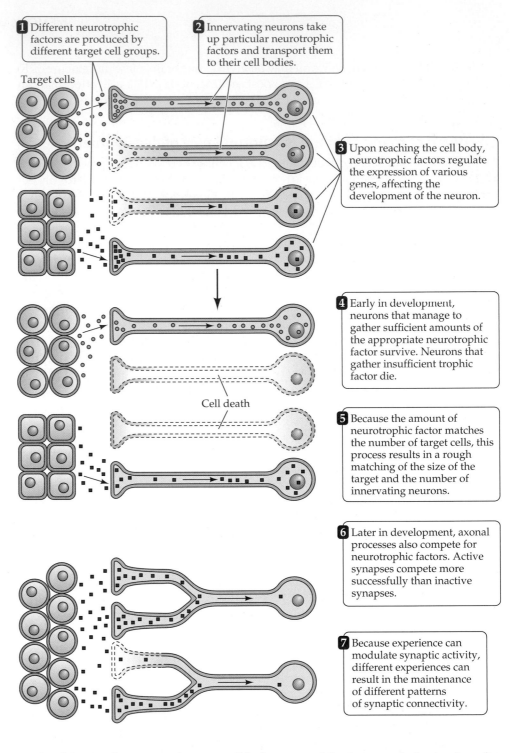

1 Different neurotrophic factors are produced by different target cell groups.

2 Innervating neurons take up particular neurotrophic factors and transport them to their cell bodies.

Target cells

3 Upon reaching the cell body, neurotrophic factors regulate the expression of various genes, affecting the development of the neuron.

4 Early in development, neurons that manage to gather sufficient amounts of the appropriate neurotrophic factor survive. Neurons that gather insufficient trophic factor die.

Cell death

5 Because the amount of neurotrophic factor matches the number of target cells, this process results in a rough matching of the size of the target and the number of innervating neurons.

6 Later in development, axonal processes also compete for neurotrophic factors. Active synapses compete more successfully than inactive synapses.

7 Because experience can modulate synaptic activity, different experiences can result in the maintenance of different patterns of synaptic connectivity.

in dendrites and synapses is responsible for most of the increase in brain size after birth (**FIGURE 13.29**). But just as not all the neurons produced by a developing individual are kept into adulthood, some of the synapses formed early in development are later retracted. Some original synapses are lost, and many, many new synapses are formed (**FIGURE 13.25F**). This **synapse rearrangement**, or *synaptic remodeling*, typically takes place after the period of cell death.

For example, as we learned already, about half of the spinal motor neurons that form die later (see Figure 13.27). By the end of the cell death period, each surviving motor neuron innervates many muscle fibers, and every muscle fiber is innervated by several motor neurons. But later the surviving motor neurons retract many of their axon collaterals, until each muscle fiber comes to be innervated by only one motor neuron. Again, which synaptic connections are retained, and which new connections

synapse rearrangement Also called *synaptic remodeling*. The loss of some synapses and the development of others.

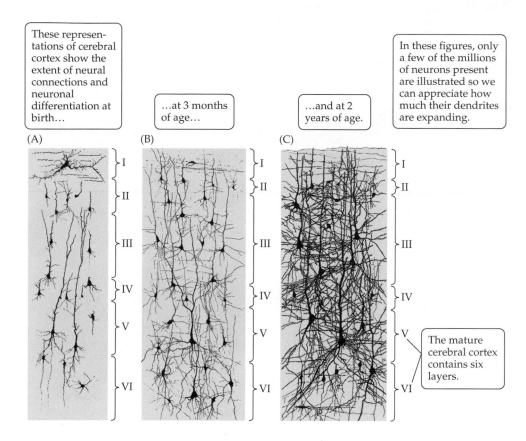

These representations of cerebral cortex show the extent of neural connections and neuronal differentiation at birth…

…at 3 months of age…

…and at 2 years of age.

In these figures, only a few of the millions of neurons present are illustrated so we can appreciate how much their dendrites are expanding.

The mature cerebral cortex contains six layers.

FIGURE 13.29 Cerebral Cortex Tissue in the Early Development of Humans (From J. L. Conel, 1939. *The postnatal development of the human cerebral cortex: Vol. 1. The cortex of the newborn*; 1947, *Vol. 3. The cortex of the three-month infant*; 1959, *Vol. 6. The cortex of the twenty-four-month infant.* Harvard University Press. Cambridge, MA.)

are formed, is thought to depend on competition for trophic factors during development (see Figure 13.28) and/or competition between Hebbian synapses (see Figure 13.22).

Similar events have been documented in several neural regions, including the cerebellum (Mariani and Changeaux, 1981), the brainstem (Jackson and Parks, 1982), the visual cortex (Hubel et al., 1977), and the autonomic nervous system (Lichtman and Purves, 1980). In human cerebral cortex there is a net loss of synapses from late childhood until midadolescence (**FIGURE 13.30**). This synaptic remodeling is evident in thinning of the cortical gray matter as pruning of dendrites and axon terminals progresses. The thinning

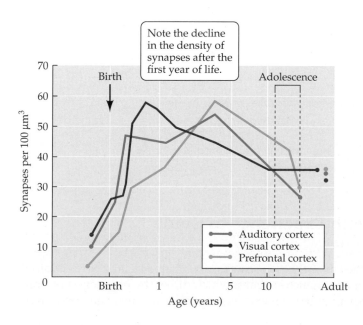

Note the decline in the density of synapses after the first year of life.

- Auditory cortex
- Visual cortex
- Prefrontal cortex

FIGURE 13.30 The Postnatal Development of Synapses in Human Cortex (After P. R. Huttenlocher and A. S. Dabholkar, 1997. *J. Comp. Neurol.* 387: 167.)

FIGURE 13.31 Synapse Rearrangement in the Developing Human Brain (From N. Gogtay et al., 2004. *Proc. Natl. Acad. Sci.* USA 101: 8174. © National Academy of Sciences, U.S.A.)

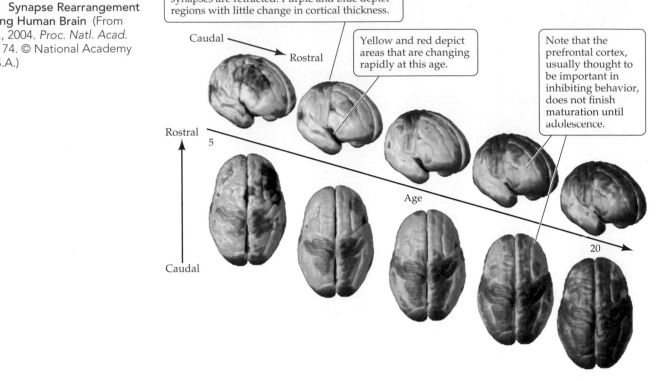

The layer of gray matter on the surface of the cortex gets thinner throughout development, as synapses are retracted. Purple and blue depict regions with little change in cortical thickness.

Yellow and red depict areas that are changing rapidly at this age.

Note that the prefrontal cortex, usually thought to be important in inhibiting behavior, does not finish maturation until adolescence.

process continues in a caudal–rostral (posterior–anterior) direction during maturation (**FIGURE 13.31**), so prefrontal cortex matures last (Gogtay et al., 2004). Since prefrontal cortex is important for inhibiting behavior (see Chapter 14), this delayed brain maturation may contribute to teenagers' impulsivity and lack of control (Paus et al., 2008).

What determines which synapses are kept and which are lost? Although we don't know all the factors, one important influence is neural activity. One theory is that active synapses take up some neurotrophic factor that maintains the synapse, while inactive synapses get too little trophic factor to remain stable (see Figure 13.28). Intellectual stimulation probably contributes, as suggested by the fact that teenagers with the highest IQ show an especially prolonged period of cortical thinning (P. Shaw et al., 2006). Another stage of brain development, the formation of myelin sheaths for axons, is discussed in **A STEP FURTHER 13.3**, on the website.

This influence of experience on the developing brain brings us to the question of how both genes and the environment affect human intelligence.

HOW'S IT GOING ❓

1. What six stages of cellular processes take place in the developing brain?
2. What is cell differentiation, and what guides this process in each cell in the developing brain?
3. What two classes of brain structures undergo loss during development?
4. Speculate about why these "regressive" events might be important.

Genes Interact with Experience to Guide Brain Development

Many factors influence the emergence of the form, arrangements, and connections of the developing brain. One influence is genes, which direct the production of every protein the cell can make. An individual who has inherited an altered gene will make an altered protein, which will affect any cell structure that includes that protein. Thus, every neuronal structure, and therefore every behavior, can be altered by changes in the appropriate gene(s). It is useful to think of genes as *intrinsic* factors—that is, factors that originate within the developing cell itself. All other influences we can consider *extrinsic*—originating outside of the developing cell.

Genotype is fixed at birth, but phenotype changes throughout life

Two terms help illustrate how these intrinsic and extrinsic factors interact. The sum of all the intrinsic, genetic information that an individual has is its **genotype**. The sum of all the physical characteristics that make up an individual is its **phenotype**. Your genotype was determined at the moment of fertilization and remains the same throughout your life. But your phenotype changes constantly, as you grow up and grow old and even, in a tiny way, as you take each breath. In other words, phenotype is determined by the interaction of genotype and extrinsic factors, including experience. Thus, as we'll see, individuals who have identical genotypes do not have identical phenotypes, because they have not received identical extrinsic influences. And since their nervous system phenotypes are somewhat different, they do not behave exactly the same.

Several hundred different genetic disorders affect the metabolism of proteins, carbohydrates, or lipids, having a profound impact on the developing brain. Characteristically, the genetic defect is the absence of a particular enzyme that controls a critical biochemical step in the synthesis or breakdown of a vital body product.

An example is *phenylketonuria* (*PKU*), a recessive hereditary disorder of protein metabolism that at one time resulted in many people with intellectual disability. About one out of 100 persons is a carrier; one in 10,000 births produces an affected victim. The basic defect is the absence of an enzyme necessary to metabolize phenylalanine, an amino acid that is present in many foods. As a result, the brain is damaged by an enormous buildup of phenylalanine, which becomes toxic.

The discovery of PKU marked the first time that an inborn error of metabolism was associated with intellectual disability. These days, the level of phenylalanine in the blood is measured in children a few days after birth. Early detection is important because brain impairment can be prevented simply by reducing phenylalanine in the diet. Such dietary control of PKU is critical during the early years of life, especially before age 2; after that, diet can be relaxed somewhat. Note this important example of the interaction of genes and the environment in PKU: the dysfunctional gene causes intellectual disability only in the presence of phenylalanine. Reducing phenylalanine consumption reduces or prevents this effect of the gene.

PKU illustrates one reason why, despite the importance of genes for nervous system development, understanding the genotype alone could never enable an understanding of the developing brain. Knowing that a baby is born with PKU doesn't tell you anything about how that child's brain will develop unless you also know something about the child's diet. Another reason why genes alone cannot tell the whole story is that experience can affect the activity of genes, as we discuss next.

Experience regulates gene expression in the developing and mature brain

Genetically identical animals, called **clones**, used to be known mainly in science fiction and horror films. But life imitates art. In pigs, genetically identical clones show as much variation in behavior and temperament as do normal siblings (G. S. Archer et al., 2003), and genetically identical mice raised in different laboratories behave very differently on a variety of tests (Finch and Kirkwood, 2000). If genes are so important to the developing nervous system, how can genetically identical individuals differ in their behavior?

Recall that although nearly all of the cells in your body have a complete copy of your genotype, each cell uses only a small subset of those genes at any one time. We mentioned earlier that when a cell uses a particular gene to make a particular protein,

genotype All the genetic information that one specific individual has inherited.

phenotype The sum of an individual's physical characteristics at one particular time.

clones Asexually produced organisms that are genetically identical.

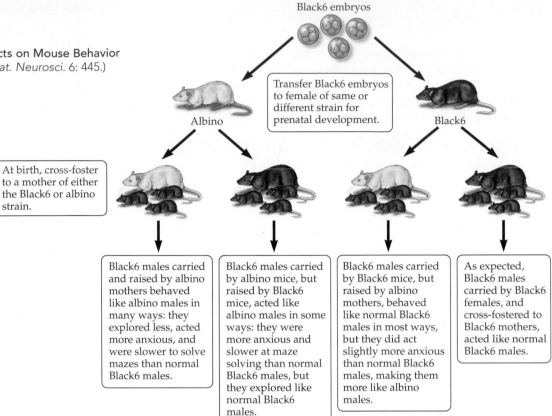

FIGURE 13.32 Epigenetic Effects on Mouse Behavior
(After D. D. Francis et al., 2003. *Nat. Neurosci.* 6: 445.)

Black6 embryos

Transfer Black6 embryos to female of same or different strain for prenatal development.

Albino

Black6

At birth, cross-foster to a mother of either the Black6 or albino strain.

Black6 males carried and raised by albino mothers behaved like albino males in many ways: they explored less, acted more anxious, and were slower to solve mazes than normal Black6 males.

Black6 males carried by albino mice, but raised by Black6 mice, acted like albino males in some ways: they were more anxious and slower at maze solving than normal Black6 males, but they explored like normal Black6 males.

Black6 males carried by Black6 mice, but raised by albino mothers, behaved like normal Black6 males in most ways, but they did act slightly more anxious than normal Black6 males, making them more like albino males.

As expected, Black6 males carried by Black6 females, and cross-fostered to Black6 mothers, acted like normal Black6 males.

we say the cell has *expressed* that gene. **Epigenetics** is the study of factors that affect gene expression without making any changes in the nucleotide sequence of the genes.

An important epigenetic factor affecting the developing brain in mice is the mothering they receive. If genetically identical embryos of one mouse strain are implanted into the womb of a foster mother of either their own strain or another strain, their behavior is affected (Francis et al., 2003). Strain Black6 males carried and raised by mothers from the albino strain show significant differences in several behaviors, including maze running and measures of anxiety (**FIGURE 13.32**). Since the various males are *genetically identical* to one another, their different behaviors must be due to the effect of different prenatal environments and postnatal experiences on how those genes are expressed.

One particular influence of mothering on gene expression has been well documented. **Methylation** is a chemical modification of DNA that does not affect the nucleotide sequence of a gene but makes that gene less likely to be expressed. Michael Meaney and colleagues demonstrated that rodent pups provided with inattentive mothers, or subjected to interruptions in maternal care, secrete more glucocorticoids in response to stress as adults (T. Y. Zhang and Meaney, 2010). Poor maternal care programs this heightened stress hormone response by inducing methylation of the glucocorticoid receptor gene in the brain, making the pups hyperresponsive to stress for the rest of their lives.

A similar mechanism may apply to humans, because this same gene is also more likely to be methylated in the postmortem brains of suicide victims than of controls, *but only in those victims who were subjected to childhood abuse.* Suicide victims who did not suffer childhood abuse were no more likely to have the gene methylated than were controls (McGowan et al., 2009). These results suggest that methylation of the gene in abused children may make them hyperresponsive to stress as adults—a condition that may lead them to take their own lives. This is a powerful demonstration of epigenetic influences on behavior. Other developmental disorders are also influenced by both genes and the environment, as we discuss in **A STEP FURTHER 13.4**, on the website.

Taken together, these studies lead us to the conclusion that the incredible intelligence of the adult human is due not only to the inheritance of genes provided us by

epigenetics The study of factors that affect gene expression without making any changes in the nucleotide sequence of the genes themselves.

methylation A chemical modification of DNA that does not affect the nucleotide sequence of a gene but makes that gene less likely to be expressed.

natural selection, but also to the effect of the environment and experience that determines where and when those genes are expressed in the brain, especially in development. Thus, the tremendous, fetal-like development of the human brain after birth (see Figure 13.24) is molded by experience and social guidance. We wish we could tell you that once your brain has been sharpened by experience (including what you gain by reading this book), you will remain brilliant forever. Sadly, development continues relentlessly toward old age. Just as our faces and bodies weaken and fade, the brain also declines, the depressing topic that concludes this chapter.

HOW'S IT GOING ?

1. Compare changes in genotype and phenotype in an individual during development and aging.
2. How does PKU illustrate an interaction between genes and the environment?
3. Describe two demonstrations of epigenetic effects on development.

The Brain Continues to Change as We Grow Older

The passage of time brings us an accumulation of joys and sorrows—perhaps riches and fame—and a progressive decline in many of our abilities. Although slower responses seem inevitable with aging, many of our cognitive abilities show little change during the adult years, until we reach an advanced age. What happens to brain structure from adolescence to the day when we all become a little forgetful and walk more hesitantly?

Memory impairment correlates with hippocampal shrinkage during aging

In a study of healthy and cognitively normal people age 55–87, investigators asked whether mild impairment in memory is specifically related to reduction in size of the hippocampal formation or is better explained by generalized shrinkage of brain tissue (Golomb et al., 1994). Volunteers took a series of memory tests, and their brains were measured from MRI images (**FIGURE 13.33**). When effects of sex, age, IQ, and overall brain atrophy were eliminated statistically, hippocampal formation volume was the only brain measure that correlated significantly with memory.

PET scans of elderly people reveal that cerebral metabolism normally remains almost constant as we age. This stability is in marked contrast to the dramatic decline of cerebral metabolism in Alzheimer's disease, which we will consider next.

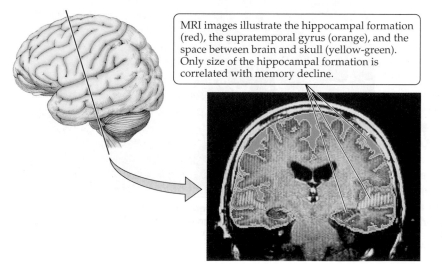

MRI images illustrate the hippocampal formation (red), the supratemporal gyrus (orange), and the space between brain and skull (yellow-green). Only size of the hippocampal formation is correlated with memory decline.

FIGURE 13.33 Hippocampal Shrinkage Correlates with Memory Decline in Aging (From J. Golomb et al., 1994. *J. Neurol. Neurosurg. Psychiatry* 57: 590. MRI courtesy of James Golumb.)

HOW'S IT GOING ❓

1. What is Alzheimer's disease, and how is it diagnosed?
2. Although genes clearly influence the risk of Alzheimer's, what environmental factors can postpone its onset?

Recommended Reading

Baddeley, A. D., Eysenck, M., and Anderson, M. C. (2015). *Memory* (2nd ed.). London, England: Psychology Press.

Breedlove, S. M. (2017). *Foundations of Neural Development*. Sunderland, MA: Oxford University Press/Sinauer.

Gilbert, S. F., and Barresi, M. J. F. (2016). *Developmental Biology* (11th ed.). Sunderland, MA: Oxford University Press/Sinauer.

Kesner, R. P., and Martinez, J. L. (Eds.). (2007). *The Neurobiology of Learning and Memory* (2nd ed.). San Diego, CA: Elsevier.

Marcus, G. (2008). *The Birth of the Mind: How a Tiny Number of Genes Creates the Complexities of Human Thought.* New York, NY: Basic Books.

Rudy, J. W. (2014). *The Neurobiology of Learning and Memory* (2nd ed.). Sunderland, MA: Oxford University Press/Sinauer.

Slotnick, S. D. (2017). *Cognitive Neuroscience of Memory*. Cambridge, UK: Cambridge University Press.

Squire, L. R., and Kandel, E. R. (2008). *Memory: From Mind to Molecules.* Greenwood Village, CO: Roberts.

13 ■ Visual Summary
3e.mindsmachine.com/vs13

You should be able to relate each summary to the adjacent illustration, including structures and processes. If you go to the website for our text (**3e.mindsmachine.com**), you can follow links to figures, animations, and activities that will help you consolidate the material.

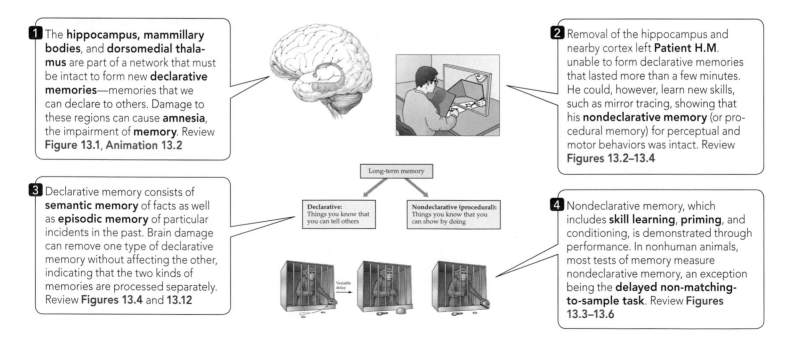

1 The **hippocampus, mammillary bodies**, and **dorsomedial thalamus** are part of a network that must be intact to form new **declarative memories**—memories that we can declare to others. Damage to these regions can cause **amnesia**, the impairment of **memory**. Review **Figure 13.1, Animation 13.2**

2 Removal of the hippocampus and nearby cortex left **Patient H.M.** unable to form declarative memories that lasted more than a few minutes. He could, however, learn new skills, such as mirror tracing, showing that his **nondeclarative memory** (or procedural memory) for perceptual and motor behaviors was intact. Review **Figures 13.2–13.4**

3 Declarative memory consists of **semantic memory** of facts as well as **episodic memory** of particular incidents in the past. Brain damage can remove one type of declarative memory without affecting the other, indicating that the two kinds of memories are processed separately. Review **Figures 13.4** and **13.12**

4 Nondeclarative memory, which includes **skill learning, priming**, and conditioning, is demonstrated through performance. In nonhuman animals, most tests of memory measure nondeclarative memory, an exception being the **delayed non-matching-to-sample task**. Review **Figures 13.3–13.6**

Long-term memory

Declarative: Things you know that you can tell others

Nondeclarative (procedural): Things you know that you can show by doing

5 Nonassociative learning includes **habituation**, while **associative learning** includes **classical conditioning** (or Pavlovian conditioning) and **instrumental conditioning** (or operant conditioning). In the slug *Aplysia*, habituation is due to a weakening of the synapse between the sensory neuron and the motor neuron. In mammals, classical conditioning happens through increases in synaptic strength in the **cerebellum**. Review **Figure 13.9, 13.18–13.19**

6 Different kinds of learning depend on different brain regions. Spatial learning requires an intact hippocampus, while skill learning relies on the **basal ganglia**, and recognition relies on the cortex. Review **Figures 13.11** and **13.12, Activities 13.1** and **13.2**

7 Memories are classified by how long they last. The **sensory buffer** is a very brief recollection of sensations. **Short-term memory (STM)** lasts for seconds to a few minutes. Then the memory is either lost or transferred to **long-term memory (LTM)**, which may last a lifetime. The successive processes transferring information from one store to the other are **encoding, consolidation**, and **retrieval**. Memories are subject to distortion during recall and reconsolidation. Strong emotion can affect the strength of memories, as in **post-traumatic stress disorder (PTSD)**. Review **Figures 13.12** and **13.13, Box 13.1**

8 **Long-term potentiation (LTP)** is a lasting increase in amplitude of the response of neurons caused by **tetanus**, a brief high-frequency stimulation of their afferents. In the hippocampus, LTP depends on the activation of **NMDA receptors**, which induces an increase in the number of postsynaptic **AMPA receptors** and greater neurotransmitter release. These are examples of changes in **Hebbian synapses**, which become stronger if they successfully drive the postsynaptic cell, and weaker if they are unsuccessful. Review **Figures 13.20–13.22, Animation 13.3, Video 13.4**

9 The brain develops in six stages: (1) **neurogenesis,** (2) **cell migration**, (3) **cell differentiation**, (4) **synaptogenesis,** (5) **cell death** (or apoptosis), and (6) **synapse rearrangement**. In adulthood, synapse rearrangement continues throughout the brain, and experience guides this process. Some neurogenesis also occurs in adults. Review **Figures 13.23–13.31, Animation 13.5, Video 13.6, Activity 13.3**

10 While genes play an important role in brain development, the environment and experience, such as mothering, can affect **gene expression**. That is, genetically identical individuals may behave very differently from one another because development is an **epigenetic** process. For example, the severe mental impairment that may accompany phenylketonuria (PKU) is avoided by controlling diet. While genes affect the buildup of **beta-amyloid** in **amyloid plaques** and therefore increase the risk of **Alzheimer's disease**, mental and physical activity postpone the onset of the disease. Review **Figures 13.32–13.35**

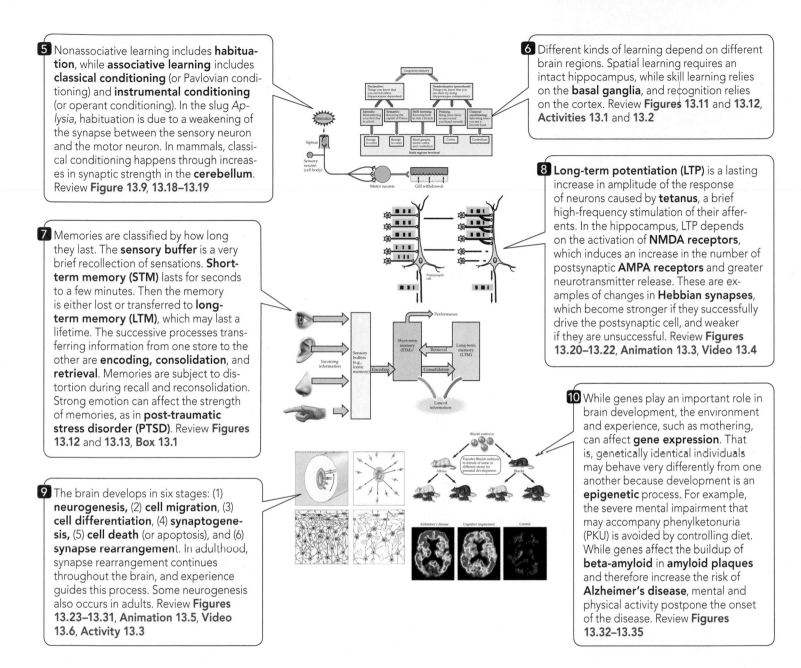

Go to **3e.mindsmachine.com** for study questions, quizzes, flashcards, and other resources.

PART I
Effects of Attention on Behavior

 THE ROAD AHEAD

The first part of this chapter is concerned with the consequences of attention processes: the ways that attention filters the world and affects our processing of sensory information. At the conclusion of this section you should be able to:

1. Provide a general definition of attention, and distinguish between overt and covert forms of attention, with examples.

2. Describe the limitations on our powers of attention, situations in which our attention may be overextended, and the behavioral manifestations of these limits on attention.

3. Speculate about the ways in which evolution may have shaped attention.

4. Distinguish between voluntary and reflexive attention, and describe general experimental designs for studying each.

5. Describe the use of focused attention to search the world for particular objects (using either a feature search or a conjunction search), and discuss the significance of the binding problem.

Attention Focuses Cognitive Processing on Specific Objects

Although she may delight in pretending otherwise, the average 5-year-old knows exactly what it means when an exasperated parent shouts, "Pay attention!" We all share an intuitive understanding of the term *attention*, but it is tricky to formally define. In general, **attention** (or *selective attention*) is the process by which we select or focus on one or more specific stimuli—either external phenomena or internal thoughts—for enhanced processing and analysis. Most of the time we direct our eyes and our attention to the same target, a process known as **overt attention**. For example, as you read this sentence, it is both the center of your visual gaze and (we hope) the main item that your brain has selected for attention. But if we choose to, we can also shift the focus of our visual attention *covertly*, keeping our eyes fixed on one location while "secretly" scrutinizing something in peripheral vision (Helmholtz, 1962; original work published in 1894). Remember that teacher who, even when looking out the window, somehow knew instantly when someone passed a note? That's an example of what is known as **covert attention** (**FIGURE 14.1**).

Selective attention isn't restricted to visual stimuli. Imagine yourself chatting with an old friend at a noisy party. Despite the background noise, you would probably find it relatively easy to focus on what your friend was saying, even if she was speaking quietly, because attention aids your sensory perception—paying close attention to your friend enhances your processing of her speech and helps filter out distracters. This phenomenon, known as the **cocktail party effect**, nicely illustrates how attention acts to *focus* cognitive processing resources on a particular target. If your attention drifts to a different stimulus—for example, if you start eavesdropping on a more interesting conversation nearby—it becomes almost impossible to simultaneously follow what your friend is saying.

There are limits on attention

The powers of attention that help you to focus on a conversation with a friend in a noisy room normally rely on cues in several different sensory modalities, such as where her speech sounds are coming from, how her face moves as she speaks, and what unique sounds her voice makes. But what if we restrict our attention to just one type of stimulus?

In **shadowing** experiments, participants must focus their attention on just one out of two or more simultaneous streams of stimuli. In a classic example of this technique,

---

To view the
Brain Explorer,
go to
3e.mindsmachine.com/av14.2

attention Also called *selective attention*. A state or condition of selective awareness or perceptual receptivity, by which specific stimuli are selected for enhanced processing.

overt attention Attention in which the focus coincides with sensory orientation (e.g., you're attending to the same thing you're looking at).

covert attention Attention in which the focus can be directed independently of sensory orientation (e.g., you're attending to one sensory stimulus while looking at another).

cocktail party effect The selective enhancement of attention in order to filter out distracters, as you might do while listening to one person talking in the midst of a noisy party.

shadowing A task in which the participant is asked to focus attention on one ear or the other while different stimuli are being presented to the two ears, and to repeat aloud the material presented to the attended ear.

FIGURE 14.1 Covert Attention

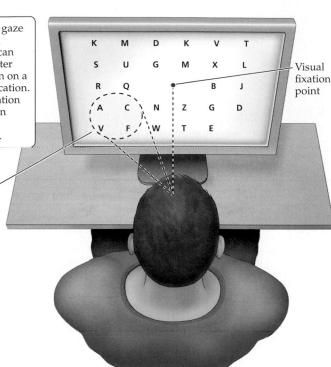

While holding our gaze steady on a central fixation point, we can independently center our visual attention on a different spatial location. This selective attention has sometimes been referred to as an *attentional spotlight*.

Visual fixation point

Location of covert spatial attention

Cherry (1953) presented different streams of speech simultaneously to people's left and right ears via headphones—the technique is called *dichotic presentation*—and asked them to focus their attention on one ear or the other and report what they heard. Participants were able to accurately report what they heard in the attended ear, but they reported very little about what was said in the *nonattended* ear, aside from simple characteristics, such as the sex of the speaker. In fact, if a shadowing task is difficult enough, people may fail to detect even their own names in the unattended ear about two-thirds of the time (N. Wood and Cowan, 1995)!

Similar restrictions of attention can be seen in other sensory modalities, such as musical notes (Zendel and Alain, 2009) and visual stimuli. Participants closely attending to one complex visual event against a background of other moving stimuli—dancers weaving through a basketball game, for example—may show **inattentional blindness**: a surprising failure to perceive nonattended stimuli. And the unperceived stimuli can be things that you might think impossible to miss, like a gorilla strolling across a movie screen out of the blue (Simons and Chabris, 1999; Simons and Jensen, 2009). Even highly trained experts can have this problem. In one study 83% of radiologists screening CT scans for lung cancer didn't notice a seemingly obvious image of a gorilla inserted into one of the scans (Drew et al., 2013) (you can see an example on our website). And even if a nonattended stimulus is highly task-relevant, it will often be missed; for example, a significant fraction of police officers and trainees will miss a gun placed in plain view during a simulated traffic stop (Simons and Schlosser, 2017).

In general, **divided-attention tasks**—in which a person is asked to process two or more simultaneous stimuli—confirm that attention is a limited resource and that it's very difficult to attend to more than one thing at a time, particularly if the stimuli are spatially separated (Bonnel and Prinzmetal, 1998). So, our limited selective attention generally acts like an **attentional spotlight** (see Figure 14.1), shifting around the environment, highlighting stimuli for enhanced processing. It's an adaptation that we share with many other species because, like us, they are confronted with the problem of extracting important signals from a noisy background (Bee and Micheyl,

To see the video
Inattentional Blindness,
go to
3e.mindsmachine.com/av14.3

inattentional blindness   The failure to perceive nonattended stimuli that seem so obvious as to be impossible to miss.

divided-attention task   A task in which the participant is asked to focus attention on two or more stimuli simultaneously.

attentional spotlight   The steerable focus of our selective attention, used to select stimuli for enhanced processing.

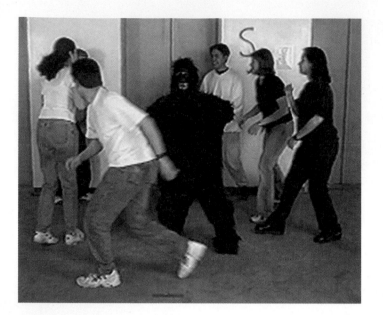

Gorillas in the Midst   Who could miss the gorilla in the video from which this still is drawn? Most people do, if they are concentrating on some other task, such as counting the number of times people in white shirts touch a ball that is being passed around. (From D. J. Simons and C. F. Chabris, 1999. *Perception* 28: 1059.)

2008). Birds, for example, must isolate the vocalizations of specific individuals from a cacophony of calls and other noises in the environment—an avian version of the cocktail party problem (Benney and Braaten, 2000). Having a single attentional spotlight helps us focus cognitive resources and behavioral responses toward the most important things in the environment at any given moment (the smell of smoke, the voice of a potential mate, a glimpse of a big spotted cat), while ignoring extraneous information.

In general, by acting as a filter, attention narrows our focus to important stimuli and protects the brain from being overwhelmed by the world. But the details of this **attentional bottleneck** have been elusive. Initial research gave evidence of an *early-selection model* of attention, in which unattended information is filtered out right away, at the level of the initial sensory input, as in the shadowing experiments (Broadbent, 1958). But other researchers noted that important but unattended stimuli (such as your name) may undergo substantial unconscious processing, right up to the level of semantic meaning and awareness, before suddenly capturing attention (N. Wood and Cowan, 1995), thus illustrating a *late-selection model* of attention. Many contemporary models of attention now combine both early- and late-selection mechanisms (e.g., Wolfe, 1994), and debate continues over their relative importance (for a classic demonstration, see **A STEP FURTHER 14.1**, on the website).

A possible resolution to this debate involves the concept of **perceptual load**—the immediate processing demands presented by a stimulus. According to this view, when we focus on a very complex stimulus, the load on our perceptual processing resources is so great that there is nothing left over. We are thus unable to process competing unattended items, so those extra stimuli are excluded right from the outset (N. Lavie, 1995; N. Lavie et al., 2004). But when we focus on stimuli that are easier to process, we may have enough perceptual resources left over to simultaneously process additional stimuli, all the way up to the level of semantic meaning and awareness. In this case the result is a late selection of stimuli to attend to (N. Lavie et al., 2009). In other words, if we view attention as a limited resource, then we only have enough of it to do one complex task at a time, or a few very simple ones. The research thus suggests that attention is continually rebalanced between early and late selection, depending on the difficulty of the task at hand. These more modern perspectives on attention are central to the development of computational models of attention in visual and auditory "scenes"; one hope is that mathematical descriptions of attentional processes will aid in the development of machine versions of vision and audition (Shic and Scassellati, 2007; Kaya and Elhilali, 2017).

HOW'S IT GOING ?

1. How do you define *attention*?
2. Distinguish between overt and covert attention, giving examples of each. What is the attentional spotlight?
3. What is inattentional blindness, and under what circumstances might it occur?
4. How do early-selection effects of attention differ from late-selection effects? What single aspect of a stimulus may determine whether early or late selection occurs?

attentional bottleneck   A filter created by the limits intrinsic to our attentional processes, whose effect is that only the most important stimuli are selected for special processing.

perceptual load   The immediate processing demands presented by a stimulus.

Attention Is Deployed in Several Different Ways

We've now seen that through an act of willpower we can direct our attention to specific stimuli without moving our eyes or otherwise reorienting. Early experiments on this phenomenon employed **sustained-attention tasks**, like the one depicted in Figure 14.1, where a single stimulus location must be held in the attentional spotlight for an extended period. Although these tasks are useful for studying basic phenomena, several key questions about attention require another approach. For example, how do we shift our attention around? How does attention enhance the processing of stimuli, and which brain regions are involved? To answer these questions, researchers devised clever tasks that employ stimulus cuing to control attention, which revealed two general categories of attention, as we'll discuss next.

RESEARCHERS AT WORK

We can choose which stimuli we will attend to

So far, our discussion of attention has focused mostly on what researchers call **voluntary attention** (or *endogenous attention*). As the name implies, voluntary shifts of attention come from within; they are the conscious, *top-down* directing of our attention toward specific aspects of the environment, according to our interests and goals. **FIGURE 14.2** features the **symbolic cuing** task, developed by Michael Posner and used extensively to study voluntary attention. Studies using cuing tasks have confirmed that consciously directing your attention to the correct location or stimulus improves processing speed and accuracy. Conversely, directing your attention to an *incorrect* location or stimulus impairs processing efficiency.

How much does it help to shift your attention to a location before a stimulus occurs there? Posner's (1980) symbolic cuing task allows us to quantify how voluntary attention benefits processing. In a symbolic cuing task, participants stare at a point in the center of a computer screen and must press a key as soon as a specific target appears on the screen (this technique thus measures reaction time, as described in **BOX 14.1**). The stimulus is preceded by a cue that briefly flashes on the screen, hinting where the stimulus will appear. Most of the time, as in **FIGURE 14.2A**, the participant is provided with a valid cue; for example, a rightward arrow flashes on the screen moments before the stimulus appears on the right side of the screen. In a few trials, like the one in **FIGURE 14.2B**, the arrow points the wrong way and thus provides an invalid cue. And in "neutral" control trials (**FIGURE 14.2C**), the cue doesn't provide any hint at all. Both the cue and the stimulus are on the screen so briefly that participants don't have time to shift their gaze (and in any case, they have been told to stare at the fixation point).

Averaged over many trials, the reaction-time data (**FIGURE 14.2D**) clearly show that people swiftly learn to use cues to predict stimulus location, shifting their attention without shifting their gaze. Compared with neutral trials, processing is significantly faster for validly cued trials, and participants pay a price for misdirecting their attention on those few trials in which the cue is invalid, pointing to the wrong side of the display. Many variants of the symbolic cuing paradigm—changing the timing of the stimuli, altering their complexity, requiring a choice between different responses (as in Box 14.1), and so on—have been used to study the neurophysiological mechanisms of attention (R. D. Wright and Ward, 2008), as we'll discuss a little later in the chapter.

(Continued)

sustained-attention task   A task in which a single stimulus source or location must be held in the attentional spotlight for a protracted period.

voluntary attention   Also called *endogenous attention*. The voluntary direction of attention toward specific aspects of the environment, in accordance with our interests and goals.

symbolic cuing   A technique for testing voluntary attention in which a visual stimulus is presented and participants are asked to respond as soon as the stimulus appears on a screen. Each trial is preceded by a meaningful symbol used as a cue to hint at where the stimulus will appear.

RESEARCHERS AT WORK   (continued)

FIGURE 14.2 Measuring the Effects of Voluntary Shifts of Attention
(After M. I. Posner, 1980. *Q. J. Exp. Psychol.* 32: 3.)

■ **Question**
Does shifting your attention to a new location, without shifting your gaze, improve the processing of stimuli that appear at the new location?

■ **Hypothesis**
Cued attention will improve subsequent processing—as measured by reaction time—if the stimulus appears at the cued location, but not if the stimulus appears elsewhere.

■ **Test**
Provide direction cues before the appearance of visual stimuli, and compare reaction times for processing validly cued vs. invalidly cued stimuli.

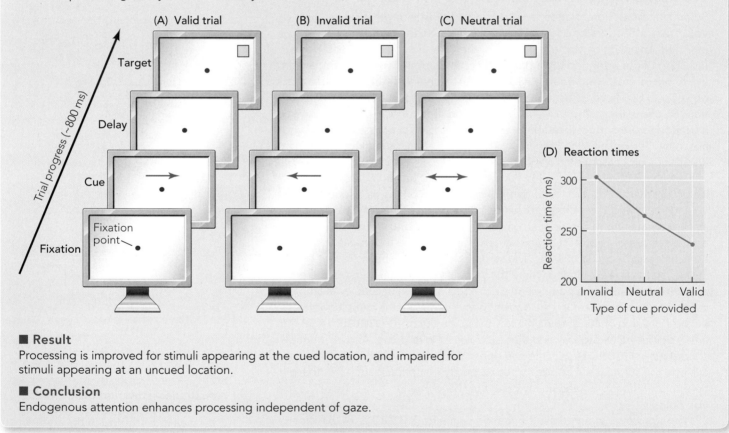

■ **Result**
Processing is improved for stimuli appearing at the cued location, and impaired for stimuli appearing at an uncued location.

■ **Conclusion**
Endogenous attention enhances processing independent of gaze.

Some stimuli grab our attention

There is a second way in which we pay attention to the world, involving more than just consciously steering our attentional spotlight around. Flashes, bangs, sudden movements—any striking or important change—can instantly snatch our attention away from whatever we're doing, unless we are very focused. Drop your glass in a restaurant, and every conversation stops, every head in the place swivels, seeking the source of the sound (you, embarrassingly). This sort of involuntary reorientation toward a sudden or important event is an example of **reflexive attention** (or *exogenous attention*). It is considered to be a *bottom-up* process, because attention is being seized by sensory inputs from lower levels of the nervous system, rather than being directed by voluntary, conscious *top-down* processes of the forebrain.

Researchers study reflexive attention using a different kind of cuing task, called **peripheral spatial cuing**. In this task, instead of a meaningful symbol like an

reflexive attention   Also called *exogenous attention*. The involuntary reorienting of attention toward a specific stimulus source, cued by an unexpected object or event.

peripheral spatial cuing   A technique for testing reflexive attention in which a visual stimulus is preceded by a simple task-irrelevant sensory stimulus either in the location where the stimulus will appear or in an incorrect location.

BOX 14.1
Reaction-Time Responses, from Input to Output

Reaction-time measures are a mainstay of cognitive neuroscience research. In tests of *simple reaction time*, participants make a single response—for example, pressing a button—in response to an experimental stimulus (the appearance of a target, the solution to a problem, a tone, or whatever the experiment is testing). In tests of *choice reaction time*, the situation is slightly more complicated: a person is presented with alternatives and has to choose among them (e.g., right versus wrong, same versus different) by pressing one of two or more buttons.

Reaction times in an uncomplicated choice-reaction-time test, in which the participant indicates whether two stimuli are the same or different, average about 300–350 milliseconds (ms). The delay between stimulus and response varies depending on the amount of neural processing required between input and output. The neural systems involved in this sort of task, and the timing of events in the response circuit, are illustrated in the figure. Brain activity proceeds from the primary visual cortex (V1) through a ventral visual object identification pathway (see Chapter 7) to prefrontal cortex, and then through premotor and primary motor cortex, down to the spinal motor neurons and out to the finger muscles. In the sequence shown in the figure—proceeding from the presentation of visual stimuli to a discrimination response—notice that it takes about 110 ms for the sensory system to recognize the stimulus (somewhere in the inferior temporal lobe), about 35 ms more for that information to reach the prefrontal cortex, and then about 30 ms more to

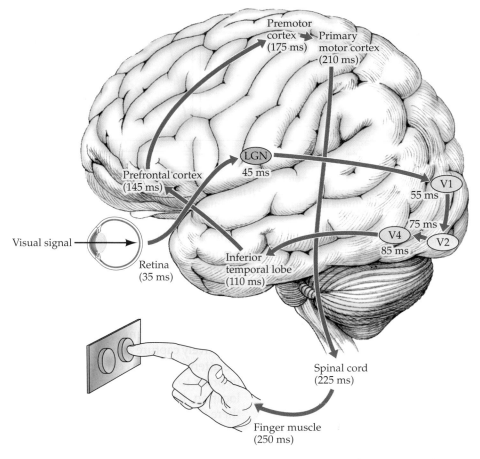

A Reaction-Time Circuit in the Brain   The sequence and timing of brain events that determine reaction time. LGN, lateral geniculate nucleus; V1, primary visual cortex; V2 and V4, extrastriate visual areas. (Timings based on S. J. Thorpe and M. Fabre Thorpe, 2001. *Science* 291: 260.)

determine which button to push. After that, it takes another 75 ms or so for the movement to be executed (that is, 75 ms of time elapses between the moment the signal from the prefrontal cortex arrives in premotor cortex and the

moment the finger pushes the button). It is fascinating to think that something like this sequence of neural events happens over and over in more-complicated behaviors, such as recognizing a long-lost friend or composing an opera.

---

arrow, the cue that is presented is a simple sensory stimulus, such as a flash of light, occurring *in the location to which attention is to be drawn*. Research with this type of simple cuing confirmed that valid reflexive cues enhance the processing of subsequent stimuli at the same location, but only when the target stimulus closely follows the cue. At longer intervals between the cue and target, starting at about 200 milliseconds, a curious phenomenon is observed: detection of stimuli at the location where the valid cue occurred is increasingly *impaired* (Posner and Cohen, 1984; R. M. Klein, 2000). It's as though attention has moved on from where the cue occurred and is reluctant to return to that location. This **inhibition of return** probably evolved because it prevented reflexively controlled attention from settling on unimportant stimuli for more than an instant.

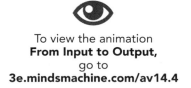

To view the animation
From Input to Output,
go to
3e.mindsmachine.com/av14.4

inhibition of return   The phenomenon, observed in peripheral spatial cuing tasks when the interval between cue and target stimulus is 200 milliseconds or more, in which the detection of stimuli at the former location of the cue is increasingly impaired.

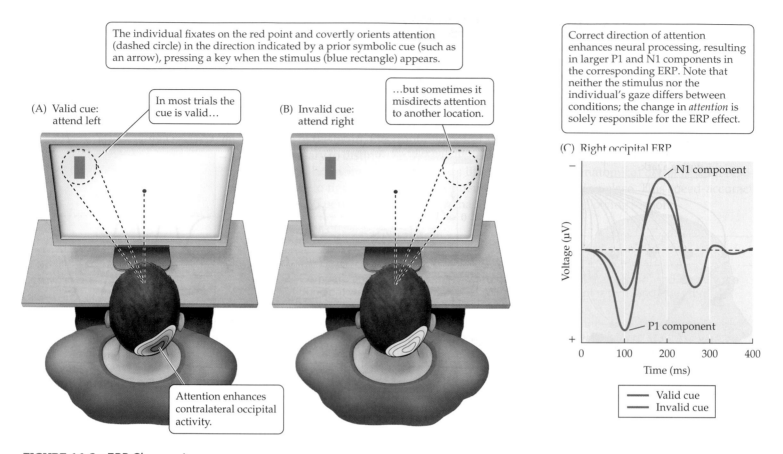

The individual fixates on the red point and covertly orients attention (dashed circle) in the direction indicated by a prior symbolic cue (such as an arrow), pressing a key when the stimulus (blue rectangle) appears.

(A) Valid cue: attend left

In most trials the cue is valid...

(B) Invalid cue: attend right

...but sometimes it misdirects attention to another location.

Correct direction of attention enhances neural processing, resulting in larger P1 and N1 components in the corresponding ERP. Note that neither the stimulus nor the individual's gaze differs between conditions; the change in *attention* is solely responsible for the ERP effect.

(C) Right occipital ERP

Voltage (μV)

N1 component

P1 component

Time (ms)

Valid cue
Invalid cue

Attention enhances contralateral occipital activity.

FIGURE 14.6 ERP Changes in Voluntary Visual Attention

visual P1 effect A positive deflection of the event-related potential, occurring 70–100 milliseconds after stimulus presentation, that is enhanced for selectively attended visual input compared with ignored input.

debating whether P3 therefore is (Dehaene and Changeux, 2011) or is not (Pitts et al., 2014) an electrophysiological marker of consciousness. Abnormal P3 responses are a reliable finding in people with schizophrenia, consistent with their difficulty in filtering out distracting information (Ford, 1999).

What about effects of attention on ERPs from *visual* stimuli? Because the neural systems involved in visual perception are different from those involved in audition, voluntary visual attention causes its own distinctive changes in the ERP. We can study these visual effects by collecting ERP data over occipital cortex—the primary visual area of the brain—while a participant performs a symbolic cuing task. **FIGURE 14.6** depicts this sort of experiment. On valid trials (remember, this is when the target appears as expected, in the location indicated by the cue, as in Figure 14.6A), electrodes over occipital cortex show a substantial enhancement of the ERP component P1, the positive wave that occurs about 70–100 milliseconds after stimulus onset, often carrying over into an enhancement of the N1 component immediately afterward (Figure 14.6C). Notice that the enhancement occurs over the *contralateral* occipital cortex; this is because information from the left visual field is processed in right occipital cortex, and vice versa, as we discussed in Chapter 7. A similar effect on P1 is evident when attention is instead oriented *reflexively* to a flash or sound (Hopfinger and Mangun, 1998; McDonald et al., 2005), but only when the interval between the cue and the appearance of the target is brief (**FIGURE 14.7**). At longer intervals, the P1 effect may actually be *reduced* as an electrophysiological manifestation of inhibition of return (McDonald et al., 1999). And for invalid trials (Figure 14.6B), where attention is being directed elsewhere, the **visual P1 effect** isn't evident at all, even though the visual stimulus is identical and in the same location as in the valid trials. Interestingly, the P1 effect is evident only in visual tasks involving manipulations of *spatial* attention (*where* is the target?)—not other features, like color, orientation, or more complex properties that would be characteristic of late-selection tasks.

The same right-sided stimulus was presented in each case, but in some trials the stimulus was preceded by an unexpected flash in the location where the stimulus then appeared (valid trials). In other trials the flash drew attention to a different location (invalid trials).

FIGURE 14.7   ERP Maps in Reflexive Visual Attention (After J. B. Hopfinger and G. R. Mangun, 1998. *Psychol. Sci.*, 9: 441.)

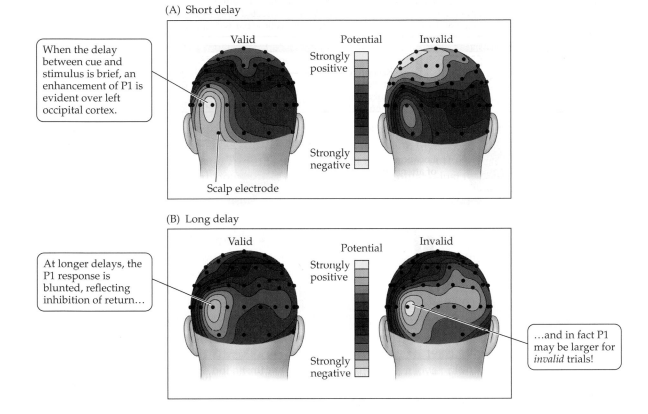

(A) Short delay

When the delay between cue and stimulus is brief, an enhancement of P1 is evident over left occipital cortex.

Valid   Potential   Invalid
Strongly positive
Strongly negative

Scalp electrode

(B) Long delay

At longer delays, the P1 response is blunted, reflecting inhibition of return…

Valid   Potential   Invalid
Strongly positive
Strongly negative

…and in fact P1 may be larger for *invalid* trials!

What happens to ERPs during visual search tasks, where we are directing attention so as to find a particular target in an array and ignore distracters? Under these conditions, a characteristic enhancement of a subcomponent of N2 (see Figure 14.5), called *N2pc,* is triggered at occipitotemporal sites contralateral to where attention is being directed (Luck and Hillyard, 1994; Hickey et al., 2009).

The neural mechanisms of visual attention may be quite plastic. Extensive experience with action video games, which heavily rely on visual attention, is associated with neural changes (S. Tanaka et al., 2013; West et al., 2015) and corresponding enhancements of longer-latency ERP components (Mishra et al., 2011; Palaus et al., 2017). Possible trade-offs for all this gaming, however, may include impaired social and emotional function (no, we're not kidding: K. Bailey and West, 2013). And of course, some people could be drawn to gaming simply because they are already good at visuospatial processing (Boot et al., 2008).

Attention affects the activity of neurons

PET and fMRI operate too slowly to track the rapid changes in brain activity that occur in reaction-time tests. Instead, researchers have used "sustained-attention tasks" to confirm that attention enhances activity in brain regions that process key aspects of the target stimulus. So, for example, when participants are presented with stimuli made up of faces overlaid on pictures of houses, and asked to focus and sustain their attention only on the faces, fMRI reveals enhanced activation of a part of the brain (called the *fusiform gyrus*) that is especially important for face processing (O'Craven et al., 1999). A different brain area (the *parahippocampal place area*) is activated if attention is focused on the houses in the stimuli, instead of the faces. Results like these suggest that attention somehow acts directly on neurons, boosting the activity of those brain regions that

FIGURE 14.10 Cortical Regions Implicated in the Top-Level Control of Attention

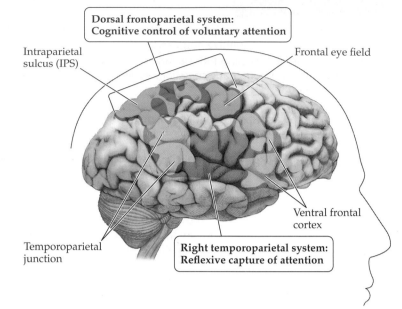

Dorsal frontoparietal system: Cognitive control of voluntary attention

Intraparietal sulcus (IPS)

Frontal eye field

Ventral frontal cortex

Temporoparietal junction

Right temporoparietal system: Reflexive capture of attention

To view the activity **Cortical Regions Implicated in the Top-Level Control of Attention,** go to **3e.mindsmachine.com/ac14.2**

lateral intraparietal area (LIP) A region in the monkey parietal lobe, homologous to the human intraparietal sulcus, that is especially involved in voluntary, top-down control of attention.

intraparietal sulcus (IPS) A region in the human parietal lobe, homologous to the monkey lateral intraparietal area, that is especially involved in voluntary, top-down control of attention.

frontal eye field (FEF) An area in the frontal lobe of the brain that contains neurons important for establishing gaze in accordance with cognitive goals (top-down processes) rather than with any characteristics of stimuli (bottom-up processes).

Dorsolateral frontal, FEF vicinity

Dorsolateral parietal, IPS vicinity

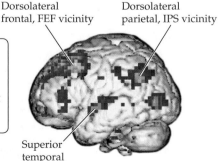

During conscious shifts of covert attention, ER-fMRI shows activation of the frontal eye field and the intraparietal sulcus (along with some activation of the temporal lobe).

Superior temporal

FIGURE 14.11 The Frontoparietal Attention Network (From J. B. Hopfinger et al., 2000. *Nat. Neurosci.* 2: 284.)

A DORSAL FRONTOPARIETAL NETWORK FOR VOLUNTARY CONTROL OF ATTENTION In monkeys, recordings from single cells show that a region called the **lateral intraparietal area**, or just **LIP**, is crucial for voluntary attention. LIP neurons increase their firing rate when attention—not gaze—is directed to particular locations, and it doesn't matter whether the voluntary attention is being directed toward visual or auditory targets (Bisley and Goldberg, 2003; Gottlieb, 2007). So it's the top-down steering of the attentional spotlight that is important to LIP neurons, not the sensory characteristics of the stimuli.

The human equivalent of this system is a region around the **intraparietal sulcus (IPS)** (**FIGURE 14.10**) that behaves much like the monkey LIP. For example, on tasks designed so that covert attention can be sustained long enough to make fMRI images, enhanced activity in the IPS is associated with the control of attention (Corbetta and Shulman, 1998). And when researchers used transcranial magnetic stimulation (see Chapter 2) to interfere with the IPS in research participants, the participants found it difficult to voluntarily shift attention (Koch et al., 2005).

People with damage to a frontal lobe region called the **frontal eye field** (**FEF**) (see Figure 14.10) struggle to prevent their gaze from being drawn away toward peripheral distracters while they're performing a voluntary attention task (Paus et al., 1991). Neurons of the FEF appear to be crucial for ensuring that our gaze is directed among stimuli according to cognitive goals rather than being guided by any characteristics of stimuli. In effect, the FEF ensures that cognitively controlled top-down attention gets priority. It's no surprise, then, that the FEF is closely connected to the superior colliculus, which, as we discussed earlier, is important for planned eye movements.

A modified form of fMRI that links rapid behavioral events to changes in activity of selected brain regions (called, unsurprisingly, *event-related fMRI,* or *ER-fMRI*) reveals network activities during top-down attentional processing (Corbetta et al., 2000; Hopfinger et al., 2000). **FIGURE 14.11** shows patterns of activation while voluntary attention is shifting in response to a symbolic cue. Enhanced activity is evident in the vicinity of the frontal eye fields (dorsolateral frontal cortex) and, simultaneously, in the IPS. Electrophysiological studies of the timing of activity in the network indicate that the attentional control–related activity is first seen in the frontal and parietal components, followed by anticipatory activation of visual cortex (if the expected stimulus is visual) or auditory cortex (if the stimulus is a sound) (McDonald and Green, 2008; Green et al., 2011). Taken together, these studies support the view that a dorsal frontoparietal network provides top-down (voluntary) control of attention.

A RIGHT TEMPOROPARIETAL NETWORK FOR REFLEXIVE SHIFTS OF ATTENTION   A second attention system, located at the border of the temporal and parietal lobes of the right hemisphere—and named, a little unimaginatively, the **temporoparietal junction (TPJ)** (see Figure 14.10)—is involved in steering attention toward novel or unexpected stimuli (flashes, color changes, and so on). ER-fMRI studies (**FIGURE 14.12**) confirm that there's a spike in right-hemisphere TPJ activity if a relevant stimulus suddenly appears in an unexpected location (Corbetta et al., 2000; Corbetta and Shulman, 2002), and people with TPJ damage may fail to react to unanticipated targets (Friedrich et al., 1998). Interestingly, the TPJ system receives direct input from the visual cortex, presumably providing direct access for information about visual stimuli. The TPJ also has strong connections with the ventral frontal cortex (VFC), a region that is involved in working memory (see Chapter 13). Because working memory tracks sensory inputs over short time frames, the VFC's contribution may be to analyze *novelty* by comparing present stimuli with those of the recent past. Overall, the ventral TPJ system seems to act as an alerting signal, or "circuit breaker," overriding our current attentional priority if something new and unexpected happens.

Ultimately, the dorsal and ventral attention-control networks need to interact extensively and function as a single interactive system. According to one influential model (Corbetta and Shulman, 2002), the more dorsal stream of processing is responsible for *voluntary* attention, enhancing neural processing of stimuli and interacting with the pulvinar and superior colliculus to steer the attentional spotlight around. At the same time, the right-sided temporoparietal system scans the environment for novel salient stimuli (which then draw *reflexive* attention), rapidly reassigning attention as interesting stimuli pop up. This basic model seems to apply across sensory modalities (Kanwisher and Wojciulik, 2000), including visual and auditory stimuli (Brunetti et al., 2008; Walther et al., 2010).

Brain disorders can cause specific impairments of attention

One way to learn about attention systems in the brain is to note the behavioral consequences of damage to specific regions of the brain. Research with neurological patients shows that damage of cortical or subcortical attention mechanisms can dramatically alter our ability to understand and interact with the environment.

RIGHT-HEMISPHERE LESIONS   We've discussed evidence that the right hemisphere normally plays a special role in attention (see Figure 14.12). Unfortunately, it is not uncommon for people to suffer strokes or other types of brain damage that particularly affect this part of the brain. The result—**hemispatial neglect**—is an extraordinary attention syndrome in which the patient tends to completely disregard the left side of the world. People and objects to the left of the person's midline may be completely ignored, as if unseen, even though the person's vision is otherwise normal (Rafal, 1994). The patient may fail to dress the left side of their body, will not notice visitors if they approach from the left, and may fail to eat the food on the left side of their dinner plate. If touched lightly on both hands at the same moment, the patient may notice only the right-hand touch—a symptom called *simultaneous extinction*. They may even

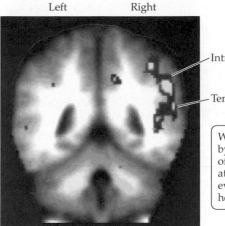

Left   Right

Intraparietal sulcus (IPS)

Temporoparietal junction (TPJ)

When attention is captured by the sudden appearance of stimuli (exogenous attention), activity is evident in this right-hemisphere system.

FIGURE 14.12   The Right Temporoparietal System and Reflexive Attention   (From M. Corbetta et al., 2000. *Nat. Neurosci.* 3: 292.)

temporoparietal junction (TPJ)   The point in the brain where the temporal and parietal lobes meet. It plays a role in shifting attention to a new location after target onset.

hemispatial neglect   Failure to pay any attention to objects presented to one side of the body.

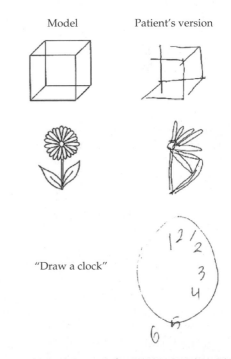

Model   Patient's version

"Draw a clock"

Diagnostic Test for Hemispatial Neglect   When asked to duplicate drawings of common symmetrical objects, people with hemispatial neglect ignore the left side of the model that they're copying. (After Parton et al., 2004. *J. Neurol. Neurosurg. Psychiatry* 75: 13.)

(A) Critical areas damaged in hemispatial neglect

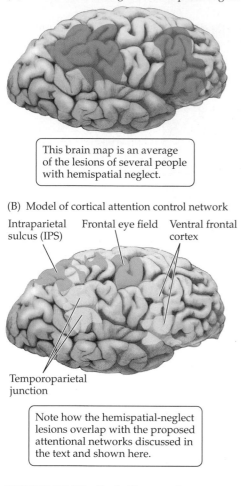

This brain map is an average of the lesions of several people with hemispatial neglect.

(B) Model of cortical attention control network

Intraparietal sulcus (IPS) Frontal eye field Ventral frontal cortex

Temporoparietal junction

Note how the hemispatial-neglect lesions overlap with the proposed attentional networks discussed in the text and shown here.

FIGURE 14.13 Brain Damage in Hemispatial Neglect

deny ownership of their left arm or leg—"My sister must've left that arm in my bed; wasn't that an awful thing to do?!"—despite normal sensory function and otherwise intact intellectual capabilities.

It is as if the normally balanced competition for attention between the two sides has become skewed and now the input from the right side overrules or extinguishes the input from the left. Lesions in patients with hemispatial neglect (**FIGURE 14.13A**) neatly overlap the frontoparietal attention network that we discussed earlier (shown again in **FIGURE 14.13B**). This overlap suggests that hemispatial neglect is a disorder of attention itself, and not a problem with processing spatial relationships, as was once thought (Mesulam, 1985; Bartolomeo, 2007). With time, hemispatial neglect can significantly improve (although simultaneous extinction often persists), and targeted therapies may help. For example, researchers are experimenting with the use of special prism glasses to shift vision to the right during intense physical therapy, in order to recalibrate the visual attention system (Barrett et al., 2012; O'Shea et al., 2017).

BILATERAL LESIONS Parminder, whom we met at the beginning of the chapter, had *bilateral* lesions of the parietal lobe regions that are implicated in the attention network. While rare, biparietal damage can result in a dramatic disorder called **Balint's syndrome**, made up of three principal symptoms. First, people with Balint's syndrome have great difficulty steering their visual gaze appropriately (a symptom called *oculomotor apraxia*). Second, they are unable to accurately reach for objects using visual guidance (*optic ataxia*). And third—the most striking symptom—people with Balint's syndrome show a profound restriction of attention, to the point that only one object or feature can be consciously observed at any moment. This problem, called **simultagnosia**, can be likened to an extreme narrowing of the attentional spotlight, to the point that it can't encompass more than one object at a time. Hold up a comb or a pencil, and Parminder has no trouble identifying the object. But hold up both the comb *and* the pencil, and she can identify only one or the other. It's as though she is simply unable to consciously experience more than one external feature at a time, despite having little or no loss of vision. Balint's syndrome thus illustrates the coordination of attention and awareness with mechanisms that orient us within our environment.

SIGNS & SYMPTOMS

Difficulty with Sustained Attention Can Sometimes Be Relieved with Stimulants

At least 5% of all children are diagnosed with **attention deficit hyperactivity disorder** (**ADHD**), characterized as difficulty with directing sustained attention to a task or activity, along with a higher degree of impulsivity than other children of the same age. About three-fourths of those diagnosed are male. Estimating the prevalence of ADHD (**FIGURE 14.14**) is complicated and very controversial; for example, there is significant variation in ADHD diagnosis and medication between different (sometimes neighboring) states within the USA, raising questions about the reliability of current diagnostic practices (Fulton et al., 2009). Nevertheless, researchers have identified several neurological changes associated with this disorder. Affected children tend to have slightly reduced overall brain volumes (about 3–4% smaller than in unaffected children), with reductions especially evident in the cerebellum and the frontal lobes

(Arnsten, 2006). As we discuss elsewhere in the chapter, frontal lobe function is important for myriad complex cognitive processes, including the inhibition of impulsive behavior. (But remember, correlational studies like these are mute with regard to causation; we don't know whether the brain differences cause, or are caused by, the behavior.)

In addition to structural changes, ADHD has been associated with abnormalities in connectivity between brain regions, such as within the default mode network (discussed in the Part III) (Cao et al., 2014). In fact, individual differences in the ability to sustain attention can be predicted with high accuracy from the strength of sets of brain connections (Rosenberg et al., 2016, 2017), even in the resting state, when the individual is not working on any particular task. Children with ADHD may have abnormal activity levels in some specific brain systems, such as the system that signals the rewarding aspects of

SIGNS & SYMPTOMS (continued)

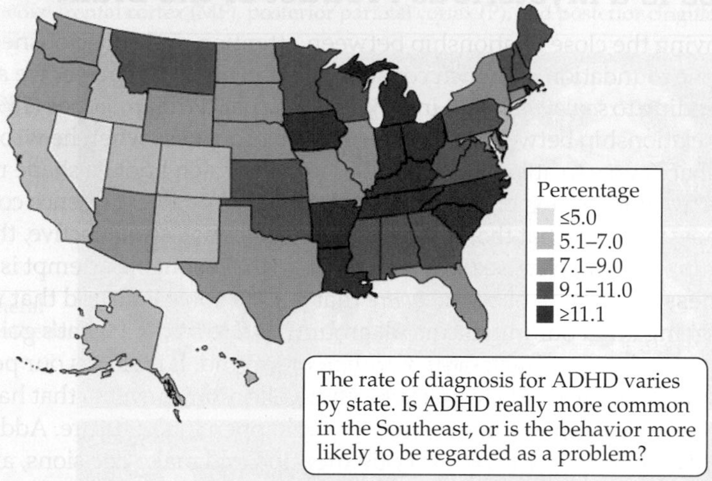

FIGURE 14.14 Prevalence of ADHD in the United States (After S. N. Visser et al., 2014. *J. Am. Acad. Child Adolesc. Psychiatry* 53: 34.)

Percentage
- ≤5.0
- 5.1–7.0
- 7.1–9.0
- 9.1–11.0
- ≥11.1

The rate of diagnosis for ADHD varies by state. Is ADHD really more common in the Southeast, or is the behavior more likely to be regarded as a problem?

activities (Furukawa et al., 2014). Based on a model of ADHD that implicates impairments in dopamine and norepinephrine neurotransmission, some researchers advocate treating these children with stimulant drugs like methylphenidate (Ritalin), which inhibits the synaptic reuptake of dopamine and norepinephrine, or with selective norepinephrine reuptake inhibitors like atomexetine (Strattera) (Schwartz and Correll, 2014). Stimulant treatment often improves the focus and performance of ADHD children in traditional school settings, but this treatment remains controversial because of the significant risk of side effects. Furthermore, stimulants improve focus in everybody, not just people with ADHD, which raises doubts about the orthodox view that impaired neurotransmission is the sole cause of ADHD (del Campo et al., 2013). An emerging alternative view is that what is diagnosed as ADHD may simply be an extreme on a continuum of normal behavior. Allowing kids diagnosed with ADHD to fidget and engage in more intense physical activity effectively reduces their symptoms and improves task performance (Hartanto et al., 2016; Den Heijer et al., 2017). You can read more about ADHD and another developmental disorder—autism spectrum disorder—in **A STEP FURTHER 13.4** (from Chapter 13), on the website.

HOW'S IT GOING ❓

1. Identify two subcortical structures that are implicated in the control of attention. What functions do they perform?
2. What is the general name for the cortical system responsible for conscious shifts of attention? What are its components, and what happens when those components are damaged?
3. Name the cortical system implicated in reflexive shifts of attention. Which specific regions are part of this system, and what happens if they are damaged?

PART III
Consciousness, Thought, and Executive Function

THE ROAD AHEAD

The final part of the chapter looks at the most enigmatic, top-level product of the brain—consciousness—and its relationships with attention, reflection, and the executive processes that direct thoughts and feelings. After reading this section, you should be able to:

1. Provide a reasonable definition of consciousness, and name the neural networks and structures that, when activated, may play a special role in coordinating conscious states.
2. Discuss the relationship between consciousness as experienced by healthy people and the diminished levels of consciousness experienced by people in comas and minimally conscious states.
3. Discuss the impediments to the scientific study of consciousness, distinguishing between the "easy" and "hard" problems of consciousness, and how free will relates to the study of consciousness.
4. Provide an overview of the organization and function of the frontal lobes, and especially prefrontal cortex, as they relate to high-level cognition and executive functions.

Balint's syndrome A disorder, caused by damage to both parietal lobes, that is characterized by difficulty in steering visual gaze (oculomotor apraxia), in accurately reaching for objects using visual guidance (optic ataxia), and in directing attention to more than one object or feature at a time (simultagnosia).

simultagnosia A profound restriction of attention, often limited to a single item or feature.

attention deficit hyperactivity disorder (ADHD) A syndrome characterized by distractibility, impulsiveness, and hyperactivity that, in children, interferes with school performance.

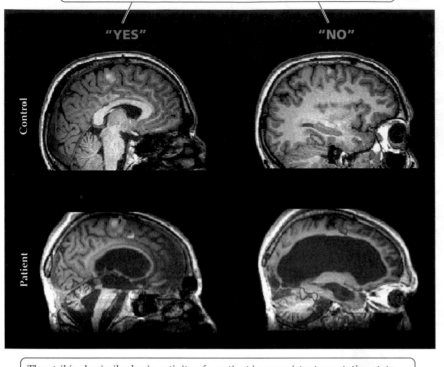

Functional MRI shows the brain activity of a healthy control participant asked to use two different mental images (playing tennis versus navigating) to signal "yes" or "no" answers to questions.

"YES" "NO"

Control

Patient

The strikingly similar brain activity of a patient in a persistent vegetative state raises questions about the definition of unconsciousness. The patient was able to correctly answer a variety of questions using this technique, despite being in a state of apparently deep unconsciousness due to profound brain damage (as evident in the grossly abnormal MRI scan) and lacking behavioral responses.

FIGURE 14.17 Communication in "Unconscious" Patients (After M. M. Monti et al., 2010. *NEJM* 362: 579.)

To see the video
Reconstructing Brain Activity,
go to
3e.mindsmachine.com/av14.5

cognitively impenetrable Referring to basic neural processing operations that cannot be experienced through introspection—in other words, that are unconscious.

easy problem of consciousness Understanding how particular patterns of neural activity create specific conscious experiences by reading brain activity directly from people's brains as they're having particular experiences.

consciousness was interrupted by bilateral electrical stimulation in lateral frontal cortex (Quraishi et al., 2017), perhaps as a result of disrupting activity in complex networks associated with consciousness.

But is clinical unconsciousness really the inverse of consciousness? Perhaps it's not that simple. For one thing, some patients in apparently deep and unresponsive coma can be instructed to use two different forms of mental imagery to create distinct "yes" and "no" patterns of activity on fMRI and then to use this mental activity to answer questions (**FIGURE 14.17**) (Monti et al., 2010; Fernández-Espejo and Owen, 2013). Most people in persistent deep coma—termed a *vegetative state*—don't respond to questions and outside stimulation, but others in *minimally conscious states* may have considerable cognitive activity and awareness with little or no overt behavior (Gosseries et al., 2014). So, it's increasingly clear that we can't simply view a coma as an exact inverse of what we experience as consciousness. In any case, there seems to be more to consciousness than just being awake, aware, and attending. How can we identify and study the additional dimensions of consciousness?

Some aspects of consciousness are easier to study than others

Most of the activity of the central nervous system is unconscious. Scientists call these brain functions **cognitively impenetrable**: they involve basic neural processing operations that cannot be experienced through introspection. For example, we see whole objects and hear whole words and can't really imagine what the primitive sensory precursors of those perceptions would feel like. Sweet food tastes sweet, and we can't mentally break it down any further. But those simpler mechanisms, operating below the surface of awareness, are the foundation that conscious experiences are built on.

In principle, then, we might someday develop technology that would let us directly reconstruct people's conscious experience—read their minds—by decoding the primitive neural activity and assembling identifiable patterns from it. This is sometimes called the **easy problem of consciousness**: understanding how particular patterns of neural activity create *specific* conscious experiences. Of course, it's almost a joke to call this problem "easy," but at least we can fairly say that, someday, the necessary technology and knowledge may be available to accomplish the task of eavesdropping on large networks of neurons, in real time.

Present-day technology offers a glimpse of that possible future. For example, if participants are repeatedly scanned while viewing several distinctive scenes, a computer can eventually learn to identify which of the scenes the participant is viewing on each trial, solely on the basis of the pattern of brain activation (**FIGURE 14.18A**) (Kay et al., 2008). Of course, this outcome relies on having the participants repeatedly view the same static images—hardly a normal state of consciousness. A much more difficult problem is to reconstruct conscious experience from neural activity during a person's first exposure to a stimulus. So far, this has been accomplished for only relatively simple visual stimuli (**FIGURE 14.18B**) (Miyawaki et al., 2008) or brief video reconstructions (**BOX 14.2**). But it's a good start, and rapid progress seems likely as technological problems are solved.

(A) Pattern identification

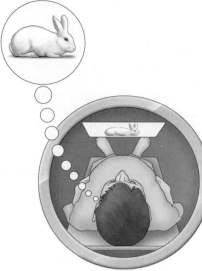

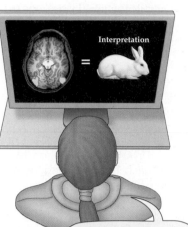

FIGURE 14.18 Easy and Hard Problems of Consciousness (Part A after K. N. Kay et al., 2008. *Nature* 452: 352; B after Y. Miyawaki et al., 2008. *Neuron* 60: 915.)

For a person in a brain scanner, repeatedly viewing the same image causes the same pattern of brain activity to occur each time. Over enough trials, researchers can develop computer models that identify which of about 20 images the participant is looking at.

"In the past, that pattern of brain activity only appeared when he was looking at the rabbit."

(B) Visual reconstruction

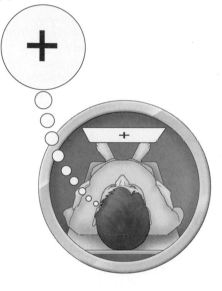

Scientists also know enough about how different parts of the brain are activated by light striking the retina that they can even predict what type of simple shapes a person is viewing.

"It looks like a 'plus' sign."

(C) Subjective experience

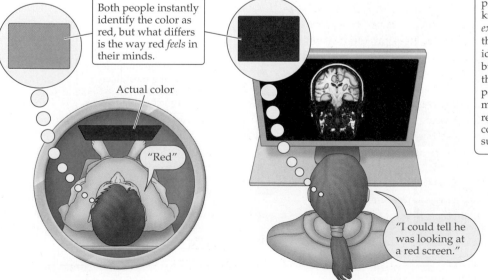

Both people instantly identify the color as red, but what differs is the way red *feels* in their minds.

Actual color

"Red"

"I could tell he was looking at a red screen."

The "hard" problem is to go beyond predicting what a person is seeing to knowing what that person's *subjective experience* is like. Here, the participant and the researcher would both immediately identify the color being viewed as "red" but, as suggested by their respective thought bubbles, the participant's personal, internal, *subjective* experience may be quite different from that of the researcher. It is difficult to see how we could ever be sure that we share any subjective experiences of consciousness.

BOX 14.2
Building a Better Mind Reader

Some sort of machine that can record and play back a person's thoughts and feelings is a staple of science fiction, but is it plausible? By tracking the activity of the retinotopic map in primary visual cortex with fMRI, researchers succeeded in detecting whether people are viewing crosses, circles, or other large and simple stimuli (Miyawaki et al., 2008; depicted in Figure 14.18B) or static pictures of faces or scenes (Naselaris et al., 2009). However, traditional fMRI is normally too slow to "read" anything more than relatively simple, static visual experiences. But of course visual perception is almost never static; it's a continuously rolling movie, directed by attention and powerfully shaping our consciousness.

So how can we sneak a look at people's internal movies? One clever approach involves building a huge library of brain responses to visual scenes and using those to reconstruct visual experiences from recordings of brain activity. Researchers in Jack Gallant's lab at UC Berkeley (Nishimoto and Gallant, 2011) began by themselves spending many, many hours watching two sets of training videos—Hollywood movie trailers—while fMRI data were recorded

from the occipitotemporal visual cortex. These data were used to develop a mathematical model that predicts how shape and motion are encoded for every voxel in the visual cortex. (*Voxel* is short for **vo**lumetric pi**xel**, and just as pixels define the two dimensions of a computer screen, voxels make up the three-dimensional volume of an imaged brain.)

Next, the researchers cut up a random assortment of YouTube videos into 18 million clips, each 1 second long, none of which were from the original training videos. This library of short clips was fed into a computer program containing the voxel-by-voxel model of brain activity for each participant. The program created a prediction for the pattern of brain activity that each of the 18 million clips would produce.

Finally, the computer compared the actual fMRI activity recorded during the second set of test videos (again, movie trailers) with the *predicted* activity associated with the YouTube clips. For each 1-second "frame" of the test videos, a computer program selected the 100 clips whose predicted activity most closely matched the actual activity recorded when the participant viewed

the original frame. These clips were then merged together into a movie reconstruction. The results of this process are shown in the figure. For each of three test video clips (A, B, and C), three individual frames are shown across the top row. The next five rows show the five best-fitting YouTube frames, as selected by the modeled brain activity of the participant. Mostly, they don't much resemble the original frames, but when averaged together, as shown in the bottom row, a blurry but pretty strong resemblance begins to emerge. The accuracy of the reconstruction is much more evident when viewing the original and reconstructed videos playing side by side, which you can see on our website. It is almost unnerving. Researchers are now developing related techniques to reconstruct participants' mental imagery of various categories of complex stimuli, such as novel faces (Nestor et al., 2016) and natural visual scenes (Lescroart et al., 2015).

As technology develops, we can expect more progress on this, the "easy" problem of consciousness.

The Mind's Eye (From S. Nishimoto et al., 2011. *Curr. Cell Biol.* 21: 1641, courtesy of Drs. Shinji Nishimoto and Jack Gallant, University of California, Berkeley.)

(A) (B) (C)

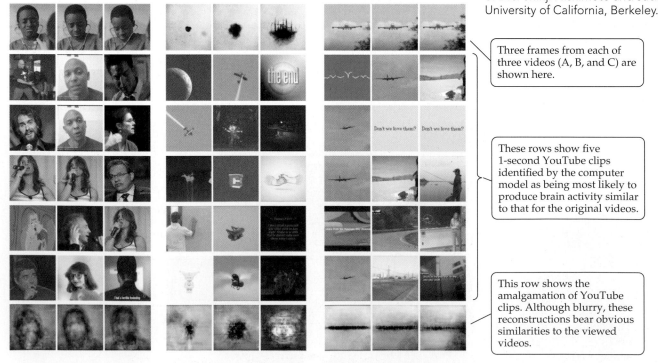

Three frames from each of three videos (A, B, and C) are shown here.

These rows show five 1-second YouTube clips identified by the computer model as being most likely to produce brain activity similar to that for the original videos.

This row shows the amalgamation of YouTube clips. Although blurry, these reconstructions bear obvious similarities to the viewed videos.

Alas, there is also the **hard problem of consciousness**, and it may prove impossible to crack. How can we understand the brain processes that produce people's *subjective experiences* of their conscious perceptions? To use a simple example, everyone with normal vision will agree that a ripe tomato is "red." That's the label that children all learn to apply to the particular pattern of information, entering consciousness from the color-processing areas of visual cortex, that is provoked by looking at something like a tomato. But that doesn't mean that your friend's internal *personal* experience of "red" is the same as yours. These purely subjective experiences of perceptions are referred to as **qualia** (singular *quale*). Because they are subjective and impossible to communicate to others—how can your friend know if "redness" feels the same in your mind as it does in hers?—qualia may prove impossible to study (**FIGURE 14.18C**). At this point, anyway, we are unable to even conceive of a technology that would make it possible.

Our subjective experience of consciousness is closely tied up with the notion of **free will**: the belief that our conscious self is unconstrained in deciding our actions and decisions and that for any given moment, given exactly the same circumstances, we *could* have chosen to engage in a different behavior. After hundreds of years of argument, there's still no agreement on whether we actually have free will, but most people behave as though there are always options, and in any event, there must be a neural substrate for the universal *feeling* of having free will. When participants *intend* to act (push a button, say), there is selective activation of the IPS (which we implicated earlier in top-down attention) and frontal regions including dorsal prefrontal cortex (Lau et al., 2004), suggesting that these regions are important for our feelings of control over our behavior. However, the conscious experience of intention may come relatively late in the process of deciding what to do. Early research (Libet, 1985), using EEG and a precise timer, found that an EEG component signaling movement preparation was evident 200 milliseconds before participants consciously decided to move. Although controversy initially surrounded this work, more recent research (**FIGURE 14.19**) found that brain activity associated with making a decision was evident in fMRI scans as much as 5–10 seconds *before* participants were consciously aware of making a choice (Soon et al., 2008)!

In any event, the earliest indications of the decision-making process are found in frontal cortex. Such involvement of prefrontal systems in most aspects of attention and consciousness, regardless of sensory modality or emotional tone, suggests that the frontal cortex is the main source of goal-driven behaviors (E. K. Miller and Cohen, 2001; Badre and Nee, 2018), as we discuss next.

hard problem of consciousness
Understanding the brain processes that produce people's subjective experiences of their conscious perceptions—that is, their qualia.

quale   A purely subjective experience of perception.

free will   The feeling that our conscious self is the author of our actions and decisions.

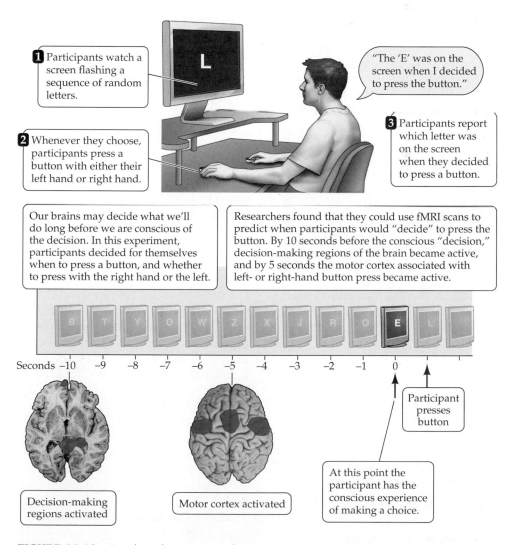

FIGURE 14.19   **Reading the Future** (After C. S. Soon et al., 2008. *Nat. Neurosci.* 11: 543.)

The human prefrontal cortex can be subdivided into a dorsolateral region (blue) and an orbitofrontal region (green). Lesions in these different areas of prefrontal cortex have different effects on behavior.

(A)

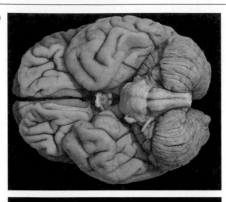

(B)

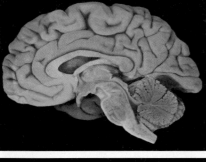

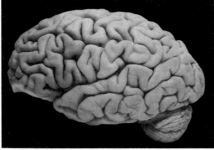

FIGURE 14.20 The Prefrontal Cortex (Images courtesy of Drs. S. Mark Williams and Dale Purves.)

prefrontal cortex The most anterior region of the frontal lobe.

executive function A neural and cognitive system that helps develop plans of action and organizes the activities of other high-level processing systems.

perseverate To continue to show a behavior repeatedly, beyond a reasonable degree.

The frontal lobes are a crucial part of the executive system that guides our thoughts, feelings, and choices

How do we decide what to do, and when to do it? Coordinated activity of a complex network of sites within the frontal lobes supports *hierarchical cognitive control*: the ability to direct shorter-term actions while simultaneously keeping longer-term goals in mind (Voytek et al., 2015; Badre and Nee, 2018). In humans, prefrontal cortex is the largest division of the brain—about a third of the entire cortex (**FIGURE 14.20A**) (Semendeferi et al., 2002). We have touched on some frontal lobe functions in earlier chapters—things like movement control, memory, language, psychopathology—but this mass of cortex also underlies other, more mysterious intellectual characteristics. Perhaps it reflects a bit of vanity about our species, but size is one reason why researchers have long viewed the frontal cortex as the source of intelligence, abstract thinking, and self-awareness. Adding to the mystery of frontal lobe function is the unusual assortment of behavioral changes that accompany damage to the frontal lobes.

The posterior portion of the frontal cortex includes motor and premotor regions (see Chapter 5). The anterior portion, usually referred to as **prefrontal cortex**, is immensely interconnected with the rest of the brain (Fuster, 1990; Mega and Cummings, 1994), and it is usually subdivided into *dorsolateral* and *orbitofrontal* regions (**FIGURE 14.20B**). The study of prefrontal cortical function began with Carlyle Jacobsen's work in the 1930s on delayed-response learning in chimpanzees. The animals were shown where food was hidden, but they had to wait before being allowed to reach for it. Chimps with prefrontal lesions were strikingly impaired on this simple task, compared with animals that sustained lesions in other brain regions. Jacobsen believed the impairment was caused by memory problems. But more recent observations, which we'll discuss next, suggest that the chimps' problems were with directing attention and formulating a plan of action.

Frontal lobe injury in humans leads to emotional, motor, and cognitive changes

Because they are large, the frontal lobes are vulnerable to injury; frontal lobe damage is a common consequence of strokes, tumors, and injuries. The exact symptoms induced by frontal lobe damage depend to some extent on the lesion location, but they include an unusual collection of emotional, motor, and cognitive changes. A common symptom in people with frontal lobe damage is a persistent strange apathy, broken by bouts of euphoria (an exalted sense of well-being). Ordinary social conventions are readily cast aside by impulsive behavior. Concern for the past or the future may be absent (Petrides and Milner, 1982; Duffy and Campbell, 1994). Forgetfulness is shown in many tasks requiring sustained attention. And yet, standard IQ test performance shows only slight changes after injury or stroke.

Clinical examination of people with frontal lesions also reveals an array of strange impairments in their behavior, especially in the realm of **executive function**, the high-level control of other cognitive functions we use to attend to important stimuli and make suitable "plans" for action. For example, a person with frontal damage who is given a simple set of errands may be unable to complete them without numerous false starts, backtracking, and confusion (Shallice and Burgess, 1991). Regions of dorsolateral prefrontal cortex, along with anterior portions of the cingulate cortex, are closely associated with executive control. Dorsolateral prefrontal cortex is also crucial for working memory, the ability to hold information in mind while processing it or using the information to solve problems.

People with frontal lobe damage often struggle with *task shifting* and tend to **perseverate** (continue beyond a reasonable degree) in any activity (B. Milner, 1963; Alvarez and Emory, 2006). Similarly, frontal lobe lesions may cause motor perseveration, repeating a simple movement over and over. However, the overall level of ordinary spontaneous motor activity is often quite diminished in people with frontal lesions. Along with movement of the head and eyes, facial expression of emotions may be greatly reduced.

Prefrontal damage site	Syndrome type	Characteristics
Dorsolateral	Dysexecutive	Diminished judgment, planning, insight, and temporal organization; reduced cognitive focus; motor programming deficits (possibly including aphasia and apraxia); diminished self-care
Orbitofrontal	Disinhibited	Stimulus-driven behavior; diminished social insight; distractibility; emotional lability
Mediofrontal	Apathetic	Diminished spontaneity; diminished verbal output; diminished motor behavior; urinary incontinence; lower-extremity weakness and sensory loss; diminished spontaneous prosody; increased response latency

TABLE 14.2 ■ Regional Prefrontal Syndromes

One explanation for these disparate effects of prefrontal lesions is that this region of cortex may be important for organizing different aspects of goal-directed behavior, including the capacity for prolonged attention and sensitivity to potential rewards and punishments. Patients with prefrontal lesions often have an inability to plan future acts and use foresight, as in the famous case of Phineas Gage. Their social skills may decline, especially the ability to inhibit inappropriate behaviors, and they may be unable to stay focused on any but short-term projects. They may agonize over even simple decisions. Some of the symptom clusters associated with damage of the major subdivisions of prefrontal cortex are summarized in **TABLE 14.2**.

The evidence suggests that prefrontal cortex—especially the orbitofrontal region—controls goal-directed behaviors. For example, monkeys that must make decisions that could lead to rewards show increased orbitofrontal activation (Matsumoto et al., 2003); in general, orbitofrontal cortex seems to link pleasant experiences (e.g., eating a delicious meal) with reward signals (dopamine release in the reward pathway) generated elsewhere in the brain (Kringelbach, 2005). In fact, some researchers believe that orbitofrontal cortex is actually more important for signaling expected outcomes (which is likewise related to reward) than for learning (Schoenbaum et al., 2009). In humans performing tasks in which some stimuli have more reward value than others, the level of activation in prefrontal cortex correlates with how rewarding the stimulus

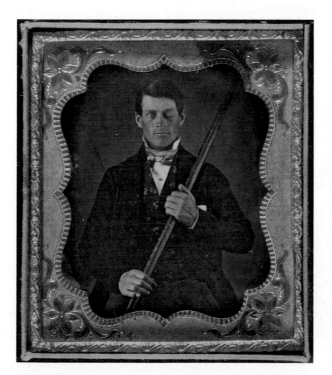

Phineas Gage Phineas P. Gage was a sober, polite, and capable member of a rail-laying crew, responsible for placing the charges used to blast rock from new rail beds. That's Gage on the left, holding a meter-long steel tamping rod. Perhaps the image on the right can help you guess why there appears to be something wrong with the left side of his face. In a horrific accident in 1848, a premature detonation blew that rod right through Gage's skull, on the trajectory shown in red, severely damaging both frontal lobes, especially in the orbitofrontal regions. Amazingly, Gage could speak shortly after the accident, and he walked to the doctor's office, although no one expected him to live (Macmillan, 2000). In fact, Gage survived another 12 years, but he was definitely a changed man, so rude and aimless, and his powers of attention so badly impaired, "that his friends and acquaintances said that he was 'no longer Gage.' " The historical account of Gage's case, now a neuroscience classic, was eventually found to closely agree with the symptoms of modern patients with frontal damage (H. Damasio et al., 1994; Wallis, 2007). (*Left* from the collection of Jack and Beverly Wilgus; *right* after J. D. Van Horn et al., 2012. *PLoS ONE* 7: e37454, courtesy of Warren Anatomical Museum, Harvard Medical School.)

is (Gottfried et al., 2003). This relationship seems to be a significant factor in gambling behavior and, more generally, is important for our decision-making processes. In fact, progress in understanding the decision-making process has spawned a new field, *neuroeconomics*, discussed in **BOX 14.3**.

We may never have a full understanding of the deepest secrets of consciousness, or an answer to the question of whether we *actually* possess the free will (or *personal agency*) that our brain seems to perceive as an element of consciousness (Haggard, 2017). But that doesn't prevent us from marveling that our consciousness has become so self-aware that it can study itself to a high degree. Perhaps it's best to allow ourselves at least one or two mysteries, if only for the sake of art. Would life seem as rich if we could predict other people's behavior, or even our own, with perfect accuracy?

BOX 14.3
Neuroeconomics Identifies Brain Regions Active during Decision Making

The waiter has brought over the dessert trolley, and it's decision time: do you go with the certain delight of the chocolate cake, or do you succumb to the glistening allure of the sticky toffee pudding? Or, do you allow yourself only a cup of black coffee, for the sake of your waistline? What happens in your brain when you finally make your difficult choice?

In the lab, researchers usually evaluate decision making by using monetary rewards (instead of desserts, darn it) because money is convenient: you can vary how much money is at stake, how great a reward is offered, and so on, to accurately gauge how we really make economic decisions. These studies show that most of us are very averse to loss and risk: we are more sensitive to losing a certain amount of money than we are to gaining that amount. In other words, losing $20 makes us feel a lot worse than gaining $20 makes us feel good. From a strictly logical point of view, the value of money, whether lost or gained, should be exactly the same. Our tendency to overemphasize loss is just one of several ways in which people fail to act rationally in the marketplace.

Neuroeconomics is the study of brain mechanisms at work during economic decision making, and our attention to environmental factors and evaluation of rewards has a tremendous impact on these decisions. In general, findings from human and animal research suggest that two main systems underlie decision processes (Kable and Glimcher, 2009). The

first, consisting of the ventromedial prefrontal cortex (including the anterior cingulate cortex) plus the dopamine-based reward system of the brain (see Chapter 4), is a *valuation system*, a network that ranks choices on the basis of their perceived worth and potential reward. Impressively, using an optogenetic technique (see Chapter 3) to selectively activate neurons that express dopamine receptor D2 in the nucleus accumbens—a central forebrain component of the brain's reward system—can instantaneously turn a risk-preferring rat into a risk-averse rat (Zalocusky et al., 2016)! Presumably, the activated cells cause the valuation system to devalue the choice relative to risk; a similar dopamine-dependent process appears to participate in human monetary decisions too (Ojala et al., 2018).

The second system, involving mostly dorsolateral prefrontal cortex, dorsal anterior cingulate cortex, and parietal regions (like the LIP or IPS discussed earlier in the chapter), is thought to be a *choice system*, sifting through the valuated alternatives and producing the conscious decision.

Neuroeconomics research is also confirming that the prefrontal cortex normally inhibits impulsive decision making as a way to avoid loss (Tom et al., 2007; Muhlert and Lawrence, 2015). As people are faced with more and more uncertainty, the prefrontal cortex becomes more and more active (Hsu et al., 2005; Huettel

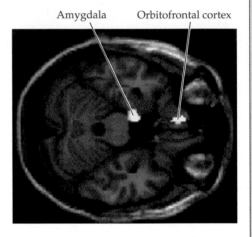

Amygdala   Orbitofrontal cortex

A Poor Choice A costly decision is associated with activation of the amygdala and orbitofrontal cortex, signaling diminished reward and aversion to loss. (From G. Coricelli et al., 2005. *Nat. Neurosci.* 8: 1255, courtesy of Angela Sirigu.)

et al., 2006), and the dorsal cingulate cortex may improve decisions by delaying action until full processing of a complex decision can be completed (Sheth et al., 2012; Heilbronner and Hayden, 2016). Likewise, when people have made wrong, costly decisions that they regret, activity increases in the amygdala and in the orbitofrontal aspect of the prefrontal cortex, as shown in the figure (Coricelli et al., 2005), probably reflecting the participant's perception of diminished reward and increasing aversion to loss.

HOW'S IT GOING ?

1. Define *consciousness* (or at least try!).
2. Discuss unconsciousness in states like deep coma. Is this unconsciousness the inverse of consciousness?
3. Contrast the easy and hard problems of consciousness, giving examples of each. What are qualia?
4. Name the main subdivisions of the prefrontal cortex. How do they differ in function?
5. What are some of the main symptoms of frontal lobe lesions?
6. What are the two main neural systems that are thought to operate in the process of decision making, as identified in neuroeconomics research?

Recommended Reading

Gazzaniga, M. S. (2018). *The Consciousness Instinct: Unraveling the Mystery of How the Brain Makes the Mind*. New York, NY: Farrar, Straus and Giroux.

Glimcher, P. W., Camerer, C., Poldrack, R. A., and Fehr, E. (2008). *Neuroeconomics: Decision Making and the Brain.* San Diego, CA: Academic Press.

Koch, C. (2012). *Consciousness: Confessions of a Romantic Reductionist.* Cambridge, MA: MIT Press.

Laureys, S., and Tononi, G. (Eds.). (2008). *The Neurology of Consciousness: Cognitive Neuroscience and Neuropathology*. New York, NY: Academic Press.

Mangun, G. R. (Ed.). (2012). *Neuroscience of Attention: Attentional Control and Selection*. Oxford, UK: Oxford University Press.

Nobre, K., and Kastner, S. (2018). *The Oxford Handbook of Attention*. Oxford, UK: Oxford University Press.

Posner, M. I. (Ed.). (2012). *Cognitive Neuroscience of Attention* (2nd ed.). New York, NY: Guilford Press.

Stuss, D. T., and Knight, R. T. (2012). *Principles of Frontal Lobe Function* (2nd ed.). Oxford, UK: Oxford University Press.

Wright, R. D., and Ward, L. M. (2008). *Orienting of Attention.* Oxford, UK: Oxford University Press.

14 ■ Visual Summary

3e.mindsmachine.com/vs14

You should be able to relate each summary to the adjacent illustration, including structures and processes. If you go to the website for our text (**3e.mindsmachine.com**), you can follow links to figures, animations, and activities that will help you consolidate the material.

1 Although we pay mostly **overt attention** to stimuli, we can also pay **covert attention** to stimuli or locations of our choosing. **Attention** has been likened to a spotlight, helping us to distinguish stimuli from distracters. Review **Figure 14.1**, **Animation 14.2**, **Video 14.3**

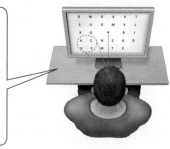

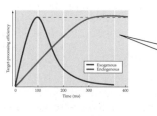

2 In **voluntary attention** we select objects to attend to; it is studied using **symbolic cuing** tasks. **Reflexive attention** is the involuntary capture of attention by stimuli, studied using **peripheral spatial cuing** tasks. Review **Figures 14.2** and **14.3**, **Animation 14.4**

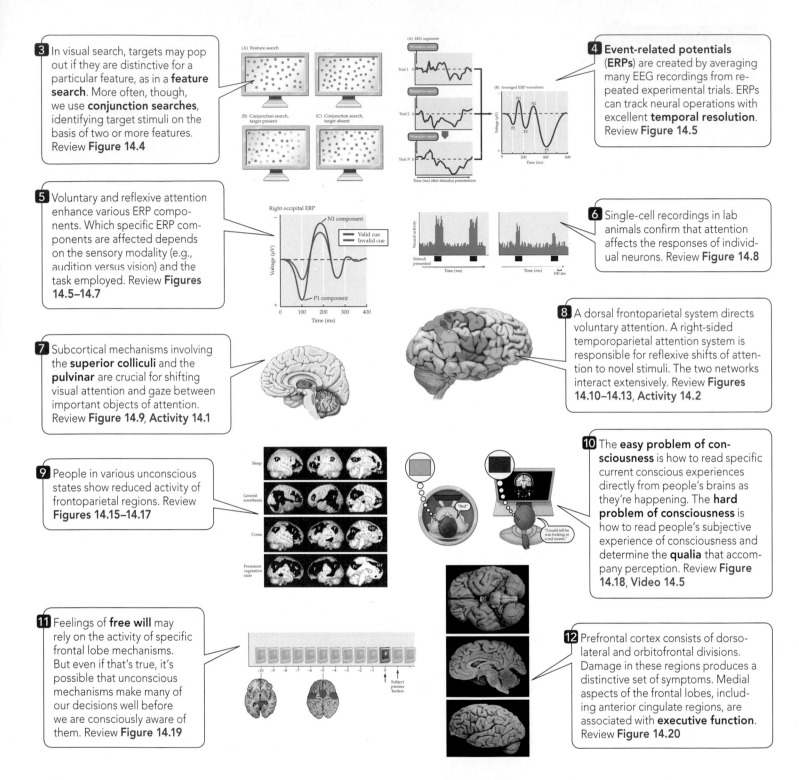

3 In visual search, targets may pop out if they are distinctive for a particular feature, as in a **feature search**. More often, though, we use **conjunction searches**, identifying target stimuli on the basis of two or more features. Review **Figure 14.4**

4 **Event-related potentials (ERPs)** are created by averaging many EEG recordings from repeated experimental trials. ERPs can track neural operations with excellent **temporal resolution.** Review **Figure 14.5**

5 Voluntary and reflexive attention enhance various ERP components. Which specific ERP components are affected depends on the sensory modality (e.g., audition versus vision) and the task employed. Review **Figures 14.5–14.7**

6 Single-cell recordings in lab animals confirm that attention affects the responses of individual neurons. Review **Figure 14.8**

7 Subcortical mechanisms involving the **superior colliculi** and the **pulvinar** are crucial for shifting visual attention and gaze between important objects of attention. Review **Figure 14.9, Activity 14.1**

8 A dorsal frontoparietal system directs voluntary attention. A right-sided temporoparietal attention system is responsible for reflexive shifts of attention to novel stimuli. The two networks interact extensively. Review **Figures 14.10–14.13, Activity 14.2**

9 People in various unconscious states show reduced activity of frontoparietal regions. Review **Figures 14.15–14.17**

10 The **easy problem of consciousness** is how to read specific current conscious experiences directly from people's brains as they're happening. The **hard problem of consciousness** is how to read people's subjective experience of consciousness and determine the **qualia** that accompany perception. Review **Figure 14.18, Video 14.5**

11 Feelings of **free will** may rely on the activity of specific frontal lobe mechanisms. But even if that's true, it's possible that unconscious mechanisms make many of our decisions well before we are consciously aware of them. Review **Figure 14.19**

12 Prefrontal cortex consists of dorsolateral and orbitofrontal divisions. Damage in these regions produces a distinctive set of symptoms. Medial aspects of the frontal lobes, including anterior cingulate regions, are associated with **executive function.** Review **Figure 14.20**

PART I
Cerebral Lateralization

THE ROAD AHEAD

The first section of the chapter looks at the functional differences between the two hemispheres of the brain. After you've read through this material, you should be able to:

1. Describe techniques for studying the left and right hemispheres independently of each other.
2. Summarize the apparent cognitive specializations of each hemisphere as revealed by behavioral testing.
3. Discuss the relationship of handedness to cerebral lateralization.
4. Itemize the types of deficits seen after left versus right hemisphere lesions, relating the deficits to specific anatomical locations within each hemisphere.
5. Provide a detailed account of the left hemisphere's language network.

The Left and Right Hemispheres of the Brain Are Different

The discovery that some brain functions are lateralized should not be especially surprising; after all, other body organs also show considerable asymmetry between the right and left sides. But when we study the *behavior* of people, cerebral lateralization of function is masked by the rich neural connections between the hemispheres: they communicate with each other so quickly and thoroughly that they seem to act as one. So researchers had to develop clever techniques to study the functioning of each hemisphere in isolation from the other.

Disconnection of the cerebral hemispheres reveals their individual specializations

Some rare and unfortunate people develop severe epilepsy that is very difficult to control with medication. Their frequent seizures start in one hemisphere and then spread to the other hemisphere through the **corpus callosum**—the huge white matter pathway consisting of hundreds of millions of axons that connect the two hemispheres. As a last resort, one treatment option is to cut the corpus callosum, preventing the spread of the seizure discharges from one hemisphere to the other. This operation, developed in the 1960s, significantly reduced the frequency and severity of seizures in affected people. It also changed their behavior in ways that presented a research opportunity: by analyzing the cognitive, perceptual, emotional, and motor behavior of these **split-brain individuals**, researchers were able to catalog the individual specializations of the newly isolated cerebral hemispheres.

In Nobel Prize–winning research, Roger Sperry and his collaborators applied techniques perfected in split-brain cats to study split-brain humans. The researchers realized that by exploiting the organization of the sensory systems, stimuli could be directed exclusively to one hemisphere or the other. For example, objects felt with the left hand, or seen only in the left visual field, are first processed in the sensory cortex of the **contralateral** (opposite side) hemisphere (in this case, the right hemisphere). Normally, information about the object would be shared with the other hemisphere immediately, via the corpus callosum. But in split-brain individuals, the sensory information remains trapped within the receiving hemisphere, so the person's response to the stimuli reflects the processing specializations of that hemisphere in isolation.

In some of these studies, words were projected visually to either the left or the right hemisphere. The results were dramatic. Split-brain individuals could easily read and verbally report words projected to the left hemisphere (via the right visual field) but not words directed to the right hemisphere (**FIGURE 15.1**). Subsequent work (Zaidel, 1976) showed that the right hemisphere does have a limited amount of linguistic

To view the
Brain Explorer,
go to
3e.mindsmachine.com/av15.2

communication   Information transfer between two individuals.

language   Communication in which arbitrary sounds or symbols are arranged according to a grammar in order to convey an almost limitless variety of concepts.

grammar   All of the rules for usage of a particular language.

spatial cognition   The ability to navigate and to understand the spatial relationships between objects.

cerebral lateralization   The divison of labor between the two cerebral hemispheres such that each hemisphere is specialized for particular types of processing.

corpus callosum   The main band of axons that connects the two cerebral hemispheres.

split-brain individual   An individual whose corpus callosum has been severed, halting communication between the right and left hemispheres.

contralateral   In anatomy, referring to a location on the opposite side of the body.

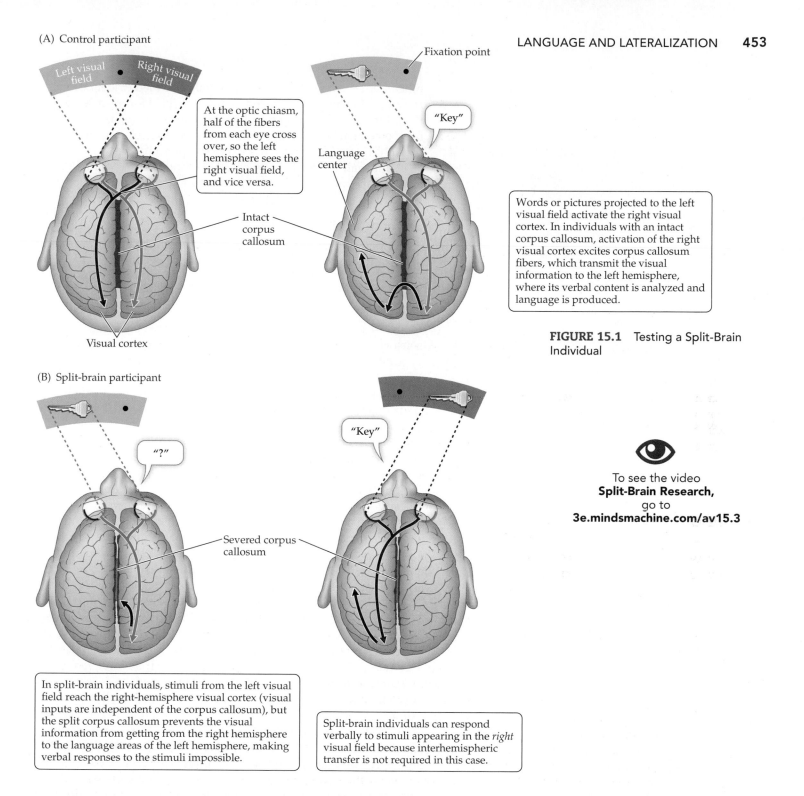

(A) Control participant

Left visual field   Right visual field

Fixation point

At the optic chiasm, half of the fibers from each eye cross over, so the left hemisphere sees the right visual field, and vice versa.

Language center

"Key"

Intact corpus callosum

Visual cortex

Words or pictures projected to the left visual field activate the right visual cortex. In individuals with an intact corpus callosum, activation of the right visual cortex excites corpus callosum fibers, which transmit the visual information to the left hemisphere, where its verbal content is analyzed and language is produced.

FIGURE 15.1 Testing a Split-Brain Individual

(B) Split-brain participant

"?"

"Key"

Severed corpus callosum

To see the video
Split-Brain Research,
go to
3e.mindsmachine.com/av15.3

In split-brain individuals, stimuli from the left visual field reach the right-hemisphere visual cortex (visual inputs are independent of the corpus callosum), but the split corpus callosum prevents the visual information from getting from the right hemisphere to the language areas of the left hemisphere, making verbal responses to the stimuli impossible.

Split-brain individuals can respond verbally to stimuli appearing in the *right* visual field because interhemispheric transfer is not required in this case.

ability; for example, it can recognize simple words and the emotional content of verbal material. But in most people, vocabulary and grammar are the exclusive domain of the left hemisphere.

The capabilities of the "mute" right hemisphere had to be tested by nonverbal means. For example, a picture of a key might be projected to the left visual field and so reach only the right visual cortex. The participant would then be asked to touch several different objects that she could not see and hold up the correct one. Such a task could be performed correctly by the left hand (controlled by the right hemisphere) but not by the right hand (controlled by the left hemisphere). So in this case, the left hemisphere literally does not know what the left hand is doing! In general, these and

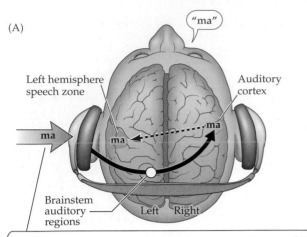

(A)

Although sounds presented to either ear reach both sides of the brain, the auditory information is mostly processed by the contralateral hemisphere (see Chapter 6). So, verbal information presented to the left ear is first processed by the right auditory cortex and then transmitted to speech systems in the left hemisphere. Participant repeats the word.

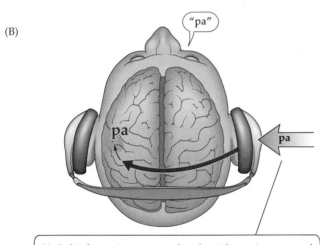

(B)

Verbal information presented to the right ear is processed by the left auditory cortex and then passed directly to speech systems within the same hemisphere.

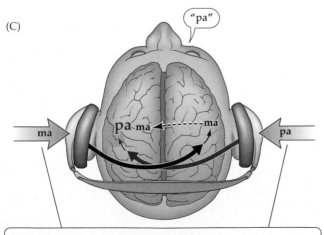

(C)

When conflicting information goes to both ears, the information to the right ear reaches the left hemisphere's speech system first. Subject repeats only the right-ear information.

other studies with split-brain individuals provided evidence that, in most people, the right hemisphere is specialized for processing spatial information. Right-hemisphere mechanisms are also crucial for face perception, for processing emotional aspects of language, and for controlling attention (as we discuss in Chapter 14).

Almost all types of behavior, from manual skills to intellectual activities, are performed better by the two hemispheres working together than by either hemisphere working alone. For this reason, and because better medical options have also been developed, the split-brain surgery has remained a very rare procedure, and the modern form of the operation generally transects only about a third of the corpus callosum.

The two hemispheres process information differently in most people

Most research on brain asymmetry in healthy people focuses on two sensory modalities: hearing and vision. That's because researchers have devised clever procedures for directing auditory or visual stimuli mostly to one hemisphere or the other and then inferring hemispheric specializations from the behavioral responses made by the participants.

THE RIGHT-EAR ADVANTAGE   Through earphones, we can present different sounds to the two ears at the same time—a technique called **dichotic presentation**. So, for example, a participant may hear a particular speech sound in one ear and, at the same time, a different vowel, consonant, or word in the other ear. The participant is asked to try to identify or recall both sounds. Although this procedure may seem designed to produce confusion, in general, right-handed people identify verbal stimuli delivered to the right ear more accurately than the stimuli simultaneously presented to the left ear. This result is described as a right-ear "advantage" for verbal information. In contrast, up to 50% of left-handed individuals may show a reduced or reversed pattern, with either no difference between the ears or a clear left-ear advantage.

As a consequence of the preferential connections between the right ear and the left hemisphere, the right-ear advantage for verbal stimuli confirms the idea that the left hemisphere is specialized for language (**FIGURE 15.2**). Although we can normally use either ear for processing speech sounds, speech presented to the right ear in dichotic presentation tests exerts stronger control over language mechanisms in the left hemisphere than does speech simultaneously presented to the left ear (Kimura, 1973). The competition between the left- and right-ear inputs is the key; presentation of speech stimuli to one ear at a time (*monaural* presentation) does not produce a right-ear advantage.

VISUAL PERCEPTION OF LINGUISTIC STIMULI   Another way to study hemispheric specialization is to use a **tachistoscope test** to pit the two hemispheres against each other, using a device (called a *tachistoscope*, surprisingly; pronounced "ta-KISS-toe-scope") that very briefly presents visual stimuli to the left or right half of the visual field

FIGURE 15.2   The Right-Ear Advantage in Dichotic Presentation (After D. Kimura, 1973. *Sci. Am.* 228: 70.)

(see Figures 7.10 and 15.1). If the stimulus exposure lasts less than 150 milliseconds or so, input is restricted to one hemisphere because there is not enough time for the eyes to shift their direction. In humans with intact brains, of course, further processing may involve the transmission of information through the corpus callosum to the other hemisphere.

Most tachistoscopic studies confirm the general verbal-spatial division of labor between the hemispheres. Verbal stimuli (words and letters) presented to the right visual field (so the left hemisphere) are recognized more accurately than the same input presented to the left visual field (right hemisphere). Conversely, nonverbal visual stimuli (such as faces or geometric forms) presented to the left visual field (right hemisphere) are better recognized than the same stimuli presented to the other side. Simpler visual processing, such as the detection of light, hue, or simple patterns, is performed equivalently by the two hemispheres.

The left and right hemispheres differ in their auditory specializations

Anatomical studies of primary auditory cortex in the left and right hemispheres are consistent with the view that the two play different roles in auditory perception. In one early postmortem study of auditory cortex, the **planum temporale**—an auditory region on the superior surface of the temporal lobe—was found to be larger in the left hemisphere than in the right in most of the brains studied (Geschwind and Levitsky, 1968) (**FIGURE 15.3A**). In only 11% of adults was the right side larger. The planum temporale includes part of a posterior cortical region called *Wernicke's area*, which we'll see a little later is important for language, so it seems likely that the larger left planum temporale is related to that hemisphere's language specialization. Direct evidence of this relationship, however, remains somewhat elusive: in one MRI study, for example, asymmetry of the planum temporale did not correlate with direct measures of language lateralization (Dorsaint-Pierre et al., 2006).

As in adults, the left planum temporale is larger than the right in the brains of infants (Wada et al., 1975). The presence of this difference in our brains before we begin to speak therefore bolsters the view that we have an inborn neural mechanism for language. In fact, by just 12–14 weeks of gestation, a variety of genes show asymmetrical expression in the fetal human brain (Sun et al., 2005). The planum temporale likewise tends to be larger on the left than on the right in chimpanzees (Gannon et al., 1998); an anterior zone implicated in speech in humans (*Broca's area*, which we'll discuss shortly) is also larger on the left in chimps, bonobos, and gorillas, as it is in

dichotic presentation The simultaneous delivery of different stimuli to both the right and left ears at the same time.

tachistoscope test A test in which stimuli are very briefly presented to either the left or right visual half field.

planum temporale An auditory region of superior temporal cortex.

FIGURE 15.3 Structural Asymmetry of the Human Planum Temporale (After G. Schlaug et al., 1995. *Science* 267: 699.)

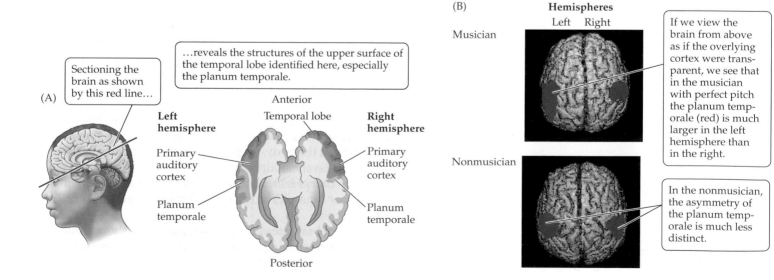

in processing faces to meet the criteria for congenital prosopagnosia (Kennerknecht et al., 2006; Duchaine et al., 2007). The congenital form of prosopagnosia appears to run in families, indicating a genetic aspect to the disorder (Grüter et al., 2008). Congenital prosopagnosia is associated with reduced activation of the fusiform gyrus, in keeping with the anatomical findings in acquired prosopagnosia that we've already discussed. At the other end of the spectrum, some people are exceptionally good with faces. These "super-recognizers," who are about as good with faces as people with prosopagnosia are bad, are actively recruited by some police forces (Russell et al., 2009; Robertson et al., 2016). (You can learn more, and test your own facial recognition ability, at www.testmybrain.org.)

Prosopagnosia of either type may be accompanied by additional forms of **agnosia**, an inability to identify individual items—makes of cars, tools, bird species, sounds, and so on—in the absence of any specific sensory deficits or memory problems (Gauthier et al., 1999). Functional-MRI studies of healthy people show that, as with face recognition, the fusiform gyrus is important for identifying individual members of large categories (e.g., faces or birds or cars) in which all members have many things in common (Gauthier et al., 2000).

HOW'S IT GOING ?

1. In general, what are the behavioral consequences of right-hemisphere damage in humans?
2. Define, compare, and contrast two of the most striking symptoms of right-hemisphere damage: astereognosis and prosopagnosia. Which areas of the brain appear to be involved in each?
3. Is prosopagnosia always associated with brain damage? What other behavioral abnormalities may co-occur with prosopagnosia?

Left Hemisphere Damage Can Cause Aphasia

For thousands of years, dating back to the earliest medical records and beyond, people have known that a selective impairment of language abilities, known as **aphasia**, could result from injury to specific regions of the brain, especially the left hemisphere (Finger, 1994). Left-hemisphere damage can impair language to varying degrees, depending on the location and extent of the injury. In cases of severe damage, people may lose the ability to produce any speech whatsoever. In less severe cases, patients may exhibit speech with **paraphasia**—insertion of incorrect sounds or words—along with labored, effortful speech production. Somewhere in the range of 25–50% of people who suffer a stroke (see Figure 2.17) will have aphasia as a primary symptom; for this reason, a sudden problem with language is considered to be one of the core warning signs of a stroke (see Figure 2.18), along with weakness or numbness on one side and dizziness, altered vision, or confusion. Most people with aphasia also show some impairment in writing, known as **agraphia**, and disturbances in reading, called **alexia**. Brain damage that produces aphasia also produces a distinctive motor impairment called **apraxia** (see Chapter 5), characterized by great difficulty in making precise *sequences* of movements, despite the absence of weakness or paralysis. In fact, as we discuss later, some theorists view aphasia as primarily a disorder of motor control. Research has distinguished several major categories of aphasia, differing from one another in the patterns of symptoms that occur (videos of people with aphasia can be seen on the website).

Damage to a left anterior speech zone causes nonfluent (or Broca's) aphasia

In the mid-1800s, French neurologist Paul Broca (1824–1880) examined a man who had lost the ability to utter more than the single syllable "tan" (**FIGURE 15.6**). Following postmortem analysis, Broca reported that this man, and other people with similar

agnosia The inability to recognize objects, despite being able to describe them in terms of form and color. Agnosia may occur after localized brain damage.

aphasia An impairment in language understanding and/or production that is caused by brain injury.

paraphasia A symptom of aphasia that is distinguished by the substitution of a word by a sound, an incorrect word, an unintended word, or a neologism (a meaningless word).

agraphia The inability to write.

alexia The inability to read.

apraxia An impairment in the ability to carry out complex sequential movements, even though there is no muscle paralysis.

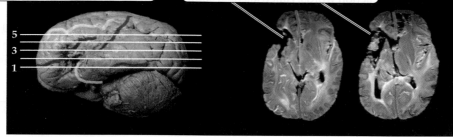

Study of this brain and similar cases led Paul Broca to identify a region in the anterior left hemisphere that is specialized for speech.

Damage in what is now known as Broca's area is clearly evident in these horizontal sections, corresponding to levels 2 and 3 on the orientation figure.

FIGURE 15.6 **The Brain of "Tan"** Photo and MRI image of the preserved brain of M. Leborgne, who could only utter the syllable "tan" after his brain injury. (From N. F. Dronkers et al., 2007. *Brain* 130: 1432.)

severe impairments of speech production, had suffered damage to a left inferior frontal region that now bears his name—**Broca's area** (**FIGURE 15.7**). Damage that includes Broca's area often produces a type of aphasia known as **nonfluent aphasia** (or *Broca's aphasia*). People with nonfluent aphasia have a lot of difficulty producing speech, talking only in a labored and hesitant manner. Reading and writing are also impaired. The ability to utter automatic speech, however, is often preserved. Such speech includes greetings ("Hello"); short, common expressions ("Oh my gosh!"); and swear words.

Compared with their difficulty with speech production, *comprehension* of language is relatively good in nonfluent aphasics. Because the primary and supplementary motor cortex is close to Broca's area (see Chapter 5), brain injuries that cause nonfluent aphasia often also cause **hemiplegia**—paralysis of one side of the body (usually the right side, which is controlled by the left hemisphere). Sometimes there is unilateral weakness, termed **hemiparesis**, rather than full paralysis.

Broca's area A region of the frontal lobe of the brain that is involved in the production of speech.

nonfluent aphasia Also called *Broca's aphasia*. A language impairment characterized by difficulty with speech production but not with language comprehension. It is related to damage in Broca's area.

hemiplegia Paralysis of one side of the body.

hemiparesis Weakness of one side of the body.

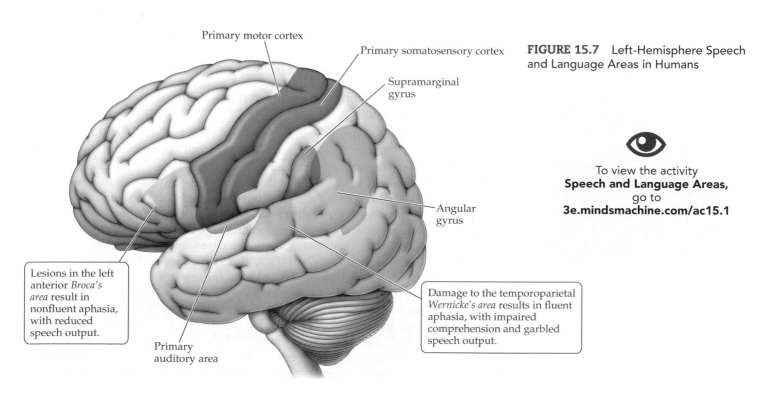

Primary motor cortex

Primary somatosensory cortex

Supramarginal gyrus

Angular gyrus

Primary auditory area

Lesions in the left anterior *Broca's area* result in nonfluent aphasia, with reduced speech output.

Damage to the temporoparietal *Wernicke's area* results in fluent aphasia, with impaired comprehension and garbled speech output.

FIGURE 15.7 Left-Hemisphere Speech and Language Areas in Humans

To view the activity **Speech and Language Areas,** go to **3e.mindsmachine.com/ac15.1**

connectionist model of aphasia
Also called the *Wernicke-Geschwind model*. A theory proposing that left-hemisphere language deficits result from disconnection between the brain regions in a language network, each of which serves a particular linguistic function.

arcuate fasciculus A fiber tract classically viewed as a connection between Wernicke's speech area and Broca's speech area.

To view the activity
The Connectionist Model of Aphasia,
go to
3e.mindsmachine.com/ac15.2

FIGURE 15.9 The Connectionist Model of Aphasia (After N. Geschwind, 1979. *Sci. Am.* 241: 180.)

neurological impairments. (Tinna and several other people with aphasia are profiled in a documentary entitled *Speechless*, by filmmaker Guillermo F. Florez; a theatrical trailer and information about the film are available at speechlessdoc.com.)

Disconnection of language regions may result in specific verbal problems

Considering how language is intertwined with so many other functions, it is not surprising that a complete description of the brain's language circuitry remains elusive, although steady progress has been made. The traditional **connectionist model of aphasia**—also known as the *Wernicke-Geschwind model* after its leading proponents—argues that language deficits result from *disconnection* between the brain regions in a language network. Each of these regions is proposed to serve a particular feature of language analysis or production. So, for example, when a word or sentence is heard, the auditory cortex transmits information about the sounds to a speech reception mechanism in Wernicke's area, where the sounds are analyzed to decode what they mean. For the word to be spoken, according to this model, Wernicke's area transmits this information, via a fiber pathway called the **arcuate fasciculus**, to the expressive mechanism in Broca's area, where a speech plan is activated. Broca's area then transmits this plan to adjacent motor cortex, which controls the muscles of the chest, throat, and mouth that are used for speech production (**FIGURE 15.9**). According to the

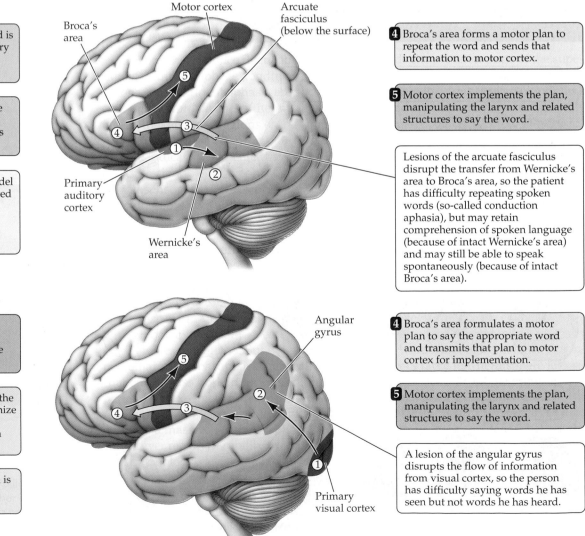

(A) Speaking a *heard* word

1 Information about the sound is analyzed by primary auditory cortex and transmitted to Wernicke's area.

2 Wernicke's area analyzes the sound information to determine the word that was said.

3 Under the connectionist model this information is transmitted via the arcuate fasciculus. (Note, however, that anatomical research casts doubt on this projection.)

4 Broca's area forms a motor plan to repeat the word and sends that information to motor cortex.

5 Motor cortex implements the plan, manipulating the larynx and related structures to say the word.

Lesions of the arcuate fasciculus disrupt the transfer from Wernicke's area to Broca's area, so the patient has difficulty repeating spoken words (so-called conduction aphasia), but may retain comprehension of spoken language (because of intact Wernicke's area) and may still be able to speak spontaneously (because of intact Broca's area).

(B) Speaking a *written* word

1 Visual cortex analyzes the image and transmits the information about the image to the angular gyrus.

2 The angular gyrus decodes the image information to recognize the word and associate this visual form with the spoken form in Wernicke's area.

3 Information about the word is transmitted via the arcuate fasciculus to Broca's area.

4 Broca's area formulates a motor plan to say the appropriate word and transmits that plan to motor cortex for implementation.

5 Motor cortex implements the plan, manipulating the larynx and related structures to say the word.

A lesion of the angular gyrus disrupts the flow of information from visual cortex, so the person has difficulty saying words he has seen but not words he has heard.

model, people with lesions that selectively disrupt the connection between the posterior speech reception zone (Wernicke's area) and the anterior speech production zone (Broca's area) will especially struggle with repetition of words and phrases that they hear, despite good speech comprehension and production—a condition termed **conduction aphasia**.

Critics of the connectionist model argue that it oversimplifies the neural mechanisms of language, and furthermore, more modern fMRI data confirms that left-hemisphere language zones are not as rigidly modular as was previously believed (Blumstein and Amso, 2013). In addition, technological advances in the visualization of white matter pathways in the living brain have raised questions about the assumptions underlying the connectionist model (**BOX 15.2**). Detailed brain-imaging research suggests that so-called conduction aphasia actually results from a specific type of lesion of superior temporal cortex, rather than the disruption of white matter pathways as proposed under the connectionist model (B. R. Buchsbaum et al., 2011). So it remains to be seen exactly how the various mechanisms of the left hemisphere collaborate to give us the verbal abilities that seem so effortless.

An alternative model of speech mechanisms—the **motor theory of language** (Lieberman, 1985; Kimura, 1993)—suggests that the anterior and posterior left-hemisphere language zones are both specialized for motor control. According to the motor theory, when we listen to speech, we simply process the speech sounds using the same neural systems that we would use to *make* those sounds: an anterior system programs simple phonemic units, and a posterior system strings speech sounds together into long sequences of movements (Kimura and Watson, 1989). Interestingly, deaf people who use American Sign Language—a language based entirely on movements—employ the same language-related regions of the left hemisphere as hearing people who use spoken language (Neville et al., 1998; Petitto et al., 2000), and they show

conduction aphasia   An impairment in the ability to repeat words and sentences.

motor theory of language   The theory that speech is perceived using the same left-hemisphere mechanisms that are used to produce the complex movements that go into speech.

diffusion tensor imaging (DTI) A modified form of MRI in which the diffusion of water in a confined space is exploited to produce images of axonal fiber tracts.

DTI tractography   Also called *fiber tracking*. Visualization of the orientation and terminations of white matter tracts in the living brain via diffusion tensor imaging."

BOX 15.2
Studying Connectivity in the Living Brain

A modern brain-imaging technology is allowing researchers to reexamine the traditional connectionist model of left-hemisphere language functions. In **diffusion tensor imaging** (**DTI**), MRI technology is used in a new way to specifically study white matter tracts—axon bundles—within the living brain.

As we discussed in Chapter 2, MRI images are created from the radio-frequency energy that is emitted by relaxing protons within water molecules. In DTI, the unique behavior of water molecules that are constrained within axons (known as *fractional anisotropy*) is exploited to create images of axonal fiber pathways between areas, a procedure called **DTI tractography**, or *fiber tracking* (Assaf and Pasternak, 2008). Although the technology doesn't have the resolution to portray individual axons, the origin, orientation, course, and termination of axonal projections can be effectively

visualized, as shown in the figure. One important discovery using this technique is that the arcuate fasciculus—long believed to connect Wernicke's area to Broca's area—appears to terminate in the precentral gyrus (motor cortex), just short of Broca's area, in most people (Bernal and Altman, 2010; E. C. Brown et al., 2014). Coupled with the clinical observation that people with purely cortical lesions sometimes have "conduction" aphasia, this finding is prompting researchers to reevaluate existing notions of language organization in the brain. The more nuanced picture of the language network emerging from this research will have implications for both fundamental understanding of brain organization and treatment of language disorders.

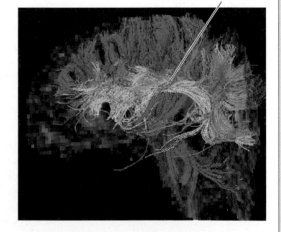

Left arcuate fasciculus

Fiber Tracking the Language Areas
In DTI tractography, the orientation, origin, and termination of fiber tracts can be visualized. Here, the left arcuate fasciculus is visualized in light green. (From M. Vandermosten et al., 2012. *Neurosci. Biobehav. Rev.* 36: 1532.)

comparable aphasia-like symptoms after focal left-hemisphere damage (Kimura, 1981; Bellugi et al., 1983).

In any event, detailed imaging studies show that the brain contains several speech-related areas well outside of the classical model (E. Bates et al., 2003; Dronkers et al., 2004), implying greater complexity than was proposed under the Wernicke-Geschwind model. Further, recent evidence that low-level aspects of speech perception occur bilaterally (Cogan et al., 2014) and that semantic processing of natural speech relies heavily on both hemispheres (Huth et al., 2016; de Heer et al., 2017) shows that much remains to be determined about exactly what is, and what is not, the exclusive domain of the left-hemisphere language network. Whatever the details may be, it seems that the answer will involve a complex network of mechanisms that link perception to action.

HOW'S IT GOING ?

1. Distinguish among aphasia, agraphia, and alexia.
2. Identify the main types of aphasia, and summarize the distinctive symptoms of each. Which type of aphasia is most often associated with paralysis?
3. Provide a brief outline of the traditional "connectionist" model of aphasia. How does it get its name, and what shortcomings of the model have been identified by critics?
4. Briefly describe the motor theory of language. Can you think of ways that this theory may relate to the evolutionary origins of language?

Brain mapping helps us understand the organization of language in the brain

In healthy people with intact language capabilities, researchers can study the brain's language network by using two general experimental approaches. In some studies, researchers stimulate discrete regions of the cortex and measure associated changes in language function. Conversely, participants may be asked to engage in specific verbal behaviors while researchers measure associated changes in brain activity, using functional brain imaging. Together, these techniques have extended our understanding of the neural bases of language.

Early studies of the organization of language areas in the brain employed electrical stimulation mapping, in which a surgeon used a handheld electrode to electrically stimulate discrete regions of cortex while the effect on behavior was observed. Most of these studies collected data from neurosurgical patients undergoing surgery to remove a tumor or epileptic tissue (as in Wilder Penfield's experiments that we described in Chapter 2). Once the brain was exposed, small stimulating electrodes were touched to the surface, disrupting the normal functioning of neurons in the immediate vicinity. Because patients were given only local anesthesia, they were conscious and able to perform various cognitive tasks (the main aim of the procedure was to identify tissue that could be removed without impairing language). Data from numerous patients were superimposed to create a map of language-related zones of the left hemisphere (**FIGURE 15.10A**) (Penfield and Roberts, 1959). Stimulation anywhere within a large anterior zone often stopped speech outright. Other forms of language interference, such as misnaming or impaired repetition of words, occurred with stimulation throughout the anterior and posterior cortical speech zones.

Later cortical stimulation studies revealed anatomical compartmentalization of linguistic systems such as naming, reading, speech production, and verbal memory (Calvin and Ojemann, 1994). An interesting example of the effects of cortical stimulation on naming is illustrated in **FIGURE 15.10B**, which shows the different places where stimulation caused naming errors in English and Spanish in a bilingual person. Note that this very fine-grained approach reveals different subregions that disrupt either English or Spanish function. People who are bilingual from an early age show

(A)

In cortical mapping studies of many patients, stimulation of these sites interfered with speech production.

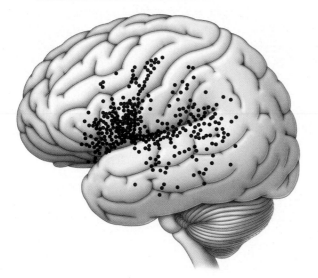

(B)

Mapping the brain of this bilingual patient indicated that stimulation of different regions interfered with either one language or the other, but not both.

○ No naming errors
● Naming errors in English only
● Naming errors in Spanish only

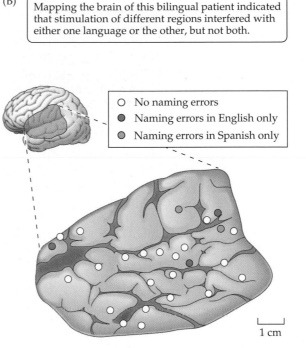

1 cm

completely overlapping organization of their two languages at the gross neuroanatomical level (Perani and Abutalebi, 2005), and evidence is mounting that early bilingualism has far-reaching beneficial effects on brain organization and resistance to cognitive decline in later life (Costa and Sebastián-Gallés, 2014; Perani et al., 2017).

More recent studies employ a noninvasive cortical stimulation technology called *transcranial magnetic stimulation* to further probe the organization of language areas in healthy volunteers. As we discuss next, these studies have confirmed the general organization of the left-hemisphere language network and have revealed new details about the compartmentalization of functions within traditional speech areas.

FIGURE 15.10 Electrical Stimulation of Some Brain Sites Can Interfere with Language (Part A after W. Penfield and L. Roberts, 1959. *Speech and brain-mechanisms.* Princeton University Press. Princeton, NJ; B after W. H. Calvin and G. Ojemann, 1994. *Conversations with Neil's brain: The neural nature of thought and language.* Addison-Wesley. Reading, MA.)

RESEARCHERS AT WORK

Noninvasive stimulation mapping reveals details of the brain's language areas

Transcranial magnetic stimulation (TMS; see Figure 2.20) allows researchers to stimulate small clusters of cortical neurons with good precision, from outside the scalp. By using MRI scans to select targets, TMS provides a noninvasive method for inducing a sort of temporary brain lesion, disrupting the activity of the selected brain region for up to an hour. Alternatively, TMS can be used along with PET or fMRI to precisely map regions of increased activity.

Using TMS mapping, researchers have generally replicated and extended the earlier findings regarding the cortical organization of language functions. For example, TMS mapping has revealed that speech production is associated with activation of not only face areas in motor cortex, but also hand areas (Meister et al., 2003), confirming the linkage and possible evolutionary relationship of hand gestures and speech. Similarly, TMS mapping has been used to

(Continued)

RESEARCHERS AT WORK (continued)

show that speech perception activates specific regions that TMS shows to be involved with speech production (Scott and Wise, 2004), providing support for the motor theory of language that we discussed earlier.

Impressively, the TMS temporary-lesion approach has revealed previously unknown functional subregions within Broca's area (**FIGURE 15.11**). In these experiments (Gough et al., 2005), researchers found that anterior parts of Broca's area are involved in the semantic meaning of words, while a more posterior part of Broca's area is important for the patterning of speech sounds. Other research has shown that the posterior speech zone likewise contributes to both word meaning and sound-related aspects of language (Stoeckel et al., 2009; Sakreida et al., 2017). So the TMS procedure is providing new insights into the fine details of the cortical organization of language, especially in conjunction with traditional neuroimaging techniques (Devlin and Watkins, 2007)

FIGURE 15.11 Subregions of Broca's Area Revealed by TMS (After P. M. Gough et al., 2005. *J. Neurosci.* 25: 8010.)

■ **Question**
How is Broca's area organized?

■ **Hypothesis**
Broca's area is made up of discrete sub-areas with differing linguistic functions.

■ **Test**
Guided by precise structural MRI scans, apply transcranial magnetic stimulation (TMS) to activate discrete regions within Broca's area.

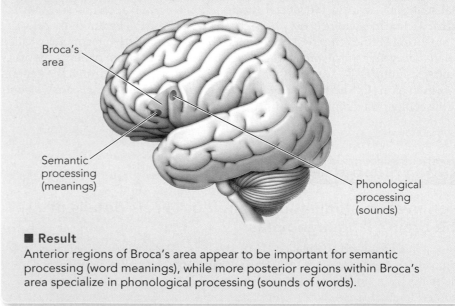

Broca's area

Semantic processing (meanings)

Phonological processing (sounds)

■ **Result**
Anterior regions of Broca's area appear to be important for semantic processing (word meanings), while more posterior regions within Broca's area specialize in phonological processing (sounds of words).

Functional neuroimaging technologies let us visualize activity in the brain's language zones during speech

Different aspects of language processing produce noticeably different patterns of brain activation, as shown in **FIGURE 15.12**. Passive *viewing* of words activates a posterior area within the left hemisphere (**FIGURE 15.12A**), but passive *hearing* of words shifts the focus of brain activation to the temporal lobes (**FIGURE 15.12B**). Repeating words orally activates the motor cortex of both sides, along with supplementary motor cortex and some of the cerebellum (**FIGURE 15.12C**). During word repetition or reading aloud, there is little activity in Broca's area. But when participants are required to generate an appropriate verb to go with a supplied noun, language-related regions in the

(A) Passively viewing words

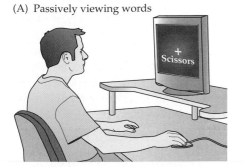

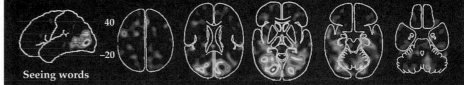

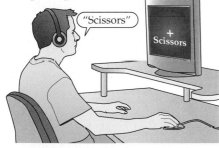

Seeing words

(B) Listening to words

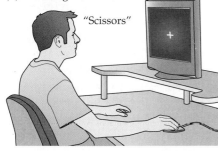

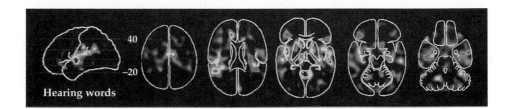

Hearing words

(C) Speaking words

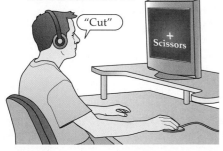

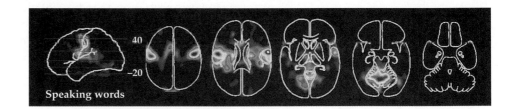

Speaking words

(D) Generating a verb associated
with each noun shown

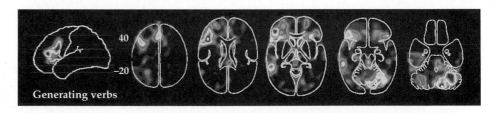

Generating verbs

FIGURE 15.12 PET Scans of Brain
Activation in Progressively More Com-
plex Language Tasks (After M. I. Posner
and M. E. Raichle, 1994. *Images of mind.*
Scientific American Library. New York, NY;
PET scans courtesy of Marcus Raichle.)

left hemisphere, including Broca's area, suddenly become markedly activate (**FIGURE
15.12D**).

Even languages that sound very, very different seem to activate much the same
brain regions in native speakers. Silbo Gomero is a very unusual whistled surrogate
language of the Canary Islands, used by shepherds (known as *silbadores*) to communicate over long distances. In Silbo, whistled notes serve as the phonemes and
morphemes of a stripped-down form of Spanish (for an audio sample of Silbo, with
translation, see **A STEP FURTHER 15.2**, on the website). Functional MRI showed
that long-term *silbadores* process Silbo using the same left-hemisphere mechanisms that they (and everyone else) use to process spoken language (Carreiras et al.,
2005). Non-*silbadore* controls, in contrast, process the whistle sounds of Silbo using

completely different regions of the brain; for these people, of course, the whistle sounds have no linguistic content. So the brain's left-hemisphere language systems appear to be sufficiently plastic to adapt to widely varying types of communication sounds, provided that they're heard early enough. In fact, while infants appear to be born with neural specializations for *speech* already in operation—they show more metabolic activity in the left hemisphere than in the right when they hear speech, even though they don't yet understand it (Dehaene-Lambertz et al., 2002)—those mechanisms don't similarly respond to the nonspeech sounds that make up Silbo Gomero (May et al., 2018). The incorporation of Silbo into the language system must therefore come about through extensive practice: the earlier the better.

Event-related potentials (ERPs; see Chapters 3 and 14) also provide hints about the brain's language network, by revealing the time base for language processing. For example, study participants can be asked to read a sentence in which there is a word that is grammatically correct but, because of its meaning, doesn't fit—such as "The man started the car engine and stepped on the pancake"—while brain electrical activity is recorded from scalp electrodes. About 400 milliseconds after the participant reads the word *pancake*, an enhancement of a distinctive ERP component called *N400* (*N* denotes "negative," and the number represents the response time in milliseconds; see Chapter 14) is detectable (Kutas and Hillyard, 1980; 1984). Such N400 responses seem to be specific to word meanings and apparently originate from temporoparietal cortex (including Wernicke's area) (Neville et al., 1992; Kutas and Federmeier, 2011). In contrast, words that are inappropriate because of grammar rather than meaning tend to elicit a *positive* potential about 600 milliseconds after they are encountered (called a *P600* response), indicating that detection of this level of error requires an extra 200 milliseconds of brain processing by other components of the language network (Osterhout, 1997). The degree to which meaning and grammar are processed independently in the brain, however, remains to be fully established and is an area of active investigation (Kuperberg, 2007; Brouwer et al., 2017).

HOW'S IT GOING ?

1. Summarize and discuss the organization of language systems in the human brain.
2. Discuss the patterns of brain activity that are observed in various verbal tasks, using functional-imaging technologies and ERPs. How well do these results align with traditional models of the organization of language areas in the brain?
3. What can we learn about general principles of language localization in the brain by studying unusual languages like Silbo?

PART II
Verbal Behavior: Speech and Reading

THE ROAD AHEAD

The second part of the chapter narrows its focus to our species' most distinctive characteristic: the everyday use of language, both in the form of speech and in the written word. After studying this section, you should be able to:

1. Provide a synopsis of the evolution and distribution of human languages.
2. Identify the principle linguistic components of speech.
3. Summarize the process of language development and the acquisition of grammar and reading skills.
4. Contrast human language with nonhuman animal communication.
5. Discuss in detail the forms of dyslexia and their possible neural underpinnings.

phoneme   A sound that is produced for language.

morpheme   The smallest grammatical unit of a language; a word or meaningful part of a word.

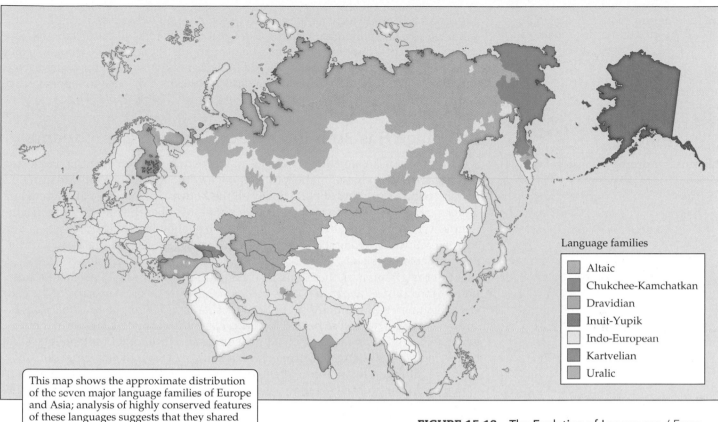

This map shows the approximate distribution of the seven major language families of Europe and Asia; analysis of highly conserved features of these languages suggests that they shared a common ancestor about 15,000 years ago—the time of the last Ice Age.

Language families

- Altaic
- Chukchee-Kamchatkan
- Dravidian
- Inuit-Yupik
- Indo-European
- Kartvelian
- Uralic

FIGURE 15.13 The Evolution of Languages (From M. Pagel et al., 2013. *Proc. Natl. Acad. Sci. U.S.A* 110: 8471; image courtesy of Dr. Mark Pagel.)

Human Languages Share Basic Features

The exact number of languages that we humans employ is unknown; our best guess is that there are 6,000–7,000 different languages, of which about 1,000 have been formally studied (Wuethrich, 2000). By applying the tools of evolutionary biology to linguistics, it is possible to track the cultural evolution of language, and this suggests a closer relation between languages than previously expected. In fact, the seven major language families found today in Europe and Asia appear to trace back to a single ancestral language in use about 15,000 years ago (**FIGURE 15.13**; Pagel et al., 2013). The subsequent explosion of new languages may have served cultural roles more than communicative ones; for example, the adoption of a new language would help a social group to identify its members and confound its rivals. But nowadays, in the increasingly globalized modern context, we seem to be inexorably sliding in the other direction as languages are lost or absorbed and we move toward a few common languages.

However we categorize them, all languages share certain basic features. Each language has basic speech sounds, or **phonemes**, that are assembled into simple units of meaning called **morphemes** (**FIGURE 15.14**). Morphemes are assembled into words (the word *unfathomable*, for example, consists of the morphemes *un*, *fathom*, and *able*), which have meaning (termed *semantics in linguistics*). In turn, the words are assembled into

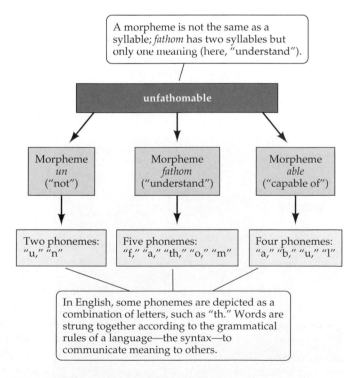

A morpheme is not the same as a syllable; *fathom* has two syllables but only one meaning (here, "understand").

unfathomable

| Morpheme *un* ("not") | Morpheme *fathom* ("understand") | Morpheme *able* ("capable of") |

| Two phonemes: "u," "n" | Five phonemes: "f," "a," "th," "o," "m" | Four phonemes: "a," "b," "u," "l" |

In English, some phonemes are depicted as a combination of letters, such as "th." Words are strung together according to the grammatical rules of a language—the syntax—to communicate meaning to others.

FIGURE 15.14 It's All in a Word

sensitive period   Also called *critical period*. The period during development in which an organism can be permanently altered by a particular experience or treatment.

stuttering   The tendency of otherwise healthy people to produce speech sounds only haltingly, tripping over certain syllables or being unable to start vocalizing certain words.

Williams syndrome   A disorder characterized by impairments of spatial cognition and IQ but superior linguistic abilities.

meaningful strings (which may be complete sentences or just phrases) according to the language's *syntax* (grammatical rules). Our speech is colored and clarified both by the context of the utterance (known as *pragmatics* in linguistics) and by the emotional tone and emphasis (called *prosody*) that we add to the things we say. But how does each of us end up with the right set of sounds and rules—the ones we need for our particular native language?

Language Has Both Inborn and Learned Components

A child's brain is an incredible linguistic machine, rapidly acquiring the phonemes, vocabulary, and grammar of the local language without need of formal instruction. Human babies start out babbling nearly all the known phonemes of all human languages, but soon come to use only those phonemes that they hear in use around themselves. And each baby's developing language abilities are especially shaped by "parentese," the singsong speech of caregivers that helps babies to attach emotion and meaning to speech sounds (Falk, 2004). By 7 months of age, infants already have a sense of the grammar of the language used in their homes, and they react to exceptions (Marcus et al., 1999).

The human brain contains specialized mechanisms for language acquisition that show a clear-cut **sensitive period** (or *critical period*): a limited span of time during which exposure and practice with language must occur in order for language skills to develop normally. This sensitive period tapers down from the maximal sensitivity of early childhood to an eventual end of special sensitivity around puberty. Individuals who are exposed to language only late in the sensitive period or after it has ended show much-reduced language development (Curtiss, 1989). And as many of us know from firsthand experience, learning a second language is much more difficult in adulthood, after the sensitive period is over. In fact, people learning a second language later than age 11 apparently use different brain regions for each language (K. H. Kim et al., 1997), unlike those who learn multiple languages early in life, as we discussed earlier.

An important genetic aspect of language acquisition was discovered by studying a most unusual family in England. Across at least three generations, about half of the members of the KE family have suffered from a severe language disorder. Affected family members take a long time to learn to speak and have difficulty with particular language tasks, such as learning verb tenses (Lai et al., 2001). Brain activation during language tasks is altered in this family too (Liégeois et al., 2003).

By studying the KE family's pedigree, researchers soon identified a gene, called *FOXP2*, that must be important for the normal acquisition of human language, because affected members of the KE family all share a mutation in this gene (**FIGURE 15.15**). In fact, multiple variants of *FOXP2* tend to produce different abnormalities in language-associated areas of the brain (Pinel et al., 2012), probably because *FOXP2* is a regulatory gene that can alter a variety of other genes (Vernes et al., 2011). **Stuttering**—the tendency of otherwise healthy people to produce speech sounds only haltingly, tripping over certain syllables or being unable to start vocalizing certain words—is likewise at least partly heritable and associated with changes in other genes (C. Kang et al., 2010).

On the flip side of the coin, children born with **Williams syndrome**—caused by the deletion of 28 genes from chromosome 7—have various intellectual deficits but excellent verbal skills. No one knows exactly what developmental mechanism results in this hyperverbal behavior (Paterson et al., 1999), but possession of *extra* copies of the identified genes on chromosome 7—rather than deletions of these genes—produces a syndrome of very poor expressive language that is, in many ways, the converse of Williams syndrome (Somerville et al., 2005).

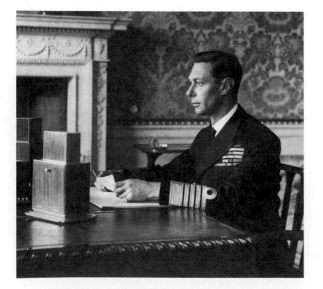

The King's Speech   England's King George VI—shown here during a wartime radio broadcast—stuttered severely. His struggle and eventual success in coping with speech difficulties, as portrayed in the film *The King's Speech*, shows that despite the possible genetic bases of the condition, effective therapy is possible. (© Hulton-Deutsch/Corbis Historical/Getty Images.)

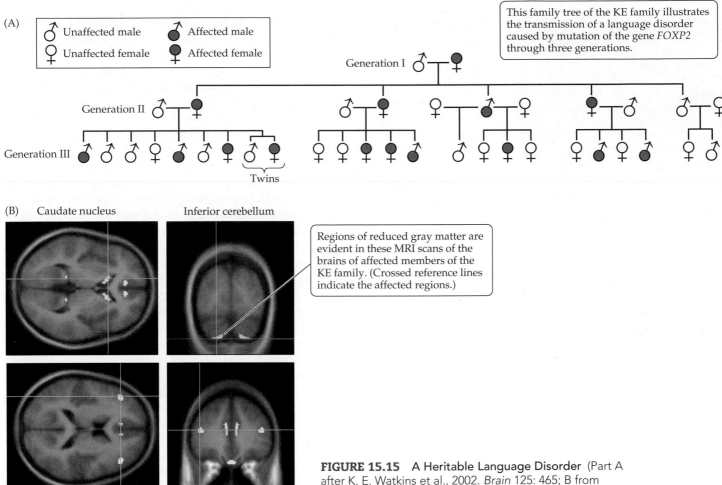

(A)

| ♂ Unaffected male | ● Affected male |
| ♀ Unaffected female | ⊕ Affected female |

This family tree of the KE family illustrates the transmission of a language disorder caused by mutation of the gene *FOXP2* through three generations.

Generation I

Generation II

Generation III

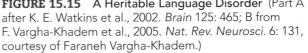

Twins

(B) Caudate nucleus   Inferior cerebellum

Regions of reduced gray matter are evident in these MRI scans of the brains of affected members of the KE family. (Crossed reference lines indicate the affected regions.)

Inferior frontal gyrus from two perspectives

FIGURE 15.15 A Heritable Language Disorder (Part A after K. E. Watkins et al., 2002. *Brain* 125: 465; B from F. Vargha-Khadem et al., 2005. *Nat. Rev. Neurosci.* 6: 131, courtesy of Faraneh Vargha-Khadem.)

Taken together, the evidence confirms that basic mechanisms of language are heritable components of the human brain, and the product of a long evolutionary history. Speech mechanisms may have evolved from more-ancient systems controlling gestures of the face and hands (Hewes, 1973; Corballis, 2002), in agreement with the motor theory of language that we discussed earlier. Even today there is a close relationship between speaking and gesturing with the hands (Krauss, 1998); in fact, most people find it difficult *not* to gesture when speaking. The use of language is one of the key adaptations of humans, so basic capabilities probably arose in an ancient ancestor of our species. For example, the Neandertals shared our version of *FOXP2* (Krause et al., 2007), so perhaps major differences in just a few genes like *FOXP2* and the stuttering genes are enough to explain why we write books and give speeches and chimps do not, despite our otherwise great genetic similarity (Fisher, 2017).

Nonhuman primates engage in elaborate vocal behavior

Every day, you utter sentences that you have never said before, yet the meaning is clear to both you and your human listener because you share an understanding of the words and grammar involved.

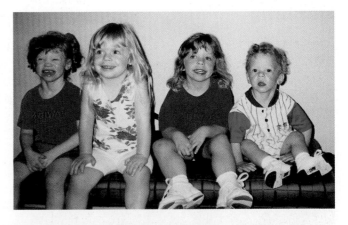

The Appearance of Williams Syndrome Children with Williams syndrome often have a characteristic facial shape, caused by the loss of a copy of the *elastin* gene. The loss of copies of other nearby genes is thought to cause mild mental disability paired with verbal fluency. (Courtesy of the Williams Syndrome Association.)

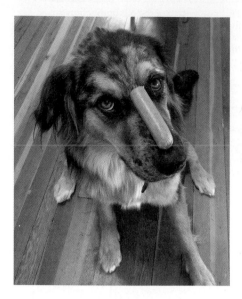

Good Dog! Dog lovers know that their willing friends can learn to associate certain words with specific actions. Maisie here knows to "wait" until she hears "okay," at which time she will enjoy both a delicious sausage and a delighted human. Dogs can learn a small collection of words with sufficient practice (lots of practice, for some dogs), enabling communication between human and nonhuman, but instilling *language* is a different matter altogether. Because most animals appear to lack a capacity for grammar—the rule for assembling units of language into new combinations—it seems that language is a uniquely human quality. (Photo by Neil Watson.)

Animals generally are incapable of similar feats, instead requiring extensive training with each specific utterance in order for communication to occur at all. Speaking to your dog ("Good dog!") reportedly activates a left hemisphere mechanism that processes meaning, as well as a right hemisphere mechanism that assigns value and reward to those words (Andics et al., 2016), but each new combination of words that you use with your dog will have to be laboriously learned from scratch. In short, dogs and most other animals appear to lack grammar. For this reason, scientists have focused the search for nonhuman language capabilities mostly on our nearest relatives, the other primate species.

Apes and monkeys employ a wide range of vocal behaviors for communication between individuals, particularly for relaying emotional information like alarm or territoriality (Ploog, 1992; Seyfarth and Cheney, 2003). The shrieking, purring, peeping, growling, and cackling sounds of squirrel monkeys, for example, can generally be related to specific social situations. Chimpanzees issue specific alarm calls to alert other members of their group to the presence of a viper (Crockford et al., 2012), and gibbons deploy a sizable repertoire of hooting calls that they recombine to communicate information about predators, social conditions, and mating opportunities (Clarke et al., 2015). But despite their apparent adaptive importance, most nonhuman primate vocalizations seem to have a somewhat "preprogrammed" quality, being repeatedly produced in much the same fashion and order. Electrical stimulation of the brain indicates that vocal behavior in monkeys and apes relies primarily on subcortical systems, especially sites in the limbic system, rather than on cortex. The vocalizations elicited by subcortical stimulation are associated with strongly emotional behaviors such as defense, attack, feeding, and sex (**FIGURE 15.16**). Vocalizations are more common if subcortical stimulation is provided to the left hemisphere, indicating a special role of the left hemisphere in the communicative behavior of monkeys and apes (Meguerditchian and Vauclair, 2006; Taglialatela et al., 2006), mirroring what we've seen for human speech.

Nonhuman primates are unlikely to ever produce human speech, as their vocal tracts and vocal repertoires are suited to their own communication needs. But can these animals be taught other forms of communication, with features similar to those of human language? Can they learn to represent objects with symbols and to manipulate those symbols according to grammatical rules? Our closest primate relatives, the great apes (chimpanzees, gorillas, orangutans) reportedly use a variety of hand gestures for communication in the wild (Hobaiter and Byrne, 2014) and are quite capable of learning hundreds of hand gestures from American Sign Language (ASL). Given enough training—it takes years—apes may learn to use ASL signs spontaneously, sometimes in novel sequences (R. A. Gardner and Gardner, 1969, 1984; F. Patterson and Linden, 1981). Through extensive practice, apes can also be trained to communicate by assembling abstract symbols, such as colored plastic chips or computerized symbols, into new sentences (Premack, 1971; Rumbaugh, 1977).

Some researchers have concluded that apes are thus able to acquire words (or equivalent symbols) and then string them together into novel, meaningful chains; that is, they seem to employ a grammar to communicate ideas. Other researchers argue that these sequences are simply subtle forms of imitation (Terrace, 1979), perhaps unconsciously

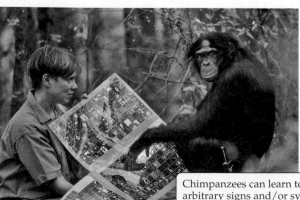

Chimpanzees can learn to use arbitrary signs and/or symbols to communicate, but it is questionable whether this usage is equivalent to human language.

Chimpanzee Using Symbols Some researchers argue that apes (chimpanzees, gorillas, and orangutans) are able to string arbitrary symbols together into meaningful, sentence-like statements. Others believe that while apes can learn subtle associations between symbols and meanings, their communicative behavior lacks the sense of grammar that is the hallmark of human language. (© Frans Lanting Studio/Alamy Stock Photo.)

cued by the experimenter who is providing the training. Observers who are native ASL users dispute the linguistic validity of the signs generated by apes, and others, such as linguist Noam Chomsky, argue that teaching primates to emulate a quintessentially human behavior in which they do not naturally engage can tell us little about the behavior, other than the obvious conclusion that ape evolution did not favor the use of language. So although the debate is far from settled, the linguistic abilities of primates have at least forced investigators to sharpen their criteria of what constitutes language.

Many different species engage in vocal communication

Many nonprimate species use vocalizations—chirps, barks, meows, songs, and more—to communicate important information to members of their own or other species. Although these communication sounds do not constitute language, in that they lack the features of language that we've discussed, such sounds nevertheless broadcast crucial signals about readiness to mate, danger, territorial defense, emotional state, and so on. Whales sing and may imitate songs that they've heard in distant oceans (Noad et al., 2000), and some seal mothers recognize their pups' vocalizations even after 4 years of separation (Insley, 2000). In fact, many species—from elephants to bats to birds to dolphins—are capable of vocal learning and use their vocalizations to help form social bonds and identify individuals (Tyack, 2003; Poole et al., 2005).

In the lab, measurement with special instruments reveals that rats and mice produce complex ultrasonic vocalizations that they use to communicate emotional information (Panksepp, 2005; Burgdorf et al., 2011). These ultrasonic vocalizations are associated with *FoxP2* gene expression (Shu et al., 2005; French and Fisher, 2014), providing an intriguing parallel to the situation in humans with *FOXP2* mutations that we discussed earlier.

Birds are particularly vocal animals. Many bird species produce only simple vocalizations, but male songbirds—canaries, zebra finches, song sparrows, etc.—produce rich and melodious vocalizations that are crucial for their social behaviors and reproductive success. Although birdsong has evolved quite independently of human speech, there are some interesting parallels between the two (Marler, 1970; Pfenning, 2014). The songbird brain contains a specialized neural system for the control of vocal behavior that, as in humans, relies principally on the left hemisphere of the brain (Moorman et al., 2012). What's more, juvenile birds must learn their songs from adult tutors during a distinct critical period in order for their own singing behavior to develop normally (DeVoogd, 1994)—a requirement that also parallels human language. And yes, as with human speech, the *FoxP2* gene is implicated in the learning and production of birdsong (Bolhuis et al., 2010). When *FoxP2* expression is blocked in parts of the song control system, young males fail to properly learn and recite their tutor's song, producing errors that in some ways resemble those in the humans with abnormal *FOXP2* described earlier (Haesler et al., 2007). (For more on birdsong and its social roles, see **A STEP FURTHER 15.3**, on the website.)

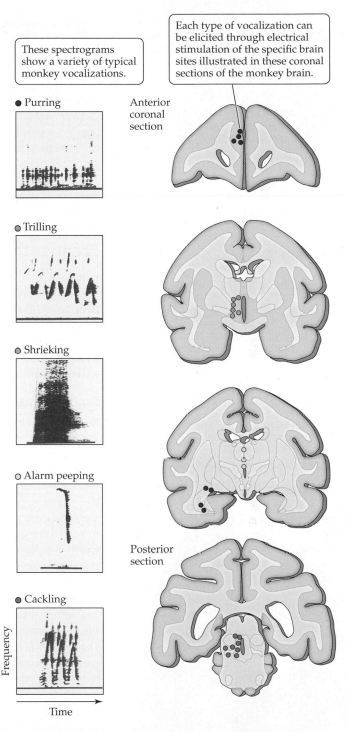

FIGURE 15.16 Electrical Stimulation of the Monkey Brain Elicits Vocalizations (After D. W. Ploog in A. Harrington, 1992. *So human a brain: Knowledge and values in the neurosciences.* Birkhauser. Boston, MA. Spectrograms courtesy of Uwe Jürgens.)

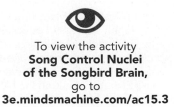

To view the activity **Song Control Nuclei of the Songbird Brain,** go to 3e.mindsmachine.com/ac15.3

dyslexia Also called *alexia*. A reading disorder attributed to brain impairment.

deep dyslexia Acquired dyslexia in which the person reads a word as another word that is semantically related.

surface dyslexia Acquired dyslexia in which the person seems to attend only to the fine details of reading.

HOW'S IT GOING ❓

1. How many languages do humans use, and how have they spread over time?
2. Why do researchers think that a capacity for language is inborn in the human brain? Briefly describe some pertinent research findings that support this position, including genetic evidence.
3. What are the basic linguistic components of spoken language?
4. Discuss the process of language acquisition in infants. What is the significance of the term sensitive period in this regard?
5. Summarize some of the ways in which studies of nonhuman animals help us understand the neural mechanisms of language.

Reading Skills Are Difficult to Acquire and Are Frequently Impaired

Why is it so much harder to learn to read and write than to speak? Compared with speech, the written word is a relatively new development, so we haven't had enough time to evolve brain mechanisms for reading and writing of the sort we have for speech. Therefore, learning the written form of a language is a slow and laborious chore of childhood that is vulnerable to developmental disruptions that result in **dyslexia** (from the Greek *dys*, "bad," and *lexis*, "word"), a mild to severe difficulty with reading.

Brain damage may cause specific impairments in reading

Sometimes people who learned to read just fine as children suddenly become dyslexic in adulthood as a result of disease or injury, usually to the left hemisphere. This *acquired dyslexia* (sometimes called *alexia*) offers hints about how the brain processes written language. One type of acquired dyslexia, known as **deep dyslexia**, is characterized by semantic errors (i.e., errors related to the *meanings* of words); for example, the printed word *cow* is read as *horse*. People with deep dyslexia are also unable to read aloud words that are abstract as opposed to concrete, and they make frequent errors in which they seem to fail to see small differences in words. It's as though they grasp words whole, without noting the details of the letters, so they have a hard time sounding out nonsense words.

In another form of acquired dyslexia, **surface dyslexia**, the person makes different types of errors when reading. These people can read nonsense words without problems, indicating that they understand which letters make which sounds. But they find it difficult to recognize words in which the letter-to-sound rules are irregular. *The Tough Coughs as He Ploughs the Dough* by Dr. Seuss (1987), for example, would utterly confound them. In contrast to people with deep dyslexia, those with surface dyslexia have difficulties that are restricted to the details and sounds of letters. Interestingly, surface dyslexia doesn't occur in native speakers of languages that are perfectly phonetic (such as Italian, where every letter is pronounced). This finding indicates that what's lost in speakers of nonphonetic languages, like English, is purely a learned aspect of language. In contrast, deep dyslexia probably involves inborn language mechanisms that are important for all languages.

Other kinds of brain damage can impair reading. For example, people with hemispatial neglect following right parietal lobe damage (discussed in Chapter 14) disregard the left half of the world, despite having otherwise normal vision. Such people thus also fail to notice the left halves of the words that they see, necessarily resulting in poor reading. In some severe cases of acquired dyslexia, the individuals exhibit *letter-by-letter reading*, a striking impairment in which the person laboriously spells out each word to herself (aloud or silently). In these cases, it seems that conscious attention to the spelling of each word is the only way by which words can be identified, so reading is dramatically slower.

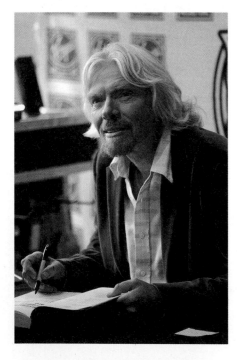

Overcoming Dyslexia Many highly intelligent, highly successful people—like Virgin Group founder Sir Richard Branson, pictured here—have coped with dyslexia on their way to fame and fortune. (© Everett Collection Inc./Alamy Stock Photo.)

Some people struggle throughout their lives to read

Some children seem to take forever to learn to read, and not even extended practice can make their reading easy and accurate. Affecting about 5% of children—especially boys and left-handers—this *developmental dyslexia* is a problem unique to written language, not a general cognitive deficit. (Indeed, children with dyslexia can have high IQs [B. Morris, 2002]; several notable examples have gone on to illustrious careers in varying fields.) Instead, the problem seems to lie in connecting reading with the more ancient brain mechanisms for speech.

Developmental dyslexia has been associated with several types of neurological abnormalities (**FIGURE 15.17**). In both postmortem investigations and anatomical studies using MRI, the brains of dyslexic people have been found to have aberrant layering of the neurons of the cerebral cortex, along with excessive cortical folding and clusters of extra neurons in unexpected locations (Galaburda, 1994; Chang et al., 2005). Cortical abnormalities are especially evident in the frontal and temporal lobes, possibly because of defective migration of newborn neurons during fetal development (Galaburda et al., 2006). Studies using fMRI confirm that people with dyslexia show impaired neural activity in left posterior speech zones (Pugh et al., 2000; Shaywitz et al., 1998, 2003) while displaying a relative overactivation of anterior regions. Abnormality in the nearby temporoparietal region has been linked to the phonological (phoneme-processing) aspects of dyslexia (Hoeft et al., 2006). And it looks like some of these abnormalities have genetic bases; for example, disruption of genes involved in brain development and the migration of neurons into adult positions are associated with developmental dyslexia (Harold et al., 2006; Gabel et al., 2010).

Taken together, imaging and behavioral studies indicate that our brains rely on two different language systems during reading: one focused on the sounds of letters, the other on the meanings of whole words (McCarthy and Warrington, 1990). Using fMRI, researchers found that people with dyslexia often have a disconnection between these systems, impairing the coordination of sounds with their meanings (Boets et al., 2013); it has been proposed that this disconnect is the result of hyperexcitability of reading-associated cortical networks (Hancock et al., 2017). Presumably, these systems are shaped by training: as with learning any highly skilled behavior, our brains mold themselves to accommodate our acquired expertise with written language, and lifelong avoidance of reading may be responsible for some of the sensory and word meaning problems that are evident in adults with dyslexia (Goswami, 2015). This could be why remedial training in people with dyslexia induces measurable changes in the left-hemisphere systems that are used for reading (Temple et al., 2003). And there are also positive findings: for example, evidence is accumulating that people with dyslexia actually outperform unaffected individuals in certain learning domains, such as aspects of spatial learning (Schneps et al., 2012). Findings like these may have important implications for developing new educational strategies in dyslexia. Perhaps,

FIGURE 15.17 Neural Disorganization in Dyslexia (After A. M. Galaburda et al., 1985. *Ann. Neurol.* 18: 222; micrographs courtesy of Albert Galaburda.)

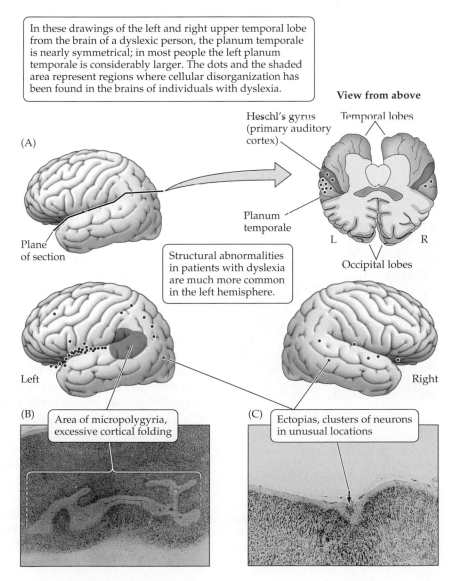

In these drawings of the left and right upper temporal lobe from the brain of a dyslexic person, the planum temporale is nearly symmetrical; in most people the left planum temporale is considerably larger. The dots and the shaded area represent regions where cellular disorganization has been found in the brains of individuals with dyslexia.

View from above

Heschl's gyrus (primary auditory cortex)   Temporal lobes

(A)

Plane of section

Planum temporale

L   R

Occipital lobes

Structural abnormalities in patients with dyslexia are much more common in the left hemisphere.

Left   Right

(B) Area of micropolygyria, excessive cortical folding

(C) Ectopias, clusters of neurons in unusual locations

recovery of function The recovery of behavioral capacity following brain damage from stroke or injury.

then, coupling education interventions with early genetic screening for dyslexia will help affected people completely overcome their trouble with words.

HOW'S IT GOING ?

1. Why do researchers believe that it is so much harder to learn to read than to learn to speak?
2. What are the two principal types of acquired dyslexia? Summarize their respective features.
3. What is developmental dyslexia, and what are some of the neurological findings associated with this form of reading disorder?

PART III
Recovery from Brain Damage

THE ROAD AHEAD

Because so much of the data on cerebral lateralization and language mechanisms has been drawn from studies of people with lateralized brain damage due to strokes and other types of brain injuries, the final section of the chapter turns to the processes by which the brain recovers at least some functions following damage. After reading this material, you should be able to:

1. Discuss the prevalence of various forms of brain damage and the reasons why so many people suffer lasting effects of brain injury.
2. Describe the typical timeline for neurological recovery from a stroke or other brain damage, and identify factors that affect this process.
3. Discuss potential therapies that can aid the process of recovery.
4. Explore how it is that children can recover from brain injury much more completely than adults can.

Stabilization and Reorganization Are Crucial for Recovery of Function

Compared with the other organs of the body, it's all too easy to seriously damage the brain. A number of factors combine to make the brain so vulnerable: extreme complexity, delicate structure, metabolic neediness, limited capacity for regrowth, and an exposed location perched atop a thin and whippy neck. In the United States alone, according to the 2016 National Health Interview Survey (Blackwell and Villarroel, 2018), almost 7.5 million adults are survivors of stroke, and many more are living with the consequences of other disease processes, such as tumors and degenerative diseases. Traumatic brain injury (TBI) has many causes: motor vehicle accidents, workplace injuries, and mishaps during activities such as horseback riding, diving, boxing, and other contact sports (**BOX 15.3**). So, while prevention is always preferable to treatment, researchers are intensively studying **recovery of function**, with the aim of developing treatments that improve outcomes for people with brain damage.

In the months following a brain injury, people often show conspicuous improvements in neural function as the injury site stabilizes, unaffected tissue reorganizes, and compensation occurs. We now know that the nervous system has much more potential for plasticity and recovery than was previously believed. For example, damaged neurons can regrow their connections under some circumstances, through a process called *collateral sprouting*. (For more information on collateral sprouting, see **A STEP FURTHER 15.4**, on the website.) And, as we've discussed in several places in this book, it has become evident that the adult brain is capable of producing new neurons; although this neurogenesis normally plays a minimal role in recovery from brain damage, perhaps we will learn how to bend these new neurons to our will and use them to replace damaged brain tissue.

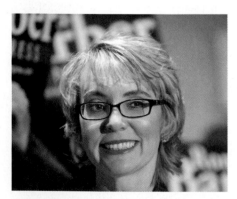

Perseverance and Plasticity Despite suffering a severe gunshot wound to the left cerebral hemisphere during an assassination attempt, former U.S. Representative Gabrielle Giffords has made striking progress in regaining her language and cognitive functions, thanks to intensive rehabilitation therapy and strategies for compensating for the damage. (© ZUMA Press, Inc./Alamy Stock Photo.)

BOX 15.3
Contact Sports Can Be Costly

Jarring blows to the head are common in a number of sports—football, hockey, boxing, and wrestling, for example—sometimes resulting in **concussion** or mild traumatic brain injury (mTBI), with a range of possible symptoms including headache, mood disturbances, confusion, memory loss, and occasionally (but not usually) a brief loss of consciousness. Even one concussion, but especially a series of concussions or minor head impacts—even seemingly mild ones—puts a person at risk of permanent brain damage. Although uncomplicated concussions generally clear up with time, up to 25% of concussions may cause persistent cognitive symptoms (Ponsford, 2005), some of which may not become evident until later in the person's life (Thornton et al., 2008; Montenigro et al., 2016). In the USA alone, mTBIs result in more than 2.2 million hospital visits per year (CDC 2015); many more go unreported.

An early large-scale CT study of 338 active boxers—athletes whose whole goal is to rain blows upon the head of an opponent—showed that scans were abnormal in 7% (showing brain atrophy) and borderline in 12% (B. D. Jordan et al., 1992). The marked cognitive impairment that results from too many concussions, once called *dementia pugilistica* (the Latin *pugil* means "boxer") or *punch-drunk*

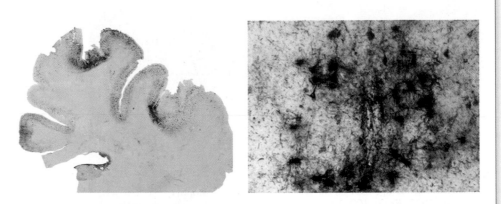

Tau Protein in the Brain of a Boxer with CTE   (*Left*) Unmagnified section of cortex. (*Right*) Cortical gray matter magnified ×350. (From McKee et al., 2009. *J. Neuropath. Exp. Neurol.* 68: 709, courtesy of Ann McKee.)

syndrome (Erlanger et al., 1999), is known today as **chronic traumatic encephalopathy (CTE)**. Evidence is mounting that CTE is also alarmingly frequent in other athletes, especially American football players (Mez et al., 2017).

Researchers have not yet agreed on a definitive diagnostic marker for CTE in living people—typically, it can be diagnosed only in postmortem analysis (McKee et al., 2016)—but one possible approach uses a special type of PET scan to detect abnormal expression of the cytostructural protein tau in the brain (Barrio et al., 2015). Neuropathological evidence indicates that, like Alzheimer's disease, CTE in athletes is a type of *tauopathy*, in which excess tau protein within neurons interferes with their

functioning (McKee et al., 2009). The photos in the figure show the brain of a former boxer who, by his mid thirties, was experiencing symptoms including memory loss, confusion, and a tendency to fall. As in other cases of CTE, an excessive amount of tau (brown in the photos) is evident in the brain, and it is found forming tangles within many neurons. CTE is a real and serious risk in contact sports, particularly where numerous blows to the head are sustained on a regular basis—which is why many researchers and physicians believe that the rules of some of these sports, especially where youths are participating, are in serious need of revision (*Nature*, 2017). And some sports, such as boxing, should perhaps retire from the ring altogether.

One of the most exciting prospects for brain repair following stroke or injury or in many other neurological conditions is the use of **embryonic stem cells** (Casarosa et al., 2014; Takahashi, 2018). Derived from embryos, these cells have not yet differentiated into specific roles and therefore are able to develop, under the control of local chemical cues, into the type of cell needed. Controversy surrounds the use of human embryos as cell donors, so researchers are working to find ways of creating stem cells from other sources, such as skin, that can then be placed in the brain and helped to survive, migrate, and mature into functioning replacement neurons (Emborg et al., 2013; Morizane et al., 2017).

Several factors determine how thoroughly a person will recover from a brain injury. One of these is simply the passage of time. Immediate medical treatment at the onset of a stroke can greatly limit the extent of damage, reducing cell death and inflammation. (Mechanisms of brain damage, and the mitigation of brain injuries, are discussed in **A STEP FURTHER 15.5**, on the website.) However, it takes months for the extent of

concussion   A form of closed head injury caused by a jarring blow to the head, resulting in damage to the tissue of the brain with short- or long-term consequences for cognitive function.

chronic traumatic encephalopathy (CTE)   A form of dementia that may develop following multiple concussions, such as in athletes engaged in contact sports.

embryonic stem cell   A cell, derived from an embryo, that has the capacity to form any type of tissue.

SIGNS & SYMPTOMS (continued)

Provided that the remaining hemisphere is healthy, children who have hemispherectomy surgery tend to show stable or improving intellectual functioning in the years following surgery (Boshuisen et al., 2010; Lew, 2014) and may have normal IQs in adulthood. So, although extensive hemispheric damage in an adult usually results in drastic and largely permanent functional and intellectual impairments, cases of childhood hemispherectomy vividly illustrate the amazing plasticity of the young brain.

HOW'S IT GOING ?

1. Just how prevalent is brain damage due to stroke, and to other diseases? Once the brain is damaged, is recovery more or less complete in a matter of hours, days, or months?

2. Discuss some of the factors that determine how thoroughly a person will recover from brain injury.

3. Is recovery better when brain damage is caused by trauma or when the damage is caused by stroke? What is believed to be responsible for the difference?

4. Discuss some of the types of therapy that appear to help maximize recovery following brain damage.

Recommended Reading

Bradbury, J. W., and Vehrencamp, S. L. (2011). *Principles of Animal Communication* (2nd ed.). Sunderland, MA: Oxford University Press/Sinauer.

Breedlove, S. M. (2017). *Foundations of Neural Development.* Sunderland, MA: Oxford University Press/Sinauer.

Ellard, C. (2009). *You Are Here: Why We Can Find Our Way to the Moon, but Get Lost in the Mall.* New York, NY: Doubleday.

Fitch, W. T. (2010). *The Evolution of Language.* Cambridge, UK: Cambridge University Press.

Gazzaniga, M. S. (2016). *Tales from Both Sides of the Brain: A Life in Neuroscience.* New York, NY: Ecco.

Harrison, D. W. (2015). *Brain Asymmetry and Neural Systems: Foundations in Clinical Neuroscience and Neuropsychology.* New York, NY: Springer.

Koelsch, S. (2012). *Brain & Music.* New York, NY: Wiley-Blackwell.

Kolb, B., and Whishaw, I. Q. (2015). *Fundamentals of Human Neuropsychology* (7th ed.). New York, NY: Worth.

Meyer, J. (2015). *Whistled Languages: A Worldwide Enquiry on Human Whistled Speech.* New York, NY: Springer.

Purves, D., Cabeza, R., Huettel, S. A., LaBar, K. S., et al. (2012). *Principles of Cognitive Neuroscience* (2nd ed.). Sunderland, MA: Oxford University Press/Sinauer.

Tomasello, M. (2010). *Origins of Human Communication.* Cambridge, MA: Bradford Books/MIT Press.

Zeigler, H. P., and Marler, P. (2008). *Neuroscience of Birdsong.* Cambridge, UK: Cambridge University Press.

15 ■ Visual Summary

You should be able to relate each summary to the adjacent illustration, including structures and processes. If you go to the website for our text (**3e.mindsmachine.com**), you can follow links to figures, animations, and activities that will help you consolidate the material.

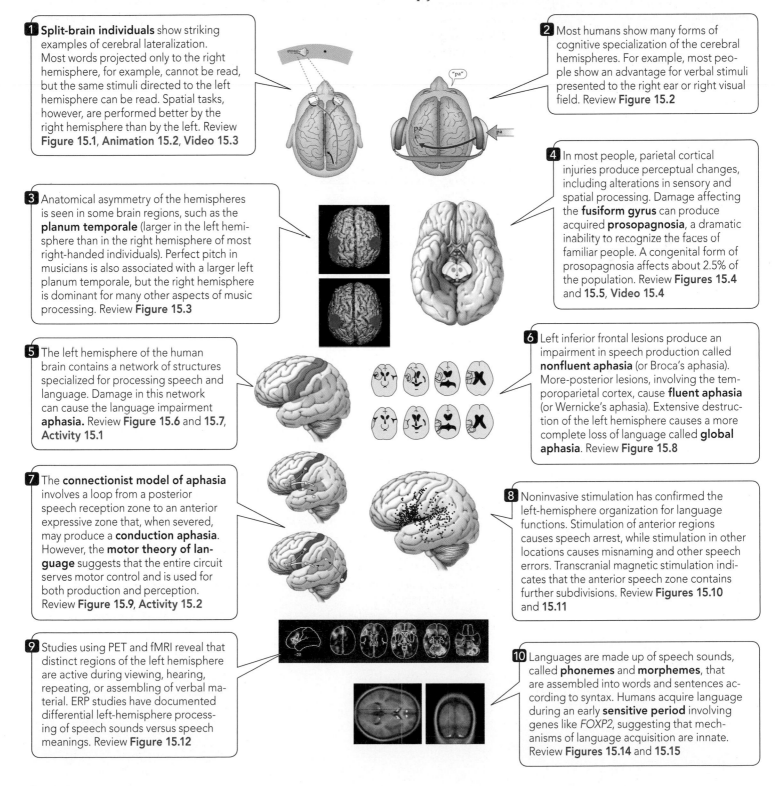

1 **Split-brain individuals** show striking examples of cerebral lateralization. Most words projected only to the right hemisphere, for example, cannot be read, but the same stimuli directed to the left hemisphere can be read. Spatial tasks, however, are performed better by the right hemisphere than by the left. Review **Figure 15.1, Animation 15.2, Video 15.3**

2 Most humans show many forms of cognitive specialization of the cerebral hemispheres. For example, most people show an advantage for verbal stimuli presented to the right ear or right visual field. Review **Figure 15.2**

3 Anatomical asymmetry of the hemispheres is seen in some brain regions, such as the **planum temporale** (larger in the left hemisphere than in the right hemisphere of most right-handed individuals). Perfect pitch in musicians is also associated with a larger left planum temporale, but the right hemisphere is dominant for many other aspects of music processing. Review **Figure 15.3**

4 In most people, parietal cortical injuries produce perceptual changes, including alterations in sensory and spatial processing. Damage affecting the **fusiform gyrus** can produce acquired **prosopagnosia**, a dramatic inability to recognize the faces of familiar people. A congenital form of prosopagnosia affects about 2.5% of the population. Review **Figures 15.4** and **15.5, Video 15.4**

5 The left hemisphere of the human brain contains a network of structures specialized for processing speech and language. Damage in this network can cause the language impairment **aphasia**. Review **Figure 15.6** and **15.7, Activity 15.1**

6 Left inferior frontal lesions produce an impairment in speech production called **nonfluent aphasia** (or Broca's aphasia). More-posterior lesions, involving the temporoparietal cortex, cause **fluent aphasia** (or Wernicke's aphasia). Extensive destruction of the left hemisphere causes a more complete loss of language called **global aphasia**. Review **Figure 15.8**

7 The **connectionist model of aphasia** involves a loop from a posterior speech reception zone to an anterior expressive zone that, when severed, may produce a **conduction aphasia**. However, the **motor theory of language** suggests that the entire circuit serves motor control and is used for both production and perception. Review **Figure 15.9, Activity 15.2**

8 Noninvasive stimulation has confirmed the left-hemisphere organization for language functions. Stimulation of anterior regions causes speech arrest, while stimulation in other locations causes misnaming and other speech errors. Transcranial magnetic stimulation indicates that the anterior speech zone contains further subdivisions. Review **Figures 15.10** and **15.11**

9 Studies using PET and fMRI reveal that distinct regions of the left hemisphere are active during viewing, hearing, repeating, or assembling of verbal material. ERP studies have documented differential left-hemisphere processing of speech sounds versus speech meanings. Review **Figure 15.12**

10 Languages are made up of speech sounds, called **phonemes** and **morphemes**, that are assembled into words and sentences according to syntax. Humans acquire language during an early **sensitive period** involving genes like *FOXP2*, suggesting that mechanisms of language acquisition are innate. Review **Figures 15.14** and **15.15**

11 Monkeys produce emotional vocalizations but cannot produce speech. Certain species of apes can learn American Sign Language, but it is not clear that this use constitutes language. Review **Figure 15.16, Activity 15.3**

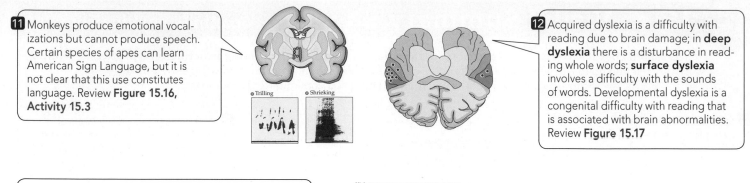

12 Acquired dyslexia is a difficulty with reading due to brain damage; in **deep dyslexia** there is a disturbance in reading whole words; **surface dyslexia** involves a difficulty with the sounds of words. Developmental dyslexia is a congenital difficulty with reading that is associated with brain abnormalities. Review **Figure 15.17**

13 The brain can show at least partial **recovery of function** after injury, especially during the first year or so, as the damaged brain stabilizes and reorganizes. Retraining is a significant part of functional recovery and may involve both compensation, by establishing new solutions to adaptive demands, and reorganization of surviving networks. Review **Figure 15.18**

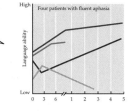

Go to **3e.mindsmachine.com** for study questions, quizzes, flashcards, and other resources.

APPENDIX
Molecular Biology
Basic Concepts and Important Techniques

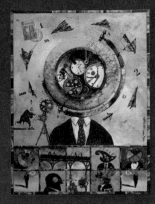

Genes Carry Information That Encodes Proteins

The most important thing about **genes** is that they are pieces of information, inherited from parents, that affect the development and function of our cells. Information carried by the genes is of a very specific sort: each gene carries the code for putting together a specific string of amino acids to form a particular **protein** molecule. This is all that genes do; they do not directly encode intelligence, or memories, or any other sort of complex behavior. The various proteins, each encoded by its own gene, make up the physical structure of the cell and most of its constituents, such as **enzymes**, which are proteins that enable chemical reactions in our cells. All these proteins make complex behavior possible, and in that context they are also the targets upon which the forces of evolution act.

Proteins are specific. For example, only cells that have liver-typical proteins will look like liver cells and be able to perform liver functions. Neurons, on the other hand, are cells that make neuron-typical proteins so that they can look and act like neurons. The genetic information for making these various proteins is crucial for an animal to live and for a nervous system to work properly.

One thing we hope this book will help you understand is that everyday experience can affect whether and when particular genetic recipes for making various proteins are used. To aid in that understanding, let's review how genetic information is stored and how proteins are made. Our discussion will be brief, but many online tutorials can provide you with more detailed information (see **A STEP FURTHER A.1**, on the website).

Genetic information is stored in molecules of DNA

The information for making all of our proteins could, in theory, be stored in any sort of format—on sheets of paper, a DVD, a smartphone—but organisms on this planet store their genetic information in a chemical called **deoxyribonucleic acid**, or **DNA**. Each molecule of DNA consists of a long strand of chemicals called **nucleotides** strung one after the other. DNA has only four nucleotides: guanine, cytosine, thymine, and adenine (abbreviated G, C, T, and A). The particular sequence of nucleotides (e.g., GCTTACC or TGGTCC or TGA) holds the information that will eventually

gene A length of DNA that encodes the information for constructing a particular protein.

protein A long string of amino acids. Proteins are the basic building material of organisms.

enzyme A complicated protein whose action increases the probability of a specific chemical reaction.

deoxyribonucleic acid (DNA) A nucleic acid that constitutes the chromosomes of cells and codes hereditary information.

nucleotide A portion of a DNA or RNA molecule that is composed of a single base and the adjoining sugar-phosphate unit of the strand.

FIGURE A.1   Duplication of DNA

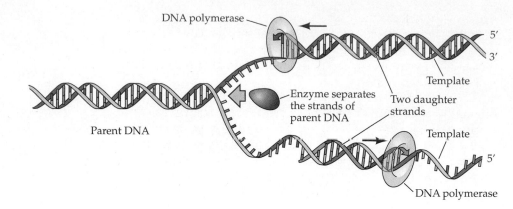

Before cell division, all of the chromosomes in the cell must be duplicated, as illustrated here, so that each daughter cell has the full complement of genetic information.

hybridization   The process by which one string of nucleotides becomes linked to a complementary series of nucleotides.

chromosome   A complex of condensed strands of DNA and associated protein molecules. Chromosomes are found in the nucleus of cells.

eukaryote   Any organism whose cells have the genetic material contained within a nuclear envelope.

cell nucleus   The spherical central structure of a cell that contains the chromosomes.

ribonucleic acid (RNA)   A nucleic acid that implements information found in DNA.

transcription   The process during which mRNA forms bases complementary to a strand of DNA. The resulting message (called a transcript) is then used to translate the DNA code into protein molecules.

messenger RNA (mRNA)   Also called *transcript* or *message*. A strand of RNA that carries the code of a section of a DNA strand to the cytoplasm.

ribosome   An organelle in the cell body where genetic information is translated to produce proteins.

translation   The process by which amino acids are linked together (directed by an mRNA molecule) to form protein molecules.

codon   A set of three nucleotides that encodes one particular amino acid.

peptide   A short string of amino acids. Longer strings of amino acids are called proteins.

make a protein. Because many millions of these nucleotides can be joined one after the other, a tremendous amount of information can be stored in very little space—on a single molecule of DNA.

A set of nucleotides that has been strung together can snuggle tightly against another string of nucleotides if it has the proper sequence: T nucleotides preferentially link with A nucleotides, and G nucleotides link with C nucleotides. Thus, T and A are said to be complementary nucleotides, and C and G are complementary nucleotides. In fact, most of the time, our DNA consists not of a single strand of nucleotides, but of two complementary strands of nucleotides wrapped around one another.

The two strands of nucleotides are said to **hybridize** with (link to) one another, coiling slightly to form the famous double helix. The double-stranded DNA twists and coils further, becoming visible in microscopes as **chromosomes**, which resemble twisted lengths of yarn. Humans and the many other organisms known as **eukaryotes** store our chromosomes in a membranous sphere called a **cell nucleus** (plural nuclei). The ability of DNA to exist as two complementary strands of nucleotides is crucial for the duplication of the chromosomes (**FIGURE A.1**), but the details of that story will not concern us. Just remember that, with very few exceptions, every cell in your body has a faithful copy of all the DNA you received from your parents.

DNA is transcribed to produce messenger RNA

The information from DNA is used to assemble another molecule—**ribonucleic acid**, or **RNA**—that serves as a template for later steps in protein synthesis. Like DNA, RNA is made up of a long string of four types of nucleotides. For RNA, those nucleotides are G and C, which you'll recall are complementary to each other, plus A and U (uracil), which are also complementary to each other. Note that the T nucleotide is found only in DNA, and the U nucleotide is found only in RNA.

When a particular gene becomes active, the double strand of DNA unwinds enough so that one strand becomes free of the other and becomes available to special cellular machinery (including an enzyme called transcriptase) that begins **transcription**—the construction of a specific string of RNA nucleotides that are complementary to the exposed strand of DNA (**FIGURE A.2**). This length of RNA goes by several names: **messenger RNA (mRNA)**, transcript, or sometimes message. Each DNA nucleotide encodes a specific RNA nucleotide (an RNA G for every DNA C, an RNA C for every DNA G, an RNA U for every DNA A, and an RNA A for every DNA T). This transcript is made in the nucleus where the DNA resides; then the mRNA molecule moves to the cytoplasm, where protein molecules are assembled.

RNA molecules direct the formation of protein molecules

In the cytoplasm, special organelles called **ribosomes** attach themselves to a molecule of RNA, "read" the sequence of RNA nucleotides, and using that information, begin linking together amino acids to form a protein molecule. The structure and function of a protein molecule depend on which particular amino acids are put together and in what order. The decoding of an RNA transcript to manufacture a particular protein is called **translation** (see Figure A.2), as distinct from transcription, the construction of the mRNA molecule.

Each trio of RNA nucleotides, or **codon**, encodes one of 20 or so different amino acids. Special molecules associated with the ribosome recognize the codon and bring a molecule of the appropriate amino acid so that the ribosome can fuse that amino acid to the previous one. If the resulting string of amino acids is short (say, 50 amino acids or less), it is called a **peptide**; if it is long, it is called a protein. Thus the ribosome assembles a very particular sequence of amino acids at the behest of a very particular sequence of RNA nucleotides, which were themselves encoded in the DNA inherited from our parents. In short, the biological secret of life is that DNA makes RNA, and RNA makes protein.

There are fascinating additions to this short story. Often the information from separate stretches of DNA is spliced together to make a single transcript; this so-called alternative splicing can create different transcripts from the same gene. Sometimes a protein is modified extensively after translation ends; special chemical processes can cleave long proteins to create one or several active peptides.

Keep in mind that each cell has the complete library of genetic information, collectively known as the **genome**, but makes only a fraction of all the proteins encoded in that DNA. In modern biology we say that each cell **expresses** only some genes; that is, the cell transcribes certain genes and makes the corresponding gene products (protein molecules). Thus, each cell must come to express all the genes needed to perform its function. Modern biologists refer to the expression of a particular subset of the genome as **cell differentiation**: the process by which different types of cells acquire their unique appearance and function. During development, individual cells appear to become more and more specialized, expressing progressively fewer genes. Many molecular biologists are striving to understand which cellular and molecular mechanisms "turn on" or "turn off" gene expression, in order to understand development and pathologies, such as cancer, or to provide crucial proteins to afflicted organs in a variety of diseases.

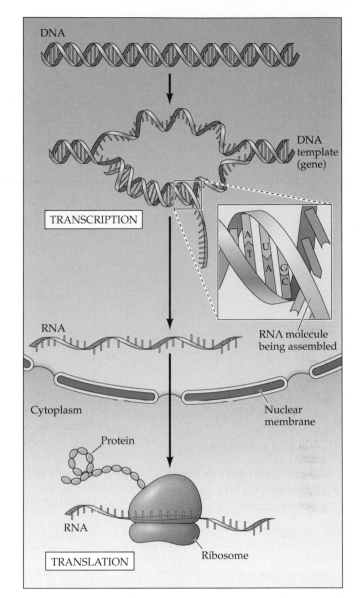

FIGURE A.2   DNA Makes RNA, and RNA Makes Protein

Molecular Biologists Have Craftily Enslaved Microorganisms and Enzymes

Many basic methods of molecular biology are not explicitly discussed in the text, so we will not describe them in detail here. However, you should understand what some of the terms mean, even if you don't know exactly how the methods are performed.

Molecular biologists have found ways to incorporate DNA from other species into the DNA of microorganisms such as bacteria and viruses. After the foreign DNA is incorporated, the microorganisms are allowed to reproduce rapidly, producing more and more copies of the (foreign) gene of interest. At this point the gene is said to be **cloned**, because researchers can make as many copies as they want. To ensure that the right gene is being cloned, the researcher generally clones many, many different genes—each into different bacteria—and then "screens" the bacteria rapidly to find the rare one that has incorporated the gene of interest.

When enough copies of the DNA have been made, the microorganisms are ground up and the DNA extracted. If sufficient DNA has been generated, chemical steps can

genome   Also called genotype. All the genetic information that one specific individual has inherited.

expression   For genes, the process by which a cell makes an mRNA transcript of a particular gene.

cell differentiation   The developmental stage in which cells acquire distinctive characteristics, such as those of neurons, as the result of expressing particular genes.

clone   Produce identical sequences of DNA or RNA, or a genetically identical organism.

then determine the exact sequence of nucleotides found in that stretch of DNA—a process known as **DNA sequencing**. Once the sequence of nucleotides has been determined, the sequence of complementary nucleotides in the messenger RNA for that gene can be inferred. The sequence of mRNA nucleotides tells the investigator the sequence of amino acids that will be made from that transcript, because biologists know which amino acid is encoded by each trio of DNA nucleotides. For example, scientists discovered the amino acid sequence of neurotransmitter receptors by this process.

The business of obtaining many copies of DNA has been boosted by a technique called the **polymerase chain reaction**, or **PCR**. This technique exploits a special type of polymerase enzyme that, like other such enzymes, induces the formation of a DNA molecule that is complementary to an existing single strand of DNA (see Figure A.1). Because this particular polymerase enzyme (called Taq polymerase) evolved in bacteria that inhabit geothermal hot springs, it can function in a broad range of temperatures. By heating double-stranded DNA, we can cause the two strands to separate, making each strand available to polymerase enzymes that, when the temperature has decreased enough, construct a new "mate" for each strand so that they are both double-stranded again. The first PCR yields only double the original number of DNA molecules; repeating the process results in 4 times as many molecules as at first. Repeatedly heating and cooling the DNA of interest in the presence of this heat-resistant polymerase enzyme soon yields millions of copies of the original DNA molecule, which is why this process is also referred to as gene amplification. In practice, PCR usually requires the investigator to provide primers—short nucleotide sequences synthesized to hybridize on either side of the gene of interest to amplify that particular gene more than others.

With PCR, sufficient quantities of DNA are produced for chemical analysis or other manipulations, such as introducing DNA into cells. For example, we might inject some of the DNA encoding a protein of interest into a fertilized mouse egg (a zygote) and then return the zygote to a pregnant mouse to grow. Occasionally the injected DNA becomes incorporated into the zygote's genome, resulting in a **transgenic** mouse that carries and expresses the foreign gene.

Southern blots identify particular genes

Suppose we want to know whether a particular individual or a particular species carries a certain gene. Because all cells contain a complete copy of the genome, we can gather DNA from just about any kind of cell population: blood, skin, or muscle, for example. After the cells are ground up, a chemical extraction procedure isolates the DNA (discarding the RNA and protein). Finding a particular gene in that DNA boils down just to finding a particular sequence of DNA nucleotides. To do that, we can exploit the tendency of nucleic acids (DNA and RNA) to hybridize with one another.

If we were looking for the DNA sequence GCT, for example, we could manufacture the sequence CGA (there are machines to do that), which would then stick to (hybridize with) any DNA sequence of GCT. The manufactured sequence CGA is called a **probe** because it is made to include a label (a colorful or radioactive molecule) that lets us track its location. Of course, such a short length of nucleotides will be found in many genes. In order for a probe to recognize one particular gene, it has to be about 15 nucleotides long.

When we extract DNA from an individual, it's convenient to let enzymes cut up the very long stretches of DNA into more manageable pieces of 1,000–20,000 nucleotides each. A process called **gel electrophoresis** uses electrical current to separate these millions of pieces more or less by size (**FIGURE A.3**). Large pieces move slowly through a tube of gelatin-like material, and small pieces move rapidly. The tube of gel is then sliced and placed on top of a sheet of paper-like material called nitrocellulose. When fluid is allowed to flow through the gel and nitrocellulose, DNA molecules are pulled out of the gel and deposited on the waiting nitrocellulose. This process of making a "sandwich" of gel and nitrocellulose and using fluid to move molecules from the former to the latter is called **blotting** (see Figure A.3).

To view the animation
Gel Electrophoresis,
go to
3e.mindsmachine.com/avA.1

DNA sequencing The process by which the order of nucleotides in a gene is identified.

polymerase chain reaction (PCR) Also called *gene amplification*. A method for reproducing a particular RNA or DNA sequence manyfold, allowing amplification for sequencing or manipulating the sequence.

transgenic Referring to an animal in which a new or altered gene has been deliberately introduced into the genome.

probe In molecular biology, a manufactured sequence of DNA that is made to include a label (a colorful or radioactive molecule) that lets us track its location.

gel electrophoresis A method of separating molecules of differing size or electrical charge by forcing them to flow through a gel.

blotting Transferring DNA, RNA, or protein fragments to nitrocellulose following separation via gel electrophoresis. The blotted substance can then be labeled.

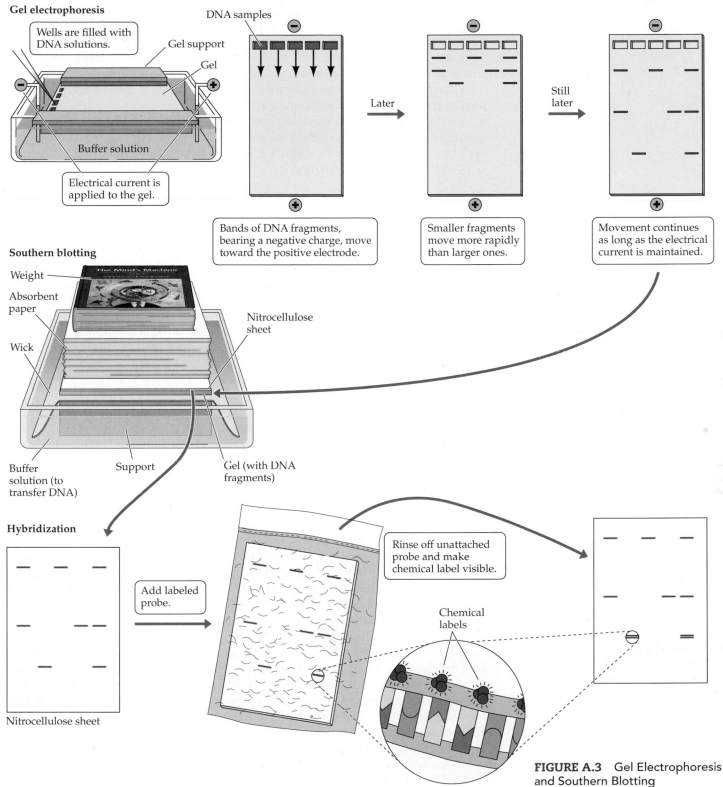

Gel electrophoresis

Wells are filled with DNA solutions.

Gel support

Gel

Electrical current is applied to the gel.

Buffer solution

DNA samples

Later →

Bands of DNA fragments, bearing a negative charge, move toward the positive electrode.

Still later →

Smaller fragments move more rapidly than larger ones.

Movement continues as long as the electrical current is maintained.

Southern blotting

Weight

Absorbent paper

Wick

Nitrocellulose sheet

Buffer solution (to transfer DNA)

Support

Gel (with DNA fragments)

Hybridization

Add labeled probe. →

Rinse off unattached probe and make chemical label visible.

Chemical labels

Nitrocellulose sheet

FIGURE A.3 Gel Electrophoresis and Southern Blotting

If the gene we're looking for is among those millions of DNA fragments sitting on the nitrocellulose, our labeled probe should recognize and hybridize with the sequence. The nitrocellulose sheet is soaked in a solution containing our labeled probe; we wait for the probe to find and hybridize with the gene of interest (if it is present), and we rinse the sheet to remove probe molecules that did not find the gene. Then we visualize the probe, either by causing the label to show its color or, if radioactive, by letting the probe expose photographic film to identify the locations where the probe has accumulated. In either case, if the probe found the gene, a labeled band will be evident, corresponding to the size of DNA fragment that contained the gene (see Figure A.3).

This process of looking for a particular sequence of DNA is called a **Southern blot**, named after the man who developed the technique, Edward Southern. Southern blots are useful for determining whether related individuals share a particular gene or for assessing the evolutionary relatedness of different species. The developed blots, with their lanes of labeled bands (see Figure A.3), are often seen in popular-media accounts of DNA fingerprinting of individuals.

Northern blots identify particular mRNA transcripts

A method more relevant for our discussions is the **Northern blot** (whimsically named as the opposite of the Southern blot). A Northern blot can identify which tissues are making a particular RNA transcript. If liver cells are making a particular protein, for example, then some transcripts for the gene that encodes that protein should be present. So we can take the liver, grind it up, and use chemical processes to isolate most of the RNA (discarding the DNA and protein). The resulting mixture consists of RNA molecules of many different sizes: long, medium, and short transcripts. Gel electrophoresis will separate the transcripts by size, and we can blot the size-sorted mRNA molecules onto nitrocellulose sheets; the process is very similar to the Southern blot procedure.

To see whether the particular transcript we're looking for is among the mRNAs, we construct a labeled probe (of either DNA nucleotides or RNA nucleotides) that is complementary to the mRNA transcript of interest and long enough that it will hybridize only with that particular transcript. We incubate the nitrocellulose in the probe, allow time for the probe to hybridize with the targeted transcript (if present), rinse off any unused probe molecules, and then visualize the probe as before. If the transcript of interest is present, we should see a band on the film (see Figure A.3). The presence of several bands indicates that the probe has hybridized to more than one transcript and we may need to make a more specific probe or alter chemical conditions to make the probe less likely to bind similar transcripts.

Because different gene transcripts have different lengths, the transcript of interest should have reached a particular point in the electrophoresis gel: small transcripts should have moved far; large transcripts should have moved only a little. If our probe has found the right transcript, the single band of labeling should be at the point that is appropriate for a transcript of that length.

In situ hybridization localizes mRNA transcripts within specific cells

Northern blots can tell us whether a particular organ has transcripts for a particular gene product. For example, Northern blot analyses have indicated that thousands of genes are transcribed only in the brain. Presumably the proteins encoded by these genes are used exclusively in the brain. But such results alone are not very informative, because the brain consists of so many different kinds of glial and neuronal cells. We can refine Northern blot analyses somewhat, by dissecting out a particular part of the brain—say, the hippocampus—to isolate mRNAs. Sometimes, though, it is important to know exactly which cells are making the transcript. In that case we use **in situ hybridization**.

With in situ hybridization we use the same sort of labeled probe, constructed of nucleotides that are complementary to (and will therefore hybridize with) the targeted transcript, as in Northern blots. Instead of using the probe to find and hybridize with the transcript on a sheet of nitrocellulose, however, we use the probe to find the transcripts in situ (Latin for "in place")—that is, on a section of tissue. After rinsing off the probe molecules that didn't find a match, we visualize the probe in the tissue section. Any cells in the section that were transcribing the gene of interest will have transcripts

Southern blot   A method of detecting a particular DNA sequence in the genome of an organism.

Northern blot   A method of detecting a particular RNA transcript in a tissue or organ.

in situ hybridization   A method for detecting particular RNA transcripts in tissue sections.

antibody   Also called *immunoglobulin*. A large protein that recognizes and permanently binds to particular shapes, normally as part of the immune system attack on foreign particles.

Western blot   A method of detecting a particular protein molecule in a tissue or organ.

immunocytochemistry (ICC)   A method for detecting a particular protein in tissues in which an antibody recognizes and binds to the protein and then chemical methods are used to leave a visible reaction product around each antibody.

in the cytoplasm that should have hybridized with our labeled probe. In situ hybridization therefore can tell us exactly which cells are expressing a particular gene (**FIGURE A.4** and Box 2.1).

Western blots identify particular proteins

Sometimes we wish to study a particular protein rather than its transcript. In such cases we can use antibodies. **Antibodies** are large, complicated molecules (proteins, in fact) that our immune system adds to the bloodstream to identify and fight invading microbes, thereby arresting and preventing disease. But if we inject a rabbit or mouse with a sample of a protein of interest, we can induce the animal to create antibodies that recognize and attach to that particular protein, just as if it were an invader.

Once these antibodies have been purified and chemically labeled, we can use them to search for the target protein. We grind up an organ, isolate the proteins (discarding the DNA and RNA), and separate them by means of gel electrophoresis. Then we blot these proteins out of the gel and onto nitrocellulose. Next we use the antibodies to tell us whether the targeted protein is among those made by that organ. If the antibodies identify only the protein we care about, there should be a single band of labeling (if there are two or more, then the antibodies may recognize more than one protein). Because proteins come in different sizes, the single band of label should be at the position corresponding to the size of the protein that we're studying. Such blots are called **Western blots**.

To review, Southern blots identify particular DNA pieces (genes), Northern blots identify particular RNA pieces (transcripts), and Western blots identify particular proteins (sometimes called products).

Antibodies can also tell us which cells possess a particular protein

If we need to know which particular cells within an organ such as the brain are making a particular protein, we can use the same sorts of antibodies that we use in Western blots, but in this case directed at that protein in tissue sections. We slice up the brain, expose the sections to the antibodies, allow time for them to find and attach to the protein, rinse off unattached antibodies, and use chemical treatments to visualize the antibodies. Cells that were making the protein will be labeled from the chemical treatments (see Box 2.1).

Because antibodies from the immune system are used to identify cells with the aid of chemical treatment, this method is called **immunocytochemistry**, or **ICC**. This technique can even tell us where, within the cell, the protein is found. Such information can provide important clues about the function of the protein. For example, if the protein is found in axon terminals, it may be a neurotransmitter.

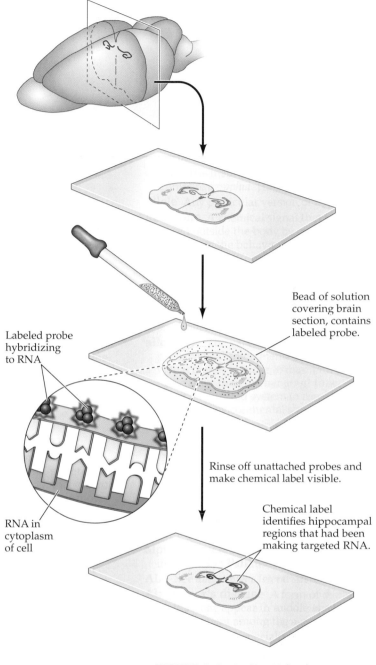

Bead of solution covering brain section, contains labeled probe.

Labeled probe hybridizing to RNA

Rinse off unattached probes and make chemical label visible.

Chemical label identifies hippocampal regions that had been making targeted RNA.

RNA in cytoplasm of cell

FIGURE A.4 In Situ Hybridization

acetylcholine, serotonin, and dopamine. See Table 4.1. Compare *amino acid neurotransmitter*, *gas neurotransmitter*, and *peptide neurotransmitter*. [4]

amino acid neurotransmitter A neurotransmitter that is itself an amino acid. Examples include GABA, glycine, and glutamate. See Table 4.1. Compare *amine neurotransmitter*, *gas neurotransmitter*, and *peptide neurotransmitter*. [4]

amnesia Severe impairment of memory. [13]

AMPA receptor A fast-acting ionotropic glutamate receptor that also binds the glutamate agonist AMPA. Compare *NMDA receptor*. [ASF 4.2, 13]

amphetamine psychosis A delusional and psychotic state, closely resembling acute schizophrenia, that is brought on by repeated use of high doses of amphetamine. [12]

amphetamine A molecule that resembles the structure of the catecholamine transmitters and enhances their activity. [4]

amplitude Also called *intensity*. The force that sound exerts per unit area, usually measured as dynes per square centimeter. In practical terms, amplitude corresponds to the volume of a sound. See Box 6.1. [6]

ampulla (pl. ampullae) An enlarged region of each semicircular canal that contains the receptor cells (hair cells) of the vestibular system. See Figure 6.14. [6]

amusia A disorder characterized by the inability to discern tunes accurately or to sing. [6]

amygdala A group of nuclei in the medial anterior part of the temporal lobe. See Figure 2.14. [2, 11]

amyloid plaque Also called *senile plaque*. A small area of the brain that has abnormal cellular and chemical patterns. Amyloid plaques correlate with dementia. See Figure 13.34. [13]

amyloid precursor protein (APP) A protein that, when cleaved by several enzymes, produces beta-amyloid, which can lead to Alzheimer's disease. [ASF 13.5]

amyotrophic lateral sclerosis (ALS) Also called *Lou Gehrig's disease*. A disease in which motor neurons and their target muscles waste away.

analgesia Absence of or reduction in pain. [5]

analgesic Having painkilling properties. [4]

anandamide An endogenous substance that binds the cannabinoid receptor molecule. [4]

androgen insensitivity syndrome (AIS) A syndrome caused by an androgen receptor gene mutation that renders tissues insensitive to androgenic hormones like testosterone. Affected XY individuals are phenotypic females, but they have internal testes and regressed internal genital structures. See Figure 8.27. [8]

androgen Any of a class of hormones that includes testosterone and similar steroids. See Figure 8.13. [8]

angel dust See *phencyclidine*. [12]

angiotensin II (AII) A hormone that is produced in the blood by the action of renin and that may play a role in the control of thirst. [9]

angular gyrus A brain region in which strokes can lead to word blindness.

anion A negatively charged ion, such as a protein or a chloride ion. Compare *cation*. [3]

anomia The inability to name persons or objects readily. [15]

anorexia nervosa A syndrome in which individuals severely deprive themselves of food. [9]

anorexigenic neurons Neurons of the hypothalamic appetite system that inhibit feeding behavior. [9]

anosmia The inability to detect odors. [6]

ANP See *atrial natriuretic peptide*. [9]

antagonist 1. A substance that blocks or attenuates the actions of a transmitter or other signaling molecule. Compare *agonist*. [3, 4] 2. A muscle that counteracts the effect of another muscle. Compare *synergist*. [5]

anterior Also called *rostral*. In anatomy, toward the head end of an organism. See Box 2.2. Compare *posterior*. [2]

anterior cerebral artery Either of two large arteries, arising from the carotid arteries, that provide blood to the anterior poles and medial surfaces of the cerebral hemispheres. Compare *middle cerebral artery* and *posterior cerebral artery*. [ASF 2.1]

anterior pituitary The front division of the pituitary gland. It secretes tropic hormones. See Figures 8.1, 8.12. Compare *posterior pituitary*. [8]

anterograde amnesia Difficulty in forming new memories beginning with the onset of a disorder. Compare *retrograde amnesia*. [13]

anterolateral system Also called *spinothalamic system*. A somatosensory system that carries most of the pain information from the body to the brain. See Figure 5.13. Compare *dorsal column system*. [5]

antibody Also called *immunoglobulin*. A large protein that recognizes and permanently binds to particular shapes, normally as part of the immune system attack on foreign particles. [ASF 11.4, App]

antidepressant A drug that relieves the symptoms of depression. Major categories include monoamine oxidase inhibitors, tricyclics, and selective serotonin reuptake inhibitors. [4]

antidiuretic hormone (ADH) See *vasopressin*. [8,9]

anti-müllerian hormone (AMH) Also called *müllerian regression hormone*. A protein hormone secreted by the fetal testes that inhibits müllerian duct development. [8]

antipsychotic Also called *neuroleptic*. Any of a class of drugs that alleviate symptoms of schizophrenia, typically by blocking dopamine receptors. [4, 12]

anxiety disorder Any of a class of psychological disorders that includes recurrent panic states and generalized persistent anxiety disorder. [12]

anxiolytic A substance that is used to reduce anxiety. Examples include alcohol, opiates, barbiturates, and the benzodiazepines. [4, 12]

aphasia An impairment in language understanding and/or production that is caused by brain injury. [15]

ApoE See *apolipoprotein E*. [ASF 13.5]

apolipoprotein E (ApoE) A protein that may help break down beta-amyloid. Individuals carrying the *ApoE4* allele are more likely to develop Alzheimer's disease. [ASF 13.5]

apoptosis See *cell death*. [13]

APP See *amyloid precursor protein*. [ASF 13.5]

appetitive behavior The second stage of mating behavior. It helps establish or maintain sexual interaction. See Figure 8.16. [8]

apraxia An impairment in the ability to carry out complex sequential movements, even though there is no muscle paralysis. [5, 15]

arachnoid The thin covering (one of the three meninges) of the brain that lies between the dura mater and the pia mater. See Figure 2.8. [2]

arcuate fasciculus A fiber tract classically viewed as a connection between Wernicke's speech area and Broca's speech area. See Figure 15.9. [15]

arcuate nucleus An arc-shaped hypothalamic nucleus implicated in appetite control. See Figure 9.15. [9]

area 17 See *primary visual cortex*.

arginine vasopressin (AVP) See *vasopressin*. [8,9]

aromatase An enzyme that converts many androgens into estrogens. [ASF 8.7]

aromatization The chemical reaction that converts testosterone to estradiol, and other androgens to other estrogens. [ASF 8.7]

aromatization hypothesis The hypothesis that testicular androgens enter the brain and are converted there into estrogens to masculinize the developing nervous system of some rodents. [ASF 8.7]

arousal The global, nonselective level of alertness of an individual.

associative learning A type of learning in which an association is formed between two stimuli or between a stimulus and a response. It includes both classical and instrumental conditioning. Compare *nonassociative learning*. [13]

astereognosis The inability to recognize objects by touching and feeling them. [15]

astrocyte A star-shaped glial cell with numerous processes (extensions) that run in all directions. See Figure 2.5. [2]

ataxia A loss of movement coordination, often caused by disease of the cerebellum. [5]

atrial natriuretic peptide (ANP) A hormone, secreted by the heart, that normally reduces blood pressure, inhibits drinking, and promotes the excretion of water and salt at the kidneys. [9]

attention Also called *selective attention*. A state or condition of selective awareness or perceptual receptivity, by which specific stimuli are selected for enhanced processing. [14]

attention deficit hyperactivity disorder (ADHD) A syndrome characterized by distractibility, impulsiveness, and hyperactivity that, in children, interferes with school performance. [14, ASF 13.4]

attentional blink The reduced ability of subjects to detect a target stimulus if it follows another target stimulus by about 200–450 milliseconds.

attentional bottleneck A filter created by the limits intrinsic to our attentional processes, whose effect is that only the most important stimuli are selected for special processing. [14]

attentional spotlight The steerable focus of our selective attention, used to select stimuli for enhanced processing. [14]

atypical antipsychotic See *second-generation antipsychotic*. [4, 12]

auditory canal See *ear canal*. [6]

auditory N1 effect A negative deflection of the event-related potential, occurring about 100 milliseconds after stimulus presentation, that is enhanced for selectively attended auditory input compared with ignored input. Compare *visual P1 effect*. [14]

auditory P300 See *P3 effect*. [14]

aura In epilepsy, the unusual sensations or premonition that may precede the beginning of a seizure. [3]

autism spectrum disorder (ASD) A disorder, arising during childhood, that is characterized by social withdrawal and perseverative behavior. Compare *Asperger's syndrome*. [ASF 13.4]

autobiographical memory See *episodic memory*. [13]

autocrine Referring to a signal that is secreted by a cell into its environment and that feeds back to the same cell.

autoimmune disorder A disorder caused when the immune system mistakenly attacks a person's own body, thereby interfering with normal functioning. [ASF 5.5]

autonomic ganglion A collection of nerve cell bodies, belonging to the autonomic division of the peripheral nervous system, that is found in any of various locations and contributes to the innervation of major organs.

autonomic nervous system A part of the peripheral nervous system that provides the main neural connections to glands and to smooth muscles of internal organs. Its two divisions (sympathetic and parasympathetic) act in opposite fashion. See Figure 2.9. [2]

autoradiography A staining technique that shows the distribution of radioactive chemicals in tissues. See Boxes 2.1, 8.1. [2, 8]

autoreceptor A receptor for a synaptic transmitter that is located in the presynaptic membrane and tells the axon terminal how much transmitter has been released. [4]

AVP See *arginine vasopressin*. [8]

axo-axonic synapse A synapse at which a presynaptic axon terminal synapses onto the axon terminal of another neuron. Compare *axo-dendritic synapse*, *axo-somatic synapse*, and *dendro-dendritic synapse*. [3]

axo-dendritic synapse A synapse at which a presynaptic axon terminal synapses onto a dendrite of the postsynaptic neuron, either via a dendritic spine or directly onto the dendrite itself. Compare *axo-axonic synapse*, *axo-somatic synapse*, and *dendro-dendritic synapse*. [3]

axon Also called *nerve fiber*. A single extension from the nerve cell that carries action potentials from the cell body toward the axon terminals. Functionally, the axon is the conduction zone of the neuron. See Figures 2.1, 2.3. [2]

axon collateral A branch of an axon. [2]

axon hillock The cone-shaped area on the cell body from which the axon originates. See Figure 2.4. [2, 3]

axon terminal Also called *synaptic bouton*. The end of an axon or axon collateral, which forms a synapse on a neuron or other target cell and thus serves as the output zone. Functionally, the axon terminals are the output zone of the neuron. See Figures 2.1, 2.3 [2]

axonal transport The transportation of materials from the neuronal cell body toward the axon terminals, and from the axon terminals back toward the cell body. [2]

axo-somatic synapse A synapse at which a presynaptic axon terminal synapses onto the cell body (soma) of the postsynaptic neuron. Compare *axo-axonic synapse*, *axo-dendritic synapse*, and *dendro-dendritic synapse*. [3]

B

B cell See *B lymphocyte*. [ASF 11.4]

B lymphocyte Also called *B cell*. An immune system cell, formed in the bone marrow (hence the *B*), that mediates humoral immunity. Compare *T lymphocyte*. [ASF 11.4]

Balint's syndrome A disorder, caused by damage to both parietal lobes, that is characterized by difficulty in steering visual gaze (oculomotor ataxia), in accurately reaching for objects using visual guidance (optic ataxia), and in directing attention to more than one object or feature at a time (simultagnosia). [14]

bar detector See *simple cortical cell*. [7]

barbiturate An early anxiolytic drug and sleep aid that has depressant activity in the nervous system. [4]

bariatrics Referring to the branch of medicine that deals with the causes, prevention, and treatment of obesity. [9]

baroreceptor A pressure receptor in the heart or a major artery that detects a change in blood pressure. [9]

basal "Toward the base" or "toward the bottom" of a structure. See Box 2.2. [2]

basal forebrain A region, ventral to the basal ganglia, that is the major source of acetylcholine in the brain and has been implicated in sleep. [4, 10]

basal ganglia A group of forebrain nuclei, including the caudate nucleus, globus pallidus, and putamen, found deep within the cerebral hemispheres. They are crucial for skill learning. See Figures 2.14, 5.28. [2, 5, 13]

basal metabolism The use of energy for processes such as heat production, maintenance of membrane potentials, and all the other basic life-sustaining functions of the body. [9]

basilar artery An artery, formed by the fusion of the vertebral arteries, that supplies blood to the brainstem and to the posterior cerebral arteries. [ASF 2.1]

basilar membrane A membrane in the cochlea that contains the principal structures involved in auditory transduction. See Figures 6.1, 6.2. [6]

behavioral intervention An approach to finding relations between body variables and behavioral variables that involves intervening in the behavior of an organism and looking for resultant changes in body structure or function. See Figure 1.10. Compare *somatic intervention*. [1]

behavioral medicine See *health psychology*. [11]

behavioral neuroscience Also called *biological psychology*, *brain and behavior*, and *physiological psychology*. The study of the biological bases of psychological processes and behavior. [1]

benzodiazepine Any of a class of anti-anxiety drugs that are noncompetitive agonists of $GABA_A$ receptors in the central nervous system. One example is diazepam (Valium). [4, 12]

beta activity See *desynchronized EEG*. [10]

beta-amyloid A protein that accumulates in amyloid plaques in Alzheimer's disease. [13]

beta-secretase An enzyme that cleaves amyloid precursor protein, forming beta-amyloid, which can lead to Alzheimer's disease. See also *presenilin*. [ASF 13.5]

between-participants experiment An experiment in which an experimental group of individuals is compared with a control group of individuals that have been treated identically in every way except that they haven't received the experimental manipulation. Compare *within-participants experiment*. [1]

binaural Pertaining to two ears. Compare *monaural*.

binding affinity Also called simply *affinity*. The propensity of molecules of a drug (or other ligand) to bind to receptors. Drugs with high affinity for their receptors are effective even at low doses. [4]

binding problem The question of how the brain understands which individual attributes blend together into a single object, when these different features are processed by different regions in the brain. [14]

binge eating The rapid intake of large quantities of food, often poor in nutritional value and high in calories. [9]

binocular Referring to two-eyed processes. [7]

binocular deprivation Depriving both eyes of form vision, as by sealing the eyelids. Compare *monocular deprivation*. [ASF 13.4]

bioavailable Referring to a substance, usually a drug, that is present in the body in a form that is able to interact with physiological mechanisms. [4]

biological rhythm A regular fluctuation in any living process. [10]

biotransformation The process in which enzymes convert a drug into a metabolite that is itself active, possibly in ways that are substantially different from the actions of the original substance. [4]

bipolar cell An interneuron in the retina that receives information from rods and cones and passes the information to retinal ganglion cells. See Figure 7.3. Compare *amacrine cell* and *horizontal cell*. [7]

bipolar disorder A psychiatric disorder characterized by periods of depression that alternate with excessive, expansive moods. [12]

bipolar neuron A nerve cell that has a single dendrite at one end and a single axon at the other end. See Figure 2.3. Compare *unipolar neuron* and *multipolar neuron*. [2]

blind spot The portion of the visual field from which light falls on the optic disc. [7]

blindsight The paradoxical phenomenon whereby, within a scotoma, a person cannot *consciously* perceive visual cues but may still be able to make some visual discrimination. [7]

blood-brain barrier The mechanisms that make the movement of substances from blood vessels into brain cells more difficult than exchanges in other body organs, thus affording the brain greater protection from exposure to some substances found in the blood. [2, 4]

blotting Transferring DNA, RNA, or protein fragments to nitrocellulose following separation via gel electrophoresis. The blotted substance can then be labeled. See Appendix Figure A.3. [App]

brain and behavior See *behavioral neuroscience*. [1]

brain self-stimulation The process in which animals will work to provide electrical stimulation to particular brain sites, presumably because the experience is very rewarding. [11]

brainstem The region of the brain that consists of the midbrain, the pons, and the medulla. [2]

brightness One of three basic dimensions of light perception, varying from dark to light. Compare *hue* and *saturation*. [7]

Broca's aphasia See *nonfluent aphasia*. [15]

Broca's area A region of the frontal lobe of the brain that is involved in the production of speech. See Figures 15.7, 15.8, 15.9. Compare *Wernicke's area*. [15]

brown fat Also called *brown adipose tissue*. A specialized type of fat tissue that generates heat through intense metabolism. [ASF 9.1]

bulimia Also called *bulimia nervosa*. A syndrome in which individuals periodically gorge themselves, usually with "junk food," and then either vomit or take laxatives to avoid weight gain. [9]

bungarotoxin A neurotoxin, isolated from the venom of the many-banded krait, that selectively blocks acetylcholine receptors. [3]

C

C fiber A small, unmyelinated axon that conducts pain information slowly and adapts slowly. [5]

caffeine A compound found in coffee and other plants that exerts a stimulant action by blocking adenosine receptors. [4]

CAH See *congenital adrenal hyperplasia*. [8]

calcium ion (Ca^{2+}) A calcium atom that carries a double positive charge. [3]

cannabidiol (CBD) One of the two major types of active compounds found in cannabis. The other is THC. [4]

cannabinoid receptors A receptor that responds to endogenous and/or exogenous cannabinoids. [4]

cannabis Also known as *marijuana*, although this name is considered pejorative. A psychoactive plant containing numerous active compounds in varying proportions. [4]

carotid artery Either of the two major arteries that ascend the left and right sides of the neck to the brain, supplying blood to the anterior and middle cerebral arteries. The branch that enters the brain is called the internal carotid artery. [ASF 2.1]

castration Removal of the gonads, usually the testes. [8]

CAT See *computerized axial tomography*. [2]

cataplexy Sudden loss of muscle tone, leading to collapse of the body without loss of consciousness. Cataplexy is sometimes a component of narcoleptic attacks. [10]

cation A positively charged ion, such as a potassium or sodium ion. Compare *anion*. [3]

cauda equina Literally, "horse's tail" (in Latin). The caudalmost spinal nerves, which extend beyond the spinal cord proper to exit the spinal column.

caudal See *posterior*. See Box 2.2. [2]

caudate nucleus One of the basal ganglia. It has a long extension or tail. See Figure 2.14. [2]

causality The relation of cause and effect, such that we can conclude that an experimental manipulation has specifically caused an observed result. [1]

CBT See *cognitive behavioral therapy*. [12]

CCK See *cholecystokinin*. [9]

cell body Also called *soma*. The region of a neuron that is defined by the presence of the cell nucleus. Functionally, the cell body is the integration zone of the neuron. See Figures 2.1, 2.3. [2]

cell death Also called *apoptosis*. The developmental process during which "surplus" cells die. See Figure 13.25. [13]

cell differentiation The developmental stage in which cells acquire distinctive characteristics, such as those of neurons, as a result of expressing particular genes. See Figure 13.25. [13, App]

cell membrane The lipid bilayer that encloses a cell. [3]

cell migration The movement of cells from site of origin to final location. See Figure 13.25. [13]

cell nucleus The spherical central structure of a cell that contains the chromosomes. [App]

cell-cell interaction The general process during development in which one cell affects the differentiation of other, usually neighboring, cells. [13]

central deafness A hearing impairment in which the auditory areas of the brain fail to process and interpret action potentials from sound stimuli in meaningful ways, usually as a consequence of damage in auditory brain areas. See Figure 6.10. Compare *conduction deafness* and *sensorineural deafness*. [6]

central modulation of sensory information The process in which higher brain centers, such as the cortex and thalamus, suppress some sources of sensory information and amplify others. [5]

central nervous system (CNS) The portion of the nervous system that includes the brain and the spinal cord. See Figures 2.6, 2.12. Compare *peripheral nervous system*. [2]

central sulcus A fissure that divides the frontal lobe from the parietal lobe. See Figure 2.10. [2]

cerebellum A structure located at the back of the brain, dorsal to the pons, that is involved in the central regulation of movement and in some forms of learning. See Figures 2.10, 2.12, 2.15, 5.28. [2, 5, 13]

cerebral arteries The three pairs of large arteries within the skull that supply blood to the cerebral cortex. [2]

cerebral cortex Also called simply *cortex*. The outer covering of the cerebral hemispheres, which consists largely of nerve cell bodies and their branches. See Figure 2.13. [2]

cerebral hemisphere One of the two halves—right or left—of the forebrain. See Figure 2.12. [2]

cerebral lateralization The division of labor between the two cerebral hemispheres such that each hemisphere is specialized for particular types of processing. [15]

cerebrocerebellum The lowermost part of the cerebellum, consisting especially of the lateral parts of each cerebellar hemisphere. It is implicated in planning complex movements. Compare *spinocerebellum* and *vestibulocerebellum*. [ASF 5.4]

cerebrospinal fluid (CSF) The fluid that fills the cerebral ventricles. See Figure 2.16. [2]

cerveau isolé See *isolated forebrain*. [10]

cervical Referring to the topmost eight segments of the spinal cord, in the neck region. See Figures 2.8, 2.9. Compare *thoracic*, *lumbar*, *sacral*, and *coccygeal*. [2]

c-fos An immediate early gene commonly used to identify activated neurons. See Box 2.1. [2]

change blindness A failure to notice changes in comparisons of two alternating static visual scenes.

ChAT See choline acetyltransferase. [ASF 4.1]

chemical transmitter See *neurotransmitter*. [2, 3]

chloride ion (Cl⁻) A chlorine atom that carries a negative charge. [3]

chlorpromazine An early antipsychotic drug that revolutionized the treatment of schizophrenia. [12]

cholecystokinin (CCK) A peptide hormone that is released by the gut after ingestion of food that is high in protein and/or fat. [9]

choline acetyltransferase (ChAT) An important enzyme involved in the synthesis of the neurotransmitter acetylcholine. [ASF 4.1]

cholinergic Referring to cells that use acetylcholine as their synaptic transmitter. [3, 4]

choroid plexus A specialized membrane lining the ventricles that produces cerebrospinal fluid by filtering blood. [2]

chromosome A complex of condensed strands of DNA and associated protein molecules. Chromosomes are found in the nucleus of cells. [App]

chronic traumatic encephalopathy (CTE) Formerly called *dementia pugilistica* or *punch-drunk syndrome*. A form of dementia that may develop following multiple concussions, such as in athletes engaged in contact sports. See Box 15.3. [15]

ciliary muscle One of the muscles that control the shape of the lens inside the eye, focusing an image on the retina. See Figure 7.1. [7]

CIMT See constraint-induced movement therapy. [15]

cingulate cortex Also called *cingulum*. A region of medial cerebral cortex that lies dorsal to the corpus callosum. [5]

cingulate gyrus Also called *cingulate cortex* or *cingulum*. A strip of cortex, found in the frontal and parietal midline, that is part of the limbic system and is implicated in many cognitive functions. See Figures 2.14, 2.15. [2]

circadian rhythm A pattern of behavioral, biochemical, or physiological fluctuation that has a 24-hour period. [10]

circle of Willis A structure at the base of the brain that is formed by the joining of the carotid and basilar arteries. [ASF 2.1]

circumventricular organ Any of multiple distinct sites that lie in the wall of a cerebral ventricle and monitor the composition of the cerebrospinal fluid. See Figure 9.8. [9]

classical conditioning Also called *Pavlovian conditioning*. A type of associative learning in which an originally neutral stimulus (the conditioned stimulus, or CS)—through pairing with another stimulus (the unconditioned stimulus, or US) that elicits a particular response—acquires the power to elicit that response when presented alone. A response elicited by the US is called an unconditioned response (UR); a response elicited by the CS alone is called a conditioned response (CR). See Figure 13.9. Compare *instrumental conditioning*. [13]

clitoris The female phallus. Compare *penis*. [8]

cloacal exstrophy A rare medical condition in which XY individuals are born completely lacking a penis. [8]

clones Asexually produced organisms that are genetically identical. [13, App]

clozapine A second-generation antipsychotic that blocks 5HT$_{2A}$ receptors. [12]

CNS See *central nervous system.* [2]

cocaine A drug of abuse, derived from the coca plant, that acts by enhancing catecholamine neurotransmission. [4]

coccygeal Referring to the lowest spinal vertebra (the coccyx, also known as the "tailbone"). See Figure 2.9. Compare *cervical, thoracic, lumbar,* and *sacral.* [2]

cochlea A snail-shaped structure in the inner ear canal that contains the primary receptor cells for hearing. See Figure 6.1. [6]

cochlear implant An electromechanical device that detects sounds and selectively stimulates nerves in different regions of the cochlea via surgically implanted electrodes. [6]

cochlear nucleus Either of two brainstem nuclei—left and right—that receive input from auditory hair cells and send output to the superior olivary nuclei. See Figure 6.5. [6]

cocktail party effect The selective enhancement of attention in order to filter out distracters, as you might do while listening to one person talking in the midst of a noisy party. [14]

codon A set of three nucleotides that encodes one particular amino acid. A series of codons determines the structure of a peptide or protein. [App]

cognitive behavioral therapy (CBT) Psychotherapy aimed at correcting negative thinking and consciously changing behaviors as a way of changing feelings. [12]

cognitive map A mental representation of the relative spatial organization of objects and information. [13]

cognitively impenetrable Referring to basic neural processing operations that cannot be experienced through introspection—in other words, that are unconscious. [14]

coitus See *copulation.* [8]

collateral sprouting The formation of a new branch on an axon, usually in response to the uncovering of unoccupied postsynaptic sites. [ASF 15.4]

co-localization The synthesis and release of more than one type of neurotransmitter by a given presynaptic neuron. [4]

communication Information transfer between two individuals. [15]

complex cortical cell A cell in the visual cortex that responds best to a bar of a particular size and orientation anywhere within a particular area of the visual field and that needs movement to make it respond actively. Compare *simple cortical cell.* [7]

complex environment See *enriched condition.* [13]

complex partial seizure In epilepsy, a type of seizure that doesn't involve the entire brain and therefore can cause a wide variety of symptoms. [3]

computerized axial tomography (CAT or CT) A noninvasive technique for examining brain structure through computer analysis of X-ray absorption at several positions around the head. See Figure 2.18. Compare *magnetic resonance imaging.* [2]

concordance Sharing of a characteristic by both individuals of a pair of twins. [12]

concussion A form of closed head injury caused by a jarring blow to the head, resulting in damage to the tissue of the brain with short- or long-term consequences for cognitive function. [15]

conduction aphasia An impairment in the ability to repeat words and sentences. [15]

conduction deafness A hearing impairment in which the ears fail to convert sound vibrations in air into waves of fluid in the cochlea. It is associated with defects of the external ear or middle ear. See Figure 6.10. Compare *central deafness* and *sensorineural deafness.* [6]

conduction velocity The speed at which an action potential is propagated along the length of an axon. [3]

conduction zone The part of a neuron—typically the axon—over which the action potential is actively propagated. See Figures 2.1, 2.3. Compare *input zone, integration zone,* and *output zone.* [2]

cone Any of several classes of photoreceptor cells in the retina that are responsible for color vision. See Figure 7.3. Compare *rod.* [7]

confabulate To fill in a gap in memory with a falsification. Confabulation is often seen in Korsakoff's syndrome. [13]

congenital adrenal hyperplasia (CAH) Any of several genetic mutations that can cause a female fetus to be exposed to adrenal androgens, resulting in partial masculinization at birth. [8]

conjunction search A search for an item that is based on two or more features (e.g., size and color) that together distinguish the target from distracters that may share some of the same attributes. Compare *feature search.* [14]

connectionist model of aphasia Also called the *Wernicke-Geschwind model.* A theory proposing that left-hemisphere language deficits result from disconnection between the brain regions in a language network, each of which serves a particular linguistic function. Compare *motor theory of language.* [15]

consciousness The state of awareness of one's own existence, thoughts, emotions, and experiences. [1, 14]

conserved In the context of evolution, referring to a trait that is passed on from a common ancestor to two or more descendant species. [1]

consolidation The second process in the memory system, in which information in short-term memory is transferred to long-term memory. See Figure 13.13. Compare *encoding* and *retrieval.* [13]

constraint-induced movement therapy (CIMT) A therapy for recovery of movement after stroke or injury in which the person's unaffected limb is constrained while they are required to perform tasks with the affected limb. [15]

contralateral In anatomy, pertaining to a location on the opposite side of the body. See Box 2.2. Compare *ipsilateral.* [2, 15]

control group In research, a group of individuals that are identical to those in an experimental (or test) group in every way except that they do not receive the experimental treatment or manipulation. The experimental group is then compared with the control group to assess the effect of the treatment. [1]

convergence The phenomenon of neural connections in which many cells send signals to a single cell. Compare *divergence.* [ASF 3.2, 7]

Coolidge effect The propensity of an animal that appears sexually satiated with a current partner to resume sexual activity when provided with a new partner. [8]

copulation Also called *coitus.* The sexual act. [8]

cornea The transparent outer layer of the eye, whose curvature is fixed. The cornea bends light rays and is primarily responsible for forming the image on the retina. See Figure 7.1. [7]

coronal plane Also called *frontal plane* or *transverse plane.* The plane that divides the body or brain into front and back parts. See Box 2.2. Compare *horizontal plane* and *sagittal plane.* [2]

corpus callosum The main band of axons that connects the two cerebral hemispheres. See Figures 2.11, 2.15. [2, 15]

corpus luteum (pl. corpora lutea) The structure that forms from the collapsed ovarian follicle after ovulation. The corpora lutea are a major source of progesterone. [8, ASF 8.4]

correlation The tendency of two measures to vary in concert, such that a change in one measure is matched by a change in the other. [1]

cortex (pl. cortices) The outer layer of a structure. See also *cerebral cortex* and *neocortex*. [2]

cortical column One of the vertical columns that constitute the basic organization of the cerebral cortex. [2]

cortical deafness A form of central deafness, caused by damage to both sides of the auditory cortex, that is characterized by difficulty in recognizing all complex sounds, whether verbal or nonverbal. [6]

corticospinal system See *pyramidal system*. [5]

cortisol A glucocorticoid stress hormone of the adrenal cortex. [11]

covert attention Attention in which the focus can be directed independently of sensory orientation (e.g., you're attending to one sensory stimulus while looking at another). Compare *overt attention*. [14]

cranial nerve One of the 12 pairs of nerves that arise directly from the brain rather than the spinal cord, supplying senory and motor connections to the head and neck. See Figure 2.7. Compare *spinal nerve*. [2]

crib death See *sudden infant death syndrome*. [10]

critical period See *sensitive period*. [15]

cross-tolerance A condition in which the development of tolerance for one drug causes an individual to develop tolerance for another drug. [4]

crystallization The final stage of birdsong formation, in which fully formed adult song is achieved. [ASF 15.3]

CSF See *cerebrospinal fluid*. [2]

CT See *computerized axial tomography*. [2]

CTE See *chronic traumatic encephalopathy*. [15]

curare A neurotoxin that causes paralysis by blocking acetylcholine receptors in muscle. [3]

Cushing's syndrome A condition in which levels of adrenal glucocorticoids are abnormally high. [ASF 12.2]

cytokine A protein that induces the proliferation of other cells, as in the immune system. Examples include interleukins and interferons. [ASF 11.4]

cytoplasm See *intracellular fluid*. [3]

D

DA See *dopamine*. [4]

dB See *decibel*. [6]

DBS See *deep brain stimulation*. [12]

deafness Hearing loss so profound that speech perception is lost. [6]

death gene A gene that is expressed only when a cell becomes committed to natural cell death (apoptosis). [13]

decibel (dB) A measure of sound intensity, perceived as loudness. See Box 6.1. [6]

declarative memory A memory that can be stated or described. See Figures 13.4, 13.12. Compare *nondeclarative memory*. [13]

decomposition of movement Difficulty of movement in which gestures are broken up into individual segments instead of being executed smoothly; it is a symptom of cerebellar lesions. [5]

decorticate rage Also called *sham rage*. Sudden intense rage characterized by actions (such as snarling and biting in dogs) that lack clear direction. [11]

deep brain stimulation (DBS) Mild electrical stimulation through an electrode that is surgically implanted deep in the brain. [12]

deep dyslexia Acquired dyslexia in which the person reads a word as another word that is semantically related. Compare *surface dyslexia*. [15]

default mode network A circuit of brain regions that is active during quiet introspective thought. [14]

degradation The chemical breakdown of a neurotransmitter into inactive metabolites. [3]

dehydration Excessive loss of water.

delayed non-matching-to-sample task A test in which the individual must respond to the unfamiliar stimulus in a pair of stimuli. See Figure 13.5. [13]

delta wave The slowest type of EEG wave, about 1/sec, characteristic of stage 3 sleep. See Figure 10.11. [10]

delta-9-tetrahydrocannabinol (THC) The major active ingredient in cannabis. [4]

delusion A false belief that is strongly held in spite of contrary evidence. [12]

dementia pugilistica See *chronic traumatic encephalopathy*. [15]

dementia Drastic failure of cognitive ability, including memory failure and disorientation. [13]

dendrite An extension of the cell body that receives information from other neurons. Functionally, the dendrites are the input zone of the neuron. See Figures 2.1, 2.3. [2]

dendritic spine An outgrowth along the dendrite of a neuron. See Figure 2.4. [2]

dendro-dendritic synapse A synapse at which a synaptic connection forms between the dendrites of two neurons. Compare *axo-axonic synapse*, *axo-dendritic synapse*, and *axo-somatic synapse*. [3]

dentate gyrus A strip of gray matter in the hippocampal formation. [13]

deoxyribonucleic acid (DNA) A nucleic acid that is present in the chromosomes of cells and codes hereditary information. Compare *ribonucleic acid*. [App]

dependent variable The factor that an experimenter measures to monitor a change in response to changes in an independent variable. [1]

depolarization A decrease in membrane potential (the interior of the neuron becomes less negative). See Figure 3.5. Compare *hyperpolarization*. [3]

depressant A drug that reduces the excitability of neurons. Compare *stimulant*. [4]

depression A psychiatric condition characterized by such symptoms as an unhappy mood; loss of interests, energy, and appetite; and difficulty concentrating. See also *bipolar disorder*. [12]

dermatome A strip of skin innervated by a particular spinal nerve. [5]

desynchronized EEG Also called *beta activity*. A pattern of EEG activity comprising a mix of many different high frequencies with low amplitude. Compare *alpha rhythm*. [10]

dexamethasone suppression test A test of pituitary-adrenal function in which the subject is given dexamethasone, a synthetic glucocorticoid hormone, which should cause a decline in the production of adrenal corticosteroids. [ASF 12.2]

DHT See *dihydrotestosterone*. [8]

diabetes mellitus A condition, characterized by excessive glucose in the blood and urine and by reduced glucose utilization by body cells, that is caused by the failure of insulin to induce glucose absorption. [9]

dichotic presentation The simultaneous delivery of different stimuli to both the right and the left ears at the same time. See Figure 15.2. [15]

diencephalon The posterior part of the fetal forebrain, which will become the thalamus and hypothalamus in the adult brain. See Figure 2.12. Compare *telencephalon*. [2]

differentiation See *cell differentiation*. [13, App]

diffusion The spontaneous spread of solute molecules from an area of high concentration to an area of low concentration through a solvent until a uniform solute concentration is achieved. See Figure 3.3. Compare *osmosis*. [3, 9]

diffusion tensor imaging (DTI) A modified form of MRI in which the diffusion of water in a confined space is exploited to produce images of axonal fiber tracts. [15]

digestion The process by which food is broken down to provide energy and nutrients. [ASF 9.3]

dihydrotestosterone (DHT) The 5-alpha-reduced metabolite of testosterone. DHT is a potent androgen that is principally responsible for the masculinization of the external genitalia in mammals. [8]

distal In anatomy, toward the periphery of an organism or toward the end of a limb. See Box 2.2. Compare *proximal*. [2]

diurnal Active during the light periods of the daily cycle. Compare *nocturnal*. [10]

divergence The phenomenon of neural connections in which one cell sends signals to many other cells. Compare *convergence*. [ASF 3.2]

divided-attention task A task in which the participant is asked to focus attention on two or more stimuli simultaneously. Compare *sustained-attention task*. [14]

dizygotic Referring to twins derived from separate eggs (fraternal twins). Compare *monozygotic*. [12]

DNA sequencing The process by which the order of nucleotides in a gene is identified. [App]

DNA See *deoxyribonucleic acid*. [App]

dopamine (DA) A monoamine transmitter found in the midbrain—especially the substantia nigra—and in the basal forebrain. See Figure 4.4; Table 4.1. [4]

dopamine hypothesis The idea that schizophrenia results from either excessive levels of synaptic dopamine or excessive postsynaptic sensitivity to dopamine. [12]

dopaminergic Referring to cells that use dopamine as their synaptic transmitter. [4]

dorsal In anatomy, toward the back of the body or the top of the brain. See Box 2.2. Compare *ventral*. [2]

dorsal column system A somatosensory system that delivers most touch stimuli via the dorsal columns of spinal white matter to the brain. See Figure 5.7. Compare *anterolateral system*. [5]

dorsomedial thalamus A limbic system structure that is connected to the hippocampus. [13]

dose-response curve (DRC) A formal graph of a drug's effects (on the y-axis) versus the dose given (on the x-axis). See Figure 4.6. [4]

down-regulation A compensatory decrease in receptor availability at the synapses of a neuron. Compare *up-regulation*. [4]

DRC See *dose-response curve*. [4]

drug tolerance Also called simply *tolerance*. A condition in which, with repeated exposure to a drug, an individual becomes less responsive to a constant dose. [4]

DTI See *diffusion tensor imaging*. [15]

DTI tractography Also called *fiber tracking*. Visualization of the orientation and terminations of white matter tracts in the living brain via diffusion tensor imaging. [15]

dualism The notion, promoted by René Descartes, that the mind has an immaterial aspect that is distinct from the material body and brain. [1]

duplex theory A theory that we localize sound by combining information about interaural intensity differences and interaural temporal differences between the two ears.

dura mater The outermost of the three meninges that surround the brain and spinal cord. See also *pia mater* and *arachnoid*. See Figure 2.8. [2]

dynorphin One of the three kinds of endogenous opioids. Compare *endorphin* and *enkephalin*. See Table 4.1. [4]

dyskinesia Difficulty or distortion in voluntary movement. See Box 12.1. [12]

dyslexia Also called *alexia*. A reading disorder attributed to brain impairment. [15]

dysphoria Unpleasant feelings; the opposite of euphoria. [4]

dystrophin A protein that is needed for normal muscle function. Dystrophin is defective in some forms of muscular dystrophy. [ASF 5.5]

E

ear canal Also called *auditory canal*. The tube leading from the pinna to the tympanic membrane. [6]

eardrum See *tympanic membrane*. [6]

easy problem of consciousness Understanding how particular patterns of neural activity create specific conscious experiences by reading brain activity directly from people's brains as they're having particular experiences. Compare *hard problem of consciousness*. [14]

EC See *enriched condition*. [13]

ecological niche The unique assortment of environmental opportunities and challenges to which each organism is adapted. [10]

Ecstasy See *MDMA*. [4]

ECT See *electroconvulsive shock therapy*. [12]

ectoderm The outer cellular layer of the developing embryo, giving rise to the skin and the nervous system. [13]

ectotherm An animal whose body temperature is regulated by, and whose heat comes mainly from, the environment. Examples include snakes and bees. Compare *endotherm*. [9]

ED$_{50}$ Effective dose 50%; the dose of a drug that is required to produce half of its maximal effect. See Figure 4.6. Compare *LD$_{50}$*.

edema A general term referring to swelling of any body tissue, including the brain. [2]

edge detector See *simple cortical cell*. [7]

EEG See *electroencephalography*. [3, 10]

efferent Carrying action potentials away from the brain, or away from one region of interest toward another region of interest. See Box 2.2. Compare *afferent*. [2]

efficacy Also called *intrinsic activity*. The extent to which a drug activates a response when it binds to a receptor. Receptor antagonist drugs have low efficacy; receptor agonists have high efficacy. See Figure 4.6. [4]

egg See *ovum*. [8]

ejaculation The forceful expulsion of semen from the penis. [8]

electrical synapse Also called *gap junction*. The region between neurons where the presynaptic and postsynaptic membranes are so close that the action potential can jump to the postsynaptic membrane without first being translated into a chemical message. [ASF 3.1]

electroconvulsive shock therapy (ECT) A last-resort treatment for unmanageable depression, in which a strong electrical current is passed through the brain, causing a seizure. [12]

electroencephalography (EEG) The recording of gross electrical activity of the brain via large electrodes placed on the scalp. The abbreviation EEG may refer either to the process of encephalography or to its product, the encephalogram. See Figures 3.15, 10.10. [3, 10]

electromyography (EMG) The electrical recording of muscle activity. See Figure 5.16. [5]

electrostatic pressure The propensity of charged molecules or ions to move toward areas with the opposite charge. [3]

embryo The earliest stage in a developing animal. Humans are considered to be embryos until 8–10 weeks after conception. Compare *fetus*. [13]

embryonic stem cell A cell, derived from an embryo, that has the capacity to form any type of tissue. [15]

EMG See *electromyography*. [5]

emotion A subjective mental state that is usually accompanied by distinctive behaviors as well as involuntary physiological changes. [11]

encéphale isolé See *isolated brain*. [10]

encoding The first process in the memory system, in which the information entering sensory channels is passed into short-term memory. See Figure 13.13. Compare *consolidation* and *retrieval*. [13]

endocannabinoid An endogenous ligand of cannabinoid receptors, thus an analog of cannabis that is produced by the brain. [4, 9]

endocrine Referring to glands that release chemicals to the interior of the body. These glands secrete the principal hormones used by the body. See Figure 8.3. [8]

endocrine gland A gland that secretes hormones into the bloodstream to act on distant targets. See Figure 8.1. [8]

endogenous Produced inside the body. Compare *exogenous*. [4]

endogenous ligand Any substance, produced within the body, that selectively binds to the type of receptor that is under study. Compare *exogenous ligand*. [4]

endogenous opioid Any of a class of opium-like peptide transmitters that have been referred to as the body's own narcotics. The three kinds are enkephalins, endorphins, and dynorphins. See Table 4.1. [4]

endorphin One of three kinds of endogenous opioids. Compare *dynorphin* and *enkephalin*. See Table 4.1. [4, 5]

endotherm An animal whose body temperature is regulated chiefly by internal metabolic processes. Examples include mammals and birds. Compare *ectotherm*. [9]

enkephalin One of the three kinds of endogenous opioids. Compare *dynorphin* and *endorphin*. See Table 4.1. [4]

enriched condition (EC) Also called *complex environment*. An environment for laboratory rodents in which animals are group-housed with a wide variety of stimulus objects. See Figure 13.15. Compare *impoverished condition* and *standard condition*. [13]

enterotype Each individual's personal composition of the gut microbiota. [9]

entrainment The process of synchronizing a biological rhythm to an environmental stimulus. See Figure 10.2. [10]

enzyme A complicated protein whose action increases the probability of a specific chemical reaction. [App]

ependymal layer See *ventricular zone*. [13]

epigenetic regulation Changes in gene expression that are due to environmental effects rather than to changes in the nucleotide sequence of the gene. [11]

epigenetic transmission The passage from one individual to another of changes in the expression of targeted genes, without modifications to the genes themselves. [9]

epigenetics The study of factors that affect gene expression without making any changes in the nucleotide sequence of the genes themselves. [1, 13]

epilepsy A brain disorder marked by major, sudden changes in the electrophysiological state of the brain that are referred to as seizures. See Figure 3.16. [3]

epinephrine Also called *adrenaline*. A compound that acts both as a hormone (secreted by the adrenal medulla under the control of the sympathetic nervous system) and as a synaptic transmitter. See Tables 4.1, 8.1. [11]

episodic memory Also called *autobiographical memory*. Memory of a particular incident or a particular time and place. Compare *semantic memory*. [13]

EPSP See *excitatory postsynaptic potential*. [3]

equilibrium potential The point at which the movement of ions across the cell membrane is balanced, as the electrostatic pressure pulling ions in one direction is offset by the diffusion force pushing them in the opposite direction. [3]

ERP See *event-related potential*. [3, 14]

estradiol Formally called *17-beta-estradiol*. The primary type of estrogen secreted by the ovary. [8]

estrogen Any of a class of steroid hormones, including estradiol, produced by female gonads. See Figure 8.13. [8]

estrus The period during which female animals are sexually receptive. [8]

eukaryote Any organism whose cells have the genetic material contained within a nuclear envelope. [App]

event-related potential (ERP) Also called *evoked potential*. Averaged EEG recordings measuring brain responses to repeated presentations of a stimulus. Components of the ERP tend to be reliable because the background noise of the cortex has been averaged out. See Figures 3.15, 14.6. [3, 14]

evoked potential See *event-related potential*. [3, 14]

evolution by natural selection The Darwinian theory that evolution proceeds by differential success in reproduction.

evolutionary psychology A field of study devoted to asking how natural selection has shaped behavior in humans and other animals. [1]

excitatory postsynaptic potential (EPSP) A depolarizing potential in a neuron that is normally caused by synaptic excitation. EPSPs increase the probability that the postsynaptic neuron will fire an action potential. See Figure 3.9. Compare *inhibitory postsynaptic potential*. [3]

excitotoxicity The property by which neurons die when overstimulated, as with large amounts of glutamate. [ASF 15.5]

executive function A neural and cognitive system that helps develop plans of action and organizes the activities of other high-level processing systems. [14]

exocytosis A cellular process that results in the release of a substance into the extracellular space. [4]

exogenous Arising from outside the body. Compare *endogenous*. [4]

exogenous ligand Any substance, originating from outside the body, that selectively binds to the type of receptor that is under study. Compare *endogenous ligand*. [4]

expression See *gene expression*. [1, 13, App]

external ear The part of the ear that we readily see (the pinna) and the canal that leads to the eardrum. See Figure 6.1. [6]

extracellular compartment The fluid space of the body that exists outside the cells. See Figure 9.6. Compare *intracellular compartment*. [9]

extracellular fluid The fluid in the spaces between cells (interstitial fluid) Compare *intracellular fluid*. [3]

extraocular muscle One of the muscles attached to the eyeball that control its position and movements. [7]

extrapyramidal system A motor system that includes the basal ganglia and some closely related brainstem structures. Axons of this system pass into the spinal cord outside the pyramids of the medulla. Compare *pyramidal system*. [5]

extrastriate cortex Visual cortex outside of the primary visual (striate) cortex. [7]

F

face blindness See *prosopagnosia*. [15]

facial feedback hypothesis The idea that sensory feedback from our facial expressions can affect our mood. [11]

fat See *lipid*. [9]

fat tissue See *adipose tissue*. [9]

fatal familial insomnia An inherited disorder in which humans sleep normally at the beginning of their life but in midlife stop sleeping and, 7–24 months later, die. [10]

fear conditioning A form of classical conditioning in which a previously neutral stimulus is repeatedly paired with an unpleasant stimulus, like foot shock, until the previously neutral stimulus alone elicits the responses seen in fear. [11, 12]

feature search A search for an item in which the target pops out right away, no matter how many distracters are present, because it possesses a unique attribute. Compare *conjunction search*. [14]

fecal transplantation A medical procedure in which gut microbiota, via fecal matter, are transplanted from a donor to a host. [9]

FEF See *frontal eye field*. [14]

fetal alcohol spectrum disorder A family of developmental disorders that vary in severity, resulting from fetal exposure to alcohol consumed by the mother. Severe cases, associated with high levels of alcohol abuse by the mother, include characteristic intellectual disability and facial abnormalities. [4]

fetus A developing individual after the embryo stage. Humans are considered to be fetuses from 10 weeks after fertilization until birth. Compare *embryo*. [13]

fiber tracking See *DTI tractography*. [15]

final common pathway The motor neurons of the brain and spinal cord, so called because they receive and integrate all motor signals from the brain to direct movement. [5]

first-generation antipsychotic Also called *typical antipsychotic* or *neuroleptic*. An antischizophrenic drug that shows antagonist activity at dopamine D_2 receptors. [4, 12]

flavor The sense of taste combined with the sense of smell. Compare *taste*. [6]

fluent aphasia Also called *Wernicke's aphasia*. A language impairment characterized by fluent, meaningless speech and little language comprehension. It is related to damage in Wernicke's area. See Figure 15.8. Compare *nonfluent aphasia*. [15]

fMRI See *functional MRI*. [2]

follicle The structure of the ovary that contains an immature ovum (egg). [8, ASF 8.4]

follicle-stimulating hormone (FSH) A gonadotropin, named for its actions on ovarian follicles. See Figure 8.13. [8, ASF 8.4]

forebrain The frontal division of the neural tube, which in the mature vertebrate contains the cerebral hemispheres, the thalamus, and the hypothalamus. See Figures 2.12, 13.23. Compare *hindbrain* and *midbrain*. [2, 13]

fornix A fiber tract that extends from the hippocampus to the mammillary body. See Figures 2.14, 2.15. [2]

Fourier analysis The mathematical decomposition of a complex pattern into a sum of sine waves. [6, ASF 7.2]

fourth ventricle The passageway within the pons that receives cerebrospinal fluid from the third ventricle and releases it to surround the brain and spinal cord. See Figure 2.16. Compare *lateral ventricle* and *third ventricle*. [2]

fovea The central portion of the retina, which is packed with the highest density of photoreceptors and is the center of our gaze. See Figure 7.1. [7]

fraternal birth order effect A phenomenon in human populations, such that the more older biological brothers a boy has, the more likely he is to grow up to be gay. [8]

free nerve ending An axon that terminates in the skin and has no specialized cell associated with it. Free nerve endings detect pain and/or changes in temperature. See Figure 5.3. [5]

free will The feeling that our conscious self is the author of our actions and decisions. [14]

free-running Referring to a rhythm of behavior shown by an animal deprived of external cues about time of day. See Figure 10.2. [10]

frequency The number of cycles per second in a sound wave, measured in hertz. See Box 6.1. [6]

frontal eye field (FEF) An area in the frontal lobe of the brain that contains neurons important for establishing gaze in accordance with cognitive goals (top-down processes) rather than with any characteristics of stimuli (bottom-up processes). [14]

frontal lobe The most anterior portion of the cerebral cortex. See Figure 2.10. Compare *occipital lobe*, *parietal lobe*, and *temporal lobe*. [2]

frontal plane See *coronal plane*. [2]

FSH See *follicle-stimulating hormone*. [8, ASF 8.4]

functional MRI (fMRI) Magnetic resonance imaging that detects changes in blood flow and therefore identifies regions of the brain that are particularly active during a given task. See Figure 2.18. Compare *positron emission tomography*. [2]

functional tolerance The form of drug tolerance that arises when repeated exposure to the drug causes receptors to be up-regulated or down-regulated. Compare *metabolic tolerance*. [4]

fundamental The predominant frequency of an auditory tone. Compare *harmonic*. See Box 6.1. [6]

fusiform gyrus A region on the inferior surface of the cortex, at the junction of the temporal and occipital lobes, that has been associated with recognition of faces. See Figure 15.5. [15]

G

GABA See *gamma-aminobutyric acid*. [4]

gamete A sex cell (sperm or ovum) that contains only unpaired chromosomes and therefore has only half of the usual number of chromosomes. [8]

gamma-aminobutyric acid (GABA) A widely distributed amino acid transmitter, the main inhibitory transmitter in the mammalian nervous system. See Table 4.1. [4]

ganglion (pl. ganglia) A collection of nerve cell bodies outside the central nervous system. Compare *nucleus* (definition 1). [2]

ganglion cell Any of a class of cells in the retina whose axons form the optic nerve. See Figure 7.15. Compare *amacrine cell*, *bipolar cell*, and *horizontal cell*. [7]

gap junction See *electrical synapse*. [ASF 3.1]

gas neurotransmitter A neurotransmitter that is a soluble gas. Examples include nitric oxide and carbon monoxide. Usually gas neurotransmitters act, in a retrograde fashion, on presynaptic neurons. See Table 4.1. Compare *amine neurotransmitter*, *amino acid neurotransmitter*, and *peptide neurotransmitter*. [4]

gel electrophoresis A method of separating molecules of differing size or electrical charge by forcing them to flow through a gel. See Appendix Figure A.3. [App]

gene A length of DNA that encodes the information for constructing a particular protein. [App]

gene amplification See *polymerase chain reaction*. [App]

gene expression The turning on or off of specific genes; the process by which a cell makes an mRNA transcript of a particular gene. [1, App]

general anesthetic A drug that renders an individual unconscious. [10]

generator potential A local change in the resting potential of a receptor cell in response to stimuli, which may initiate an action potential. [5]

genital tubercle In the early fetus, a "bump" between the legs that can develop into either a clitoris or a penis. [8]

genome See *genotype*. [App]

genotype Also called *genome*. All the genetic information that one specific individual has inherited. Compare *phenotype*. [13, App]

GH See *growth hormone*. [8, ASF 8.4]

ghrelin A peptide gut hormone believed to act on the hypothalamic appetite system to increase hunger. See Figure 9.15. Compare PYY_{3-36}. [9]

glial cells Also called *glia*. Nonneuronal brain cells that provide structural, nutritional, and other types of support to the brain. See Figure 2.5. [2]

global aphasia The total loss of ability to understand language, or to speak, read, or write. See Figure 15.8. [15]

globus pallidus One of the basal ganglia. See Figure 2.14. [2]

glomerulus (pl. glomeruli) A complex arbor of dendrites from a group of olfactory cells. [6]

glucagon A pancreatic hormone that converts glycogen to glucose and thus increases blood glucose. Compare *insulin*. [9]

glucocorticoid Any of a class of steroid hormones, released by the adrenal cortex, that affect carbohydrate metabolism and inflammation. [8]

glucodetector A specialized type of liver cell that detects and informs the nervous system about levels of circulating glucose. [9]

glucose An important sugar molecule used by the body and brain for energy. [9]

glutamate An amino acid transmitter, the most common excitatory transmitter. See Table 4.1. [4, 13]

glutamate hypothesis The idea that schizophrenia may be caused, in part, by understimulation of glutamate receptors. [12]

glutamatergic Referring to cells that use glutamate as their synaptic transmitter.

glycine An amino acid transmitter, often inhibitory. See Table 4.1. [4]

glycogen A complex carbohydrate made by the combining of glucose molecules for a short-term store of energy. [9]

glymphatic system A lymphatic system in the brain that participates in removal of wastes and the movement of nutrients and signaling compounds. [2]

GnRH See *gonadotropin-releasing hormone*. [8]

Golgi stain A tissue stain that completely fills a small proportion of neurons with a dark, silver-based precipitate. See Box 2.1. [2]

Golgi tendon organ A type of receptor found within tendons that sends impulses to the central nervous system

when a muscle contracts. See Figure 5.21. Compare *muscle spindle*. [5]

gonad Any of the sexual organs (ovaries in females, testes in males) that produce gametes for reproduction. See Figure 8.1. [8]

gonadotropin An anterior pituitary tropic hormone that selectively stimulates the cells of the gonads to produce sex steroids and gametes. See *luteinizing hormone* and *follicle-stimulating hormone*. [8, ASF 8.4]

gonadotropin-releasing hormone (GnRH) A hypothalamic hormone that controls the release of luteinizing hormone and follicle-stimulating hormone from the pituitary. See Figure 8.13. [8]

grammar All of the rules for usage of a particular language. [15]

grand mal seizure See *tonic-clonic seizure*. [3]

gray matter Areas of the brain that are dominated by cell bodies and are devoid of myelin. Gray matter mostly receives and processes information. See Figure 2.11. Compare *white matter*. [2]

gross neuroanatomy Anatomical features of the nervous system that are apparent to the naked eye. [2]

growth hormone (GH) Also called *somatotropin* or *somatotropic hormone*. A tropic hormone, secreted by the anterior pituitary, that promotes the growth of cells and tissues. [8, ASF 8.4]

guevedoces Literally "eggs at 12" (in Spanish). A nickname for individuals who are raised as girls but at puberty change appearance and begin behaving as boys. [8]

gustatory system The sensory system that detects taste. See Figure 6.18. [6]

gut microbiota The microorgansims that normally inhabit the digestive system. [9]

gyrus (pl. gyri) A ridged or raised portion of a convoluted brain surface. Compare *sulcus*. [2]

H

habituation A form of nonassociative learning in which an organism becomes less responsive following repeated presentations of a stimulus. See Figure 13.18. [13]

hair cell One of the receptor cells for hearing in the cochlea, named for the stereocilia that protrude from the top of the cell and transduce vibrational energy in the cochlea into neural activity. See Figure 6.1. [6]

hallucinogen A drug that alters sensory perception and produces peculiar experiences. Compare *dissociative*. [4]

hard problem of consciousness Understanding the brain processes that

produce people's subjective experiences of their conscious perceptions—that is, their qualia. Compare *easy problem of consciousness*. [14]

harmonic A multiple of a particular frequency called the *fundamental*. See Box 6.1. [6]

health psychology Also called *behavioral medicine*. A field of study that focuses on psychological influences on health-related processes. [11]

hearing loss Decreased sensitivity to sound, in varying degrees. [6]

Hebbian synapse A synapse that is strengthened when it successfully drives the postsynaptic cell. [13, ASF 13.4]

hemiparesis Weakness of one side of the body. Compare *hemiplegia*. [15]

hemiplegia Paralysis of one side of the body. Compare *hemiparesis*. [15]

hemispatial neglect Failure to pay any attention to objects presented to one side of the body. [14]

hermaphrodite An individual possessing the reproductive organs of both sexes, either simultaneously or at different points in time. [ASF 8.6]

heroin Diacetylmorphine, an artificially modified, very potent form of morphine. [4]

hertz (Hz) Cycles per second, as of an auditory stimulus. Hertz is a measure of frequency. See Box 6.1. [6]

hindbrain The rear division of the brain, which in the mature vertebrate contains the cerebellum, pons, and medulla. See Figures 2.12, 13.23. Compare *forebrain* and *midbrain*. [2, 13]

hippocampus (pl. hippocampi) A medial temporal lobe structure that is important for spatial cognition, learning, and memory. See Figures 2.14, 13.1, 13.20. [2, 13]

histology The study of tissue structure.

homeostasis The maintenance of a relatively constant internal physiological environment. [9]

horizontal cell A specialized retinal cell that contacts both photoreceptors and bipolar cells. Compare *amacrine cell* and *ganglion cell*. [7]

horizontal plane The plane that divides the body or brain into upper and lower parts. See Box 2.2. Compare *coronal plane* and *sagittal plane*. [2]

hormone A chemical, usually secreted by an endocrine gland, that is conveyed by the bloodstream and regulates target organs or tissues. See Table 8.1. [8]

horseradish peroxidase (HRP) An enzymatic label, originating in horseradish and other plants, that is used to determine the cells of origin of a particular set of axons. See Box 2.1. [2]

HRP See *horseradish peroxidase*. [2]

hue One of three basic dimensions of light perception, varying through the spectrum from blue to red. Compare *brightness* and *saturation*. [7]

hunger The internal state of an animal seeking food. Compare *satiety*. [9]

huntingtin A protein produced by a gene (called *HTT*) that, when containing too many trinucleotide repeats, results in Huntington's disease in a carrier. [ASF 5.5]

Huntington's disease A genetic disorder, with onset in middle age, in which the destruction of basal ganglia results in a syndrome of abrupt, involuntary writhing movements and changes in mental functioning. Compare *Parkinson's disease*. [5]

hybridization The process by which one string of nucleotides becomes linked to a complementary series of nucleotides. [App]

hydrocephalus A ballooning of the ventricles, at the expense of the surrounding brain, which may occur when the circulation of CSF is blocked. [2]

hyperpolarization An increase in membrane potential (the interior of the neuron becomes even more negative). See Figure 3.5. Compare *depolarization*. [3]

hypertonic Referring to a solution with a higher concentration of salt than that found in interstitial fluid and blood plasma (more than about 0.9% salt). Compare *hypotonic* and *isotonic*. [9]

hypocretin See *orexin*. [9, 10]

hypofrontality hypothesis The idea that schizophrenia may reflect underactivation of the frontal lobes. [12]

hypothalamic-pituitary portal system An elaborate bed of blood vessels leading from the hypothalamus to the anterior pituitary. [8]

hypothalamus Part of the diencephalon, lying ventral to the thalamus. See Figures 2.12, 2.14, 2.15. [2]

hypotonic Referring to a solution with a lower concentration of salt than that found in interstitial fluid and blood plasma (less than about 0.9% salt). Compare *hypertonic* and *isotonic*. [9]

hypovolemic thirst A desire to ingest fluids that is stimulated by a reduction in volume of the extracellular fluid. Compare *osmotic thirst*. [9]

Hz See *hertz*. [6]

I

IC See *impoverished condition*. [13]

ICC See *immunocytochemistry*. [2, 8, App]

iconic memory See *sensory buffer*. [13]

IEG See *immediate early gene*. [2]

IHC See *inner hair cell*. [6]

immediate early gene (IEG) A gene that shows rapid but temporary increases in expression in cells that have become activated. See Box 2.1. [2]

immunocytochemistry (ICC) A method for detecting a particular protein in tissues in which an antibody recognizes and binds to the protein and then chemical methods are used to leave a visible reaction product around each antibody. See Boxes 2.1, 8.1. [2, 8, App]

immunoglobulin See *antibody*. [ASF 11.4, App]

impoverished condition (IC) Also called *isolated condition*. An environment for laboratory rodents in which each animal is housed singly in a small cage without complex stimuli. See Figure 13.15. Compare *enriched condition* and *standard condition*. [13]

in situ hybridization A method for detecting particular RNA transcripts in tissue sections by providing a nucleotide probe that is complementary to, and will therefore hybridize with, the transcript of interest. See Boxes 2.1, 8.1; Appendix Figure A.4. [2, 8, App]

in vitro Literally "in glass" (in Latin). Usually, in a laboratory dish; outside the body.

inattentional blindness The failure to perceive nonattended stimuli that seem so obvious as to be impossible to miss. [14]

incus Latin for "anvil." A middle-ear bone situated between the malleus (attached to the tympanic membrane) and the stapes (attached to the cochlea). It is one of the three ossicles that conduct sound across the middle ear. See Figure 6.1. [6]

independent variable The factor that is manipulated by an experimenter. Compare *dependent variable*. [1]

indifferent gonads The undifferentiated gonads of the early mammalian fetus, which will eventually develop into either testes or ovaries. See Figure 8.24. See also *gonad*. [8]

indoleamines A class of monoamines that serve as neurotransmitters, including serotonin and melatonin. See Table 4.1. [4]

inferior colliculi (sing. colliculus) Paired gray matter structures of the dorsal midbrain that process auditory information. See Figure 2.15. Compare *superior colliculi*. [2, 6]

inferior In anatomy, below. See Box 2.2. Compare *superior*. [2]

infradian Referring to a rhythmic biological event with a period longer than a day. Compare *ultradian*. [10]

infrasound Very low frequency sound; in general, below the threshold for human hearing, at about 20 Hz. Compare *ultrasound*. [6]

infundibulum See *pituitary stalk*. [8]

inhibition of return The phenomenon, observed in peripheral spatial cuing tasks when the interval between cue and target stimulus is 200 milliseconds or more, in which the detection of stimuli at the former location of the cue is increasingly impaired. [14]

inhibitory postsynaptic potential (IPSP) A hyperpolarizing potential in a neuron. IPSPs decrease the probability that the postsynaptic neuron will fire an action potential. See Figure 3.9. Compare *excitatory postsynaptic potential*. [3]

inner ear The cochlea and vestibular apparatus. See Figure 6.1. [6]

inner hair cell (IHC) One of the two types of receptor cells for hearing in the cochlea. Compared with outer hair cells, IHCs are positioned closer to the central axis of the coiled cochlea. See Figure 6.1. [6]

innervate To provide neural input to. [2]

input zone The part of a neuron that receives information from other neurons or from specialized sensory structures. This zone usually corresponds to the cell's dendrites. See Figures 2.1, 2.3. Compare *conduction zone, integration zone*, and *output zone*. [2]

instrumental conditioning Also called *operant conditioning*. A form of associative learning in which the likelihood that an act (instrumental response) will be performed depends on the consequences (reinforcing stimuli) that follow it. Compare *classical conditioning*. [13]

insula A region of cortex lying below the surface, within the lateral sulcus, of the frontal, temporal, and parietal lobes. [4]

insulin A pancreatic hormone that lowers blood glucose, promotes energy storage, and facilitates glucose utilization by cells. Compare *glucagon*. [9]

integration zone The part of a neuron that initiates neural electrical activity. This zone usually corresponds to the neuron's cell body. See Figures 2.1, 2.3. Compare *conduction zone, input zone*, and *output zone*. [2]

intensity See *amplitude*. [6]

interaural intensity difference (IID) A perceived difference in loudness between the two ears, which the nervous system can use to localize a sound source. [6]

interaural temporal difference (ITD) A difference between the two ears in the time of arrival of a sound, which the nervous system can use to localize a sound source. [6]

intermale aggression Aggression between males of the same species. [11]

interneuron A nerve cell that is neither a sensory neuron nor a motor neuron; interneurons receive input from and send output to other neurons. Compare *motor neuron* and *sensory neuron*. [2]

intersex Referring to an individual with atypical genital development and sexual differentiation, whose genitalia are generally intermediate in form between typical male and typical female genitalia. [8]

intracellular compartment The fluid space of the body that is contained within cells. See Figure 9.6. Compare *extracellular compartment*. [9]

intracellular fluid Also called *cytoplasm*. The watery solution found within cells. Compare *extracellullar fluid*. [3]

intrafusal fiber Any of the small muscle fibers that lie within each muscle spindle. See Figure 5.21. [5]

intraparietal sulcus (IPS) A region in the human parietal lobe, homologous to the monkey lateral intraparietal area, that is especially involved in voluntary, top-down control of attention. [14]

intrinsic activity See *efficacy*. [4]

intromission Insertion of the penis into the vagina during copulation. [8]

inverse agonist A substance that binds to a receptor and causes it to do the opposite of what the naturally occurring transmitter does.

ion An atom or molecule that has acquired an electrical charge by gaining or losing one or more electrons. [3]

ion channel A pore in the cell membrane that permits the passage of certain ions through the membrane when the channels are open. See Figure 3.2. [3]

ionotropic receptor Also called *ligand-gated ion channel*. A receptor protein containing an ion channel that opens when the receptor is bound by an agonist. See Figure 4.2. Compare *metabotropic receptor*. [4]

IPS See *intraparietal sulcus*. [14]

ipsilateral In anatomy, pertaining to a location on the same side of the body. See Box 2.2. Compare *contralateral*. [2]

IPSP See *inhibitory postsynaptic potential*. [3]

iris (pl. irides) The circular structure of the eye that provides an opening to form the pupil. See Figure 7.1. [7]

isocortex See *neocortex*.

isolated condition See *impoverished condition*. [13]

isotonic Referring to a solution with a concentration of salt that is the same as that found in interstitial fluid and blood plasma (about 0.9% salt). Compare *hypertonic* and *hypotonic*. [9]

K

K complex A sharp, negative EEG potential that is seen in stage 2 sleep. [10]

kcal See *kilocalorie*. [ASF 9.1]

ketamine A dissociative anesthetic drug, similar to PCP, that acts as an NMDA receptor antagonist. [12]

ketone An organic molecule, derived from the breakdown of fat, that can be used by cells as an energy source. [9]

khat Also spelled *qat*. An African shrub that, when chewed, acts as a stimulant. [4]

kilocalorie (kcal) A measure of energy commonly applied to food; formally defined as the quantity of heat required to raise the temperature of 1 kilogram of water by 1°C. [ASF 9.1]

Klüver-Bucy syndrome A condition, brought about by bilateral amygdala damage, that is characterized by dramatic emotional changes including reduction in fear and anxiety. [11]

knee jerk reflex A variant of the stretch reflex in which stretching of the tendon beneath the knee leads to an upward kick of the leg. See Figure 3.14. [3]

knockout organism An individual in which a particular gene has been disabled by an experimenter. See Box 8.1. [8]

Korsakoff's syndrome A memory disorder, caused by thiamine deficiency, that is generally associated with chronic alcoholism. [13]

L

labeled lines The concept that each nerve input to the brain reports only a particular type of information. [5]

lamellated corpuscle See *Pacinian corpuscle*. [5]

language Communication in which arbitrary sounds or symbols are arranged according to a grammar in order to convey an almost limitless variety of concepts. [15]

lateral In anatomy, toward one side. See Box 2.2. Compare *medial*. [2]

lateral geniculate nucleus (LGN) The part of the thalamus that receives information from the optic tract and

sends it to visual areas in the occipital cortex. [7]

lateral hypothalamus (LH) A hypothalamic region involved in the control of appetite and other functions. See Figure 9.12. [9]

lateral inhibition The phenomenon by which interconnected neurons inhibit their neighbors, producing contrast at the edges of regions. See Figure 7.15. [7]

lateral intraparietal area (LIP) A region in the monkey parietal lobe, homologous to the human intraparietal sulcus, that is especially involved in voluntary, top-down control of attention. [14]

lateral sulcus See *Sylvian fissure*. [2]

lateral tegmental area A brainstem region that provides some of the norepinephrine-containing projections of the brain. [4]

lateral ventricle A complex C-shaped lateral portion of the ventricular system within each hemisphere of the brain. See Figure 2.16. Compare *fourth ventricle* and *third ventricle*. [2]

lateralization The tendency for the right and left halves of a system to differ from one another. [15]

LD$_{50}$ Lethal dose 50%; the dose of a drug at which half the treated animals will die. See Figure 4.6. Compare *ED$_{50}$*. [4]

L-dopa The immediate precursor of the transmitter dopamine. It is known to markedly reduce symptoms in patients with Parkinson's, decreasing tremors and increasing the speed of movements. [ASF 5.5]

learned helplessness A learning paradigm in which individuals are subjected to inescapable, unpleasant conditions. [12]

learning The process of acquiring new and relatively enduring information, behavior patterns, or abilities, characterized by modifications of behavior as a result of practice, study, or experience. [13]

lens A structure in the eye that helps focus an image on the retina. See Figure 7.1. [7]

leptin A peptide hormone released by fat cells. [9]

level of analysis The scope of an experimental approach. A scientist may try to understand behavior by monitoring molecules, nerve cells, brain regions, or social environments or using some combination of these levels of analysis. [1]

LGN See *lateral geniculate nucleus*. [7]

LH 1. See *lateral hypothalamus*. [9] 2. See *luteinizing hormone*. [8, ASF 8.4]

lie detector See *polygraph*. [11]

ligand A substance that binds to receptor molecules, such as a neurotransmitter or drug that binds postsynaptic receptors. [3, 4]

ligand-gated ion channel See *ionotropic receptor*. [4]

limbic system A loosely defined, widespread group of brain nuclei that innervate each other and form a network. These nuclei are implicated in emotions. See Figure 2.14. [2, 11]

LIP See *lateral intraparietal area*. [14]

lipid A large molecule (frequently a fat) that consists of fatty acids and glycerol. Lipids are insoluble in water. [9]

liposuction The surgical removal of fat tissue. [9]

lithium An element that, administered to people with bipolar disorder, often relieves the symptoms of bipolar disorder. [12]

lobotomy The surgical separation of a portion of the frontal lobes from the rest of the brain, once used as a treatment for schizophrenia and many other ailments. [12]

local anesthetic A drug, such as procaine or lidocaine, that blocks sodium channels to stop neural transmission in pain fibers.

local potential An electrical potential that is initiated by stimulation at a specific site, which is a graded response that spreads passively across the cell membrane, decreasing in strength with time and distance. [3]

localization of function The concept that different brain regions specialize in specific behaviors. [1]

locus coeruleus A small nucleus in the brainstem whose neurons produce norepinephrine and modulate large areas of the forebrain. Compare *substantia nigra*. [4, 10]

long-term memory (LTM) An enduring form of memory that lasts days, weeks, months, or years. LTM has a very large capacity. Compare *sensory buffer* and *short-term memory*. See Figure 13.13. [13]

long-term potentiation (LTP) A stable and enduring increase in the effectiveness of synapses following repeated strong stimulation. See Figures 13.20, 13.21. [13]

lordosis A female receptive posture in four-legged animals in which the hindquarters are raised and the tail is turned to one side, facilitating intromission by the male. See Figures 8.17, 8.20. [8]

Lou Gehrig's disease See *amyotrophic lateral sclerosis*. [ASF 5.5]

LSD Also called *acid*. Lysergic acid diethylamide, a hallucinogenic drug. [4]

LTM See *long-term memory*. [13]

LTP See long-term potentiation. [13]

lumbar Referring to the five spinal segments in the upper part of the lower back. See Figures 2.8, 2.9. Compare *cervical, thoracic, sacral,* and *coccygeal*. [2]

luteinizing hormone (LH) A gonadotropin, named for its stimulatory effects on the ovarian corpora lutea. See Figure 8.13. [8, ASF 8.4]

lysergic acid diethylamide See *LSD*. [4]

M

M1 See *primary motor cortex*. [5]

magnetic resonance imaging (MRI) A noninvasive brain-imaging technology that uses magnetism and radio-frequency energy to create images of the gross structure of the living brain. See Figure 2.18. Compare *computerized axial tomography*. [2]

magnetoencephalography (MEG) A noninvasive brain-imaging technology that creates maps of brain activity during cognitive tasks by measuring tiny magnetic fields produced by active neurons. Compare *transcranial magnetic stimulation*. [2]

malleus Latin for "hammer." A middle-ear bone that is connected to the tympanic membrane. It is one of the three ossicles that conduct sound across the middle ear. See Figure 6.1. Compare *incus* and *stapes*. [6]

mammillary body One of a pair of limbic system structures that are connected to the hippocampus. See Figure 2.14. [13]

MAO See *monoamine oxidase*. [4, ASF 4.1, 12]

maternal aggression Aggression of a mother defending her nest or offspring. [11]

maternal behavior Behavior of adult females that has the goal of enhancing the well-being of their own offspring, often at some cost to the parents. [8]

MDMA Also called *Ecstasy* or *Molly*. 3,4-Methylenedioxymethamphetamine, a drug of abuse. [4]

medial In anatomy, toward the middle. See Box 2.2. Compare *lateral*. [2]

medial amygdala A portion of the amygdala that receives olfactory and pheromonal information. [8, 11]

medial forebrain bundle A collection of axons traveling in the midline region of the forebrain. [11]

medial geniculate nucleus Either of two nuclei—left and right—in the thalamus that receive input from the inferior colliculi and send output to the auditory cortex. See Figure 6.6. [6]

medial preoptic area (mPOA) A region of the anterior hypothalamus implicated in the control of many behaviors, includ-

ing sexual behavior, gonadotropin secretion, and thermoregulation. [8]

median eminence A midline feature on the base of the brain that marks the point at which the pituitary stalk exits the hypothalamus to connect to the pituitary. The median eminence contains one end of the hypothalamic-pituitary portal system. See Figure 8.12. [8]

medulla The posterior part of the hindbrain, continuous with the spinal cord. See Figures 2.12, 2.15. [2]

MEG See *magnetoencephalography*. [2]

Meissner's corpuscle Also called *tactile corpuscle*. A skin receptor cell type that detects light touch, responding especially to changes in stimuli. See Figure 5.3. Compare *Merkel's disc, Pacinian corpuscle,* and *Ruffini corpuscle*. [5]

melanopsin A photopigment found in those retinal ganglion cells that project to the suprachiasmatic nucleus. See Figure 10.5. [10]

melatonin An amine hormone that is secreted by the pineal gland at night, thereby signaling day length to the brain. See Table 4.1. [10, ASF 8.1]

memory 1. The ability to learn and neurally encode information, consolidate the information for longer-term storage, and retrieve or reactivate the consolidated information at a later time. 2. The specific information that is stored in the brain. [13]

memory trace Also called an *engram*. A persistent change in the brain that reflects the storage of memory. [13]

meninges The three protective membranes—dura mater, pia mater, and arachnoid—that surround the brain and spinal cord. See Figure 2.8. [2]

meningioma A noninvasive tumor of the meninges. [2]

meningitis An acute inflammation of the meninges, usually caused by a viral or bacterial infection. [2]

Merkel's disc A skin receptor cell type that detects light touch, responding especially to edges and isolated points on a surface. See Figure 5.3. Compare *Meissner's corpuscle, Pacinian corpuscle,* and *Ruffini corpuscle*. [5]

message See *messenger RNA*. [App]

messenger RNA (mRNA) Also called *transcript* or *message*. A strand of RNA that carries the code of a section of a DNA strand to the cytoplasm. [App]

meta-analysis A type of quantitative review of a field of research, in which the results of multiple previous studies are combined in order to identify overall patterns that are consistent across studies. [12]

metabolic tolerance The form of drug tolerance that arises when repeated exposure to the drug causes the metabolic machinery of the body to become more efficient at clearing the drug. Compare *functional tolerance*. [4]

metabolism The breakdown of complex molecules into smaller molecules. [ASF 9.1]

metabotropic receptor A receptor protein that does not contain ion channels but may, when activated, use a second-messenger system to open nearby ion channels or to produce other cellular effects. See Figure 4.2. Compare *ionotropic receptor*. [4]

methylation A chemical modification of DNA that does not affect the nucleotide sequence of a gene but makes that gene less likely to be expressed. [13]

microbiome The collective term for the population of microorganisms that inhabit the body. [9]

microelectrode An especially small electrode used to record electrical potentials in living cells. [3]

microglial cells Also called *microglia*. Extremely small motile glial cells that remove cellular debris from injured or dead cells. [2]

midbrain The middle division of the brain. See Figures 2.12, 13.23. Compare *forebrain* and *hindbrain*. [2, 13]

middle canal See *scala media*. See Figure 6.1.

middle cerebral artery Either of two large arteries, arising from the carotid arteries, that provide blood to most of the forebrain. Compare *anterior cerebral artery* and *posterior cerebral artery*. [ASF 2.1]

middle ear The cavity between the tympanic membrane and the cochlea. See Figure 6.1. [6]

milk letdown reflex The reflexive release of milk by the mammary glands of a nursing female in response to suckling or to stimuli associated with suckling. See Figure 8.9. [8]

millivolt (mV) A thousandth of a volt. [3]

mirror neuron A neuron that is active both when an individual makes a particular movement and when that individual sees another individual make the same movement. [5]

mitochondrion (pl. mitochondria) A cellular organelle that provides metabolic energy for the cell's processes. See Figure 2.4. [2]

mitosis The process of division of somatic cells that involves duplication of DNA. [13]

monaural Pertaining to one ear. Compare *binaural*.

monoamine hormone See *amine hormone*. [8]

monoamine oxidase (MAO) An enzyme that breaks down monoamine neurotransmitters, thereby inactivating them. [4, 12, ASF 4.1]

monocular deprivation Depriving one eye of form vision. Compare *binocular deprivation*. [ASF 13.4]

monopolar neuron See *unipolar neuron*. [2]

monozygotic Referring to twins derived from a single fertilized egg (identical twins). Such individuals share an identical set of genes. Compare *dizygotic*. [12]

morpheme The smallest grammatical unit of a language; a word or meaningful part of a word. [15]

morphine An opiate compound derived from the poppy flower. [4]

motion sickness The experience of nausea brought on by unnatural passive movement, as may occur in a car or boat. [6]

motivation The psychological process that induces or sustains a particular behavior. [9]

motoneuron See *motor neuron*.

motor nerve A nerve that transmits information from the central nervous system to the muscles and glands. Compare *sensory nerve*. [2]

motor neuron Also called *motoneuron*. A neuron that transmits neural messages to muscles (or glands). See Figure 5.20. Compare *interneuron* and *sensory neuron*. [2, 5]

motor plan Also called *motor program*. A plan for a series of muscular contractions, established in the nervous system prior to its execution. [5]

motor theory of language The theory that speech is perceived using the same left-hemisphere mechanisms that are used to produce the complex movements that go into speech. Compare *connectionist model of aphasia*. [15]

motor unit A single motor axon and all the muscle fibers that it innervates. [5]

movement A single relocation of a body part, usually resulting from a brief muscle contraction. It is less complex than an act. [5]

mPOA See *medial preoptic area*. [8]

MRI See *magnetic resonance imaging*. [2]

mRNA See *messenger RNA*. [App]

müllerian duct A duct system in the embryo that will develop into female reproductive structures (oviducts, uterus, and upper vagina) in the absence of AMH. See Figure 8.24. Compare *wolffian duct*. [8]

müllerian regression hormone See *anti-müllerian hormone*. [8]

multiple sclerosis (MS) Literally "many scars." A disorder characterized by the widespread degeneration of myelin. [2, 3, ASF 13.3]

multipolar neuron A nerve cell that has many dendrites and a single axon. See Figure 2.3. Compare *bipolar neuron* and *unipolar neuron*. [2]

multisensory See *polymodal*. [ASF 6.3]

muscarinic Referring to cholinergic receptors that respond to the chemical muscarine as well as to acetylcholine. Muscarinic receptors mediate chiefly the inhibitory activities of acetylcholine. Compare *nicotinic*.

muscle fiber Large, cylindrical cells, making up most of a muscle, that can contract in response to neurotransmitter released from a motor neuron. See Figures 5.20, 5.21. See *intrafusal fiber*. [5]

muscle spindle A muscle receptor that lies parallel to a muscle and sends impulses to the central nervous system when the muscle is stretched. See Figure 5.20. Compare *Golgi tendon organ*. [5]

muscular dystrophy (MD) A disease that leads to degeneration of and functional changes in muscles. See ASF 5.5 for more information.

musth An annual period of heightened aggressiveness and sexual activity in male elephants. See ASF 8.7 for more information.

mV See *millivolt*. [3]

myasthenia gravis A disorder characterized by a profound weakness of skeletal muscles. It is caused by a loss of acetylcholine receptors. See ASF 5.5 for more information.

myelin The fatty insulation around an axon, formed by glial cells. This myelin sheath boosts the speed at which action potentials are conducted. See Figures 2.5, 3.8. [2, 3]

myelination The process by which myelin sheaths develop around axons. See Figure 2.5. [ASF 13.3]

myopia Nearsightedness; the inability to focus the retinal image of objects that are far away. [7]

N

N1 effect See *auditory N1 effect*. [14]

naloxone A potent antagonist of opiates that is often administered to people who have taken drug overdoses. It blocks receptors for endogenous opioids. [5]

narcolepsy A disorder that involves frequent, intense episodes of sleep, which last from 5 to 30 minutes and can occur anytime during the usual waking hours. [10]

NE See *norepinephrine*. [4, 11]

negative feedback The process whereby a system monitors its own output and reduces its activity when a set point is reached. [8, 9]

negative symptom In psychiatry, an abnormality that reflects insufficient functioning. Examples include emotional and social withdrawal, and blunted affect. Compare *positive symptom*. [12]

neocortex Also called simply *cortex*. Cerebral cortex that is made up of six distinct layers. [2]

neonatal Referring to newborns. [8]

nerve A collection of axons bundled together outside the central nervous system. See Figures 2.6, 2.7. Compare *tract*. [2]

nerve cell See *neuron*. [1, 2]

nerve fiber See *axon*. [2]

neural chain A simple kind of neural circuit in which neurons are attached linearly, end-to-end. [ASF 3.2]

neural groove In the developing embryo, the groove between the neural folds. See Figure 13.23.

neural plasticity See *neuroplasticity*. [1, 2, 13]

neural tube An embryonic structure with subdivisions that correspond to the future forebrain, midbrain, and hindbrain. The cavity of this tube will include the cerebral ventricles and the passages that connect them. See Figure 13.23. [2, 13]

neuroeconomics The study of brain mechanisms at work during economic decision making. [1, 14]

neuroendocrine cell A neuron that releases hormones into local or systemic circulation. [8]

neurofibrillary tangle An abnormal whorl of neurofilaments within nerve cells that is seen in Alzheimer's disease. See Figure 13.34. [13]

neurogenesis The mitotic division of nonneuronal cells to produce neurons. See Figure 13.25. [13]

neuroleptic See *antipsychotic*. [4, 12]

neuromuscular junction The region where the motor neuron terminal meets its target muscle fiber. It is the point where the nerve transmits its message to the muscle fiber. [5]

neuron Also called *nerve cell*. The basic unit of the nervous system, each composed of receptive extensions called *dendrites*, an integrating cell body, a conducting axon, and a transmitting axon terminal. See Figures 2.2, 2.3. [1, 2]

neuron doctrine The hypothesis that the brain is composed of separate cells

that are distinct structurally, metabolically, and functionally.

neuropathic pain Pain that persists long after the injury that started it has healed. [5]

neuropeptide See peptide neurotransmitter. [4]

neurophysiology The study of the life processes of neurons. [3]

neuroplasticity Also called *neural plasticity*. The ability of the nervous system to change in response to experience or the environment. [1, 2, 13]

neuroscience The scientific study of the nervous system. [1]

neurotransmitter Also called *synaptic transmitter*, *chemical transmitter*, or simply *transmitter*. A signaling chemical, released by a presynaptic axon terminal, that diffuses across the synaptic cleft to alter the functioning of the postsynaptic neuron. It serves as the basis of communication between neurons. See Figure 3.11; Table 4.1. [2, 3, 4]

neurotransmitter receptor Also called simply *receptor*. A specialized protein, embedded in the cell membrane, that selectively senses and reacts to molecules of a corresponding neurotransmitter or hormone. [2, 3, 4]

neurotrophic factor Also called simply *trophic factor*. A target-derived chemical that acts as if it "feeds" certain neurons to help them survive. See Figure 13.28. [13]

nicotine A compound found in plants, including tobacco, that acts as an agonist on a large class of cholinergic receptors. [4]

nicotinic Referring to cholinergic receptors that respond to nicotine as well as to acetylcholine. Nicotinic receptors mediate chiefly the excitatory activities of acetylcholine, including at the neuromuscular junction. Compare *muscarinic*.

night terror A sudden arousal from stage 3 sleep that is marked by intense fear and autonomic activation. Compare *nightmare*. [10]

nightmare A long, frightening dream that awakens the sleeper from REM sleep. Compare *night terror*. [10]

Nissl stain A tissue stain that outlines all cell bodies because the dyes are attracted to RNA, which encircles the nucleus. See Box 2.1. [2]

NMDA receptor A glutamate receptor that also binds the glutamate agonist NMDA (*N*-*m*ethyl-d-*a*spartate) and that is both ligand-gated and voltage-sensitive. Compare *AMPA receptor*. [13, ASF 4.2]

nociceptor A receptor that responds to stimuli that produce tissue damage or pose the threat of damage. [5]

nocturnal Active during the dark periods of the daily cycle. Compare *diurnal*. [10]

node of Ranvier A gap between successive segments of the myelin sheath where the axon membrane is exposed. See Figures 2.5, 3.8. [2, 3]

non-REM sleep Sleep, divided into stages 1–3, that is defined by the presence of distinctive EEG activity that differs from that seen in REM sleep. [10]

nonassociative learning A type of learning in which presentation of a particular stimulus alters the strength or probability of a response. It includes habituation and sensitization. See Figure 13.18. Compare *associative learning*. [13]

noncompetitive ligand A drug that affects a transmitter receptor while binding at a site other than that bound by the endogenous ligand.

nondeclarative memory Also called *procedural memory*. A memory that is shown by performance rather than by conscious recollection. See Figures 13.4, 13.12. Compare *declarative memory*. [13]

nonfluent aphasia Also called *Broca's aphasia*. A language impairment characterized by difficulty with speech production but not with language comprehension. It is related to damage in Broca's area. See Figure 15.8. Compare *fluent aphasia*. [15]

nonprimary motor cortex Frontal lobe regions adjacent to the primary motor cortex that contribute to motor control and modulate the activity of the primary motor cortex. See Figure 5.26. [5]

nonprimary sensory cortex Also called *secondary sensory cortex*. For a given sensory modality, the cortical regions receiving direct projections from primary sensory cortex for that modality. Compare *primary sensory cortex*. [5]

noradrenaline See *norepinephrine*. [4, 11]

noradrenergic Referring to cells using norepinephrine (noradrenaline) as a transmitter. [4]

norepinephrine (NE) Also called *noradrenaline*. A neurotransmitter produced and released by sympathetic postganglionic neurons to accelerate organ activity. It is also produced in the brainstem and found in projections throughout the brain. See Figure 4.4; Table 4.1. [4, 11]

Northern blot A method of detecting a particular RNA transcript in a tissue or organ by separating RNA from that source with gel electrophoresis, blotting the separated RNA molecules onto nitrocellulose, and then using a nucleotide probe to hybridize with, and highlight, the transcript of interest. Compare *Southern blot* and *Western blot*. [App]

NPY neuron A neuron, involved in the hypothalamic appetite control system, that produces both neuropeptide Y and agouti-related peptide. Compare *POMC neuron*. [9]

NST See *nucleus of the solitary tract*. [9]

nucleotide A portion of a DNA or RNA molecule that is composed of a single base and the adjoining sugar-phosphate unit of the strand. [App]

nucleus (pl. nuclei) 1. A collection of neuronal cell bodies within the central nervous system (e.g., the caudate nucleus). Compare *ganglion*. [2] 2. See *cell nucleus*. [App]

nucleus accumbens A region of the forebrain that receives dopaminergic innervation from the ventral tegmental area, often associated with reward and pleasurable sensations. [4, 11]

nucleus of the solitary tract (NST) A complicated brainstem nucleus that receives visceral and taste information via several cranial nerves. See Figure 9.15. [9]

nutrient A chemical that is needed for effective functioning, growth, maintenance, and repair of the body. [9]

O

obsessive-compulsive disorder (OCD) An anxiety disorder in which the affected individual experiences recurrent unwanted thoughts and engages in repetitive behaviors without reason or the ability to stop. [12]

occipital cortex Also called *visual cortex*. Cortex of the occipital lobe of the brain, corresponding to the primary visual area of the cortex. See Figure 7.10. [7]

occipital lobe A large region of cortex that covers much of the posterior part of each cerebral hemisphere. See Figure 2.10. Compare *frontal lobe, parietal lobe*, and *temporal lobe*. [2]

OCD See *obsessive-compulsive disorder*. [12]

ocular dominance histogram A graph that plots how strongly a brain neuron responds to stimuli presented to either the left eye or the right eye. Ocular dominance histograms are used to determine the effects of manipulating visual experience. [ASF 13.4]

odor The sensation of smell. [6]

off-center bipolar cell A retinal bipolar cell that is inhibited by light in the center of its receptive field. See Figures 7.13, 7.14. Compare *on-center bipolar cell*. [7]

off-center ganglion cell A retinal ganglion cell that is activated when light is presented to the periphery, rather than the center, of the cell's receptive field.

See Figures 7.13, 7.14. Compare *on-center ganglion cell*. [7]

off-center/on-surround Referring to a concentric receptive field in which stimulation of the center inhibits the cell of interest while stimulation of the surround excites it. See Figure 7.14. Compare *on-center/off-surround*. [7]

OHC See *outer hair cell*. [6]

olfaction The sensory system that detects smell; the act of smelling. [6]

olfactory bulb An anterior projection of the brain that terminates in the upper nasal passages and, through small openings in the skull, provides receptors for smell. See Figures 2.10, 2.15, 6.19. [2, 6]

olfactory epithelium (pl. epithelia) A sheet of cells, including olfactory receptors, that lines the dorsal portion of the nasal cavities and adjacent regions. See Figures 6.19, 6.20. [6]

oligodendrocyte A type of glial cell that forms myelin in the central nervous system. See Figure 2.5. Compare *Schwann cell*. [2]

on-center bipolar cell A retinal bipolar cell that is excited by light in the center of its receptive field. See Figures 7.13, 7.14. Compare *off-center bipolar cell*. [7]

on-center ganglion cell A retinal ganglion cell that is activated when light is presented to the center, rather than the periphery, of the cell's receptive field. See Figures 7.13, 7.14. Compare *off-center ganglion cell*. [7]

on-center/off-surround Referring to a concentric receptive field in which stimulation of the center excites the cell of interest while stimulation of the surround inhibits it. See Figure 7.14. Compare *off-center/on-surround*. [7]

ontogeny The process by which an individual changes in the course of its lifetime—that is, grows up and grows old. [1]

Onuf's nucleus The human homolog of the spinal nucleus of the bulbocavernosus (SNB) in rats. [8]

operant conditioning See *instrumental conditioning*. [13]

opiate Any of a class of compounds that exert an effect like that of opium, including reduced pain sensitivity. [4]

opioid peptide A type of endogenous peptide that mimics the effects of morphine in binding to opioid receptors and producing marked analgesia and reward. See Table 4.1. [4]

opioid receptor A receptor that responds to endogenous opioids and/or exogenous opiates. [4]

opium An extract of the opium poppy, *Papaver somniferum*. Drugs based on opium are potent painkillers. [4]

opponent-process hypothesis A hypothesis of color perception stating that different systems produce opposite responses to light of different wavelengths. See Figures 7.23, 7.24. [7]

optic ataxia Spatial disorientation in which the patient is unable to accurately reach for objects using visual guidance. [7]

optic chiasm The point at which parts of the two optic nerves cross the midline. See Figure 7.10. [7]

optic disc The region of the retina that is devoid of photoreceptors because ganglion cell axons and blood vessels exit the eyeball there. See Figure 7.7. [7]

optic nerve Cranial nerve II; the collection of ganglion cell axons that extend from the retina to the brain. See Figures 2.7, 7.10. [7]

optic radiation Axons from the lateral geniculate nucleus that terminate in the primary visual areas of the occipital cortex. See Figure 7.10. [7]

optic tract The axons of retinal ganglion cells after they have passed the optic chiasm. Most of these axons terminate in the lateral geniculate nucleus. See Figure 7.10. [7]

optogenetics The use of light to excite or inhibit neurons expressing light-sensitive membrane channels, typically in transgenic mice. [11]

oral contraceptive A birth control pill, typically consisting of steroid hormones to prevent ovulation. [8]

orexigenic neurons Neurons of the hypothalamic appetite system that promote feeding behavior. [9]

orexin Also called *hypocretin*. A neuropeptide produced in the hypothalamus that is involved in switching between sleep states, in narcolepsy, and in the control of appetite. [9, 10]

organ of Corti A structure in the inner ear that lies on the basilar membrane of the cochlea and contains the hair cells and terminations of the auditory nerve. See Figure 6.1. [6]

organizational effect A permanent alteration of the nervous system, and thus permanent change in behavior, resulting from the action of a steroid hormone on an animal early in its development. Compare *activational effect*. [8]

orgasm The climax of sexual behavior, marked by extremely pleasurable sensations. [8]

osmosensory neuron A specialized neuron that monitors the concentration of the extracellular fluid by measuring the movement of water into and out of the intracellular compartment. See Figures 9.6, 9.8. [9]

osmosis The passive movement of a solvent, usually water, through a semipermeable membrane until a uniform concentration of solute (often salt) is achieved on both sides of the membrane. See Figure 9.5. Compare *diffusion*. [9]

osmotic pressure The tendency of a solvent to move across a membrane in order to equalize the concentration of solute on both sides of the membrane. [9]

osmotic thirst A desire to ingest fluids that is stimulated by a high concentration of solute (like salt) in the extracellular compartment. Compare *hypovolemic thirst*. [9]

ossicles Three small bones (*incus, malleus,* and *stapes*) that transmit vibrations across the middle ear, from the tympanic membrane to the oval window. See Figure 6.1. [6]

otolith A small crystal on the gelatinous membrane in the vestibular system.

outer hair cell (OHC) One of the two types of receptor cells for hearing in the cochlea. Compared with inner hair cells, OHCs are positioned farther from the central axis of the coiled cochlea. See Figure 6.1. [6]

output zone The part of a neuron at which the cell sends information to another cell. This zone usually corresponds to the axon terminals. See Figures 2.1, 2.3. Compare *conduction zone, input zone,* and *integration zone*. [2]

oval window The opening from the middle ear to the inner ear. See Figure 6.1. [6]

ovaries The female gonads, which produce eggs (ova) for reproduction. See Figure 8.1. Compare *testes*. [8]

overt attention Attention in which the focus coincides with sensory orientation (e.g., you're attending to the same thing you're looking at). Compare *covert attention*. [14]

ovulation The production and release of an egg (ovum). [8]

ovulatory cycle The periodic occurrence of ovulation in females. See Figure 8.19. [8]

ovum (pl. ova) An egg, the female gamete. Compare *sperm*. [8]

oxytocin A peptide hormone, released from the posterior pituitary, that triggers milk letdown in the nursing female but is also associated with a variety of complex behaviors. See Figures 8.8, 8.9. [8]

P

P1 effect See *visual P1 effect*. [14]

P3 effect Also called *auditory P300*. A positive deflection of the event-related potential, occurring about 300 milliseconds after stimulus presentation, that is associated with higher-order auditory stimulus processing and late attentional selection. [14]

Pacinian corpuscle Also called *lamellated corpuscle*. A skin receptor cell type that detects vibration and pressure. See Figures 5.3, 5.4. Compare *Meissner's corpuscle, Merkel's disc,* and *Ruffini corpuscle*. [5]

pain The discomfort normally associated with tissue damage. [5]

pair-bond A durable and exclusive relationship between two individuals. [8]

Papez circuit A group of brain regions within the limbic system.

papilla (pl. papillae) A small bump that projects from the surface of the tongue. Papillae contain most of the taste receptor cells. See Figures 6.15, 6.16. [6]

parabiotic Referring to a surgical preparation that joins two animals to share a single blood supply. [8]

paradoxical sleep See *rapid-eye-movement sleep (REM)* sleep. [10]

paraphasia A symptom of aphasia that is distinguished by the substitution of a word by a sound, an incorrect word, an unintended word, or a neologism (a meaningless word). [15]

parasympathetic nervous system The part of the autonomic nervous system that generally prepares the body to relax and recuperate. See Figure 2.9. Compare *sympathetic nervous system*. [2, 11]

paraventricular nucleus (PVN) A nucleus of the hypothalamus involved in the release of peptide hormones and in the control of feeding and other behaviors. [9]

paresis Muscular weakness, often the result of damage to motor cortex. Compare *plegia*. [5]

parietal lobe The large region of cortex lying between the frontal and occipital lobes in each cerebral hemisphere. See Figure 2.10. Compare also *temporal lobe*. [2]

Parkinson's disease A degenerative neurological disorder, characterized by tremors at rest, muscular rigidity, and reduction in voluntary movement, caused by loss of the dopaminergic neurons of the substantia nigra. Compare *Huntington's disease*. [5]

partial agonist A drug that, when bound to a receptor, has less effect than the endogenous ligand would. The term *partial antagonist* is equivalent. [4]

Patient H.M. The late Henry Molaison, a man who was unable to encode new declarative memories because of surgical removal of medial temporal lobe structures. See Figure 13.1. [13]

Patient K.C. The late Kent Cochrane, who sustained damage to the cortex that rendered him unable to form and retrieve episodic memories. [13]

Patient N.A. A still-living man who is unable to encode new declarative memories, because of damage to the dorsomedial thalamus and the mammillary bodies. [13]

Pavlovian conditioning See *classical conditioning*. [13]

PCP See *phencyclidine*. [12]

PCR See *polymerase chain reaction*. [App]

penis The male phallus. Compare *clitoris*. [8]

peptide A short string of amino acids. Longer strings of amino acids are called *proteins*. [App]

peptide hormone Also called *protein hormone*. A hormone that consists of a string of amino acids. [8]

peptide neurotransmitter Also called *neuropeptide*. A neurotransmitter consisting of a short chain of amino acids. See Table 4.1. Compare *amine neurotransmitter, amino acid neurotransmitter,* and *gas neurotransmitter*. [4]

perceptual load The immediate processing demands presented by a stimulus. [14]

periaqueductal gray A midbrain region involved in pain perception. [2, 4, 8]

period The interval of time between two similar points of successive cycles, such as sunset to sunset. [10]

peripheral nervous system The portion of the nervous system that includes all the nerves and neurons outside the brain and spinal cord. See Figures 2.6, 2.12. Compare *central nervous system*. [2]

peripheral spatial cuing A technique for testing reflexive attention in which a visual stimulus is preceded by a simple task-irrelevant sensory stimulus either in the location where the stimulus will appear or in an incorrect location. Compare *symbolic cuing*. [14]

perseverate To continue to show a behavior repeatedly, beyond a reasonable degree. [14, ASF 13.4]

PET See *positron emission tomography*. [2]

phagocyte An immune system cell that engulfs invading molecules or microbes. [ASF 11.4]

phallus The clitoris or penis. [8]

pharmacokinetics Collective name for all the factors that affect the movement of a drug into, through, and out of the body. [4]

phase shift A shift in the activity of a biological rhythm, typically provided by a synchronizing environmental stimulus, such as light. [10]

phasic receptor A receptor in which the frequency of action potentials drops rapidly as stimulation is maintained. Compare *tonic receptor*. [5]

phencyclidine (PCP) Also called *angel dust*. An anesthetic agent that is also a psychedelic drug. PCP makes many people feel dissociated from themselves and their environment. [12]

phenotype The sum of an individual's physical characteristics at one particular time. Compare *genotype*. [13]

phenylketonuria (PKU) An inherited disorder of protein metabolism in which the absence of an enzyme leads to a toxic buildup of certain compounds, causing intellectual disability. [13]

pheromone A chemical signal that is released outside the body of an animal and affects other members of the same species. See Figure 8.3. Compare *allomone*. [6, 8]

phoneme A sound that is produced for language. [15]

photopic system A system in the retina that operates at high levels of light, shows sensitivity to color, and involves the cones. See Table 7.1. Compare *scotopic system*. [7]

photoreceptor A neural cell in the retina that responds to light. [7]

photoreceptor adaptation The tendency of rods and cones to adjust their light sensitivity to match current levels of illumination. [7]

phrenology The belief that bumps on the skull reflect enlargements of brain regions responsible for certain behavioral faculties. See Figure 1.4. [1]

physiological psychology See *behavioral neuroscience*. [1]

pia mater The innermost of the three meninges that surround the brain and spinal cord. See also *dura mater* and *arachnoid*. See Figure 2.8. [2]

pineal gland A secretory gland in the brain midline that is the source of melatonin release. See Figure 8.1. [8, ASF 8.1]

pinna (pl. pinnae) The external part of the ear. [6]

pitch A dimension of auditory experience in which sounds vary from low to high. See Box 6.1. [6]

pituitary gland A small, complex endocrine gland located in a socket at the base of the skull. See Figures 2.15, 8.8, 8.12. [8]

pituitary stalk Also called *infundibulum*. A thin piece of tissue that connects the pituitary gland to the hypothalamus. [8]

place cell A neuron in the hippocampus that selectively fires when the animal is in a particular location. [13]

place coding theory Theory that the pitch of a sound is determined by the location of activated hair cells along the length of the basilar membrane. Compare *temporal coding theory*. [6]

placebo effect Relief of a symptom, such as pain, that results following a treatment that is known to be ineffective or inert. [5]

planum temporale An auditory region of superior temporal cortex. See Figure 15.3. [15]

plegia Paralysis; the loss of the ability to move. Compare *paresis*. [5]

polarized Exhibiting a difference in electrical charge between the inside and outside of the cell. [3]

poliovirus A virus that destroys motor neurons of the spinal cord and brainstem, causing permanent paralysis. See ASF 5.5 for more information.

polygraph Popularly known as a *lie detector*. A device that measures several bodily responses, such as heart rate and blood pressure. See Box 11.1. [11]

polymerase chain reaction (PCR) Also called *gene amplification*. A method for reproducing a particular RNA or DNA sequence manyfold, allowing amplification for sequencing or manipulating the sequence. [App]

polymodal Also called *multisensory*. Involving several sensory modalities. [ASF 6.3]

polymodal neuron A neuron upon which information from more than one sensory system converges. [5]

POMC neuron A neuron, involved in the hypothalamic appetite control system, that produces both pro-opiomelanocortin and cocaine- and amphetamine-regulated transcript. Compare *NPY neuron*. [9]

pons The portion of the brainstem that connects the midbrain to the medulla. See Figures 2.12, 2.15. [2]

positive symptom In psychiatry, an abnormal behavioral state. Examples include hallucinations, delusions, and excited motor behavior. Compare *negative symptom*. [12]

positron emission tomography (PET) A brain-imaging technology that tracks the metabolism of injected radioactive substances in the brain, in order to map brain activity. See Figure 2.18. Compare *functional MRI*. [2]

post-traumatic stress disorder (PTSD) A disorder in which memories of an unpleasant episode repeatedly plague the victim. See Box 13.1. [12, 13]

postcentral gyrus The strip of parietal cortex, just posterior to (behind) the central sulcus, that receives somatosensory information from the entire contralateral side of the body. See Figure 2.10. Compare *precentral gyrus*. [2]

postcopulatory behavior The final stage in mating behavior. Species-specific postcopulatory behaviors include rolling (in the cat) and grooming (in the rat). See Figure 8.16. [8]

posterior Also called *caudal*. In anatomy, toward the tail end of an organism. See Box 2.2. Compare *anterior*. [2]

posterior cerebral artery Either of two large arteries, arising from the basilar artery, that provide blood to posterior aspects of the cerebral hemispheres, cerebellum, and brainstem. Compare *anterior cerebral artery* and *middle cerebral artery*. [ASF 2.1]

posterior pituitary The rear division of the pituitary gland. See Figures 8.1, 8.8. Compare *anterior pituitary*. [8]

postpartum depression A bout of depression that afflicts a woman either immediately before or after giving birth. [12]

postsynaptic Referring to the region of a synapse that receives and responds to neurotransmitter. See Figure 2.4. Compare *presynaptic*. [2, 3, 4]

postsynaptic membrane The specialized membrane on the surface of a neuron that receives information by responding to neurotransmitter from a presynaptic neuron. See Figure 2.4. Compare *presynaptic membrane*. [2]

postsynaptic potential A local potential that is initiated by stimulation at a synapse, which can vary in amplitude, and spreads passively across the cell membrane, decreasing in strength with time and distance. Compare *all-or-none property*. [3]

potassium ion (K$^+$) A potassium atom that carries a positive charge. [3]

precentral gyrus The strip of frontal cortex, just anterior to (in front of) the central sulcus, that is crucial for motor control of the contralateral side of the body. See Figure 2.10. Compare *postcentral gyrus*. [2, 5]

prefrontal cortex The most anterior region of the frontal lobe. [14]

premotor cortex A region of nonprimary motor cortex just anterior to the primary motor cortex. See Figure 5.26. [5]

presenilin An enzyme that cleaves amyloid precursor protein, forming beta-amyloid, which can lead to Alzheimer's disease. See *beta-secretase*. [ASF 13.5]

presynaptic Located on the "transmitting" side of a synapse. See Figure 2.4. Compare *postsynaptic*. [2, 3, 4]

presynaptic membrane The specialized membrane on the axon terminal of a nerve cell that transmits information by releasing neurotransmitter. See Figure 2.4. [2]

primacy effect The superior performance seen in a memory task for items at the start of a list. It is usually attributed to long-term memory. Compare *recency effect*. [13]

primary auditory cortex Also called *A1*. The cortical region, located on the superior surface of the temporal lobe, that processes complex sounds transmitted from lower auditory pathways. [6]

primary motor cortex (M1) The apparent executive region for the initiation of movement. It is primarily the precentral gyrus. Compare *nonprimary motor cortex*. [5]

primary sensory cortex For a given sensory modality, the region of cortex that receives most of the information about that modality from the thalamus (or, in the case of olfaction, directly from the secondary sensory neurons). Compare *nonprimary sensory cortex*. See Figure 5.8. [5]

primary somatosensory cortex Also called *somatosensory 1* or *S1*. Primarily the postcentral gyrus of the parietal lobe, where sensory inputs from the body surface are mapped. See Figure 5.7. [5]

primary visual cortex (V1) Also called *striate cortex* or *area 17*. The region of the occipital cortex where most visual information first arrives. See Figures 7.10, 7.11, 7.20. [7]

priming Also called *repetition priming*. In memory, the phenomenon by which exposure to a stimulus facilitates subsequent responses to the same or a similar stimulus. [13]

probe In molecular biology, a manufactured sequence of DNA that is made to include a label (a colorful or radioactive molecule) that lets us track its location. [App]

procedural memory See *nondeclarative memory*. [13]

proceptive Referring to a state in which a female advertises her readiness to mate through species-typical behaviors. [8]

progesterone The primary type of progestin secreted by the ovary. See Figure 8.13. [8]

progestin Any of a major class of steroid hormones that are produced by the ovary, including progesterone. See Figure 8.13. [8]

progressive supranuclear palsy (PSP) A rare, degenerative disease of the brain that begins with marked, persistent visual symptoms and leads to more widespread intellectual deterioration.

prolactin A protein hormone, produced by the anterior pituitary, that promotes mammary development for lactation in female mammals. [ASF 8.4]

proprioception Body sense; information about the position and movement of the body. [5]

prosody The perception of emotional tone-of-voice aspects of language. [15]

prosopagnosia Also called *face blindness*. A condition characterized by the inability to recognize faces. [15]

protein A long string of amino acids. Proteins are the basic building material of organisms. Compare *peptide*. [App]

protein hormone See *peptide hormone*.

proximal In anatomy, near the trunk or center of an organism. See Box 2.2. Compare *distal*. [2]

psychoneuroimmunology The study of the immune system and its interaction with the nervous system and behavior. [11]

psychopath An individual incapable of experiencing remorse. [11]

psychosocial dwarfism A syndrome of stunted growth in children subjected to social stress, such as abusive caregivers. [8]

psychosomatic medicine A field of study that emphasizes the role of psychological factors in disease. [11]

psychosurgery Surgery in which brain lesions are produced to modify severe psychiatric disorders.

psychotomimetic A drug that induces a state resembling schizophrenia. [12]

PTSD See *post-traumatic stress disorder*. [12, 13]

pulvinar In humans, the posterior portion of the thalamus. It is heavily involved in visual processing and direction of attention. [14]

punch-drunk syndrome See *chronic traumatic encephalopathy*. [15]

pupil The opening, formed by the iris, that allows light to enter the eye. See Figures 7.1, 7.6. [7]

pure tone A tone with a single frequency of vibration. See Box 6.1. [6]

Purkinje cell A type of large nerve cell in the cerebellar cortex.

putamen One of the basal ganglia. See Figure 2.14. [2]

pyramidal cell A type of large nerve cell that has a roughly pyramid-shaped cell body and is found in the cerebral cortex. See Figure 2.13. [2]

pyramidal system Also called *corticospinal system*. The motor system that includes neurons within the cerebral cortex and their axons, which form the pyramidal tract. See Figure 5.23. Compare *extrapyramidal system*. [5]

PYY$_{3-36}$ A peptide gut hormone believed to act on the hypothalamic appetite system to suppress appetite. Compare *ghrelin*. [9]

Q

quale (pl. qualia) A purely subjective experience of perception. [14]

R

range fractionation The means by which sensory systems cover a wide range of intensity values, as each sensory receptor cell specializes in just one part of the overall range of intensities. [7]

raphe nuclei A string of nuclei in the midline of the midbrain and brainstem that contain most of the serotonergic neurons of the brain. [4]

rapid-eye-movement (REM) sleep Also called *paradoxical sleep*. A stage of sleep characterized by small-amplitude, fast EEG waves, no postural tension, and rapid eye movements. *REM* rhymes with "gem." See Figure 10.10. Compare *stage 3 sleep*. [10]

RBD See *REM behavior disorder*. [10]

recency effect The superior performance seen in a memory task for items at the end of a list. It is usually attributed to short-term memory. Compare *primacy effect*. [13]

receptive field The stimulus region and features that affect the activity of a cell in a sensory system. See Figures 5.5, 7.14, 7.17. [5, 7]

receptor See *neurotransmitter receptor*. [2, 3, 4]

receptor cell A specialized cell that responds to a particular energy or substance in the internal or external environment and converts this energy into a change in the electrical potential across its membrane. [5]

receptor subtype Any type of receptor having functional characteristics that distinguish it from other types of receptors for the same neurotransmitter. For example, at least 15 different subtypes of receptor molecules respond to serotonin.

reconsolidation The return of a memory trace to stable long-term storage after it has been temporarily made changeable during the process of recall. [13]

recovery of function The recovery of behavioral capacity following brain damage from stroke or injury. [15]

reductionism The scientific strategy of breaking a system down into increasingly smaller parts in order to understand it. [1]

reflex A simple, highly stereotyped, and unlearned response to a particular stimulus (e.g., an eye blink in response to a puff of air). See Figures 3.14, 5.22. [5]

reflexive attention Also called *exogenous attention*. The involuntary reorienting of attention toward a specific stimulus source, cued by an unexpected object or event. Compare *voluntary attention*. [14]

refraction The bending of light rays by a change in the density of a medium, such as the cornea and the lens of the eyes. [7]

refractory Temporarily unresponsive or inactivated. [3]

refractory phase 1. A period during and after an action potential in which the responsiveness of the axonal membrane is reduced. A brief period of complete insensitivity to stimuli (absolute refractory phase) is followed by a longer period of reduced sensitivity (relative refractory phase) during which only strong stimulation produces an action potential. [3] 2. A period following copulation during which an individual does not recommence copulation. See Figure 8.23. [8]

relative refractory phase A period of reduced sensitivity during which only strong stimulation produces an action potential. Compare *absolute refractory phase*. [3]

releasing hormone Any of a class of hormones, produced in the hypothalamus, that traverse the hypothalamic-pituitary portal system to control the pituitary's release of tropic hormones. See Figure 8.12. [8]

REM behavior disorder (RBD) A sleep disorder in which a person physically acts out a dream. [10]

REM sleep See *rapid-eye-movement (REM) sleep*. [10]

repetition priming See *priming*. [13]

repetitive transcranial magnetic stimulation (rTMS) A noninvasive treatment in which repeated pulses of focused magnetic energy are used to stimulate the cortex through the scalp. [12]

resting potential The difference in electrical potential across the membrane of a nerve cell at rest. See Figures 3.1, 3.5. [3]

reticular formation Also called *reticular activating system*. An extensive region

of the brainstem, extending from the medulla through the thalamus, that is involved in arousal (waking). See Figure 10.19. [2, 10]

retina The receptive surface inside the eye that contains photoreceptors and other neurons. See Figures 7.1, 7.3. [7]

retinohypothalamic pathway The route by which specialized retinal ganglion cells send their axons to the suprachiasmatic nuclei. [10]

retrieval The third process of the memory system, in which a stored memory is used by an organism. See Figure 13.13. Compare *encoding* and *consolidation*. [13]

retrograde amnesia Difficulty in retrieving memories formed before the onset of amnesia. Compare *anterograde amnesia*. [13]

retrograde transmitter A neurotransmitter that is released by the postsynaptic neuron, diffuses back across the synapse, and alters the functioning of the presynaptic neuron. [4, 13]

reuptake The reabsorption of molecules of neurotransmitter by the neurons that released them, thereby ending the signaling activity of the transmitter molecules. [3, 4]

rhodopsin The photopigment in rods that responds to light. [7]

ribonucleic acid (RNA) A nucleic acid that implements information found in DNA. Compare *deoxyribonucleic acid*. [App]

ribosome An organelle in the cell body where genetic information is translated to produce proteins. See Appendix Figure A.2. [App]

RNA See *ribonucleic acid (RNA)*. [App]

rod A photoreceptor cell in the retina that is most active at low levels of light. See Figure 7.3. Compare *cone*. [7]

root Either of two distinct branches of a spinal nerve, each of which serves a separate function. The dorsal root enters the dorsal horn of the spinal cord and carries sensory information, the ventral root arises from the ventral horn of the spinal cord and carries motor messages. See Figure 2.8. [2]

rostral See *anterior*. [2]

round window A membrane separating the tympanic canal from the middle ear. See Figure 6.1. [6]

Ruffini corpuscle A skin receptor cell type that detects stretching of the skin. See Figure 5.3. Compare *Meissner's corpuscle*, *Merkel's disc*, and *Pacinian corpuscle*. [5]

S

S1 See *primary somatosensory cortex*. [5]

sacral Referring to the five spinal segments in the lower part of the lower back. See Figures 2.8, 2.9. Compare *cervical*, *thoracic*, *lumbar*, and *coccygeal*. [2]

SAD See *seasonal affective disorder*. [ASF 12.3]

sagittal plane The plane that divides the body or brain into right and left portions. See Box 2.2. Compare *coronal plane* and *horizontal plane*. [2]

saltatory conduction The form of conduction that is characteristic of myelinated axons, in which the action potential jumps from one node of Ranvier to the next. [3]

saturation One of three basic dimensions of light perception, varying from rich to pale. Compare *brightness* and *hue*. [7]

SC See *standard condition*. [13]

scala media Also called *middle canal*. The central of the three spiraling canals inside the cochlea, situated between the *scala vestibuli* and the *scala tympani*. See Figure 6.1. [6]

scala tympani Also called *tympanic canal*. One of three principal canals running along the length of the cochlea. Compare *scala media* and *scala vestibuli*. See Figure 6.1. [6]

scala vestibuli Also called *vestibular canal*. One of three principal canals running along the length of the cochlea. Compare *scala media* and *scala tympani*. See Figure 6.1. [6]

schizophrenia A severe psychopathological disorder characterized by negative symptoms such as emotional withdrawal and flat affect, by positive symptoms such as hallucinations and delusions, and by cognitive symptoms such as poor attention span. [12]

Schwann cell A type of glial cell that forms myelin in the peripheral nervous system. Compare *oligodendrocyte*. [2]

SCN See *suprachiasmatic nucleus*. [10]

scotoma A region of blindness within the visual fields, caused by injury to the visual pathway or brain. [7]

scotopic system A system in the retina that operates at low levels of light and involves the rods. See Table 7.1. Compare *photopic system*. [7]

SDN-POA See *sexually dimorphic nucleus of the preoptic area*. [8]

seasonal affective disorder (SAD) A depression putatively brought about by the short days of winter. [ASF 12.3]

second messenger A slow-acting substance in a target cell that amplifies the effects of synaptic or hormonal activity and regulates activity within the target cell. [8]

second-generation antipsychotic Also called *atypical antipsychotic* and *atypical neuroleptic*. An antipsychotic drug that has primary actions other than or in addition to the dopamine D_2 receptor antagonism that characterizes the first-generation antipsychotics. [4, 12]

secondary sensory cortex See *non-primary sensory cortex*. [5]

seizure A wave of abnormally synchronous electrical activity in the brain. See Figure 3.16. [3]

selective attention See *attention*. [14]

selective permeability The property of a membrane that allows some substances to pass through, but not others. [3]

selective serotonin reuptake inhibitor (SSRI) An antidepressant drug that blocks the reuptake of transmitter at serotonergic synapses. [4, 12]

semantic memory Generalized declarative memory, such as knowing the meaning of a word. Compare *episodic memory*. [13]

semantics The meanings or interpretation of words and sentences in a language.

semen A mixture of fluid and sperm that is released during ejaculation. [8]

semicircular canal Any one of the three fluid-filled tubes in the inner ear that are part of the vestibular system. Each of the tubes, which are at right angles to each other, detects angular acceleration in a particular direction. See Figure 6.14. [6]

senile dementia A neurological disorder of the aged that is characterized by progressive behavioral deterioration, including personality change and profound intellectual decline. It includes, but is not limited to, Alzheimer's disease.

senile plaque See *amyloid plaque*. [13]

sensitive period Also called *critical period*. The period during development in which an organism can be permanently altered by a particular experience or treatment. [8, 15, ASF 13.4]

sensorineural deafness A hearing impairment most often caused by the permanent damage or destruction of hair cells or by interruption of the vestibulocochlear nerve that carries auditory information to the brain. See Figure 6.10. Compare *central deafness* and *conduction deafness*. [6]

sensory adaptation The progressive loss of receptor response as stimulation is maintained. See Figure 5.6. [5]

sensory buffer A very brief type of memory that stores the sensory impression of a scene. In vision, it is sometimes called *iconic memory*. See Figure 13.13. [13]

sensory nerve A nerve that conveys information from the body to the central nervous system. Compare *motor nerve*. [2]

sensory neuron A nerve cell that is directly affected by changes in the environment, such as light, odor, or touch. Compare *interneuron* and *motor neuron*. [2]

sensory transduction The process in which a receptor cell converts the energy in a stimulus into a change in the electrical potential across its membrane. [5]

serotonergic Referring to cells that use serotonin as their synaptic transmitter. [4]

serotonin (5-HT) A synaptic transmitter that is produced in the raphe nuclei and is active in structures throughout the central nervous system. See Figure 4.4; Table 4.1. [4, 11]

set point The point of reference in a feedback system. An example is the temperature at which a thermostat is set. Compare *set zone*. [9]

set zone The optimal range of a variable that a feedback system tries to maintain. Compare *set point*. [9]

sex determination The process that normally establishes whether a fetus will develop as a male or a female. [8]

sexual attraction The first step in the mating behavior of many animals, in which animals emit stimuli that attract members of the opposite sex. See Figure 8.16. [8]

sexual differentiation The process by which individuals develop either male-like or female-like bodies and behavior. See Figure 8.24. [8]

sexual dimorphism The condition in which males and females of the same species show pronounced sex differences in appearance. [8]

sexually dimorphic nucleus of the preoptic area (SDN-POA) A region of the preoptic area that is 5 to 6 times larger in volume in male than in females rats. See Figure 8.30. [8]

sexually receptive Referring to the state in which an individual (in mammals, typically the female) is willing to copulate. [8]

shadowing A task in which the participant is asked to focus attention on one ear or the other while different stimuli are being presented to the two ears, and to repeat aloud the material presented to the attended ear. [14]

sham rage See *decorticate rage*. [11]

shivering Rapid involuntary muscle contractions that generate heat in hypothermic animals. [ASF 9.1]

short-term memory (STM) Also called *working memory*. A form of memory that usually lasts only seconds, or as long as rehearsal continues. Working memory can be considered a portion of STM where information can be manipulated. See Figure 13.13. Compare *sensory buffer* and *long-term memory*. [13]

SIDS See *sudden infant death syndrome*. [10]

simple cortical cell Also called *bar detector* or *edge detector*. A cell in the visual cortex that responds best to an edge or a bar that has a particular width, as well as a particular orientation and location in the visual field. Compare *complex cortical cell*. [7]

simple partial seizure Also called *petit mal seizure* or *absence attack*. A seizure that is characterized by a spike-and-wave EEG and often involves a loss of awareness and inability to recall events surrounding the seizure. [3]

simultagnosia A profound restriction of attention, often limited to a single item or feature. Simultagnosia is one of the three primary symptoms of Balint's syndrome. [14]

skeletal muscle A muscle that is used for movement of the skeleton, typically under our conscious control. [5]

skill learning The process of learning to perform a challenging task simply by repeating it over and over. [13]

sleep apnea A sleep disorder in which respiration slows or stops periodically, waking the patient. Excessive daytime sleepiness results from the frequent nocturnal awakening. [10]

sleep cycle A period of slow-wave sleep followed by a period of REM sleep. In humans, a sleep cycle lasts 90–110 minutes. [10]

sleep deprivation The partial or total prevention of sleep. [10]

sleep enuresis Bed-wetting. [10]

sleep paralysis A state, during the transition to or from sleep, in which the ability to move or talk is temporarily lost. [10]

sleep recovery The process of sleeping more than normally after a period of sleep deprivation, as though in compensation. [10]

sleep spindle A characteristic 12–14 Hz wave in the EEG of a person said to be in stage 2 sleep. See Figure 10.10. [10]

sleep state misperception Commonly, a person's perception that they have not been asleep when in fact they have. It typically occurs at the start of a sleep episode. [10]

sleep-maintenance insomnia Difficulty in staying asleep. Compare *sleep-onset insomnia*. [10]

sleep-onset insomnia Difficulty in falling asleep. Compare *sleep-maintenance insomnia*. [10]

slow wave sleep (SWS) Also called *non-REM sleep*. Sleep, divided into stages 1–3, that is defined by the presence of slow-wave EEG activity. See Figure 10.10. Compare *rapid-eye-movement (REM) sleep*. [10]

SMA See *supplementary motor area*. [5]

SNB See *spinal nucleus of the bulbocavernosus*. [8]

social neuroscience A field of study that uses the tools of neuroscience to discover both the biological bases of social behavior and the effects of social circumstances on brain activity. [1]

sodium ion (Na⁺) A sodium atom that carries a positive charge. [3]

sodium-potassium pump The energetically expensive mechanism that pushes sodium ions out of a cell, and potassium ions in. [3]

solute A solid compound that is dissolved in a liquid. Compare *solvent*.

solvent The liquid (often water) in which a compound is dissolved. Compare *solute*.

soma (pl. somata) See *cell body* [2]

somatic intervention An approach to finding relations between body variables and behavioral variables that involves manipulating body structure or function and looking for resultant changes in behavior. See Figure 1.10. Compare *behavioral intervention*. [1]

somatic nerve See *spinal nerve*. [2]

somatic nervous system A part of the peripheral nervous system that supplies neural connections mostly to the skeletal muscles and sensory systems of the body. It consists of cranial nerves and spinal nerves. [2]

somatosensory 1 (S1) See *primary somatosensory cortex*. [5]

somatosensory system A set of specialized receptors and neural mechanisms responsible for body sensations such as touch and pain. [5]

somatotropic hormone Also called *somatotropin*. See *growth hormone*. [8]

somnambulism Sleepwalking. [10]

Southern blot A method of detecting a particular DNA sequence in the genome of an organism by separating DNA with gel electrophoresis, blotting the separated DNA molecules onto nitrocellulose, and then using a nucleotide probe to hybridize with, and highlight, the gene of interest. See Appendix Figure A.3. Compare *Northern blot* and *Western blot*. [App]

spasticity Markedly increased rigidity in response to forced movement of the limbs.

spatial cognition The ability to navigate and to understand the spatial relationships between objects. [15]

spatial resolution The ability to observe the detailed structure of the brain. Compare *temporal resolution*. [14]

spatial summation The summation of postsynaptic potentials that reach the axon hillock from different locations across the cell body. If this summation reaches threshold, an action potential is triggered. See Figure 3.10. Compare *temporal summation*. [3]

spatial-frequency model A model of visual perception that emphasizes the analysis of the different spatial frequencies present in various orientations and in various parts of a visual scene. [7, ASF 7.2]

spectral filtering The process by which the hills and valleys of the external ear alter the amplitude of some, but not all, frequencies in a sound. [6]

spectrally opponent cell Also called *color-opponent cell*. A visual system neuron that has opposite firing responses to different regions of the spectrum. See Figures 7.26, 7.27. [7]

sperm The gamete produced by males for the fertilization of eggs (ova). [8]

spike See *action potential*. [3]

spinal nerve Also called *somatic nerve*. A nerve that emerges from the spinal cord. There are 31 pairs of spinal nerves. Compare *cranial nerve*. See Figure 2.8. [2]

spinal nucleus of the bulbocavernosus (SNB) A group of motor neurons in the spinal cord of rats that innervate muscles controlling the penis. See Figure 8.32. See also *Onuf's nucleus*. [8]

spinocerebellum The uppermost part of the cerebellum, consisting mostly of the vermis and the anterior lobe. It receives sensory information about the current spatial location of the parts of the body and anticipates subsequent movement. Compare *cerebrocerebellum* and *vestibulocerebellum*. [ASF 5.4]

spinothalamic system See *anterolateral system*. [5]

split-brain individual An individual whose corpus callosum has been severed, halting communication between the right and left hemispheres. [15]

SRY gene A gene on the Y chromosome that directs the developing gonads to become testes. The name *SRY* stands for **s**ex-determining **r**egion on the **Y** chromosome. [8]

SSRI See *selective serotonin reuptake inhibitor*. [4, 12]

stage 1 sleep The initial stage of non-REM sleep, which is characterized by small-amplitude EEG waves of irregular frequency, slow heart rate, and reduced muscle tension. See Figure 10.10. [10]

stage 2 sleep A stage of sleep that is defined by bursts of regular 12- to 14-hertz EEG waves called *sleep spindles*. See Figure 10.10. [10]

stage 3 sleep Also called *slow wave sleep (SWS)*. A stage of non-REM sleep that is defined by the presence of large-amplitude, slow delta waves. See Figure 10.10. [10]

standard condition (SC) The usual environment for laboratory rodents, with a few animals in a cage and adequate food and water, but no complex stimulation. See Figure 13.15. Compare *enriched condition* and *impoverished condition*. [13]

stapedius A middle-ear muscle that is attached to the stapes. See Figure 6.1. [6]

stapes Latin for "stirrup." A middle-ear bone that is connected to the oval window. It is one of the three ossicles that conduct sounds across the middle ear. See Figure 6.1. [6]

stem cell A cell that is undifferentiated and therefore can take on the fate of any cell that a donor organism can produce. [13]

stereocilium (pl. stereocilia) A tiny bristle that protrudes from a hair cell in the auditory or vestibular system. See Figure 6.1. [6]

steroid hormone Any of a class of hormones, each of which is composed of four interconnected rings of carbon atoms. Compare *amine hormone* and *peptide hormone*. [8]

stimulant A drug that enhances the excitability of neurons. Compare *depressant*. [4]

stimulus (pl. stimuli) A physical event that triggers a sensory response. [5]

stimulus cuing A technique for testing reaction time to sensory stimuli, in which a cue to where the stimulus will be presented is provided before the stimulus itself.

STM See *short-term memory*. [13]

stress Any circumstance that upsets homeostatic balance. [11]

stress immunization The concept that mild stress early in life makes an individual better able to handle stress later in life. The benefits seem to be due to effective comforting after stressful events, not the stressful events themselves. [11]

stretch reflex The contraction of a muscle in response to stretch of that muscle. See Figure 5.22. [5]

striate cortex See *primary visual cortex*. [7]

striate muscle A type of muscle that has a striped appearance. It is generally under voluntary control.[5]

striatum The caudate nucleus and putamen together.

stroke Damage to a region of brain tissue that results from the blockage or rupture of vessels that supply blood to that region. [2]

stuttering The tendency of otherwise healthy people to produce speech sounds only haltingly, tripping over certain syllables or being unable to start vocalizing certain words. [15]

substance P A peptide transmitter that is involved in pain transmission. [5]

substantia nigra A brainstem structure that innervates the basal ganglia and is a major source of dopaminergic projections to the basal ganglia. Compare *locus coeruleus*. [2, 4, 5]

sudden infant death syndrome (SIDS) Also called *crib death*. The sudden, unexpected death of an apparently healthy human infant who simply stops breathing, usually during sleep. [10]

sulcus (pl. sulci) A crevice or valley of a convoluted brain surface. Compare *gyrus*. [2]

superior In anatomy, above. See Box 2.2. Compare *inferior*. [2]

superior colliculi (sing. superior colliculus) Paired gray matter structures of the dorsal midbrain that process visual information and are involved in direction of visual gaze and visual attention to intended stimuli. See Figures 2.15, 7.10. Compare *inferior colliculi*. [2, 7, 14]

superior olivary nucleus Either of two brainstem nuclei—left and right—that receive input from both right and left cochlear nuclei and provide the first binaural analysis of auditory information. See Figure 6.6. [6]

supersensitivity psychosis An exaggerated "rebound" psychosis that may emerge when doses of antipsychotic medication are reduced, probably as a consequence of the up-regulation of receptors that occurred during drug treatment. See Box 12.1. [12]

supplementary motor area (SMA) A region of nonprimary motor cortex that receives input from the basal ganglia and modulates the activity of the primary motor cortex. See Figure 5.26. [5]

suprachiasmatic nucleus (SCN) A small region of the hypothalamus above the optic chiasm that is the location of a circadian clock. [10]

surface dyslexia Acquired dyslexia in which the person seems to attend only to the fine details of reading. Compare *deep dyslexia*. [15]

sustained-attention task A task in which a single stimulus source or location must be held in the attentional spotlight for a protracted period. Compare *divided-attention task*. [14]

SWS See *stage 3 sleep*. [10]

Sylvian fissure Also called *lateral sulcus*. A deep fissure that demarcates the temporal lobe. See Figure 2.10. [2]

symbolic cuing A technique for testing voluntary attention in which a visual stimulus is presented and participants are asked to respond as soon as the stimulus appears on a screen. Each trial is preceded by a meaningful symbol used as a cue to hint at where the stimulus will appear. Compare *peripheral spatial cuing*. [14]

sympathetic nervous system The part of the autonomic nervous system that acts as the fight-or-flight system, generally preparing the body for action. See Figure 2.9. Compare *parasympathetic nervous system*. [2, 11]

synapse The cellular location at which information is transmitted from a neuron to another cell. See Figure 2.4. [2, 4, 8]

synapse rearrangement Also called *synaptic remodeling*. The loss of some synapses and the development of others; a refinement of synaptic connections that is often seen in development. See Figure 13.25. [13]

synaptic bouton See *axon terminal*. [2]

synaptic cleft The space between the presynaptic and postsynaptic neurons at a synapse. This gap measures about 20–40 nm. See Figures 2.2, 2.4, 3.11. [2, 3]

synaptic delay The brief delay between the arrival of an action potential at the axon terminal and the creation of a postsynaptic potential. [3]

synaptic remodeling See *synapse rearrangement*. [13]

synaptic transmitter See *neurotransmitter*. [2, 3]

synaptic vesicle A small, spherical structure that contains molecules of neurotransmitter. See Figure 2.4. [2, 3]

synaptogenesis The establishment of synaptic connections as axons and dendrites grow. See Figure 13.25. [13]

synergist A muscle that acts together with another muscle. Compare *antagonist* (definition 2). [5]

synesthesia A condition in which stimuli in one modality evoke the involuntary experience of an additional sensation in another modality. [5]

syrinx The vocal organ in birds. [ASF 15.3]

T

T cell See *T lymphocyte*. [ASF 11.4]

T lymphocyte Also called *T cell*. An immune system cell, formed in the thymus (hence the *T*), that attacks foreign microbes or tissue; "killer cell." Compare *B lymphocyte*. [ASF 11.4]

T1R A family of taste receptor proteins that, when particular members bind together, form taste receptors for sweet flavors and umami flavors. Compare *T2R*. [6]

T2R A family of bitter taste receptors. Compare *T1R*. [6]

TAAR See *trace amine–associated receptor*. [6]

tachistoscope test A test in which stimuli are very briefly presented to either the left or right visual half field. [15]

tactile corpuscle See *Meissner's corpuscle*. [5]

tactile Referring to touch. [5]

tailbone See *coccygeal*. [2]

tardive dyskinesia A disorder associated with first-generation antipsychotic use and characterized by involuntary movements, especially of the face and mouth. See Box 12.1. [12]

taste bud A cluster of 50–150 cells that detects tastes. Taste buds are found in papillae. See Figures 6.15, 6.16. [6]

taste Any of the five basic sensations detected by the tongue: sweet, salty, sour, bitter, and umami. Compare *flavor*. [6]

tau A protein associated with neurofibrillary tangles in Alzheimer's disease.

tectorial membrane A membrane that sits atop the organ of Corti in the cochlear duct. See Figure 6.1. [6]

tectum The dorsal portion of the midbrain consisting of the inferior and superior colliculi. [2]

tegmentum The main body of the midbrain, containing the substantia nigra, periaqueductal gray, part of the reticular formation, and multiple fiber tracts. [2]

telencephalon The anterior part of the fetal forebrain, which will become the cerebral hemispheres in the adult brain. See Figure 2.12, 13.23. Compare *diencephalon*. [2, 13]

temporal coding theory Theory that the pitch of a sound is determined by the rate of firing of auditory neurons. Compare *place coding theory*. [6]

temporal lobe The large lateral region of cortex in each cerebral hemisphere. It is continuous with the parietal lobe posteriorly and separated from the frontal lobe by the Sylvian fissure. See Figure 2.10. Compare *occipital lobe*. [2]

temporal resolution The ability to track changes in the brain that occur very quickly. Compare *spatial resolution*. [14]

temporal summation The summation of postsynaptic potentials that reach the axon hillock at different times. The closer in time the potentials occur, the more complete the summation is. See Figure 3.10. Compare *spatial summation*. [3]

temporoparietal junction (TPJ) The point in the brain where the temporal and parietal lobes meet. It plays a role in shifting attention to a new location after target onset. [14]

TENS See *transcutaneous electrical nerve stimulation*. [5]

testes (sing. testis) The male gonads, which produce sperm and androgenic steroid hormones. See Figure 8.1. Compare *ovaries*. [8]

testosterone A hormone, produced by male gonads, that controls a variety of bodily changes that become visible at puberty. It is one of a class of hormones called *androgens*. See Figure 8.13. [8, 11]

tetanus An intense volley of action potentials. [13]

tetrahydrocannabinol (THC) See *delta-9-tetrahydrocannabinol*. [4]

thalamus (pl. thalami) Paired structures to either side of the third ventricle that direct the flow of sensory information to and from the cortex. See Figures 2.14, 2.15. [2, 5]

THC See *delta-9-tetrahydrocannabinol*. [4]

therapeutic index The margin of safety for a given drug, expressed as the distance between effective doses and toxic doses. See Figure 4.6. [4]

thermoregulation The active process of maintaining a relatively constant internal temperature through behavioral and physiological adjustments. [9]

third ventricle The midline ventricle that conducts cerebrospinal fluid from the lateral ventricles to the fourth ventricle. See Figure 2.16. Compare *fourth ventricle* and *lateral ventricle*. [2]

thoracic Referring to the 12 spinal segments below the cervical (neck) portion of the spinal cord, in the torso. See Figures 2.8, 2.9. Compare *cervical, lumbar, sacral*, and *coccygeal*. [2]

threshold Here, the stimulus intensity that is just adequate to trigger an action potential in a sensory cell. [3, 5]

thrombolytic A substance that is used to unblock blood vessels and restore circulation. [ASF 15.5]

thyroid-stimulating hormone (TSH) A tropic hormone, released by the anterior pituitary gland, that signals the thyroid gland to secrete its hormones. [ASF 8.4]

timbre The characteristic sound quality of a musical instrument, as determined by the relative intensities of its various harmonics. See Box 6.1. [6]

tinnitus A sensation of noises or ringing in the ears not caused by external sound. [6]

tip link A fine, threadlike fiber that runs along and connects the tips of stereocilia. [6]

TMS See *transcranial magnetic stimulation*. [2]

tolerance See *drug tolerance*. [4]

tonic receptor A receptor in which the frequency of action potentials declines slowly or not at all as stimulation is maintained. Compare *phasic receptor*. [5]

tonic-clonic seizure Also called *grand mal seizure*. A type of generalized epileptic seizure in which nerve cells fire in high-frequency bursts, usually accompanied by involuntary rhythmic contractions of the body. [3]

tonotopic organization A major organizational feature in auditory systems, in which neurons are arranged as an orderly map of stimulus frequency, with cells responsive to high frequencies located at a distance from those responsive to low frequencies. [6]

topographic projection A mapping that preserves the point-to-point correspondence between neighboring parts of space. For example, a topographical projection extends from the retina to the cortex. [7]

Tourette's syndrome A disorder that is characterized by heightened sensitivity to sensory stimuli that may be accompanied by the buildup of an urge to emit verbal or phonic tics. See Box 12.2. [12]

TPJ See *temporoparietal junction*. [14]

trace amine–associated receptor (TAAR) Any one of a family of probable pheromone receptors produced by neurons in the main olfactory epithelium. [6]

tract A bundle of axons found within the central nervous system. Compare *nerve*. [2]

transcranial magnetic stimulation (TMS) A noninvasive technique for examining brain function that applies strong magnetic fields to stimulate cortical neurons, in order to identify discrete areas of the brain that are par-

ticularly active during specific behaviors. Compare *magnetoencephalography*. [2]

transcript See *messenger RNA*. [App]

transcription The process during which mRNA forms bases complementary to a strand of DNA. The resulting message (called a *transcript*) is then used to translate the DNA code into protein molecules. See Appendix Figure A.2. Compare *translation*. [App]

transcutaneous electrical nerve stimulation (TENS) The delivery of electrical pulses through electrodes attached to the skin, which excite nerves that supply the region to which pain is referred. [5]

transduction The conversion of one form of energy to another, such as conversion of light to neuronal activity. [6, 7]

transgenic Referring to an animal in which a new or altered gene has been deliberately introduced into the genome. [App]

transient ischemic attack (TIA) A temporary blood restriction to part of the brain that causes stroke-like symptoms that quickly resolve, serving as a warning of elevated stroke risk. [2]

transient receptor potential type M3 (TRPM3) A receptor, found in some free nerve endings, that opens its channel in response to rising temperatures. [5]

translation The process by which amino acids are linked together (directed by an mRNA molecule) to form protein molecules. See Appendix Figure A.2. Compare *transcription*. [App]

transmitter See *neurotransmitter*. [2, 3, 4]

transporter A specialized membrane component that returns transmitter molecules to the presynaptic neuron for reuse. [3, 4]

transverse plane See *coronal plane*. [2]

trichromatic hypothesis A hypothesis of color perception stating that there are three different types of cones, each excited by a different region of the spectrum and each having a separate pathway to the brain. [7]

tricyclic antidepressant An antidepressant that acts by increasing the synaptic accumulation of serotonin and norepinephrine. [4]

trinucleotide repeat Repetition of the same three nucleotides within a gene, which can lead to dysfunction, as in Huntington's disease. See ASF 5.5 for more information.

trophic factor See *neurotrophic factor*. [13]

tropic hormone Any of a class of anterior pituitary hormones that affect the secretion of hormones by other endocrine glands. See Figure 8.12. [8]

TSH See *thyroid-stimulating hormone*. [ASF 8.4]

tuberomammillary nucleus A region of the basal hypothalamus, near the pituitary stalk, that plays a role in generating slow wave sleep. [10]

tuning curve A graph of the responses of a single auditory nerve fiber or neuron to sounds that vary in frequency and intensity. See Figure 6.4. [6]

Turner's syndrome A condition, seen in individuals carrying a single X chromosome but no other sex chromosome, in which an apparent female has underdeveloped but recognizable ovaries. [8]

tympanic canal See *scala tympani*. [6]

tympanic membrane Also called *eardrum*. The partition between the external ear and the middle ear. See Figure 6.1. [6]

U

ultradian Referring to a rhythmic biological event with a period shorter than a day, usually from several minutes to several hours long. Compare *infradian*. [10]

ultrasound High-frequency sound; in general, above the threshold for human hearing, at about 20,000 Hz. Compare *infrasound*. [6]

umami One of the five basic tastes—the meaty, savory flavor. (The other four tastes are salty, sour, sweet, and bitter.) [6]

unipolar neuron Also called *monopolar neuron*. A nerve cell with a single branch that leaves the cell body and then extends in two directions; one end is the input zone, and the other end is the output zone. See Figure 2.3. Compare *bipolar neuron* and *multipolar neuron*. [2]

up-regulation A compensatory increase in receptor availability at the synapses of a neuron. Compare *down-regulation*. [4]

V

V1 See *primary visual cortex*. [7]

vagina The opening from the outside of the body to the cervix and uterus in females. [8]

vagus nerve Cranial nerve X, which provides extensive innervation of the viscera (organs). The vagus both regulates visceral activity and transmits signals from the viscera to the brain. See Figures 2.7, 9.15. [2, 9]

vasopressin Also called *arginine vasopressin (AVP)* or *antidiuretic hormone (ADH)*. A peptide hormone from the posterior pituitary that promotes water conservation and increases blood pressure. [8, 9]

ventral tegmental area (VTA) A portion of the midbrain that projects dopaminergic fibers to the nucleus accumbens. [4]

ventral In anatomy, toward the belly or front of the body, or the bottom of the brain. See Box 2.2. Compare *dorsal*. [2]

ventricular system A system of fluid-filled cavities inside the brain. See Figure 2.16. [2]

ventricular zone Also called *ependymal layer*. A region lining the cerebral ventricles that displays mitosis, providing neurons early in development and glial cells throughout life. See Figure 13.25. [13]

ventromedial hypothalamus (VMH) A hypothalamic region involved in sexual behaviors, eating, and aggression. See Figures 8.20, 9.12. [8, 9, 11]

vertex spike A sharp-wave EEG pattern that is seen during stage 1 sleep. See Figure 10.10. [10]

vestibular canal See *scala vestibuli*. See Figure 6.1. [6]

vestibular nucleus A brainstem nucleus that receives information from the vestibular organs through cranial nerve VIII (the vestibulocochlear nerve). [6]

vestibular system The sensory system that detects balance. It consists of several small inner-ear structures that adjoin the cochlea. [6]

vestibulocerebellum The middle portion of the cerebellum, sandwiched between the spinocerebellum and the cerebrocerebellum and consisting of the nodule and the flocculus. It helps the motor systems to maintain posture and appropriate orientation toward the external world. [ASF 5.4]

vestibulocochlear nerve Cranial nerve VIII, which runs from the cochlea to the brainstem auditory nuclei. See Figures 2.7, 6.1. [6]

visual acuity Sharpness of vision. [7]

visual cortex See *occipital cortex*. [7]

visual field The whole area that you can see without moving your head or eyes. [7]

visual P1 effect A positive deflection of the event-related potential, occurring 70–100 milliseconds after stimulus presentation, that is enhanced for selectively attended visual input compared with ignored input. Compare *auditory N1 effect*. [14]

VMH See *ventromedial hypothalamus*. [8, 9, 11]

VNO See *vomeronasal organ*. [6, 8]

voltage-gated Na+ channel A Na+-selective channel that opens or closes in response to changes in the voltage of the local membrane potential. It mediates the action potential. Compare *ionotropic receptor*. [3]

voluntary attention Also called *endogenous attention*. The voluntary direction of attention toward specific aspects of the environment, in accordance with our interests and goals. Compare *reflexive attention*. [14]

vomeronasal organ (VNO) A collection of specialized receptor cells, near to but separate from the olfactory epithelium, that detect pheromones and send electrical signals to the accessory olfactory bulb in the brain. [6, 8]

vomeronasal system A specialized sensory system that detects pheromones and transmits information to the brain. [6]

VTA See *ventral tegmental area*. [4]

W

Wada test A test in which a short-lasting anesthetic is delivered into one carotid artery to determine which cerebral hemisphere principally mediates language. See Box 15.1. [15]

wavelength The length between two peaks in a repeated stimulus such as a wave, light, or sound. See Figure 7.23. [7]

Wernicke-Geschwind model See *connectionist model of aphasia*. [15]

Wernicke's aphasia See *fluent aphasia*. [15]

Wernicke's area A region of temporoparietal cortex in the brain that is involved in the perception and production of speech. See Figure 15.7. Compare *Broca's area*. [15]

Western blot A method of detecting a particular protein molecule in a tissue or organ by separating proteins from that source with gel electrophoresis, blotting the separated proteins onto nitrocellulose, and then using an antibody that binds, and highlights, the protein of interest. Compare *Northern blot* and *Southern blot*. [App]

white matter A light-colored layer of tissue, consisting mostly of myelin-sheathed axons, that lies underneath the gray matter of the cortex. White matter mostly transmits information. See Figures 2.8, 2.11. Compare *gray matter*. [2]

Williams syndrome A disorder characterized by impairments of spatial cognition and IQ but superior linguistic abilities. [15]

withdrawal symptom An uncomfortable symptom that arises when a person stops taking a drug that they have used frequently, especially at high doses. [4]

within-participants experiment
An experiment in which the same set of individuals is compared before and after an experimental manipulation. The experimental group thus serves as its own control group. Compare *between-participants experiment*. [1]

wolffian duct A duct system in the embryo that will develop into male reproductive structures (epididymis, vas deferens, and seminal vesicle) if androgens are present. See Figure 8.24. Compare *müllerian duct*. [8]

word blindness A selective inability to understand written words. [15]

word deafness 1. A form of central deafness that is characterized by the specific inability to hear words, although other sounds can be detected. [6] 2. A selective inability to understand spoken words. [15]

working memory See *short-term memory*. [13]

Z

zeitgeber Literally "time-giver" (in German). The stimulus (usually the light-dark cycle) that entrains circadian rhythms. [10]

zygote The fertilized egg. [8]

References

A

Abbott, S. M., and Videnovic, A. (2014). Sleep disorders in atypical parkinsonism. *Movement Disorders Clinical Practice (Hoboken), 1*, 89–96.

Abe, N., Suzuki, M., Mori, E., Itoh, M., et al. (2007). Deceiving others: Distinct neural responses of the prefrontal cortex and amygdala in simple fabrication and deception with social interactions. *Journal of Cognitive Neuroscience, 19*, 287–295.

Aben, B., Stapert, S., and Blokland, A. (2012). About the distinction between working memory and short-term memory. *Frontiers in Psychology, 3*, 301. doi:10.3389/fpsyg.2012.00301

Abramowitz, J. S., Blakey, S. M., Reuman, L., and Buchholz, J. L. (2018). New directions in the cognitive-behavioral treatment of OCD: Theory, research, and practice. *Behavior Therapy, 49*(3), 311–322.

Absil, P., Pinxten, R., Balthazart, J., and Eens, M. (2003). Effect of age and testosterone on autumnal neurogenesis in male European starlings (*Sturnus vulgaris*). *Behavioural Brain Research, 143*, 15–30.

Ackermann, S., and Rasch, B. (2018). Differential effects of non-REM and REM sleep on memory consolidation? *Current Neurology and Neuroscience Reports, 14*(2), 430.

Ader, R. (2001). Psychoneuroimmunology. *Current Directions in Psychological Science, 10*(3), 94–98.

Adler, E., Hoon, M. A., Mueller, K. L., Chandrashekar, J., et al. (2000). A novel family of mammalian taste receptors. *Cell, 100*, 693–702.

Adolphs, R., Gosselin, F., Buchanan, T. W., Tranel, D., et al. (2005). A mechanism for impaired fear recognition after amygdala damage. *Nature, 433*, 68–72.

Agarwal, N., Pacher, P., Tegeder, I., Amay, F., et al. (2007). Cannabinoids mediate analgesia largely via peripheral type cannabinoid receptors in nociceptors. *Nature Neuroscience, 10*, 870–878.

Agmon-Snir, H., Carr, C. E., and Rinzel, J. (1998). The role of dendrites in auditory coincidence detection. *Nature, 393*, 268–272.

Ahn, S., and Phillips, A. G. (2002). Modulation by central and basolateral amygdalar nuclei of dopaminergic correlates of feeding to satiety in the rat nucleus accumbens and medial prefrontal cortex. *Journal of Neuroscience, 22*, 10958–10965.

Ajslev, T. A., Andersen, C. S., Gamborg, M., Sørensen, T. I., et al. (2011). Childhood overweight after establishment of the gut microbiota: The role of delivery mode, pre-pregnancy weight and early administration of antibiotics. *International Journal of Obesity (London), 35*(4), 522–529.

Al-Barazanji, K. A., Buckingham, R. E., Arch, J. R., Haynes, A., et al. (1997). Effects of intracerebroventricular infusion of leptin in obese Zucker rats. *Obesity Research, 5*, 387–394.

Albers, G. W., Marks, M. P., Kemp, S., Christensen, S., et al. (2018). Thrombectomy for stroke at 6 to 16 hours with selection by perfusion imaging. *New England Journal of Medicine*. PubMed PMID: 29364767. [Epub ahead of print] doi:10.1056/NEJMoa1713973

Alberts, J. R. (1978). Huddling by rat pups: Multisensory control of contact behavior. *Journal of Comparative and Physiological Psychology, 92*, 220–230.

Aldrich, M. A. (1993). The neurobiology of narcolepsy-cataplexy. *Progress in Neurobiology, 41*, 533–541.

Almer, G., Hainfellner, J. A., Brücke, T., Jellinger, K., et al. (1999). Fatal familial insomnia: A new Austrian family. *Brain, 122*, 5–16.

Almutairi, N., Kundart, J., Muthuramalingam, N., Hayes, J., et al. (2017). *Assessment of Enchroma filter for correcting color vision deficiency* (Dissertation). Retrieved from College of Optometry. 21. (http://commons.pacificu.edu/opt/21)

Altemus, M., Sarvaiya, N., and Neill Epperson, C. (2014). Sex differences in anxiety and depression clinical perspectives. *Frontiers in Neuroendocrinology, 35*(3), 320–330.

Altschuler, E. L., Wisdom, S. B., Stone, L., Foster, C., et al. (1999). Rehabilitation of hemiparesis after stroke with a mirror. *Lancet, 353*, 2035–2036.

Alvarez, J. A., and Emory, E. (2006). Executive function and the frontal lobes: A meta-analytic review. *Neuropsychology Review, 16*, 17–42.

American Psychiatric Association. (2013). *Diagnostic and statistical manual of mental disorders: DSM-5*. Washington, DC: American Psychiatric Association.

Amici, R., Bastianini, S., Berteotti, C., Cerri, M., et al. (2014). Sleep and bodily functions: The physiological interplay between body homeostasis and sleep homeostasis. *Archives Italiennes de Biologie, 152*, 66–78.

Amunts, K., Schlaug, G., Jaencke, L., Steinmetz, H., et al. (1997). Motor cortex and hand motor skills: Structural compliance in the human brain. *Human Brain Mapping, 5*, 206–215.

Anacker, C., Luna, V. M., Stevens, G. S., Millette, A., et al. (2018). Hippocampal neurogenesis confers stress resilience by inhibiting the ventral dentate gyrus. *Nature, 559*(7712), 98–102.

Anand, B. K., and Brobeck, J. R. (1951). Localization of a "feeding center" in the hypothalamus of the rat. *Proceedings of the Society for Experimental Biology and Medicine, 77*, 323–324.

Andersen, B. B., Korbo, L., and Pakkenberg, B. (1992). A quantitative study of the human cerebellum with unbiased stereological techniques. *Journal of Comparative Neurology, 326*, 549–560.

Andersen, P. M., Nilsson, P., Ala-Hurula, V., Keranen, M. L., et al. (1995). Amyotrophic lateral sclerosis associated with homozygosity for an Asp90Ala mutation in CuZn-superoxide dismutase. *Nature Genetics, 10*, 61–66.

Andics, A., Gábor, A., Gácsi, M., Faragó, T., et al. (2016). Neural mechanisms for lexical processing in dogs. *Science, 353*(6303), 1030–1032.

Andreasen, N., Nassrallah, H. A., Dunn, V., Olson, S. C., et al. (1986). Structural abnormalities in the frontal system in schizophrenia. *Archives of General Psychiatry, 43*, 136–144.

Anstey, M. L., Rogers, S. M., Ott, S. R., Burrows, M., et al. (2009). Serotonin mediates behavioral gregarization underlying swarm formation in desert locusts. *Science, 323*(5914), 627–630.

Apkarian, A. V., Sosa, Y., Sonty, S., Levy, R. M., et al. (2004). Chronic back pain is associated with decreased prefrontal and thalamic gray matter density. *Journal of Neuroscience, 24*, 10410–10415.

Archer, G. S., Friend, T. H., Piedrahita, J., Nevill, C. H., et al. (2003). Behavioral variation among cloned pigs. *Applied Animal Behaviour Science, 82*, 151–161.

Archer, J. (2006). Testosterone and human aggression: An evaluation of the challenge hypothesis. *Neuroscience and Biobehavioral Reviews, 30,* 319–345.

Argyll-Robertson, D. M. C. L. (1869). On an interesting series of eye symptoms in a case of spinal disease, with remarks on the action of belladonna on the iris. *Edinburgh Medical Journal, 14,* 696–708.

Arnold, A. P. (1980). Sexual differences in the brain. *American Scientist, 68,* 165–173.

Arnold, A. P., and Schlinger, B. A. (1993). Sexual differentiation of brain and behavior: The zebra finch is not just a flying rat. *Brain, Behavior and Evolution, 42,* 231–241.

Arnone, D., Cavanagh, J., Gerber, D., Lawrie, S. M., et al. (2009). Magnetic resonance imaging studies in bipolar disorder and schizophrenia: Meta-analysis. *British Journal of Psychiatry, 195,* 194–201.

Arnsten, A. F. (2006). Fundamentals of attention-deficit/hyperactivity disorder: Circuits and pathways. *Journal of Clinical Psychiatry, 67,* 7–12.

Asberg, M., Nordstrom, P., and Traskman-Bendz, L. (1986). Cerebrospinal fluid studies in suicide. An overview. *Annals of the New York Academy of Sciences, 487,* 243–255.

Aschner, M., and Ceccatelli, S. (2010). Are neuropathological conditions relevant to ethylmercury exposure? *Neurotoxicity Research, 18,* 59–68.

Aschwanden, C. (2013, March 9). The curious lives of people who feel no fear. *New Scientist,* 2907, 36–40.

Aserinsky, E., and Kleitman, N. (1953). Regularly occurring periods of eye motility, and concomitant phenomena, during sleep. *Science, 118,* 273–274.

Ashmore, J. F. (1994). The cellular machinery of the cochlea. *Experimental Physiology, 79,* 113–134.

Ashtari, M., Kumra, S., Bhaskar, S. L., Clarke, T., et al. (2005). Attention-deficit/hyperactivity disorder: A preliminary diffusion tensor imaging study. *Biological Psychiatry, 57,* 448–455.

Assaf, Y., and Pasternak, O. (2008). Diffusion tensor imaging (DTI)-based white matter mapping in brain research: A review. *Journal of Molecular Neuroscience, 34,* 51–61.

Audero, E., Coppi, E., Mlinar, B., Rossetti, T., et al. (2008). Sporadic autonomic dysregulation and death associated with excessive serotonin autoinhibition. *Science, 321,* 130–133.

Augustine, V., Gokce, S. K., Lee, S., Wang, B., et al. (2018). Hierarchical neural architecture underlying thirst regulation. *Nature, 555*(7695), 204–209.

Aungst, J. L., Heyward, P. M., Puche, A. C., Karnup, S. V., et al. (2003). Centre-surround inhibition among olfactory bulb glomeruli. *Nature, 426,* 623–629.

Avila, M. T., Hong, L. E., Moates, A., Turano, K. A., et al. (2006). Role of anticipation in schizophrenia-related pursuit initiation deficits. *Journal of Neurophysiology, 95,* 593–601.

B

Baars, B. J., Ramsøy, T. Z., and Laureys, S. (2003). Brain, conscious experience and the observing self. *Trends in Neuroscience, 26,* 671–675.

Badre, D., and Nee, D. E. (2018). Frontal cortex and the hierarchical control of behavior. *Trends in Cognitive Sciences, 22*(2), 170–188.

Bagemihl, B. (1999). *Biological exuberance: Animal homosexuality and natural diversity.* New York, NY: St. Martin's Press.

Bailey, C. H., and Chen, M. (1983). Morphological basis of long-term habituation and sensitization in *Aplysia. Science, 220,* 91–93.

Bailey, J. M., Pillard, R. C., Neale, M. C., and Agyei, Y. (1993). Heritable factors influence sexual orientation in women. *Archives of General Psychiatry, 50,* 217–223.

Bailey, K., and West, R. (2013). The effects of an action video game on visual and affective information processing. *Brain Research, 1504,* 35–46.

Baillet, S. (2017). Magnetoencephalography for brain electrophysiology and imaging. *Nature Neuroscience, 20*(3), 327–339.

Bakker, J., De Mees, C., Douhard, Q., Balthazart, J., et al. (2006). Alpha-fetoprotein protects the developing female mouse brain from masculinization and defeminization by estrogens. *Nature Neuroscience, 9,* 220–226.

Baldermann, J. C., Schüller, T., Huys, D., Becker, I., et al. (2016). Deep brain stimulation for Tourette-syndrome: A systematic review and meta-analysis. *Brain Stimulation, 9*(2), 296–304.

Baldwin, M. W, Toda, Y., Nakagita, T., O'Connell, M. J., et al. (2014). Sensory biology: Evolution of sweet taste perception in hummingbirds by transformation of the ancestral umami receptor. *Science, 345,* 929–933.

Ball, G. F., and Hulse, S. H. (1998). Birdsong. *American Psychologist, 53,* 37–58.

Ban, T. A. (2007). Fifty years chlorpromazine: A historical perspective. *Neuropsychiatric Disease and Treatment, 3*(4), 495–500.

Bancaud, J., Brunet-Bourgin, F., Chauvel, P., and Halgren, E. (1994). Anatomical origin of deja vu and vivid "memories" in human temporal lobe. *Brain, 117,* 71–90.

Bao, S., Chan, V. T., and Merzenich, M. M. (2001). Cortical remodelling induced by activity of ventral tegmental dopamine neurons. *Nature, 412,* 79–83.

Baptista, L. F. (1996). Nature and its nurturing in avian vocal development. In D. E.

Kroodsma and E. H. Miller (Eds.), *Ecology and evolution of acoustic communication in birds* (pp. 39–60). Ithaca, NY: Cornell University Press.

Baptista, L., and Petrinovich, L. (1986). Song development in the white-crowned sparrow: Social factors and sex differences. *Animal Behaviour, 34,* 1359–1371.

Barbeau, H., Norman, K., Fung, J., Visintin, M., et al. (1998). Does neurorehabilitation play a role in the recovery of walking in neurological populations? *Annals of the New York Academy of Sciences, 860,* 377–392.

Bark, N. (2002). Did schizophrenia change the course of English history? The mental illness of Henry VI. *Medical Hypotheses, 59,* 416–421.

Barkow, J. H., Cosmides, L., and Tooby, J. (1992). *The adapted mind: Evolutionary psychology and the generation of culture.* New York, NY: Oxford University Press.

Barnea, G., O'Donnell, S., Mancia, F., Sun, X., et al. (2004). Odorant receptors on axon termini in the brain. *Science, 304,* 1468.

Baron-Cohen, S. (2003). *The essential difference: Men, women and the extreme male brain.* London, UK: Allen Lane.

Barnett, S.A. (1975). *The rat: A study in behavior.* Chicago: University of Chicago Press.

Barrett, A. M., Goedert, K. M., and Basso, J. C. (2012). Prism adaptation for spatial neglect after stroke: Translational practice gaps. *Nature Reviews Neurology, 8*(10), 567–577.

Barrio, J. R., Small, G. W., Wong, K. P., Huang, S. C., et al. (2015). In vivo characterization of chronic traumatic encephalopathy using [F-18]FDDNP PET brain imaging. *Proceedings of the National Academy of Sciences, USA, 112*(16), E2039–E2047.

Bartels, A., and Zeki, S. (2000). The neural basis of romantic love. *NeuroReport, 11,* 3829–3834.

Bartfai, T. (2001). Telling the brain about pain. *Nature, 410,* 425–426.

Bartolomeo, P. (2007). Visual neglect. *Current Opinion in Neurology, 20,* 381–386.

Bartoshuk, L. M. (1993). Genetic and pathological taste variation: What can we learn from animal models and human disease? In D. Chadwick, J. Marsh, and J. Goode (Eds.), *The molecular basis of smell and taste transduction* (pp. 251–267). New York, NY: Wiley.

Bartoshuk, L. M., and Beauchamp, G. K. (1994). Chemical senses. *Annual Review of Psychology, 45,* 419–449.

Basson, R. (2001). Human sex-response cycles. *Journal of Sex & Marital Therapy, 27,* 33–43.

Basson, R. (2008). Women's sexual function and dysfunction: Current uncertainties, future directions. *International Journal of Impotence Research, 20,* 466–478.

Bates, E., Wilson, S. M., Saygin, A. P., Dick, F., et al. (2003). Voxel-based lesion-symptom mapping. *Nature Neuroscience, 6*, 448–450.

Batterham, R. L., and Bloom, S. R. (2003). The gut hormone peptide YY regulates appetite. *Annals of the New York Academy of Sciences, 994*, 162–168.

Bautista, D. M., Siemens, J., Glazer, J. M., Tsuruda, P. R., et al. (2007). The menthol receptor TRPM8 is the principal detector of environmental cold. *Nature, 448*, 204–208.

Baynes, K. C., Dhillo, W. S., and Bloom, S. R. (2006). Regulation of food intake by gastrointestinal hormones. *Current Opinion in Gastroenterology, 22*, 626–631.

Beach, F. A. (1976). Sexual attractivity, proceptivity, and receptivity in female mammals. *Hormones and Behavior, 7*, 105–138.

Beach, F. A. (1977). *Human sexuality in four perspectives*. Baltimore, MD: Johns Hopkins University Press.

Bedrosian, T. A., Vaughn, C. A., Galan, A., Daye, G., et al. (2013). Nocturnal light exposure impairs affective responses in a wavelength-dependent manner. *Journal of Neuroscience, 33*, 13081–13087.

Bee, M. A., and Micheyl, C. (2008). The cocktail party problem: What is it? How can it be solved? And why should animal behaviorists study it? *Journal of Comparative Psychology, 122*, 235–251.

Beeli, G., Esslen, M., and Jäncke, L. (2005). When coloured sounds taste sweet. *Nature, 434*, 38.

Beggs, S., Trang, T., and Salter, M. W. (2012). P2X4R+ microglia drive neuropathic pain. *Nature Neuroscience, 15*, 1068–1073.

Beggs, W. D., and Foreman, D. L. (1980). Sound localization and early binaural experience in the deaf. *British Journal of Audiology, 14*, 41–48.

Bellinger, D. L., Ackerman, K. D., Felten, S. Y., and Felten, D. L. (1992). A longitudinal study of age-related loss of noradrenergic nerves and lymphoid cells in the rat spleen. *Experimental Neurology, 116*, 295–311.

Bellugi, U., Poizner, H., and Klima, E. S. (1983). Brain organization for language: Clues from sign aphasia. *Human Neurobiology, 2*, 155–171.

Bennett, A. F., and Ruben, J. A. (1979). Endothermy and activity in vertebrates. *Science, 206*, 649–654.

Bennett, M. V. (2000). Electrical synapses, a personal perspective (or history). *Brain Research Reviews, 32*, 16–28.

Bennett, W. (1983). The nicotine fix. *Rhode Island Medical Journal, 66*, 455–458.

Benney, K. S., and Braaten, R. F. (2000). Auditory scene analysis in estrildid finches (*Taeniopygia guttata* and *Lonchura striata domestica*): A species advantage for detection of conspecific song. *Journal of Comparative Psychology, 114*, 174–182.

Benson, P. J., Beedie, S. A., Shephard, E., Giegling, I., et al. (2012). Simple viewing tests can detect eye movement abnormalities that distinguish schizophrenia cases from controls with exceptional accuracy. *Biological Psychiatry, 72*(9), 716–724.

Berenbaum, S. A. (2001). Cognitive function in congenital adrenal hyperplasia. *Endocrinology and Metabolism Clinics of North America, 30*, 173–192.

Berman, K. F., Torrey, E. F., Daniel, D. G., and Weinberger, D. R. (1992). Regional cerebral blood flow in monozygotic twins discordant and concordant for schizophrenia. *Archives of General Psychiatry, 49*(12), 927–934.

Bermon, S., Garnier, P. Y., Hirschberg, A. L., Robinson, N., et al. (2014). Serum androgen levels in elite female athletes. *Journal of Clinical Endocrinology and Metabolism, 99*(11), 4328–4335.

Bernal, B., and Altman, N. (2010). The connectivity of the superior longitudinal fasciculus: A tractography DTI study. *Magnetic Resonance Imaging, 28*, 217–225.

Bernhardt, P. C. (1997). Influences of serotonin and testosterone in aggression and dominance: Convergence with social psychology. *Current Directions in Psychological Science, 2*(6), 44–48.

Bernhardt, P. C., Dabbs, J. M., Jr., Fielden, J. A., and Lutter, C. D. (1998). Testosterone changes during vicarious experiences of winning and losing among fans at sporting events. *Physiology & Behavior, 65*, 59–62.

Bernstein, I. S., and Gordon, T. P. (1974). The function of aggression in primate societies. *American Scientist, 62*, 304–311.

Bernstein, L. E., Auer, E. T., Jr., Moore, J. K., Ponton, C. W., et al. (2002). Visual speech perception without primary auditory cortex activation. *NeuroReport, 13*, 311–315.

Bernstein-Goral, H., and Bregman, B. S. (1993). Spinal cord transplants support the regeneration of axotomized neurons after spinal cord lesions at birth: A quantitative double-labeling study. *Experimental Neurology, 123*, 118–132.

Berthold, A. (1849). Transplantation der Hoden. *Archiv für Anatomie, Physiologie und Wissenschaftliche Medicin, 16*, 42–46.

Bertram, L., and Tanzi, R. E. (2008). Thirty years of Alzheimer's disease genetics: The implications of systematic meta-analyses. *Nature Reviews Neuroscience, 9*, 768–778.

Besedovsky, H. O., and del Rey, A. (1992). Immune-neuroendocrine circuits: Integrative role of cytokines. *Frontiers of Neuroendocrinology, 13*, 61–94.

Binder, J. R., Rao, S. M., Hammeke, T. A., Yetkin, F. Z., et al. (1994). Functional magnetic resonance imaging of human auditory cortex. *Annals of Neurology, 35*, 662–672.

Birch, L. L., Fisher, J. O., and Davison, K. K. (2003). Learning to overeat: Maternal use of restrictive feeding practices promotes girls' eating in the absence of hunger. *American Journal of Clinical Nutrition, 78*, 215–220.

Birnbaum, R., and Weinberger, D. R. (2017). Genetic insights into the neurodevelopmental origins of schizophrenia. *Nature Reviews Neuroscience, 18*(12), 727–740.

Bisley, J. W., and Goldberg, M. E. (2003). Neuronal activity in the lateral intraparietal area and spatial attention. *Science, 299*, 81–86.

Blackwell, D. L, Lucas, J. W, and Clarke, T. C. (2014). Summary health statistics for U.S. adults: National Health Interview Survey, 2012. *Vital and Health Statistics 10*(260), 1–161.

Blackwell, D. L., and Villarroel, M. A. (2018). Tables of Summary Health Statistics (for U.S. Adults: 2016 National Health Interview Survey), www.cdc.gov/nchs/nhis/SHS/tables.htm.

Blake, D. J., Weir, A., Newey, S. E., and Davies, K. E. (2002). Function and genetics of dystrophin and dystrophin-related proteins in muscle. *Physiology Review, 82*, 291–329.

Blake, D. T., Heiser, M. A., Caywood, M., and Merzenich, M. M. (2006). Experience-dependent adult cortical plasticity requires cognitive association between sensation and reward. *Neuron, 52*, 371–381.

Blakemore, C., and Campbell, F. W. (1969). On the existence of neurones in the human visual system selectively sensitive to the orientation and size of retinal images. *Journal of Physiology (London), 203*, 237–260.

Blanchard, R., Cantor, J. M., Bogaert, A. F., Breedlove, S. M., et al. (2006). Interaction of fraternal birth order and handedness in the development of male homosexuality. *Hormones and Behavior, 49*, 405–414.

Blehar, M. C., and Rosenthal, N. E. (1989). Seasonal affective disorders and phototherapy. Report of a National Institute of Mental Health–sponsored workshop. *Archives of General Psychiatry, 46*, 469–474.

Bleuler, E. (1950). *Dementia praecox; or, The group of schizophrenias* (J. Zinkin, Trans.). New York, NY: International Universities Press.

Bliss, T. V. P., and Gardner-Medwin, A. R. (1973). Long-lasting potentiation of synaptic transmission in the dentate area of the unanaesthetized rabbit following stimulation of the perforant path. *Journal of Physiology (London), 232*, 357–374.

Bliss, T. V. P., and Lømo, T. (1973). Long-lasting potentiation of synaptic transmission in the dentate area of the anaesthetized rabbit following stimulation of the perforant path. *Journal of Physiology (London), 232,* 331–356.

Bliwise, D. L. (1989). Neuropsychological function and sleep. *Clinics in Geriatric Medicine, 5,* 381–394.

Bloom, F. E., and Lazerson, A. (1988). *Brain, Mind, and Behavior* (2nd ed.). New York: W. H. Freeman and Company.

Blum, I. D., Bell, B., and Wu, M. N. (2018). Time for bed: Genetic mechanisms mediating the circadian regulation of sleep. *Trends in Genetics, 34*(5), 379–388.

Blumberg, M. S., Sokoloff, G., and Kirby, R. F. (1997). Brown fat thermogenesis and cardiac rate regulation during cold challenge in infant rats. *American Journal of Physiology, 272,* R1308–R1313.

Blumberger, D. M., Hsu, J. H., and Daskalakis, Z. J. (2015). A review of brain stimulation treatments for late-life depression. *Current Treatment Options in Psychiatry, 2*(4), 413–421.

Blumstein, S. E., and Amso, D. (2013). Dynamic functional organization of language: Insights from functional neuroimaging. *Perspectives on Psychological Science, 8*(1), 44–48.

Boddhula, S. K., Boddhula, S., Gunasekaran, K., and Bischof, E. (2018). An unusual cause of thunderclap headache after eating the hottest pepper in the world—"The Carolina Reaper." *BMJ Case Reports,* pii: bcr-2017-224085. doi:10.1136/bcr-2017-224085

Boets, B., Op de Beeck, H. P., Vandermosten, M., Scott, S. K., et al. (2013). Intact but less accessible phonetic representations in adults with dyslexia. *Science, 342*(6163), 1251–1254.

Bogaert, A. F. (2006). Biological versus nonbiological older brothers and men's sexual orientation. *Proceedings of the National Academy of Sciences, USA, 103,* 10771–10774.

Bogaert, A. F. (2007). Extreme right-handedness, older brothers, and sexual orientation in men. *Neuropsychology, 21,* 141–148.

Bogaert, A. F., Skorska, M. N., Wang, C., Gabrie, J., et al. (2018). Male homosexuality and maternal immune responsivity to the Y-linked protein NLGN4Y. *Proceedings of the National Academy of Sciences, USA, 115*(2), 302–306.

Bogenschutz, M. P., and Johnson, M. W. (2016). Classic hallucinogens in the treatment of addictions. *Progress in Neuro-Psychopharmacology and Biological Psychiatry, 64,* 250–258.

Bogin, B. (1997). Evolutionary hypotheses for human childhood. *Yearbook of Physical Anthropology, 40,* 63–89.

Boldrini, M., Fulmore, C. A., Tartt, A. N., Simeon, L. R., et al. (2018). Human hippocampal neurogenesis persists throughout aging. *Cell Stem Cell, 22*(4), 589–599.

Bolhuis, J. J., and Gahr, M. (2006). Neural mechanisms of birdsong memory. *Nature Reviews Neuroscience, 7,* 347–357.

Bolhuis, J. J., Okanoya, K., and Scharff, C. (2010). Twitter evolution: Converging mechanisms in birdsong and human speech. *Nature Reviews Neuroscience, 11,* 747–759.

Bonaz, B., Bazin, T., and Pellissier, S. (2018). The vagus nerve at the interface of the microbiota-gut-brain axis. *Frontiers in Neuroscience, 12,* 49. doi:10.3389/fnins.2018.00049

Bonnel, A. M., and Prinzmetal, W. (1998). Dividing attention between the color and the shape of objects. *Perception & Psychophysics, 60,* 113–124.

Boolell, M., Gepi-Attee, S., Gingell, J. C., and Allen, M. J. (1996). Sildenafil, a novel effective oral therapy for male erectile dysfunction. *British Journal of Urology, 78,* 257–261.

Boot, W. R., Kramer, A. F., Simons, D. J., Fabiani, M., et al. (2008). The effects of video game playing on attention, memory, and executive control. *Acta Psychologica (Amsterdam), 129,* 387–398.

Borgstein, J., and Grootendorst, C. (2002). Clinical picture: Half a brain. *Lancet, 359,* 473.

Borota, D., Murray, E., Keceli, G., Chang, A., et al. (2014). Post-study caffeine administration enhances memory consolidation in humans. *Nature Neuroscience, 17*(2), 201–203.

Boshuisen, K., van Schooneveld, M. M., Leijten, F. S., de Kort, G. A., et al. (2010). Contralateral MRI abnormalities affect seizure and cognitive outcome after hemispherectomy. *Neurology, 75,* 1623–1630.

Boström, P., Wu, J., Jedrychowski, M. P., Korde, A., et al. (2012). A PGC1-α-dependent myokine that drives brown-fat-like development of white fat and thermogenesis. *Nature, 481,* 463–846.

Bottjer, S. W., Miesner, E. A., and Arnold, A. P. (1984). Forebrain lesions disrupt development but not maintenance of song in passerine birds. *Science, 224,* 901–903.

Bourke, C. H., Stowe, Z. N., and Owens, M. J. (2014). Prenatal antidepressant exposure: Clinical and preclinical findings. *Pharmacological Reviews, 66,* 435–465.

Bourque, C. W. (2008). Central mechanisms of osmosensation and systemic osmoregulation. *Nature Reviews Neuroscience, 9,* 519–531.

Bourque, J., Afzali, M. H., O'Leary-Barrett, M., and Conrod P. (2017). Cannabis use and psychotic-like experiences trajectories during early adolescence: The coevolution and potential mediators. *Journal of Child Psychology and Psychiatry, 58*(12), 1360–1369.

Bouwknecht, J. A., Hijzen, T. H., van der Gugten, J., Maes, R. A., et al. (2001).

Absence of 5-HT(1B) receptors is associated with impaired impulse control in male 5-HT(1B) knockout mice. *Biological Psychiatry, 49,* 557–568.

Bower, B. (2006). Prescription for controversy: Medications for depressed kids spark scientific dispute. *Science News, 169,* 168–172.

Bowman, M. L. (1997). *Individual differences in posttraumatic response.* Mahwah, NJ: Erlbaum.

Boyce, R., Glasgow, S. D., Williams, S., and Adamantidis, A. (2016). Causal evidence for the role of REM sleep theta rhythm in contextual memory consolidation. *Science, 352*(6287), 812–816.

Brady, T. F., Konkle, T., Alvarez, G. A., and Oliva, A. (2014). Visual long-term memory has a massive storage capacity for object details. *Proceedings of the National Academy of Sciences, USA, 105,* 14325–14329.

Brainard, D. H., Roorda, A., Yamauchi, Y., Calderone, J. B., et al. (2000). Functional consequences of the relative numbers of L and M cones. *Journal of the Optical Society of America. Part A, Optics, Image Science and Vision, 17,* 607–614.

Brandlistuen, R. E., Ystrom, E., Eberhard-Gran, M., Nulman, I., et al. (2015). Behavioural effects of fetal antidepressant exposure in a Norwegian cohort of discordant siblings. *International Journal of Epidemiology, 44*(4), 1397–1407.

Brasser, S. M., Mozhui, K., and Smith, D. V. (2005). Differential covariation in taste responsiveness to bitter stimuli in rats. *Chemical Senses, 30,* 793–799.

Bray, G. A. (1969). Effect of caloric restriction on energy expenditure in obese patients. *Lancet, 2,* 397–398.

Breier, A., Malhotra, A. K., Pinals, D. A., Weisenfeld, N. I., et al. (1997). Association of ketamine-induced psychosis with focal activation of the prefrontal cortex in healthy volunteers. *American Journal of Psychiatry, 154*(6), 805–811.

Breitner, J. C., Wyse, B. W., Anthony, J. C., Welsh-Bohmer, K. A., et al. (1999). APOE-epsilon4 count predicts age when prevalence of AD increases, then declines: The Cache County Study. *Neurology, 53,* 321–331.

Bremer, F. (1938). L'activité électrique de l'écorce cérébrale. *Actualités Scientifiques et Industrielles, 658,* 3–46.

Bremner, J. D., Randall, P., Scott, T. M., Bronen, R. A., et al. (1995). MRI-based measurement of hippocampal volume in patients with combat-related posttraumatic stress disorder. *American Journal of Psychiatry, 152,* 973–981.

Brennan, P., Kaba, H., and Keverne, E. B. (1990). Olfactory recognition: A simple memory system. *Science, 250,* 1223–1226.

Brennan, S. C., Davies, T. S., Schepelmann, M., and Riccardi, D. (2014). Emerging roles of the extracellular calcium-sensing receptor in nutrient sensing: Control of taste modulation and intestinal hormone secretion. *British Journal of Nutrition, 111*(Suppl. 1), S16–22.

Brigande, J. V., and Heller, S. (2009). Quo vadis, hair cell regeneration? *Nature Neuroscience, 12*, 679–685.

Briggs, F., Mangun, G. R., and Usrey, W. M. (2013). Attention enhances synaptic efficacy and the signal-to-noise ratio in neural circuits. *Nature, 499*(7459), 476–480.

Broadbent, D. A. (1958). *Perception and communication.* New York, NY: Pergamon Press.

Broberg, D. J., and Bernstein, I. L. (1989). Cephalic insulin release in anorexic women. *Physiology & Behavior, 45*, 871–874.

Brouwer, H., Crocker, M. W., Venhuizen, N. J., and Hoeks, J. C. J. (2017). A neurocomputational model of the N400 and the P600 in language processing. *Cognitive Science, 41*(Suppl. 6), 1318–1352.

Brown, A. S. (2011). The environment and susceptibility to schizophrenia. *Progress in Neurobiology, 93*, 23–58.

Brown, C. (2003, February 2). The man who mistook his wife for a deer. *The New York Times*, Section 6, p. 32.

Brown, E. C., Jeong, J. W., Muzik, O., Rothermel, R., et al. (2014). Evaluating the arcuate fasciculus with combined diffusion-weighted MRI tractography and electrocorticography. *Human Brain Mapping, 35*, 2333–2347.

Brown, J. (1958). Some tests of the decay theory of immediate memory. *Quarterly Journal of Experimental Psychology, 10*, 12–21.

Brown, R. E., and Milner, P. M. (2003). The legacy of Donald O. Hebb: More than the Hebb synapse. *Nature Reviews Neuroscience, 4*(12), 1013–1019.

Brown, S. P., Mathur, B. N., Olsen, S. R., Luppi, P. H., et al. (2017). New breakthroughs in understanding the role of functional interactions between the neocortex and the claustrum. *Journal of Neuroscience, 37*(45), 10877–10881.

Brownlee, S., and Schrof, J. M. (1997). The quality of mercy. Effective pain treatments already exist. Why aren't doctors using them? *U.S. News & World Report, 122*, 54–67.

Bruel-Jungerman, E., Davis, S., Rampon, C., and Laroche, S. (2006). Long-term potentiation enhances neurogenesis in the adult dentate gyrus. *The Journal of Neuroscience, 26*, 5888–5893.

Bruel-Jungerman, E., Rampon, C., and Laroche, S. (2007). Adult hippocampal neurogenesis, synaptic plasticity and memory: Facts and hypotheses. *Review in the Neurosciences, 18*, 93–114.

Brunetti, M., Della Penna, S., Ferretti, A., Del Gratta, C., et al. (2008). A fronto-parietal network for spatial attention reorienting in the auditory domain: A human fMRI/MEG study of functional and temporal dynamics. *Cerebral Cortex, 18*, 1139–1147.

Bryant, P., Trinder, J., and Curtis, N. (2004). Sick and tired: Does sleep have a vital role in the immune system? *Nature Reviews Immunology, 4*, 457–467.

Bu, G. (2009). Apolipoprotein E and its receptors in Alzheimer's disease: Pathways, pathogenesis and therapy. *Nature Reviews Neuroscience, 10*, 333–344.

Buccino, G., Lui, F., Canessa, N., Patteri, I., et al. (2004). Neural circuits involved in the recognition of actions performed by nonconspecifics: An fMRI study. *Journal of Cognitive Neuroscience, 16*, 114–126.

Buccino, G., Solodkin, A., and Small, S. L. (2006). Functions of the mirror neuron system: Implications for neurorehabilitation. *Cognitive and Behavioral Neurology, 19*, 55–63.

Buchsbaum, B. R., Baldo, J., Okada, K., Berman, K. F., et al. (2011). Conduction aphasia, sensory-motor integration, and phonological short-term memory—An aggregate analysis of lesion and fMRI data. *Brain and Language, 119*, 119–128.

Buchsbaum, M. S., Buchsbaum, B. R., Chokron, S., Tang, C., et al. (2006). Thalamocortical circuits: fMRI assessment of the pulvinar and medial dorsal nucleus in normal volunteers. *Neuroscience Letters, 404*, 282–287.

Buchsbaum, M. S., Mirsky, A. F., DeLisi, L. E., Morihisa, J., et al. (1984) The Genain quadruplets: Electrophysiological, positron emission and X-ray tomographic studies. *Psychiatry Research, 13*, 95–108.

Buck, L., and Axel, R. (1991). A novel multigene family may encode odorant receptors: A molecular basis for odor recognition. *Cell, 65*, 175–187.

Buckner, R. L., and Koutstaal, W. (1998). Functional neuroimaging studies of encoding, priming, and explicit memory retrieval. *Proceedings of the National Academy of Sciences, USA, 95*(3), 891–898.

Burgdorf, J., Kroes, R. A., Moskal, J. R., Pfaus, J. G., et al. (2008). Ultrasonic vocalizations of rats (*Rattus norvegicus*) during mating, play, and aggression: Behavioral concomitants, relationship to reward, and self-administration of playback. *Journal of Comparative Psychology, 122*, 357–367.

Burgdorf, J., Panksepp, J., and Moskal, J. R. (2011). Frequency-modulated 50 kHz ultrasonic vocalizations: A tool for uncovering the molecular substrates of positive affect. *Neuroscience & Biobehavioral Reviews, 35*, 1831–1836.

Burgess, H. J., and Emens, J. S. (2018). Drugs used in circadian sleep-wake rhythm disturbances. *Sleep Medicine Clinics, 13*(2), 231–241.

Bushdid, C., Magnasco, M. O., Vosshall, L. B., and Keller, A. (2014). Humans can discriminate more than 1 trillion olfactory stimuli. *Science, 343*(6177), 1370–1372.

Bushman, J. D., Ye, W., and Liman, E. R. (2015). A proton current associated with sour taste: Distribution and functional properties. *FASEB Journal, 29*, 3014–3026.

Buss, D. (2013). *Evolutionary psychology: The new science of the mind.* New York, NY: Psychology Press.

Butler, A. C., Chapman, J. E., Forman, E. M., and Beck, A. T. (2006). The empirical status of cognitive-behavioral therapy: A review of meta-analyses. *Clinical Psychology Review, 26*, 17–31.

Byne, W., Tobet, S., Mattiace, L. A., Lasco, M. S., et al. (2001). The interstitial nuclei of the human anterior hypothalamus: An investigation of variation with sex, sexual orientation, and HIV status. *Hormones and Behavior, 40*, 86–92.

C

Cade, J. F. (1949). Lithium salts in the treatment of psychotic excitement. *Medical Journal of Australia, 2*(10), 349–352.

Cahill, L. (2014). Equal ≠ the same: Sex differences in the human brain. *Cerebrum.* Apr 1, 5. eCollection 2014 (http://www.dana.org/Cerebrum/2014/Equal_%E2%89%A0_The_Same__Sex_Differences_in_the_Human_Brain/).

Cahill, L., and McGaugh, J. L. (1991). NMDA-induced lesions of the amygdaloid complex block the retention-enhancing effect of posttraining epinephrine. *Psychobiology, 19*, 206–210.

Cahill, L., Prins, B., Weber, M., and McGaugh, J. L. (1994). Beta-adrenergic activation and memory for emotional events. *Nature, 371*, 702–704.

Calder, A. J., Keane, J., Manes, F., Antoun, N., et al. (2000). Impaired recognition and experience of disgust following brain injury. *Nature Neuroscience, 3*, 1077.

Calvert, G. A., Bullmore, E. T., Brammer, M. J., Campbell, R., et al. (1997). Activation of auditory cortex during silent lipreading. *Science, 276*, 593–596.

Calvin, W. H., and Ojemann, G. A. (1994). *Conversation's with Neil's brain: The neural nature of thought and language.* Reading, MA: Adison-Wesley.

Cameron, J. L., Eagleson, K. L., Fox, N. A., Hensch, T. K., et al. (2017). Social origins of developmental risk for mental and physical illness. *Journal of Neuroscience, 37*(45), 10783–10791.

Campbell, F. W., and Robson, J. G. (1968). Application of Fourier analysis to the visibility of gratings. *Journal of Physiology (London), 197*, 551–566.

Cannon, T. D., Chung, Y., He, G., Sun, D., et al. (2015). Progressive reduction in cortical thickness as psychosis develops:

A multisite longitudinal neuroimaging study of youth at elevated clinical risk. *Biological Psychiatry, 77,* 147–157.

Cannon, W. B. (1929). *Bodily changes in pain, hunger, fear and rage.* New York, NY: Appleton.

Cantalupo, C., and Hopkins, W. D. (2001). Asymmetric Broca's area in great apes. *Nature, 414,* 505.

Cantor, J. M., Blanchard, R., Paterson, A. D., and Bogaert, A. F. (2002). How many gay men owe their sexual orientation to fraternal birth order? *Archives of Sexual Behavior, 31,* 63–71.

Cao, M., Shu, N., Cao, Q., Wang, Y., et al. (2014). Imaging functional and structural brain connectomics in attention-deficit/hyperactivity disorder. *Molecular Neurobiology, 50,* 1111–1123.

Cao, Y. Q., Mantyh, P. W., Carlson, E. J., Gillespie, A. M., et al. (1998). Primary afferent tachykinins are required to experience moderate to intense pain. *Nature, 392,* 390–394.

Caramazza, A., Anzellotti, S., Strnad, L., and Lingnau, A. (2014). Embodied cognition and mirror neurons: A critical assessment. *Annual Review of Neuroscience, 37,* 1–15.

Cardno, A. G., and Gottesman, I. I. (2000). Twin studies of schizophrenia: From bow-and-arrow concordances to Star Wars Mx and functional genomics. *American Journal of Medical Genetics, 97,* 12–17.

Carey, B. (2018, June 8). How suicide quietly morphed into a public health crisis. *The New York Times,* p. A21.

Carhart-Harris, R. L., Bolstridge, M., Rucker, J., Day, C. M., et al. (2016). Psilocybin with psychological support for treatment-resistant depression: An open-label feasibility study. *Lancet Psychiatry, 3*(7), 619–627.

Carhart-Harris, R. L., Erritzoe, D., Williams, T., Stone, J. M., et al. (2012). Neural correlates of the psychedelic state as determined by fMRI studies with psilocybin. *Proceedings of the National Academy of Sciences, USA, 109,* 2138–2143.

Carlson, P. J., Diazgranados, N., Nugent, A. C., Ibrahim, L., et al. (2013). Neural correlates of rapid antidepressant response to ketamine in treatment-resistant unipolar depression: A preliminary positron emission tomography study. *Biological Psychiatry, 73*(12), 1213–1221.

Carmichael, M. S., Warburton, V. L., Dixen, J., and Davidson, J. M. (1994). Relationships among cardiovascular, muscular, and oxytocin responses during human sexual activity. *Archives of Sexual Behavior, 23,* 59–79.

Carreiras, M., Lopez, J., Rivero, F., and Corina, D. (2005). Linguistic perception: Neural processing of a whistled language. *Nature, 433,* 31–32.

Carretié, L. (2014). Exogenous (automatic) attention to emotional stimuli: A review. *Cognitive, Affective, & Behavioral Neuroscience, 14*(4), 1228–1258.

Carroll, J., McMahon, C., Neitz, M., and Neitz, J. (2000). Flicker-photometric electroretinogram estimates of L:M cone photoreceptor ratio in men with photopigment spectra derived from genetics. *Journal of the Optical Society of America. Part A, Optics, Image Science, and Vision, 17,* 499–509.

Carter, C. S. (1992). Oxytocin and sexual behavior. *Neuroscience and Biobehavioral Reviews, 16,* 131–144.

Cartwright, R. D. (1979). The nature and function of repetitive dreams: A survey and speculation. *Psychiatry, 42,* 131–137.

Casarosa, S., Bozzi, Y., and Conti, L. (2014). Neural stem cells: Ready for therapeutic applications? *Molecular and Cellular Therapies, 2,* 31.

Castellanos, F. X., Lee, P. P., Sharp, W., Jeffries, N. O., et al. (2002). Developmental trajectories of brain volume abnormalities in children and adolescents with attention-deficit/hyperactivity disorder. *Journal of the American Medical Association, 288,* 1740–1748.

Caterina, M. J., Leffler, A., Malmberg, A. B., Martin, W. J., et al. (2000). Impaired nociception and pain sensation in mice lacking the capsaicin receptor. *Science, 288,* 306–313.

Caterina, M. J., Schumacher, M. A., Tominaga, M., Rosen, T. A., et al. (1997). The capsaicin receptor: A heat-activated ion channel in the pain pathway. *Nature, 389,* 816–824.

CDC (Centers for Disease Control and Prevention). (2010). Current depression among adults—United States, 2006 and 2008. *Morbidity and Mortality Weekly Report, 59,* 1229–1235 (www.cdc.gov/mmwr/preview/mmwrhtml/mm5938a2.htm).

CDC (Centers for Disease Control and Prevention). (2015). *Report to Congress on traumatic brain injury in the United States: Epidemiology and rehabilitation.* Atlanta, GA: National Center for Injury Prevention and Control, Division of Unintentional Injury Prevention.

CDC (Centers for Disease Control and Prevention). (2016). Fetal alcohol spectrum disorders (FASDs), www.cdc.gov/ncbddd/fasd/alcohol-use.html.

Celeghin, A., de Gelder, B., and Tamietto, M. (2015). From affective blindsight to emotional consciousness. *Consciousness and Cognition, 36,* 414–425.

Centerwall, B. S., and Criqui, M. H. (1978). Prevention of the Wernicke-Korsakoff syndrome: A cost-benefit analysis. *New England Journal of Medicine, 299,* 285–289.

Chamberlain, S. R., Menzies, L., Hampshire, A., Suckling, J., et al. (2008). Orbitofrontal dysfunction in patients with obsessive-compulsive disorder and their unaffected relatives. *Science, 321,* 421–422.

Champagne, F., Diorio, J., Sharma, S., and Meaney, M. J. (2001). Naturally occurring variations in maternal behavior in the rat are associated with differences in estrogen-inducible central oxytocin receptors. *Proceedings of the National Academy of Sciences, USA, 98,* 12736–12741.

Chan, M. Y., Na, J., Agres, P. F., Savalia, N. K., et al. (2018). Socioeconomic status moderates age-related differences in the brain's functional network organization and anatomy across the adult lifespan. *Proceedings of the National Academy of Sciences, USA, 115*(22), E5144–E5153.

Chandrashekar, J., Hoon, M. A., Ryba, N. J., and Zuker, C. S. (2006). The receptors and cells for mammalian taste. *Nature, 444,* 288–294.

Chandrashekar, J., Mueller, K. L., Hoon, M. A., Adler, E., et al. (2000). T2Rs function as bitter taste receptors. *Cell, 100,* 703–711.

Chandrashekar, J., Yarmolinsky, D., von Buchholtz, L., Oka, Y., et al. (2009). The taste of carbonation. *Science, 326,* 443–445.

Chang, B. S., Ly, J., Appignani, B., Bodell, A., et al. (2005). Reading impairment in the neuronal migration disorder of periventricular nodular heterotopia. *Neurology, 64,* 799–803.

Chapman, C. D., Dono, L. M., French, M. C., Weinberg, Z. Y., et al. (2012). Paraventricular nucleus anandamide signaling alters eating and substrate oxidation. *NeuroReport, 23,* 425–429.

Charney, D. S., Deutch, A. Y., Krystal, J. H., Southwick, S. M., et al. (1993). Psychobiologic mechanisms of posttraumatic stress disorder. *Archives of General Psychiatry, 50,* 295–305.

Charpentier, P., Gailliot, P., Jacob, R., Gaudechon, J., et al. (1952). Recherches sur les diméthylaminopropyl-N phénothiazines substituées. *Comptes rendus de l'Académie des Sciences (Paris), 235,* 59–60.

Chaudhari, N., Landin, A. M., and Roper, S. D. (2000). A metabotropic glutamate receptor variant functions as a taste receptor. *Nature Neuroscience, 3,* 113–119.

Chelikani, P. K., Haver, A. C., and Reidelberger, R. D. (2005). Intravenous infusion of peptide YY(3-36) potently inhibits food intake in rats. *Endocrinology, 146,* 879–888.

Chemelli, R. M., Willie, J. T., Sinton, C. M., Elmquist, J. K., et al. (1999). Narcolepsy in orexin knockout mice: Molecular genetics of sleep regulation. *Cell, 98,* 437–451.

Chen, L., and Feany, M. B. (2005). α-Synuclein phosphorylation controls neurotoxicity and inclusion formation in a Drosophila model of Parkinson disease. *Nature Neuroscience, 8,* 657–663.

Cherdieu, M., Versace, R., Rey, A. E., Vallet, G. T., et al. (2018). Sleep on your memory traces: How sleep effects can be explained by Act-In, a functional memory model. *Sleep Medicine Reviews, 39,* 155–163.

Cherry, E. C. (1953). Some experiments on the recognition of speech, with one and with two ears. *Journal of the Acoustical Society of America, 25,* 975–979.

Cheyne, J. A. (2002). Situational factors affecting sleep paralysis and associated hallucinations: Position and timing effects. *Journal of Sleep Research, 11,* 169–177.

Cho, I., Yamanishi, S., Cox, L., Methé, B. A., et al. (2012). Antibiotics in early life alter the murine colonic microbiome and adiposity. *Nature, 488*(7413), 621–626.

Choquet, D., and Triller, A. (2013). The dynamic synapse. *Neuron, 80*(3), 691–703.

Chung, W. S., Clarke, L. E., Wang, G. X., Stafford, B. K., et al. (2013). Astrocytes mediate synapse elimination through *MEGF10* and *MERTK* pathways. *Nature, 504*(7480), 394–400.

Chung, W. S., Welsh, C. A., Barres, B. A., and Stevens, B. (2015). Do glia drive synaptic and cognitive impairment in disease? *Nature Neuroscience, 18*(11), 1539–1545.

Chung, Y., Haut, K. M., He, G., van Erp, T. G. M., et al. (North American Prodrome Longitudinal Study Consortium). (2017). Ventricular enlargement and progressive reduction of cortical gray matter are linked in prodromal youth who develop psychosis. *Schizophrenia Research, 189,* 169–174.

Ciccocioppo, R., Martin-Fardon, R., and Weiss, F. (2004). Stimuli associated with a single cocaine experience elicit long-lasting cocaine-seeking. *Nature Neuroscience, 7,* 495–496.

Clapham, J. C., Arch, J. R. S., Chapman, H., Haynes, A., et al. (2000). Mice overexpressing human uncoupling protein-3 in skeletal muscle are hyperphagic and lean. *Nature, 406,* 415–418.

Clarke, E., Reichard, U. H., and Zuberbühler, K. (2015). Context-specific close-range "hoo" calls in wild gibbons (*Hylobates lar*). *BMC Evolutionary Biology, 15,* 56.

Clarke, M. C., Tanskanen, A., Huttunen, M., Leon, D. A., et al. (2011). Increased risk of schizophrenia from additive interaction between infant motor developmental delay and obstetric complications: Evidence from a population-based longitudinal study. *American Journal of Psychiatry, 168,* 1295–1302.

Classen, J., Liepert, J., Wise, S. P., Hallett, M., et al. (1998). Rapid plasticity of human cortical movement representation induced by practice. *Journal of Neurophysiology, 79,* 1117–1123.

Clemente, C. D., and Sterman, M. B. (1967). Limbic and other forebrain mechanisms in sleep induction and behavioral inhibition. *Progress in Brain Research, 27,* 34–37.

Cogan, G. B., Thesen, T., Carlson, C., Doyle, W., et al. (2014). Sensory-motor transformations for speech occur bilaterally. *Nature, 507*(7490), 94–98.

Coghill, R. C., McHaffie, J. G., and Yen, Y.-F. (2003). Neural correlates of interindividual differences in the subjective experience of pain. *Proceedings of the National Academy of Sciences, USA, 100,* 8538–8542.

Cohen, A. H., Baker, M. T., and Dobrov, T. A. (1989). Evidence for functional regeneration in the adult lamprey spinal cord following transection. *Brain Research, 496,* 368–372.

Cohen, S., Alper, C. M., Doyle, W. H., Treanor, J. J., et al. (2006). Positive emotional style predicts resistance to illness after experimental exposure to rhinovirus or influenza A virus. *Psychosomatic Medicine, 68,* 809–815.

Cohen, S., Doyle, W. J., Alper, C. M., Janicki-Deverts, D., et al. (2009). Sleep habits and susceptibility to the common cold. *Archive of Internal Medicine, 169,* 62–67.

Cohen, S., Janicki-Deverts, D., Turner, R. B., and Doyle, W. J. (2015). Does hugging provide stress-buffering social support? A study of susceptibility to upper respiratory infection and illness. *Psychological Science, 26*(2), 135–147.

Cohen, S., Lichtenstein, E., Prochaska, J. O., Rossi, J. S., et al. (1989). Debunking myths about quitting. Evidence from 10 perspective studies of persons who attempt to quit smoking by themselves. *American Psychologist, 44,* 1355–1365.

Cole, J. (1995). *Pride and a daily marathon.* Cambridge, MA: MIT Press.

Colman, R. J., Beasley, T. M., Kemnitz, J. W., Johnson, S. C., et al. (2014). Caloric restriction reduces age-related and all-cause mortality in rhesus monkeys. *Nature Communications, 5,* 3557.

Colom, R., Haier, R. J., Head, K., Álvarez-Linera, J., et al. (2009). Gray matter correlates of fluid, crystallized, and spatial intelligence: Testing the P-FIT model. *Intelligence, 37,* 124–135.

Conel, J. L. (1939). *The postnatal development of the human cerebral cortex: Vol. 1. The cortex of the newborn.* Cambridge, MA: Harvard University Press.

Conel, J. L. (1947). *The postnatal development of the human cerebral cortex: Vol. 3. The cortex of the three-month infant.* Cambridge, MA: Harvard University Press.

Conel, J. L. (1959). *The postnatal development of the human cerebral cortex: Vol. 6. The cortex of the twenty-four-month infant.* Cambridge, MA: Harvard University Press.

Conrad, A. J., Abebe, T., Austin, R., Forsythe, S., et al. (1991). Hippocampal pyramidal cell disarray in schizophrenia as a bilateral phenomenon. *Archives of General Psychiatry, 48,* 413–417.

Cooke, B. M., Breedlove, S. M., and Jordan, C. L. (2003). Both estrogen receptors and androgen receptors contribute to testosterone-induced changes in the morphology of the medial amygdala and sexual arousal in male rats. *Hormones and Behavior, 43,* 336–346.

Cooke, B. M., Chowanadisai, W., and Breedlove, S. M. (2000). Post-weaning social isolation of male rats reduces the volume of the medial amygdala and leads to deficits in adult sexual behavior. *Behavioural Brain Research, 117,* 107–113.

Cooke, J. R., and Ancoli-Israel, S. (2011). Normal and abnormal sleep in the elderly. *Handbook of Clinical Neurology, 98,* 653–665.

Corballis, M. C. (2002). *From hand to mouth: The origins of language.* Princeton, NJ: Princeton University Press.

Corballis, M. C. (2014). Left brain, right brain: Facts and fantasies. *PLOS Biology, 12*(1), e1001767.

Corbetta, M., and Shulman, G. L. (1998). Human cortical mechanisms of visual attention during orienting and search. *Philosophical Transactions of the Royal Society of London. Series B: Biological Sciences, 353,* 1353–1362.

Corbetta, M., and Shulman, G. L. (2002). Control of goal-directed and stimulus-driven attention in the brain. *Nature Reviews Neuroscience, 3,* 201–215.

Corbetta, M., Kincade, J. M., Ollinger, J. M., McAvoy, M. P., et al. (2000). Voluntary orienting is dissociated from target detection in human posterior parietal cortex. *Nature Neuroscience, 3,* 292–297.

Coricelli, G., Critchley, H. D., Joffily, M., O'Doherty, J. P., et al. (2005). Regret and its avoidance: A neuroimaging study of choice behavior. *Nature Neuroscience, 8,* 1255–1262.

Corkin, S. (2002). What's new with the amnesic patient H.M.? *Neuroscience, 3,* 153–159.

Corkin, S., Amaral., D. G., Gonzalez, R. G., Johnson, K. A., et al. (1997). H.M.'s medial temporal lobe lesion: Findings from magnetic resonance imaging. *Journal of Neuroscience, 17,* 3964–3979.

Coryell, W., Noyes, R., Jr., and House, J. D. (1986). Mortality among outpatients with anxiety disorders. *American Journal of Psychiatry, 143,* 508–510.

Costa, A., and Sebastián-Gallés, N. (2014). How does the bilingual experience sculpt the brain? *Nature Reviews Neuroscience, 15*(5), 336–345.

Costanzo, R. M. (1991). Regeneration of olfactory receptor cells. *CIBA Foundation Symposium, 160,* 233–242.

Counotte, D. S., Goriounova, N. A., Li, K. W., Loos, M., et al. (2011). Lasting synaptic changes underlie attention deficits caused by nicotine exposure during adolescence. *Nature Neuroscience, 14,* 417–419.

Cox, J. H., Seri, S., and Cavanna, A. E. (2018). Sensory aspects of Tourette syndrome. *Neuroscience & Biobehavioral Reviews, 88,* 170–176.

Cox, J. J., Reimann, F., Nicholas, A. K., Thornton, G., et al. (2006). An *SCN9A* channelopathy causes congenital inability to experience pain. *Nature, 444,* 894–898.

Cox, L. M., and Blaser, M. J. (2015). Antibiotics in early life and obesity. *Nature Reviews Endocrinology, 11*(3), 182–190.

Cox, S. S., Speaker, K. J., Beninson, L. A., Craig, W. C., et al. (2014). Adrenergic and glucocorticoid modulation of the sterile inflammatory response. *Brain, Behavior, and Immunity, 36,* 183–192.

Cragg, B. G. (1975). The development of synapses in the visual system of the cat. *Journal of Comparative Neurology, 160,* 147–166.

Crews, F. T., Vetreno, R. P., Broadwater, M. A., and Robinson, D. L. (2016). Adolescent alcohol exposure persistently impacts adult neurobiology and behavior. *Pharmacological Reviews, 68*(4), 1074–1109.

Crick, F. C., and Koch, C. (2005). What is the function of the claustrum? *Philosophical Transactions of the Royal Society of London. Series B: Biological Sciences, 360*(1458), 1271–1279.

Crivelli, C., Russell, J. A., Jarillo, S., and Fernández-Dols, J. M. (2016). The fear gasping face as a threat display in a Melanesian society. *Proceedings of the National Academy of Sciences, USA, 113*(44), 12403–12407.

Crockford, C., Wittig, R. M., Mundry, R., and Zuberbühler, K. (2012). Wild chimpanzees inform ignorant group members of danger. *Current Biology, 22,* 142–146.

Crossley, N. A., Constante, M., McGuire, P., and Power, P. (2010). Efficacy of atypical v. typical antipsychotics in the treatment of early psychosis: Meta-analysis. *British Journal of Psychiatry, 196*(6), 434–439.

Crow, T. J. (1980). Positive and negative schizophrenic symptoms and the role of dopamine. *British Journal of Psychiatry, 137,* 383–386.

Cruce, J. A. F., Greenwood, M. R. C., Johnson, P. R., and Quartermain, D. (1974). Genetic versus hypothalamic obesity: Studies of intake and dietary manipulation in rats. *Journal of Comparative and Physiological Psychology, 87,* 295–301.

Cummings, D. E. (2006). Ghrelin and the short- and long-term regulation of appetite and body weight. *Physiology & Behavior, 89,* 71–84.

Cummings, J. L. (1995). Dementia: The failing brain. *Lancet, 345,* 1481–1484.

Curcio, C. A., Sloan, K. R., Packer, O., Hendrickson, A. E., et al. (1987). Distribution of cones in human and monkey retina:

Individual variability and radial asymmetry. *Science, 236,* 579–582.

Curran, H. V., Freeman, T. P., Mokrysz, C., Lewis, D. A, et al. (2016). Keep off the grass? Cannabis, cognition and addiction. *Nature Reviews Neuroscience, 17*(5), 293–306.

Curtis, V., Aunger, R., and Rabie, T. (2004). Evidence that disgust evolved to protect from risk of disease. *Proceedings of the Royal Society of London. Series B: Biological Sciences, 271*(Suppl. 4), S131–S133.

Curtiss, S. (1989). The independence and task-specificity of language. In M. H. Bornstein and J. S. Bruner (Eds.), *Interaction in human development* (pp. 105–137). Hillsdale, NJ: Erlbaum.

Cussotto, S., Sandhu, K. V., Dinan, T. G., and Cryan, J. F. (2018, May 14). The neuroendocrinology of the microbiota-gut-brain axis: A behavioural perspective. *Frontiers in Neuroendocrinology,* pii: S0091-3022(18)30039-6.

Cytowic, R. E., and Eagleman, D. M. (2009). *Wednesday is indigo blue: Discovering the brain of synesthesia.* Cambridge, MA: MIT Press.

D

Dabbs, J. M., and Morris, R. (1990). Testosterone, social class, and antisocial behavior in a sample of 4,462 men. *Psychological Science, 1,* 209–211.

Dabbs, J. M., Jr., and Hargrove, M. F. (1997). Age, testosterone, and behavior among female prison inmates. *Psychosomatic Medicine, 59,* 477–480.

Dabbs, J. M., Ruback, R. B., Frady, R. L., Hopper, C. H., et al. (1988). Saliva testosterone and criminal violence among women. *Personality and Individual Differences, 9,* 269–275.

Dale, R. C., Heyman, I., Giovannoni, G., and Church, A. W. (2005). Incidence of anti-brain antibodies in children with obsessive-compulsive disorder. *British Journal of Psychiatry, 187,* 314–319.

Dalton, K. M., Nacewicz, B. M., Johnstone, T., Schaefer, H. S., et al. (2005). Gaze fixation and the neural circuitry of face processing in autism. *Nature Neuroscience, 8,* 519–526.

Damasio, A. R., Grabowski, T. J., Bechara, A., Damasio, H., et al. (2000). Subcortical and cortical brain activity during the feeling of self-generated emotions. *Nature Neuroscience, 3,* 1049–1056.

Damasio, H., Grabowski, T., Frank, R., Galaburda, A. M., et al. (1994). The return of Phineas Gage: Clues about the brain from the skull of a famous patient. *Science, 264,* 1102–1105.

Damassa, D. A., Smith, E. R., Tennent, B., and Davidson, J. M. (1977). The relationship between circulating testosterone

levels and male sexual behavior in rats. *Hormones and Behavior, 8,* 275–286.

Dantz, B., Edgar, D. M., and Dement, W. C. (1994). Circadian rhythms in narcolepsy: Studies on a 90 minute day. *Electroencephalography and Clinical Neurophysiology, 90,* 24–35.

Dantzer, R., O'Connor, J. C., Freund, G. G., Johnson, R. W., et al. (2008). From inflammation to sickness and depression: When the immune system subjugates the brain. *Nature Reviews Neuroscience, 9,* 46–56.

Dapretto, M., Davies, M. S., Pfeifer, J. H., Scott, A. A., et al. (2006). Understanding emotions in others: Mirror neuron dysfunction in children with autism spectrum disorders. *Nature Neuroscience, 9,* 28–30.

Darwin, C. (1872). *The expression of the emotions in man and animals.* London, UK: J. Murray.

Davalos, D., Grutzendler, J., Yang, G., Kim, J. V., et al. (2005). ATP mediates rapid microglial response to local brain injury in vivo. *Nature Neuroscience, 8,* 752–758.

Davey-Smith, G., Frankel, S., and Yarnell, J. (1997). Sex and death: Are they related? Findings from the Caerphilly Cohort Study. *British Medical Journal (Clinical Research Edition), 315,* 1641–1644.

David, L. A., Maurice, C. F., Carmody, R. N., Gootenberg, D. B., et al. (2014). Diet rapidly and reproducibly alters the human gut microbiome. *Nature, 505*(7484), 559–563.

Davidson, J. M., Camargo, C. A., and Smith, E. R. (1979). Effects of androgen on sexual behavior in hypogonadal men. *Journal of Clinical Endocrinology and Metabolism, 48,* 955–958.

Davis, J. I., Senghas, A., and Ochsner, K. N. (2009). How does facial feedback modulate emotional experience? *Journal of Research in Personality, 43,* 822–829.

Davis, J. I., Senghas, A., Brandt, F., and Ochsner, K. N. (2010). The effects of BOTOX injections on emotional experience. *Emotion, 10,* 433–440.

Davis, M. C., Horan, W. P., and Marder, S. R. (2014). Psychopharmacology of the negative symptoms: Current status and prospects for progress. *European Neuropsychopharmacology, 24*(5), 788–799.

Davis, N. (2018, April 10). Man eats world's hottest chilli pepper—and ends up in hospital. *Guardian.* ww.theguardian.com/science/2018/apr/09/competitive-eater-taken-to-hospital-after-eating-worlds-hottest-chilli-pepper.

Dawson, T. M., and Dawson, V. L. (2003). Molecular pathways of neurodegeneration in Parkinson's disease. *Science, 302,* 819–822.

De Boeck, P., and Jeon, M. (2018). Perceived crisis and reforms: Issues, explanations, and remedies. *Psychological Bulletin, 144*(7), 757–777.

De Felipe, C., Herrero, J. F., O'Brien, J. A., Palmer, J. A., et al. (1998). Altered nociception, analgesia and aggression in mice lacking the receptor for substance P. *Nature, 392*, 394–397.

de Gelder, B., Hortensius, R., and Tamietto, M. (2012). Attention and awareness each influence amygdala activity for dynamic bodily expressions: A short review. *Frontiers in Integrative Neuroscience, 6*, 54.

de Gelder, B., Tamietto, M., van Boxtel, G., Goebel, R., et al. (2008). Intact navigation skills after bilateral loss of striate cortex. *Current Biology, 18*, R1128–R1129.

De Groot, C. M., Janus, M. D., and Bornstein, R. A. (1995). Clinical predictors of psychopathology in children and adolescents with Tourette syndrome. *Journal of Psychiatric Research, 29*, 59–70.

de Groot, J. H., Semin, G. R., and Smeets, M. A. (2017). On the communicative function of body odors. *Perspectives on Psychological Science, 12*(2), 306–324.

de Heer, W. A., Huth, A. G., Griffiths, T. L., Gallant, J. L., et al. (2017). The hierarchical cortical organization of human speech processing. *Journal of Neuroscience, 37*(27), 6539–6557.

de Kloet, E. R., and Joëls, M. (2017). Brain mineralocorticoid receptor function in control of salt balance and stress-adaptation. *Physiology & Behavior, 178*, 13–20.

de Kluiver, H., Buizer-Voskamp, J. E., Dolan, C. V., and Boomsma, D. I. (2017). Paternal age and psychiatric disorders: A review. *American Journal of Medical Genetics Part B: Neuropsychiatric Genetics, 174*(3), 202–213.

de Quervain, D., Schwabe, L., and Roozendaal, B. (2017). Stress, glucocorticoids and memory: Implications for treating fear-related disorders. *Nature Reviews Neuroscience, 18*(1), 7–19.

De Valois, K. K., De Valois, R. L., and Yund, E. W. (1979). Responses of striate cortex cells to grating and checkerboard patterns. *Journal of Physiology (London), 291*, 483–505.

De Valois, R. L., and De Valois, K. K. (1980). Spatial vision. *Annual Review of Psychology, 31*, 309–341.

De Valois, R. L., and De Valois, K. K. (1988). *Spatial vision.* New York, NY: Oxford University Press.

De Valois, R. L., and De Valois, K. K. (1993). A multi-stage color model. *Vision Research, 33*, 1053–1065.

De Waal, F. B. M. (2003). Darwin's legacy and the study of primate visual communication. *Annals of the New York Academy of Sciences, 1000*, 7–31.

De Win, M. M., Jager, G., Booij, J., Reneman, L., et al. (2008). Sustained effects of ecstasy on the human brain: A prospective neuroimaging study in novel users. *Brain, 131*(Pt. 11), 2936–2945.

Dearborn, G. V. N. (1932). A case of congenital general pure analgesia. *Journal of Nervous and Mental Disease, 75*, 612–615.

Dehaene, S., and Changeux, J. P. (2011). Experimental and theoretical approaches to conscious processing. *Neuron, 70*(2), 200–227.

Dehaene-Lambertz, G., Dehaene, S., and Hertz-Pannier, L. (2002). Functional neuroimaging of speech perception in infants. *Science, 298*, 2013–2015.

del Campo, N., Fryer, T. D., Hong, Y. T., Smith, R., et al. (2013). A positron emission tomography study of nigro-striatal dopaminergic mechanisms underlying attention: Implications for ADHD and its treatment. *Brain, 136*(Pt. 11), 3252–3270.

Delgado, J. M. R. (1969). *Physical control of the mind: Toward a psychocivilized society.* New York, NY: Harper & Row.

Dement, W. C. (1974). *Some must watch while some must sleep.* San Francisco, CA: W.H. Freeman.

Den Heijer, A. E., Groen, Y., Tucha, L., Fuermaier, A. B., et al. (2017). Sweat it out? The effects of physical exercise on cognition and behavior in children and adults with ADHD: A systematic literature review. *Journal of Neural Transmission (Vienna), 124*(Suppl. 1), 3–26.

Dennis, S. G., and Melzack, R. (1983). Perspectives on phylogenetic evolution of pain expression. In R. L. Kitchell, H. H. Erickson, E. Carstens, and L. E. Davis (Eds.), *Animal pain* (pp. 151–161). Bethesda, MD: American Physiological Society.

Denton, D., Shade, R., Zamarippa, F., Egan, G., et al. (1999). Neuroimaging of genesis and satiation of thirst and an interoceptor-driven theory of origins of primary consciousness. *Proceedings of the National Academy of Sciences, USA, 96*, 5304–5309.

Depaepe, V., Suarez-Gonzalez, N., Dufour, A., Passante, L., et al. (2005). Ephrin signalling controls brain size by regulating apoptosis of neural progenitors. *Nature, 435*, 1244–1250.

DeRubeis, R. J., Siegle, G. J., and Hollon, S. D. (2008). Cognitive therapy versus medication for depression: Treatment outcomes and neural mechanisms. *Nature, 9*, 788–796.

Devane, W. A., Dysarz, F. A., Johnson, M. R., Melvin, L. S., et al. (1988). Determination and characterization of a cannabinoid receptor in rat brain. *Molecular Pharmacology, 34*, 605–613.

Devane, W. A., Hanus, L., Breuer, A., Pertwee, R. G., et al. (1992). Isolation and structure of a brain constituent that binds the cannabinoid receptor. *Science, 258*, 1946–1949.

Devlin, J. T., and Watkins, K. E. (2007). Stimulating language: Insights from TMS. *Brain, 130*(Pt. 3), 610–622.

DeVoogd, T. J. (1994). Interactions between endocrinology and learning in the avian song system. *Annals of the New York Academy of Sciences, 743*, 19–41.

Dewan, A., Pacifico, R., Zhan, R., Rinberg, D., et al. (2013). Non-redundant coding of aversive odours in the main olfactory pathway. *Nature, 497*(7450), 486–489.

Dewsbury, D. A. (1972). Patterns of copulatory behavior in male mammals. *Quarterly Review of Biology, 47*, 1–33.

Dhabhar, F. S. (2018). The short-term stress response: Mother nature's mechanism for enhancing protection and performance under conditions of threat, challenge, and opportunity. *Frontiers in Neuroendocrinology, 49*, 175–192.

Di Marzo, V., and Matias, I. (2005). Endocannabinoid control of food intake and energy balance. *Nature Neuroscience, 8*, 585–589.

Diamond, J., Cooper, E., Turner, C., and Macintyre, L. (1976). Trophic regulation of nerve sprouting. *Science, 193*, 371–377.

Diamond, M. C. (1967). Extensive cortical depth measurements and neuron size increases in the cortex of environmentally enriched rats. *Journal of Comparative Neurology, 131*, 357–364.

Diamond, M. C., Lindner, B., Johnson, R., Bennett, E. L., et al. (1975). Differences in occipital cortical synapses from environmentally enriched, impoverished, and standard colony rats. *Journal of Neuroscience Research, 1*, 109–119.

Diana, M., Raij, T., Melis, M., Nummenmaa, A., et al. (2017). Rehabilitating the addicted brain with transcranial magnetic stimulation. *Nature Reviews Neuroscience, 18*(11), 685–693.

Dichgans, J. (1984). Clinical symptoms of cerebellar dysfunction and their topodiagnostical significance. *Human Neurobiology, 2*, 269–279.

Dietz, P. M., Williams, S. B., Callaghan, W. M., Bachman, D. J., et al. (2007). Clinically identified maternal depression before, during, and after pregnancies ending in live births. *American Journal of Psychiatry, 164*, 1457–1459.

Dittmann, R. W., Kappes, M. E., and Kappes, M. H. (1992). Sexual behavior in adolescent and adult females with congenital adrenal hyperplasia. *Psychoneuroendocrinology, 17*, 153–170.

Do, M. T. H., Kang, S. H., Xue, T., Zhong, H., et al. (2009). Photon capture and signalling by melanopsin retinal ganglion cells. *Nature, 457*, 281–287.

Dohanich, G. (2003). Ovarian steroids and cognitive function. *Current Directions in Psychological Science, 12*, 57–61.

Dohrenwend, B. P., Turner, J. B., Turse, N. A., Adams, B. G., et al. (2006). The psychological risks of Vietnam for U.S. veterans:

A revisit with new data and methods. *Science, 313*, 979–982.

Dolan, R. J. (2002). Emotion, cognition, and behavior. *Science, 298*, 1191–1194.

Dolder, C. R., and Nelson, M. H. (2008). Hypnosedative-induced complex behaviours: Incidence, mechanisms and management. *CNS Drugs, 22*, 1021–1036.

Domjan, M., and Purdy, J. E. (1995). Animal research in psychology: More than meets the eye of the general psychology student. *American Psychologist, 50*, 496–503.

Donaldson, Z. R., and Young, L. J. (2008). Oxytocin, vasopressin, and the neurogenetics of sociality. *Science, 322*, 900–903.

Dorsaint-Pierre, R., Penhune, V. B., Watkins, K. E., Neelin, P., et al. (2006). Asymmetries of the planum temporale and Heschl's gyrus: Relationship to language lateralization. *Brain, 129*, 1164–1176.

Drea, C. M., Weldele, M. L., Forger, N. G., Coscia, E. M., et al. (1998). Androgens and masculinization of genitalia in the spotted hyaena (*Crocuta crocuta*). 2. Effects of prenatal anti-androgens. *Journal of Reproduction and Fertility, 113*, 117–127.

Dreger, A. (2018, April 27). Track's absurd new rules for women. *New York Times* (https://www.nytimes.com/2018/04/27/opinion/caster-semenya-intersex-athletes.html).

Drevets, W. C. (1998). Functional neuroimaging studies of depression: The anatomy of melancholia. *Annual Review of Medicine, 49*, 341–361.

Drew, T., Võ, M. L., and Wolfe, J. M. (2013). The invisible gorilla strikes again: Sustained inattentional blindness in expert observers. *Psychological Science, 24*(9), 1848–1853.

Drickamer, L. C. (1992). Behavioral selection of odor cues by young female mice affects age of puberty. *Developmental Psychobiology, 25*, 461–470.

Dronkers, N. F., Plaisant, O., Iba-Zizen, M. T., and Cabanis, E. A. (2007). Paul Broca's historic cases: High resolution MR imaging of the brains of Leborgne and Lelong. *Brain, 130* (Pt. 5), 1432–1441.

Dronkers, N. F., Wilkins, D. P., Van Valin, R. D., Jr., Redfern, B. B., et al. (2004). Lesion analysis of the brain areas involved in language comprehension. *Cognition, 92*, 145–177.

Druckman, D., and Bjork, R. A. (1994). *Learning, remembering, believing: Enhancing human performance*. Washington, DC: National Academies Press.

Du, J. L., and Poo, M. M. (2004). Rapid BDNF-induced retrograde synaptic modification in a developing retinotectal system. *Nature, 429*, 878–882.

Du, L., Bakish, D., Lapierre, Y. D., Ravindran, A. V., et al. (2000). Association of polymorphism of serotonin 2A receptor gene with suicidal ideation in major depressive disorder. *American Journal of Medical Genetics, 96*, 56–60.

Duchaine, B., Germine, L., and Nakayama, K. (2007). Family resemblance: Ten family members with prosopagnosia and within-class object agnosia. *Cognitive Neuropsychology, 24*, 419–430.

Duchamp-Viret, P., Chaput, M. A., and Duchamp, A. (1999). Odor response properties of rat olfactory receptor neurons. *Science, 284*, 2171–2174.

Duffy, J. D., and Campbell, J. J. (1994). The regional prefrontal syndromes: A theoretical and clinical overview. *Journal of Neuropsychiatry and Clinical Neurosciences, 6*, 379–387.

Dulac, C., and Torello, A. T. (2003). Molecular detection of pheromone signals in mammals, from genes to behaviour. *Nature Reviews Neuroscience, 4*, 551–562.

Dulak, J., Szade, K., Szade, A., Nowak, W., et al. (2015). Adult stem cells: Hopes and hypes of regenerative medicine. *Acta Biochimica Polonica, 62*(3), 329–337.

Dully, H., and Fleming, C. (2007). *My lobotomy*. New York, NY: Crown. ISBN: 978-0307381262

Dunah, A. W., Hyunkyung, J., Griffin, A., Kim, Y.-M., et al. (2002). Sp1 and TAFII130 transcriptional activity disrupted in early Huntington's disease. *Science, 296*, 2238–2242.

E

Eapen, V., Cavanna, A. E., and Robertson, M. M. (2016). Comorbidities, social impact, and quality of life in Tourette syndrome. *Frontiers in Psychiatry, 7*, 97.

Earnest, D. J., Liang, F. Q., Ratcliff, M., and Cassone, V. M. (1999). Immortal time: Circadian clock properties of rat suprachiasmatic cell lines. *Science, 283*, 693–695.

Ebbinghaus, H. (1908). *Psychology: An elementary textbook*. Boston: Heath.

Edelsohn, G. A. (2006). Hallucinations in children and adolescents: Considerations in the emergency setting. *American Journal of Psychiatry, 163*, 781–785.

Edwards, R. R., Grace, E., Peterson, S., Klick, B., et al. (2009). Sleep continuity and architecture: Associations with pain-inhibitory processes in patients with temporomandibular joint disorder. *European Journal of Pain, 13*, 1043–1047.

Egaas, B., Courchesne, E., and Saitoh, O. (1995). Reduced size of corpus callosum in autism. *Archives of Neurology, 52*, 794–801.

Eklund, A., Nichols, T. E., and Knutsson, H. (2016). Cluster failure: Why fMRI inferences for spatial extent have inflated false-positive rates. *Proceedings of the National Academy of Sciences, USA, 113*(28), 7900–7905.

Elbert, T., Pantev, C., Wienbruch, C., Rockstroh, B., et al. (1995). Increased cortical representation of the fingers of the left hand in string players. *Science, 270*, 305–307.

Ellenbogen, J. M., Hu, P. T., Payne, J. D., Titone, D., et al. (2007). Human relational memory requires time and sleep. *Proceedings of the National Academy of Sciences, USA, 104*, 7317–7318.

Ellis, H. D., and Lewis, M. B. (2001). Capgras delusion: A window on face recognition. *Trends in Cognitive Sciences, 5*(4), 149–156.

Emborg, M. E., Liu, Y., Xi, J., Zhang, X., et al. (2013). Induced pluripotent stem cell–derived neural cells survive and mature in the nonhuman primate brain. *Cell Reports, 3*(3), 646–650.

Emery, N. J., Capitanio, J. P., Mason, W. A., Machado, C. J., et al. (2001). The effects of bilateral lesions of the amygdala on dyadic social interactions in rhesus monkeys (*Macaca mulatta*). *Behavioral Neuroscience, 115*, 515–544.

Engel, J., Jr. (1992). Recent advances in surgical treatment of temporal lobe epilepsy. *Acta Neurologica Scandinavica. Supplementum, 140*, 71–80.

English, P. J., Ghatei, M. A., Malik, I. A., Bloom, S. R., et al. (2002). Food fails to suppress ghrelin levels in obese humans. *Journal of Clinical Endocrinology and Metabolism, 87*, 2984–2987.

Epstein, A. N., Fitzsimons, J. T., and Rolls, B. J. (1970). Drinking induced by injection of angiotensin into the brain of the rat. *Journal of Physiology (London), 210*, 457–474.

Eriksson, A., and Lacerda, F. (2007). Charlantry in forensic speech science: A problem to be taken seriously. *International Journal of Speech Language and the Law, 14*, 169–193.

Erlanger, D. M., Kutner, K. C., Barth, J. T., and Barnes, R. (1999). Neuropsychology of sports-related head injury: Dementia pugilistica to post concussion syndrome. *Clinical Neuropsychologist, 13*, 193–209.

Ernst, T., Chang, L., Leonido-Yee, M., and Speck, O. (2000). Evidence for long-term neurotoxicity associated with methamphetamine abuse: A 1H MRS study. *Neurology, 54*, 1344–1349.

Erren, T. C., Morfeld, P., Stork, J., Knauth, P., et al. (2009). Shift work, chronodisruption and cancer?—The IARC 2007 challenge for research and prevention and 10 theses from the Cologne Colloquium 2008. *Scandinavian Journal of Work, Environment & Health, 35*, 74–79.

Everitt, B. J., and Stacey, P. (1987). Studies of instrumental behavior with sexual reinforcement in male rats (*Rattus norvegicus*): II. Effects of preoptic area lesions, castration, and testosterone. *Journal of Comparative Psychology, 101*, 407–419.

Everson, C. A. (1993). Sustained sleep deprivation impairs host defense. *American Journal of Physiology, 265*, R1148–R1154.

Everson, C. A., Bergmann, B. M., and Rechtschaffen, A. (1989). Sleep deprivation in the rat: III. Total sleep deprivation. *Sleep, 12,* 13–21.

Eybalin, M. (1993). Neurotransmitters and neuromodulators of the mammalian cochlea. *Physiological Reviews, 73,* 309–373.

F

Falk, D. (2004). Prelinguistic evolution in early hominins: Whence motherese? *Behavioral and Brain Sciences, 27,* 491–503.

Falkner, A. L., Grosenick, L., Davidson, T. J., Deisseroth, K., et al. (2016). Hypothalamic control of male aggression-seeking behavior. *Nature Neuroscience, 19*(4), 596–604.

Faraone, S. V., Glatt, S. J., Su, J., and Tsuang, M. T. (2004). Three potential susceptibility loci shown by a genome-wide scan for regions influencing the age at onset of mania. *American Journal of Psychiatry, 161,* 625–630.

Farbman, A. I. (1994). The cellular basis of olfaction. *Endeavour, 18,* 2–8.

Farrell, A. K., Slatcher, R. B., Tobin, E. T., Imami, L., et al. (2018). Socioeconomic status, family negative emotional climate, and anti-inflammatory gene expression among youth with asthma. *Psychoneuroendocrinology, 91,* 62–67.

Fay, R. R. (1988). *Hearing in vertebrates: A psychophysics databook.* Winnetka, IL: Hill-Fay Associates.

Feder, H. H., and Whalen, R. E. (1965). Feminine behavior in neonatally castrated and estrogen-treated male rats. *Science, 147,* 306–307.

Feinstein, J. S., Adolphs, R., Damasio, A., and Tranel, D. (2011). The human amygdala and the induction and experience of fear. *Current Biology, 21,* 34–38.

Feinstein, J. S., Buzza, C., Hurelmann, R., Follmer, R. L., et al. (2013). Fear and panic in humans with bilateral amygdala damage. *Nature Neuroscience, 16,* 270–272. doi:10.1038/nn.3323

Felitti, V. J., Anda, R. F., Nordenberg, D., Williamson, D. F., et al. (1998). Relationship of childhood abuse and household dysfunction to many of the leading causes of death in adults. The Adverse Childhood Experiences (ACE) Study. *American Journal of Preventive Medicine, 14*(4), 245–258.

Felleman, D. J., and Van Essen, D. C. (1991). Distributed hierarchical processing in the primate cerebral cortex. *Cerebral Cortex 1*(1), 1–47. https://doi.org/10.1093/cercor/1.1.1-a

Feng, W., Störmer, V. S., Martinez, A., McDonald, J. J., et al. (2017). Involuntary orienting of attention to a sound desynchronizes the occipital alpha rhythm and improves visual perception. *NeuroImage, 150,* 318–328.

Fenstemaker, S. B., Zup, S. L., Frank, L. G., Glickman, S. E., et al. (1999). A sex difference in the hypothalamus of the spotted hyena. *Nature Neuroscience, 2,* 943–945.

Ferguson, J. N., Young, L. J., Hearn, E. F., Matzuk, M. M., et al. (2000). Social amnesia in mice lacking the oxytocin gene. *Nature Genetics, 25,* 284–288.

Fernández-Espejo, D., and Owen, A. M. (2013). Detecting awareness after severe brain injury. *Nature Reviews Neuroscience, 14*(11), 801–809.

Fields, R. D., and Stevens-Graham, B. (2002). New insights into neuron-glia communication. *Science, 298,* 556–562.

Finch, C. E., and Kirkwood, T. B. L. (2000). *Chance, development, and aging.* New York, NY: Oxford University Press.

Finger, S. (1994). *Origins of neuroscience: A history of explorations into brain function.* New York, NY: Oxford University Press.

Fink, H., Rex, A., Voits, M., and Voigt, J. P. (1998). Major biological actions of CCK—A critical evaluation of research findings. *Experimental Brain Research, 123,* 77–83.

Fink, M., and Taylor, M. A. (2007). Electroconvulsive therapy: Evidence and challenges. *JAMA, 298,* 330–332.

Fisher, S. E. (2017). Evolution of language: Lessons from the genome. *Psychonomic Bulletin & Review, 24*(1), 34–40.

Fishman, R. B., Chism, L., Firestone, G. L., and Breedlove, S. M. (1990). Evidence for androgen receptors in sexually dimorphic perineal muscles of neonatal male rats. Absence of androgen accumulation by the perineal motoneurons. *Journal of Neurobiology, 21,* 694–704.

Fitzsimmons, J. T. (1998). Angiotensin, thirst, and sodium appetite. *Physiological Reviews, 78,* 583–686.

Flegal, K. M., Carroll, M. D., Ogden, C. L., and Johnson, C. L. (2002). Prevalence and trends in obesity among US adults, 1999-2000. *JAMA, 288,* 1723–1727.

Fleming, A. S., Kraemer, G. W., Gonzalez, A., Lovic, V., et al. (2002). Mothering begets mothering: The transmission of behavior and its neurobiology across generations. *Pharmacology, Biochemistry, and Behavior, 73,* 61–75.

Fleming, A. S., Ruble, D., Krieger, H., and Wong, P. Y. (1997). Hormonal and experiential correlates of maternal responsiveness during pregnancy and the puerperium in human mothers. *Hormones and Behavior, 31,* 145–158.

Florence, S. L., Taub, H. B., and Kaas, J. H. (1998). Large-scale sprouting of cortical connections after peripheral injury in adult macaque monkeys. *Science, 282,* 1117–1121.

Fluharty, S. J., and Epstein, A. N. (1983). Sodium appetite elicited by intracerebroventricular infusion of angiotensin II

in the rat: II. Synergistic interaction with systemic mineralocorticoids. *Behavioral Neuroscience, 97*(5), 746–758.

Foerster, O., and Penfield, W. (1930). The structural basis of traumatic epilepsy and results of radical operation. *Brain, 53,* 8–119.

Foley, C., Corvin, A., and Nakagome, S. (2017). Genetics of schizophrenia: Ready to translate? *Current Psychiatry Reports, 19*(9), 61.

Ford, J. M. (1999). Schizophrenia: The broken P300 and beyond. *Psychophysiology, 36,* 667–682.

Forger, N. G., and Breedlove, S. M. (1987). Motoneuronal death during human fetal development. *The Journal of Comparative Neurology, 264,* 118–122.

Forger, N. G., and Breedlove, S. M. (1986). Sexual dimorphism in human and canine spinal cord: Role of early androgen. *Proceedings of the National Academy of Sciences, USA, 83,* 7527–7531.

Forger, N. G., and Breedlove, S. M. (1987). Seasonal variation in mammalian striated muscle mass and motoneuron morphology. *Journal of Neurobiology, 18,* 155–165.

Forger, N. G., Frank, L. G., Breedlove, S. M., and Glickman, S. E. (1996). Sexual dimorphism of perineal muscles and motoneurons in spotted hyenas. *Journal of Comparative Neurology, 375,* 333–343.

Foster, G. D., Wyatt, H. R., Hill, J. O., McGuckin, B. G., et al. (2003). A randomized trial of a low-carbohydrate diet for obesity. *New England Journal of Medicine, 348,* 2082–2090.

Foster, R. G., and Soni, B. G. (1998). Extraretinal photoreceptors and their regulation of temporal physiology. *Reproduction, 3,* 145–150.

Foster, R. G., Peirson, S. N., Wulff, K., Winnebeck, E., et al. (2013). Sleep and circadian rhythm disruption in social jetlag and mental illness. *Progress in Molecular Biology and Translational Science, 119,* 325–346.

Fothergill, E., Guo, J., Howard, L., Kerns, J. C., et al. (2016). Persistent metabolic adaptation 6 years after "The Biggest Loser" competition. *Obesity (Silver Spring), 24*(8), 1612–1619. doi:10.1002/oby.21538

Fournier, J. C., DeRubeis, R. J., Hollon, S. D., Dimidjian, S., et al. (2010). Antidepressant drug effects and depression severity: A patient-level meta-analysis. *JAMA, 303,* 47–53.

Francis, D. D., Szegda, K., Campbell, G., Martin, W. D., et al. (2003). Epigenetic sources of behavioral differences in mice. *Nature Neuroscience, 6,* 445–446.

Frank, L. G., Glickman, S. E., and Licht, P. (1991). Fatal sibling aggression, precocial development, and androgens in neonatal spotted hyenas. *Science, 252,* 702–704.

Frank, M. J., Samanta, J., Moustafa, A. A., and Sherman, S. J. (2007). Hold your horses: Impulsivity, deep brain stimulation, and medication in parkinsonism. *Science, 318,* 1309–1312.

Frankenhaeuser, M. (1978). Psychoneuroendocrine approaches to the study of emotion as related to stress and coping. *Nebraska Symposium on Motivation, 26,* 123–162.

Franklin, T. R., Acton, P. D., Maldjian, J. A., Gray, J. D., et al. (2002). Decreased gray matter concentration in the insular, orbitofrontal, cingulate, and temporal cortices of cocaine patients. *Biological Psychiatry, 51,* 134–142.

Franks, N. P. (2008). General anaesthesia: From molecular targets to neuronal pathways of sleep and arousal. *Nature, 9,* 370–386.

Franssen, C. L., Bardi, M., Shea, E. A., Hampton, J. E., et al. (2011). Fatherhood alters behavioural and neural responsiveness in a spatial task. *Journal of Neuroendocrinology, 23,* 1177–1187.

Freed, C. R., Greene, P. E., Breeze, R. E., Tsai, W.-Y., et al. (2001). Transplantation of embryonic dopamine neurons for severe Parkinson's disease. *New England Journal of Medicine, 344,* 710–719.

Freedman, M. S., Lucas, R. J., Soni, B., von Schantz, M., et al. (1999). Regulation of mammalian circadian behavior by non-rod, non-cone, ocular photoreceptors. *Science, 284,* 502–504.

Freitag, J., Ludwig, G., Andreini, P., Roessler, P., et al. (1998). Olfactory receptors in aquatic and terrestrial vertebrates. *Journal of Comparative Physiology, 183,* 635–650.

Freiwald, W. A., Tsao, D. Y., and Livingstone, M. S. (2009). A face feature space in the macaque temporal lobe. *Nature Neuroscience, 12,* 1187–1196.

French, C. A., and Fisher, S. E. (2014). What can mice tell us about Foxp2 function? *Current Opinion in Neurology, 28,* 72–79.

Frey, S. H., Bogdanov, S., Smith, J. C., Watrous, S., et al. (2008). Chronically deafferented sensory cortex recovers a grossly typical organization after allogenic hand transplantation. *Current Biology, 18,* 1530–1534.

Fried, I., Wilson, C. L., MacDonald, K. A., and Behnke, E. J. (1998). Electric current stimulates laughter. *Nature, 391,* 650.

Friedman, L., and Jones, B. E. (1984). Study of sleep-wakefulness states by computer graphics and cluster analysis before and after lesions of the pontine tegmentum in the cat. *Electroencephalography and Clinical Neurophysiology, 57,* 43–56.

Friedrich, F. J., Egly, R., Rafal, R. D., and Beck, D. (1998). Spatial attention deficits in humans: A comparison of superior parietal and temporal-parietal junction lesions. *Neuropsychology, 12,* 193–207.

Fritz, J., Shamma, S., Elhilali, M., and Klein, D. (2003). Rapid task-related plasticity of spectrotemporal receptive fields in primary auditory cortex. *Nature Neuroscience, 6,* 1216–1223.

Fryar, C. D., Carroll, M. D., and Ogden, C. L. (2016). Prevalence of overweight and obesity among children and adolescents aged 2–19 years: United States, 1963–1965 through 2013–2014. National Center for Health Statistics. July 2016. Available from: http://www.cdc.gov/nchs/products/hestats.htm

Fukuda, K., Ogilvie, R. D., Chilcott, L., Vendittelli, A.-M., et al. (1998). The prevalence of sleep paralysis among Canadian and Japanese college students. *Dreaming: Journal of the Association for the Study of Dreams, 8*(2), 59–66.

Fulton, B. D., Scheffler, R. M., Hinshaw, S. P., Levine, P., et al. (2009). National variation of ADHD diagnostic prevalence and medication use: Health care providers and education policies. *Psychiatric Services, 60,* 1075–1083.

Fung, T. C., Olson, C. A., and Hsiao, E. Y. (2017). Interactions between the microbiota, immune and nervous systems in health and disease. *Nature Neuroscience, 20*(2), 145–155.

Furukawa, E., Bado, P., Tripp, G., Mattos, P., et al. (2014). Abnormal striatal BOLD responses to reward anticipation and reward delivery in ADHD. *PLOS ONE, 9*(2), e89129.

Fuster, J. M. (1990). Prefrontal cortex and the bridging of temporal gaps in the perception-action cycle. *Annals of the New York Academy of Sciences, 608,* 318–336.

G

Gabel, L. A., Gibson, C. J., Gruen, J. R., and LoTurco, J. J. (2010). Progress towards a cellular neurobiology of reading disability. *Neurobiology of Disease, 38*(2), 173–180.

Galaburda, A. M. (1994). Developmental dyslexia and animal studies: At the interface between cognition and neurology. *Cognition, 56,* 833–839.

Galaburda, A. M., LoTurco, J., Ramus, F., Fitch, R. H., et al. (2006). From genes to behavior in developmental dyslexia. *Nature Neuroscience, 9,* 1213–1217.

Galaburda, A. M., Sherman, G. F., Rosen, G. D., Aboitiz, F., et al. (1985). Developmental dyslexia: four consecutive patients with cortical anomalies. *Annals of Neurology, 18,* 222–233.

Gallant, J. L., Braun, J., and Van Essen, D. C. (1993). Selectivity for polar, hyperbolic, and Cartesian gratings in macaque visual cortex. *Science, 259,* 100–103.

Gallese, V., and Sinigaglia, C. (2011). What is so special about embodied simulation? *Trends in Cognitive Sciences, 15,* 512–519.

Gallopin, T., Fort, P., Eggermann, E., Cauli, B., et al. (2000). Identification of sleep-promoting neurons in vitro. *Nature, 404,* 992–995.

Gangwisch, J. E., Heymsfield, S. B., Boden-Albala, B., Buijs, R. M., et al. (2007). Sleep duration as a risk factor for diabetes incidence in a large U.S. sample. *Sleep, 30,* 1667–1673.

Gannon, P. J., Holloway, R. L., Broadfield, D. C., and Braun, A. R. (1998). Asymmetry of chimpanzee planum temporale: Human-like pattern of brain language area homolog. *Science, 279,* 220–222.

Gardner, R. A., and Gardner, B. T. (1969). Teaching sign language to a chimpanzee. *Science, 165,* 664–672.

Gardner, R. A., and Gardner, B. T. (1984). A vocabulary test for chimpanzees (*Pan troglodytes*). *Journal of Comparative Psychology, 98,* 381–404.

Gardner, T. J., Naef, F., and Nottebohm, F. (2005). Freedom and rules: The acquisition and reprogramming of a bird's learned song. *Science, 308,* 1046–1049.

Garfield, A. S., Li, C., Madara, J. C., Shah, B. P., et al. (2015). A neural basis for melanocortin-4 receptor-regulated appetite. *Nature Neuroscience, 18*(6), 863–871.

Garver, D. L., Holcomb, J. A., and Christensen, J. D. (2000). Heterogeneity of response to antipsychotics from multiple disorders in the schizophrenia spectrum. *Journal of Clinical Psychiatry, 61,* 964–972.

Gasser, P., Holstein, D., Michel, Y., Doblin, R., et al. (2014). Safety and efficacy of lysergic acid diethylamide-assisted psychotherapy for anxiety associated with life-threatening diseases. *Journal of Nervous and Mental Disease, 202*(7), 513–520.

Gates, N. J, and Sachdev, P. (2014). Is cognitive training an effective treatment for preclinical and early Alzheimer's disease? *Journal of Alzheimer's Disease, 42,* S551–S559.

Gaulin, S. J. C, and Fitzgerald, R. W. (1989). Sexual selection for spatial-learning ability. *Animal Behaviour, 37,* 322–331.

Gauthier, I., Behrmann, M., and Tarr, M. J. (1999). Can face recognition really be dissociated from object recognition? *Journal of Cognitive Neuroscience, 11,* 349–370.

Gauthier, I., Skudlarski, P., Gore, J. C., and Anderson, A. W. (2000). Expertise for cars and birds recruits brain areas involved in face recognition. *Nature Neuroscience, 3,* 191–197.

Gazzaniga, M. S., and Smylie, C. S. (1983). Facial recognition and brain asymmetries: Clues to underlying mechanisms. *Annals of Neurology, 13,* 536–540.

Geers, A. E., Mitchell, C. M., Warner-Czyz, A., Wang, N. Y., et al. (2017). Early sign language exposure and cochlear implantation benefits. *Pediatrics, 140*(1), pii: e20163489.

Gelber, R. P., Redline, S., Ross, G. W., Petrovitch, H., et al. (2015). Associations of brain lesions at autopsy with polysomnography features before death. *Neurology, 84*, 296–303.

Gelstein, S., Yeshurun, Y., Rozenkrantz, L., Shushan, S., et al. (2011). Human tears contain a chemosignal. *Science, 331*, 226–230.

Geniole, S. N., and Carré, J. M. (2018). Human social neuroendocrinology: Review of the rapid effects of testosterone. *Hormones and Behavior*, pii: S0018-506X(18)30066-7. [Epub ahead of print] doi:10.1016/j.yhbeh.2018.06.001

George, D. T., Phillips, M. J., Lifshitz, M., Lionetti, T. A., et al. (2011). Fluoxetine treatment of alcoholic perpetrators of domestic violence: A 12-week, double-blind, randomized, placebo-controlled intervention study. *Journal of Clinical Psychiatry, 72*(1), 60–65.

Georgiadis, J. R., Reinders, A. A., Paans, A. M., Renken, R., et al. (2009). Men versus women on sexual brain function: Prominent differences during tactile genital stimulation, but not during orgasm. *Human Brain Mapping, 10*, 3089–3101.

Georgopoulos, A. P., Kalaska, J. F., Caminiti, R., and Massey, J. T. (1982). On the relations between the direction of two-dimensional arm movements and cell discharge in primate motor cortex. *Journal of Neuroscience, 2*, 1527–1537.

Georgopoulos, A. P., Taira, M., and Lukashin, A. (1993). Cognitive neurophysiology of the motor cortex. *Science, 260*, 47–52.

Gerashchenko, D., Kohls, M. D., Greco, M. A., Waleh, N. S., et al. (2001). Hypocretin-2-saporin lesions of the lateral hypothalamus produce narcoleptic-like sleep behavior in the rat. *Neuroscience, 21*, 7273–7283.

Gerkin, R. C., and Castro, J. B. (2015). The number of olfactory stimuli that humans can discriminate is still unknown. *eLife, 4*, e08127.

Geschwind, N. (1976). Language and cerebral dominance. In T. N. Chase (Ed.), *Nervous system: Vol. 2. The clinical neurosciences* (pp. 433–439). New York, NY: Raven Press.

Geschwind, N. (1979). Specializations of the human brain. *Scientific American, 241*, 180–199.

Geschwind, N., and Levitsky, W. (1968). Human brain: Left-right asymmetries in temporal speech region. *Science, 161*, 186–187.

Gibbons, R. D., Hur, K., Brown, C. H., Davis, J. M., et al. (2012). Benefits from antidepressants: Synthesis of 6-week patient-level outcomes from double-blind placebo-controlled randomized trials of fluoxetine and venlafaxine. *Archives of General Psychiatry, 69*, 572–579.

Gilbertson, M. W., Shenton, M. E., Ciszewski, A., Kasai, K., et al. (2002). Smaller hippocampal volume predicts pathologic vulnerability to psychological trauma. *Nature Neuroscience, 5*, 1242–1247.

Gildersleeve, K., Haselton, M. G., and Fales, M. R. (2014). Do women's mate preferences change across the ovulatory cycle? A meta-analytic review. *Psychological Bulletin, 140*(5), 1205–1259.

Gill, R. E., Tibbitts, T. L., Douglas, D. C., Hanel, C. M., et al. (2009). Extreme endurance flights by landbirds crossing the Pacific Ocean: Ecological corridor rather than barrier? *Proceedings of the Royal Society of London. Series B: Biological Sciences, 276*, 447–457.

Gillin, J. C., Duncan, W. C., Murphy, D. L., Post, R. M., et al. (1981). Age-related changes in sleep in depressed and normal subjects. *Psychiatry Research, 4*, 73–78.

Giustino, T. F., Fitzgerald, P. J., and Maren, S. (2016). Revisiting propranolol and PTSD: Memory erasure or extinction enhancement? *Neurobiology of Learning and Memory, 130*, 26–33.

Glaser, R., Rice, J., Speicher, C. E., Stout, J. C., et al. (1986). Stress depresses interferon production by leukocytes concomitant with a decrease in natural killer cell activity. *Behavioral Neuroscience, 100*, 675–678.

Glasser, M. F., Smith, S. M., Marcus, D. S., Andersson, J. L., et al. (2016). The Human Connectome Project's neuroimaging approach. *Nature Neuroscience, 19*(9), 1175–1187.

Glenn, A. L., and Raine, A. (2014). Neurocriminology: Implications for the punishment, prediction and prevention of criminal behaviour. *Nature Reviews Neuroscience, 15*(1), 54–63.

Glickman, S. E. (1977). Comparative psychology. In P. Mussen and M. R. Rosenzweig (Eds.), *Psychology: An introduction* (2nd ed., pp. 625–703). Lexington, MA: Heath.

Glickman, S. E., Frank, L. G., Davidson, J. M., Smith, E. R., et al. (1987). Androstenedione may organize or activate sex-reversed traits in female spotted hyenas. *Proceedings of the National Academy of Sciences, USA, 84*, 344–347.

Goel, V., and Dolan, R. J. (2001). The functional anatomy of humor: Segregating cognitive and affective components. *Nature Neuroscience, 4*, 237–238.

Gogtay, N., Giedd, J. N., Lusk, L., Hayashi, K. M., et al. (2004). Dynamic mapping of human cortical development during childhood through early adulthood. *Proceedings of the National Academy of Sciences, USA, 101*, 8174–8179.

Golden, R. N., Gaynes, B. N., Ekstrom, R. D., Hamer, R. M., et al. (2005). The efficacy of light therapy in the treatment of mood disorders: A review and meta-analysis of the evidence. *American Journal of Psychiatry, 162*, 656–662.

Goldin, P. R., and Gross, J. J. (2010). Effects of mindfulness-based stress reduction (MBSR) on emotion regulation in social anxiety disorder. *Emotion, 10*, 83–91.

Goldstein, J. M., Seidman, L. J., Horton, N. J., Makris, N., et al. (2001). Normal sexual dimorphism of the adult human brain assessed by in vivo magnetic resonance imaging. *Cerebral Cortex, 11*, 490–497.

Golomb, J., de Leon, M. J., George, A. E., Kluger, A., et al. (1994). Hippocampal atrophy correlates with severe cognitive impairment in elderly patients with suspected normal pressure hydrocephalus. *Journal of Neurology, Neurosurgery and Psychiatry, 57*, 590–593.

Gonçalves, T. C., Londe, A. K., Albano, R. I., et al. (2014). Cannabidiol and endogenous opioid peptide-mediated mechanisms modulate antinociception induced by transcutaneous electrostimulation of the peripheral nervous system. *Journal of Neurological Sciences, 347*, 82–89.

Gooch, C. L., Pracht, E., and Borenstein, A. R. (2017). The burden of neurological disease in the United States: A summary report and call to action. *Annals of Neurology, 81*(4), 479–484.

Goodale, M. A., Milner, A. D., Jakobson, L. S., and Carey, D. P. (1991). A neurological dissociation between perceiving objects and grasping them. *Nature, 349*, 154–156.

Gooley, J. J., Rajaratnam, S. M., Brainard, G. C., Kronauer, R. E., et al. (2010). Spectral responses of the human circadian system depend on the irradiance and duration of exposure to light. *Science Translational Medicine, 2*, 31ra33.

Gordon, N. S., Burke, S., Akil, H., Watson, S. J., et al. (2003). Socially-induced brain "fertilization": Play promotes brain derived neurotrophic factor transcription in the amygdala and dorsolateral frontal cortex in juvenile rats. *Neuroscience Letters, 341*, 17–20.

Gorski, R. A., Gordon, J. H., Shryne, J. E., and Southam, A. M. (1978). Evidence for a morphological sex difference within the medial preoptic area of the rat brain. *Brain Research, 148*, 333–346.

Gorzalka, B. B., Mendelson, S. D., and Watson, N. V. (1990). Serotonin receptor subtypes and sexual behavior. *Annals of the New York Academy of Sciences, 600*, 435–444.

Gosseries, O., Di, H., Laureys, S., and Boly, M. (2014). Measuring consciousness in severely damaged brains. *Annual Review of Neuroscience, 37*, 457–478.

Goswami, U. (2015). Sensory theories of developmental dyslexia: Three challenges for research. *Nature Reviews Neuroscience, 16*(1), 43–54.

Gottesman, I. I. (1991). *Schizophrenia genesis: The origins of madness*. New York, NY: Freeman.

Neurobiological and functional considerations. *Progress in Neurobiology, 98*, 82–98.

Hodgkin, A. L., and Katz, B. (1949). The effect of sodium ions on the electrical activity of the giant axon of the squid. *Journal of Physiology (London), 108*, 37–77.

Hoeft, F., Hernandez, A., McMillon, G., Taylor-Hill, H., et al. (2006). Neural basis of dyslexia: A comparison between dyslexic and nondyslexic children equated for reading ability. *Journal of Neuroscience, 26*, 10700–10708.

Hoekzema, E., Barba-Müller, E., Pozzobon, C., Picado, M., et al. (2017). Pregnancy leads to long-lasting changes in human brain structure. *Nature Neuroscience, 20*(2), 287–296.

Hofmann, S. G., Sawyer, A. T., Witt, A. A., and Oh, D. (2010). The effect of mindfulness-based therapy on anxiety and depression: A meta-analytic review. *Journal of Consulting and Clinical Psychology, 78*, 169–183.

Hohmann, A. G., Suplita, R. L., Bolton, N. M., Neely, M. H., et al. (2005). An endocannobinoid mechanism for stress-induced analgesia. *Nature, 435*, 1108–1112.

Hohmann, G. W. (1966). Some effects of spinal cord lesions on experienced emotional feelings. *Psychophysiology, 3*, 143–156.

Hollon, S. D., Thase, M. E., and Markowitz, J. C. (2002). Treatment and prevention of depression. *Psychological Science in the Public Interest, 3*, 39–77.

Holmes, C., Boche, D., Wilkinson, D., Yadegarfar, G., et al. (2008). Long-term effects of Abeta42 immunisation in Alzheimer's disease: Follow-up of a randomized, placebo-controlled phase I trial. *Lancet, 372*, 216–223.

Honey, G. D., Bullmore, E. T., Soni, W., Varatheesan, M., et al. (1999). Differences in frontal cortical activation by a working memory task after substitution of risperidone for typical antipsychotic drugs in patients with schizophrenia. *Proceedings of the National Academy of Sciences, USA, 96*, 13432–13437.

Hopfinger, J. B., Buonocore, M. H., and Mangun, G. R. (2000). The neural mechanisms of top-down attentional control. *Nature Neuroscience, 3*, 284–291.

Hopfinger, J., and Mangun, G. (1998). Reflexive attention modulates processing of visual stimuli in human extrastriate cortex. *Psychological Science, 6*, 441–447.

Hopkins, W. D., Misiura, M., Pope, S. M., and Latash, E. M. (2015). Behavioral and brain asymmetries in primates: A preliminary evaluation of two evolutionary hypotheses. *Annals of the New York Academy of Sciences, 1359*, 65–83.

Horton, J. C., and Adams, D. L. (2005). The cortical column: A structure without a function. *Philosophical Transactions of the Royal Society of London. Series B: Biological Sciences, 360*, 837–862.

Howard-Jones, P. A. (2014). Neuroscience and education: Myths and messages. *Nature Reviews Neuroscience, 15*(12), 817–824.

Howland, R. H. (2007). Lithium: Underappreciated and underused? *Journal of Psychosocial Nursing and Mental Health Services, 45*(8), 13–17.

Hsu, M., Bhatt, M., Adolphs, R., Tranel, D., et al. (2005). Neural systems responding to degrees of uncertainty in human decision-making. *Science, 310*, 1680–1683.

Hua, J. T., Hildreth, K. L., and Pelak, V. S. (2016). Effects of testosterone therapy on cognitive function in aging: A systematic review. *Cognitive and Behavioral Neurology, 29*(3), 122–138.

Huang, A. L., Chen, X., Hoon, M. A., Chandrashekar, J., et al. (2006). The cells and logic for mammalian sour taste detection. *Nature, 442*, 934–938.

Huang, G., and Basaria, S. (2018). Do anabolic-androgenic steroids have performance-enhancing effects in female athletes? *Molecular and Cellular Endocrinology, 464*, 56–64.

Huang, Z. J., and Luo, L. (2015). It takes the world to understand the brain. *Science, 350*(6256), 42–44.

Hubel, D. H., and Wiesel, T. N. (1959). Receptive fields of single neurones in the cat's striate cortex. *Journal of Physiology (London), 148*, 573–591.

Hubel, D. H., and Wiesel, T. N. (1962). Receptive fields, binocular interaction and functional architecture in the cat's visual cortex. *Journal of Physiology (London), 160*, 106–154.

Hubel, D. H., and Wiesel, T. N. (1965). Binocular interaction in striate cortex of kittens reared with artificial squint. *Journal of Neurophysiology, 28*, 1041–1059.

Hubel, D. H., Wiesel, T. N., and LeVay, S. (1977). Plasticity of ocular dominance in monkey striate cortex. *Philosophical Transactions of the Royal Society of London. Series B: Biological Sciences, 278*, 377–409.

Hudspeth, A. J. (2014). Integrating the active process of hair cells with cochlear function. *Nature Reviews Neuroscience, 15*, 600–614.

Hudspeth, A. J., Choe, Y., Mehta, A. D., and Martin, P. (2000). Putting ion channels to work: Mechanoelectrical transduction, adaptation, and amplification by hair cells. *Proceedings of the National Academy of Sciences, USA, 97*, 11765–11772.

Huedo-Medina, T. B., Kirsch, I., Middlemass, J., Klonizakis, M., et al. (2012). Effectiveness of non-benzodiazepine hypnotics in treatment of adult insomnia: Meta-analysis of data submitted to the Food and Drug Administration. *BMJ, 345*, e8343.

Huettel, S. A., Stowe, C. J., Gordon, E. M., Warner, B. T., et al. (2006). Neural signatures of economic preferences for risk and ambiguity. *Neuron, 49*, 765–775.

Hughes, I. A., Houk, C., Ahmed, S. F., Lee, P. A., et al. (2006). Consensus statement on management of intersex disorders. *Journal of Pediatric Urology, 2*(3), 148–162.

Hughes, J., Smith, T. W., Kosterlitz, H. W., Fothergill, L. A., et al. (1975). Identification of two related pentapeptides from the brain with potent opiate agonist activity. *Nature, 258*, 577–580.

Hülsheger, U. R., and Schewe, A. F. (2011). On the costs and benefits of emotional labor: A meta-analysis of three decades of research. *Journal of Occupational Health Psychology, 16*(3), 361–389.

Human Rights Watch. (2017). *"I want to be like nature made me": Medically unnecessary surgeries on intersex children in the US.* New York, NY (https://www.hrw.org/sites/default/files/report_pdf/lgbtintersex0717_web_0.pdf).

Huntington, G. (1872). On chorea. *Medical and Surgical Reporter, 26*, 317–321.

Hurtado, M. D., Sergeyev, V. G., Acosta, A., Spegele, M., et al. (2013). Salivary peptide tyrosine-tyrosine 3-36 modulates ingestive behavior without inducing taste aversion. *Journal of Neuroscience, 33*, 18368–18380.

Hussain, S. J., and Cole, K. J. (2015). No enhancement of 24-hour visuomotor skill retention by post-practice caffeine administration. *PLOS ONE, 10*(6), e0129543.

Huth, A. G., de Heer, W. A., Griffiths, T. L., Theunissen, F. E., et al. (2016). Natural speech reveals the semantic maps that tile human cerebral cortex. *Nature, 532*(7600), 453–458.

Huttenlocher, P. R., and Dabholkar, A. S. (1997). Regional differences in synaptogenesis in human cerebral cortex. *Journal of Comparative Neurology, 387*, 167–178.

Huttenlocher, P. R., deCourten, C., Garey, L. J., and Van der Loos, H. (1982). Synaptogenesis in human visual cortex—Evidence for synapse elimination during normal development. *Neuroscience Letters, 33*, 247–252.

Hyde, K. L., and Peretz I. (2004). Brains that are out of tune but in time. *Psychological Science, 15*, 356–360.

Hyde, K. L., Zatorre, R. J., Griffiths, T. D., Lerch, J. P., et al. (2006). Morphometry of the amusic brain: A two-site study. *Brain, 129*, 2562–2570.

Hyde, T. M., and Weinberger, D. R. (1990). The brain in schizophrenia. *Seminars in Neurology, 10*, 276–286.

Hyman, S. E. (2018). The daunting polygenicity of mental illness: Making a new map. *Philosophical Transactions of the Royal Society of London. Series B: Biological Sciences, 373*(1742), pii: 20170031.

I

Imai, T., Yamazaki, T., Kobayakawa, R., Kobayakawa, K., et al. (2009). Pre-target axon sorting establishes the neural map topography. *Science, 325*, 585–590.

Imeri, L., and Opp, M. R. (2009). How (and why) the immune system makes us sleep. *Nature Reviews Neuroscience, 10*, 199–210.

Imperato-McGinley, J., Guerrero, L., Gautier, T., and Peterson, R. E. (1974). Steroid 5α-reductase deficiency in man: An inherited form of male pseudohermaphroditism. *Science, 86*, 1213–1215.

Infurna, F. J., and Luthar, S. S. (2016). Resilience to major life stressors is not as common as thought. *Perspectives on Psychological Science, 11*(2), 175–194.

Insley, S. J. (2000). Long-term vocal recognition in the northern fur seal. *Nature, 406*, 404–405.

Institute of Medicine. (1990). *Broadening the base of treatment for alcohol problems.* Washington, DC: National Academies Press.

Institute of Medicine. (2010). *Gulf War and health: Vol. 8. Update of health effects of serving in the Gulf War.* Washington, DC: National Academies Press.

Isacson, O., Bjorklund, L., and Sanchez Pernaute, R. (2001). Parkinson's disease: Interpretations of transplantation study erroneous. *Nature Neuroscience, 4*, 533.

Isles, A. R., Baum, M. J., Ma, D., Keverne, E. B., et al. (2001). Urinary odour preferences in mice. *Nature, 409*, 783–784.

Izumikawa, M., Minoda, R., Kawamoto, K., Abrashkin, K. A., et al. (2005). Auditory hair cell replacement and hearing improvement by *Atoh1* gene therapy in deaf mammals. *Nature Medicine, 11*, 271–276.

J

Jackson, H., and Parks, T. N. (1982). Functional synapse elimination in the developing avian cochlear nucleus with simultaneous reduction in cochlear nerve axon branching. *Journal of Neuroscience, 2*, 1736–1743.

Jacobs, G. H. (1993). The distribution and nature of colour vision among the mammals. *Biological Reviews of the Cambridge Philosophical Society, 68*, 413–471.

Jacobs, G. H., Williams, G. A., Cahill, H., and Nathans, J. (2007). Emergence of novel color vision in mice engineered to express a human cone photopigment. *Science, 315*, 1723–1725.

Jacobs, J., Weidemann, C. T., Miller, J. F., Solway, A., et al. (2013). Direct recordings of grid-like neuronal activity in human spatial navigation. *Nature Neuroscience, 16*(9), 1188–1190.

Jacobs, L. F., and Spencer, W. D. (1994). Natural space-use patterns and hippocampal size in kangaroo rats. *Brain, Behavior and Evolution, 44*, 125–132.

Jacobs, L. F., Gaulin, S. J., Sherry, D. F., and Hoffman, G. E. (1990). Evolution of spatial cognition: Sex-specific patterns of spatial behavior predict hippocampal size. *Proceedings of the National Academy of Sciences, USA, 87*, 6349–6352.

Jain, R., and Correll, C. U. (2018). Tardive dyskinesia: Recognition, patient assessment, and differential diagnosis. *Journal of Clinical Psychiatry, Mar/Apr*(2), pii: nu17034ah1c.

James, T. W., Culham, J., Humphery, G. K., Milner, A. D., et al. (2003). Ventral occipital lesions impair object recognition but not object-directed grasping: An fMRI study. *Brain, 126*, 2464–2475.

James, W. (1890). *Principles of psychology.* New York, NY: Holt.

Jamieson, D., and Roberts, A. (2000). Responses of young *Xenopus laevis* tadpoles to light dimming: Possible roles for the pineal eye. *Journal of Experimental Biology, 203*, 1857–1867.

Janak, P. H., and Tye, K. M. (2015). From circuits to behaviour in the amygdala. *Nature, 517*(7534), 284–292.

Jaskiw, G. E., and Popli, A. P. (2004). A meta-analysis of the response to chronic l-dopa in patients with schizophrenia: Therapeutic and heuristic implications. *Psychopharmacology (Berlin), 171*, 365–374.

Jasper, H., and Penfield, W. (1954). *Epilepsy and the functional anatomy of the human brain* (2nd ed.). New York, NY: Little, Brown.

Jeffress, L. A. (1948). A place theory of sound localization. *Journal of Comparative and Physiological Psychology, 41*, 35–39.

Jenkins, J., and Dallenbach, K. (1924). Oblivescence during sleep and waking. *American Journal of Psychology, 35*, 605–612.

Jentsch, J. D., Redmond, D. E., Jr., Elsworth, J. D., Taylor, J. R., et al. (1997). Enduring cognitive deficits and cortical dopamine dysfunction in monkeys after long-term administration of phencyclidine. *Science, 277*, 953–955.

Jessen, N. A., Munk, A. S., Lundgaard, I., and Nedergaard, M. (2015). The glymphatic system: A beginner's guide. *Neurochemical Research, 40*(12), 2583–2599.

Johansson, R. S., and Flanagan, J. R. (2009). Coding and use of tactile signals from the fingertips in object manipulation tasks. *Nature Reviews Neuroscience, 10*, 345–358.

Johnson, L. C. (1969). Psychological and physiological changes following total sleep deprivation. In A. Kales (Ed.), *Sleep: Physiology & pathology; a symposium* (pp. 206–220). Philadelphia, PA: Lippincott.

Jones, H. J., Gage, S. H., Heron, J., Hickman, M., et al. (2018). Association of combined patterns of tobacco and cannabis use in adolescence with psychotic experiences. *JAMA Psychiatry.* [Epub ahead of print] doi:10.1001/jamapsychiatry.2017.4271

Jones, P. B., Barnes, T. R. E., Davies, L., Dunn, G., et al. (2006). Randomized controlled trial of the effect on Quality of Life of second- vs first-generation antipsychotic drugs in schizophrenia. *Archives of General Psychiatry, 39*, 1079–1087.

Jones, T. A. (2017). Motor compensation and its effects on neural reorganization after stroke. *Nature Reviews Neuroscience, 18*(5), 267–280.

Jordan, B. D., Jahre, C., Hauser, W. A., Zimmerman, R. D., et al. (1992). CT of 338 active professional boxers. *Radiology, 185*, 509–512.

Jordan, C. L., Breedlove, S. M., and Arnold, A. P. (1991). Ontogeny of steroid accumulation in spinal lumbar motoneurons of the rat: Implications for androgen's site of action during synapse elimination. *Journal of Comparative Neurology, 313*, 441–448.

Jordt, S.-E., Bautista, D. M., Chuang, H., McKemy, D. D., et al. (2004). Mustard oils and cannabinoids excite sensory nerve fibres through the TRP channel ANKTM1. *Nature, 427*, 260–265.

Joseph, J. (2013b). "Schizophrenia" and heredity: Why the emperor (still) has no genes. In J. Read and J. Dillon (Eds.), *Models of madness: Psychological, social and biological approaches to psychosis* (2nd ed., pp. 72–89). London, UK: Routledge.

Joseph, J. S., Chun, M. M., and Nakayama, K. (1997). Attentional requirements in a "preattentive" feature search task. *Nature, 387*, 805–807.

Julian, T., and McKenry, P. C. (1979). Relationship of testosterone to men's family functioning at mid-life: A research note. *Aggressive Behavior, 15*, 281–289.

K

Kaar, G. F., and Fraher, J. P. (1985). The development of alpha and gamma motoneuron fibres in the rat. I. A comparative ultrastructural study of their central and peripheral axon growth. *Journal of Anatomy, 141*, 77–88.

Kaas, J. H., Nelson, R. J., Sur, M., Lin, C. S., et al. (1979). Multiple representations of the body within the primary somatosensory cortex of primates. *Science, 204*, 521–523.

Kable, J. W., and Glimcher, P. W. (2009). The neurobiology of decision: Consensus and controversy. *Neuron, 63*, 733–745.

Kaiser, D. (2013). Infralow frequencies and ultradian rhythms. *Seminars in Pediatric Neurology, 20*, 242–245.

Kajimura, S., and Saito, M. (2014). A new era in brown adipose tissue biology: Molecular control of brown fat development and energy homeostasis. *Annual Review of Physiology, 76*, 225–249.

Kales, A., and Kales, J. (1970). Evaluation, diagnosis and treatment of clinical conditions related to sleep. *JAMA, 213,* 2229–2235.

Kales, A., and Kales, J. D. (1974). Sleep disorders. Recent findings in the diagnosis and treatment of disturbed sleep. *New England Journal of Medicine, 290,* 487–499.

Kandel, E. R. (1976). *Cellular basis of behavior.* San Francisco: Freeman.

Kandel, E. R. (2009). The biology of memory: A forty-year perspective. *Journal of Neuroscience, 29,* 12748–12756.

Kandler, K., Clause, A., and Noh, J. (2009). Tonotopic reorganization of developing auditory brainstem circuits. *Nature Neuroscience, 12,* 711–716.

Kane, J. M., and Correll, C. U. (2010). Past and present progress in the pharmacologic treatment of schizophrenia. *Journal of Clinical Psychiatry, 71*(9), 1115–1124.

Kang, C., Riazuddin, S., Mundorff, J., Krasnewich, D., et al. (2010). Mutation in the lysosomal enzyme–targeting pathway and persistent stuttering. *New England Journal of Medicine, 362,* 677–685.

Kang, J.-E., Lim, M. M., Bateman, R. J., Lee, J. J., et al. (2009). Amyloid-β dynamics are regulated by orexin and the sleep-wake cycle. *Science, 326,* 1005–1007.

Kanwisher, N., and Wojciulik, E. (2000). Visual attention: Insights from brain imaging. *Nature Reviews Neuroscience, 1,* 91–100.

Karch, S. B. (2006). *Drug abuse handbook* (2nd ed.). Boca Raton, FL: CRC Press.

Karlin, A. (2002). Emerging structure of the nicotinic acetylcholine receptors. *Nature Reviews Neuroscience, 3,* 102–114.

Karni, A., Tanne, D., Rubenstein, B. S., Askenasy, J. J., et al. (1994). Dependence on REM sleep of overnight improvement of a perceptual skill. *Science, 265,* 679–682.

Karpicke, J. D., and Roediger, H. L., III. (2008). The critical importance of retrieval for learning. *Science, 319,* 966–968.

Karra, E., Chandarana, K., and Batterham, R. L. (2009). The role of peptide YY in appetite regulation and obesity. *Journal of Physiology, 587,* 19–25.

Kass, A. E., Kolko, R. P., and Wilfley, D. E. (2013). Psychological treatments for eating disorders. *Current Opinion in Psychiatry, 26,* 549–555.

Katz, D. B., and Steinmetz, J. E. (2002). Psychological functions of the cerebellum. *Behavioral Cognitive Neuroscience Review, 1,* 229–241.

Katzenberg, D., Young, T., Finn, L., Lin, L., et al. (1998). A CLOCK polymorphism associated with human diurnal preference. *Sleep, 21,* 569–576.

Kaushall, P. I., Zetin, M., and Squire, L. R. (1981). A psychosocial study of chronic, circumscribed amnesia. *Journal of Nervous and Mental Disease, 169,* 383–389.

Kay, K. N., Naselaris, T., Prenger, R. J., and Gallant, J. L. (2008). Identifying natural images from human brain activity. *Nature, 452,* 352–355.

Kaya, E. M., and Elhilali, M. (2017). Modelling auditory attention. *Philosophical Transactions of the Royal Society of London. Series B: Biological Sciences, 372*(1714), 1–10.

Kaye, W. H., Fudge, J. L., and Paulus, M. (2009). New insights into symptoms and neurocircuit function of anorexia nervosa. *Nature Reviews Neuroscience, 10,* 573–584.

Keane, T. M. (1998). Psychological and behavioral treatments of post-traumatic stress disorder. In P. E. Nathan and J. M. Gorman (Eds.), *A guide to treatments that work* (pp. 398–407). New York, NY: Oxford University Press.

Kee, N., Teixeira, C. M., Wang, A. H., and Frankland, P. W. (2007). Preferential incorporation of adult-generated granule cells into spatial memory networks in the dentate gyrus. *Nature Neuroscience, 10,* 355–362.

Keenan, J. P., Nelson, A., O'Connor, M., and Pascual-Leone, A. (2001). Self-recognition and the right hemisphere. *Nature, 409,* 305.

Keesey, R. E. (1980). A set-point analysis of the regulation of body weight. In A. J. Stunkard (Ed.), *Obesity* (pp. 144–165). Philadelphia, PA: Saunders.

Keesey, R. E., and Boyle, P. C. (1973). Effects of quinine adulteration upon body weight of LH-lesioned and intact male rats. *Journal of Comparative and Physiological Psychology, 84,* 38–46.

Keesey, R. E., and Corbett, S. W. (1984). Metabolic defense of the body weight set-point. *Research Publications—Association for Research in Nervous and Mental Disease, 62,* 87–96.

Keesey, R. E., and Powley, T. L. (1986). The regulation of body weight. *Annual Review of Psychology, 37,* 109–133.

Kelly, J. P. (2011). Cathinone derivatives: A review of their chemistry, pharmacology and toxicology. *Drug Testing and Analysis, 3*(7–8), 439–453.

Keltner, D., and Ekman, P. (2000). Facial expression of emotion. In M. Lewis and J. M. Haviland-Jones (Eds.), *Handbook of emotions* (2nd ed., pp. 236–250). New York, NY: Guilford Press.

Kemp, J. A., and McKernan, R. M. (2002). NMDA receptor pathways as drug targets. *Nature Neuroscience, 5*(Suppl.), 1039–1042.

Kempermann, G., Kuhn, H. G., and Gage, F. H. (1997). More hippocampal neurons in adult mice living in an enriched environment. *Nature, 386,* 493–495.

Kendler, K. S., Gardner, C. O., and Prescott, C. A. (1999). Clinical characteristics of major depression that predict risk of depression in relatives. *Archives of General Psychiatry, 56,* 322–327.

Kenis, G., and Maes, M. (2002). Effects of antidepressants on the production of cytokines. *International Journal of Neuropsychopharmacology, 5,* 401–412.

Kennedy, D. P., Gläscher, J., Tyszka, J. M., and Adolphs, R. (2009). Personal space regulation by the human amygdala. *Nature Neuroscience, 12*(10), 1226–1227.

Kennedy, J. L., Farrer, L. A., Andreasen, N. C., Mayeux, R., et al. (2003). The genetics of adult-onset neuropsychiatric disease: Complexities and conundra? *Science, 302,* 822–826.

Kennerknecht, I., Grueter, T., Welling, B., Wentzek, S., et al. (2006). First report of prevalence of non-syndromic hereditary prosopagnosia (HPA). *American Journal of Medical Genetics Part A, 140,* 1617–1622.

Kerns, J. C., Guo, J., Fothergill, E., Howard, L., et al. (2017). Increased physical activity associated with less weight regain six years after "The Biggest Loser" competition. *Obesity (Silver Spring), 25*(11), 1838–1843.

Kertesz, A., Harlock, W., and Coates, R. (1979). Computer tomographic localization, lesion size, and prognosis in aphasia and nonverbal impairment. *Brain and Language, 8,* 34–50.

Kertesz, A. and McCabe, P. (1977). Recovery patterns and prognosis in aphasia. *Brain, 100,* 1–18.

Kessels, H. W., and Malinow, R. (2009). Synaptic AMPA receptor plasticity and behavior. *Neuron, 61,* 340–350.

Kessler, R. C., Angermeyer, M., Anthony, J. C., de Graaf, R., et al. (2007). Lifetime prevalence and age-of-onset distributions of mental disorders in the World Health Organization's World Mental Health Survey Initiative. *World Psychiatry, 6,* 168–176.

Kessler, R. C., Berglund, P., Demler, O., Jin, R., et al. (2005). Lifetime prevalence and age-of-onset distributions of *DSM-IV* disorders in the National Comorbidity Survey Replication. *Archives of General Psychiatry, 62,* 593–602.

Kety, S. S., Wender, P. H., Jacobsen, B., Ingraham, L. J., et al. (1994). Mental illness in the biological and adoptive relatives of schizophrenic adoptees. Replication of the Copenhagen Study in the rest of Denmark. *Archives of General Psychiatry, 51,* 442–455.

Kheirbek, M. A., Klemenhagen, K. C., Sahay, A., and Hen, R. (2012). Neurogenesis and generalization: A new approach to stratify and treat anxiety disorders. *Nature Neuroscience, 15,* 1613–1620.

Kiang, N. Y. S. (1965). *Discharge patterns of single fibers in the cat's auditory nerve.* Cambridge, MA: MIT Press.

Kim, D. R., Pesiridou, A., and O'Reardon, J. P. (2009). Transcranial magnetic stimulation in the treatment of psychiatric disorders. *Current Psychiatry Reports, 11,* 447–452.

Kim, J. S., Kornhuber, H. H., Schmid-Burgk, W., and Holzmüller, B. (1980). Low cerebrospinal fluid glutamate in schizophrenic patients and a new hypothesis on schizophrenia. *Neuroscience Letters, 20*(3), 379–382.

Kim, K. H., Relkin, N. R., Lee, K. M., and Hirsch, J. (1997). Distinct cortical areas associated with native and second languages. *Nature, 388,* 171–174.

Kimura, D. (1973). The asymmetry of the human brain. *Scientific American, 228*(3), 70–78.

Kimura, D. (1981). Neural mechanisms in manual signing. *Sign Language Studies, 33,* 291–312.

Kimura, D. (1993). *Neuromotor mechanisms in human communication.* Oxford, UK: Oxford University Press.

Kimura, D., and Watson, N. V. (1989). The relation between oral movement control and speech. *Brain and Language, 37,* 565–590.

Kindt, M., Soeter, M., and Vervliet, B. (2009). Beyond extinction: Erasing human fear responses and preventing the return of fear. *Nature Neuroscience, 12,* 256–258.

King, A. (2013). The nose knows: How to train a canine conservationist. *New Scientist, 219,* 40–43.

King, S., St-Hilaire, A., and Heidkamp, D. (2010). Prenatal factors in schizophrenia. *Current Directions in Psychological Science, 19,* 209–213.

Kingsbury, S. J., and Garver, D. L. (1998). Lithium and psychosis revisited. *Progress in Neuro-Psychopharmacology & Biological Psychiatry, 22,* 249–263.

Kinney, H. C. (2009). Brainstem mechanisms underlying the sudden infant death syndrome: Evidence from human pathologic studies. *Developmental Psychobiology, 51,* 223–233.

Kinsey, A. C., Pomeroy, W. B., and Martin, C. E. (1948). *Sexual behavior in the human male.* Philadelphia, PA: Saunders.

Kinsey, A. C., Pomeroy, W. B., Martin, C. E., and Gebhard, P. H. (1953). *Sexual behavior in the human female.* Philadelphia, PA: Saunders.

Kinsley, C. H., and Lambert, K. G. (2006). The maternal brain. *Scientific American, 294,* 72–79.

Kirik, D., Georgievska, B., and Björklund, A. (2004). Localized striatal delivery of GDNF as a treatment for Parkinson disease. *Nature Neuroscience, 7,* 105–110.

Kisely, S., Li, A., Warren, N., and Siskind, D. (2018). A systematic review and meta-analysis of deep brain stimulation for depression. *Depression and Anxiety, 35*(5), 468–480.

Klar, A. J. (2003). Human handedness and scalp hair-whorl direction develop from a common genetic mechanism. *Genetics, 165,* 269–276.

Kleiber, M. (1947). Body size and metabolic rate. *Physiological Reviews, 15,* 511–541.

Klein, B. A. (2003). Signatures of sleep in a paper wasp. *Sleep, 26,* A115–A116.

Klein, M., Shapiro, K. M., and Kandel, E. R. (1980). Synaptic plasticity and the modulation of the Ca²⁺ current. *Journal of Experimental Biology, 89,* 117–157.

Klein, R. M. (2000). Inhibition of return. *Trends in Cognitive Science, 4,* 138–147.

Kleitman, N., and Engelmann, T. (1953). Sleep characteristics of infants. *Journal of Applied Physiology, 6,* 269–282.

Kluger, M. J. (1978). The evolution and adaptive value of fever. *American Scientist, 66,* 38–43.

Klüver, H., and Bucy, P. C. (1938). An analysis of certain effects of bilateral temporal lobectomy in the rhesus monkey, with special reference to "psychic blindness." *Journal of Psychology, 5,* 33–54.

Knecht, S., Flöel, A., Dräger, B., Breitenstein, C., et al. (2002). Degree of language lateralization determines susceptibility to unilateral brain lesions. *Nature Neuroscience, 5,* 695–699.

Knibestol, M., and Valbo, A. B. (1970). Single unit analysis of mechanoreceptor activity from the human glabrous skin. *Acta Physiologica Scandinavica, 80,* 178–195.

Knudsen, E. I. (1982). Auditory and visual maps of space in the optic tectum of the owl. *Journal of Neuroscience, 2,* 1177–1194.

Knudsen, E. I. (1984). The role of auditory experience in the development and maintenance of sound localization. *Trends in Neurosciences, 7,* 326–330.

Knudsen, E. I., and Konishi, M. (1978). A neural map of auditory space in the owl. *Science, 200,* 795–797.

Knudsen, E. I., Knudsen, P. F., and Esterly, S. D. (1984). A critical period for the recovery of sound localization accuracy following monaural occlusion in the barn owl. *Journal of Neuroscience, 4,* 1012–1020.

Knudsen, E., and Knudsen, P. (1985). Vision guides adjustment of auditory localization in young barn owls. *Science, 230,* 545–548.

Koch, G., Oliveri, M., Torriero, S., and Caltagirone, C. (2005). Modulation of excitatory and inhibitory circuits for visual awareness in the human right parietal cortex. *Experimental Brain Research, 160,* 510–516.

Kodama, T., Lai, Y. Y., and Siegel, J. M. (2003). Changes in inhibitory amino acid release linked to pontine-induced atonia: An in vivo microdialysis study. *Journal of Neuroscience, 23,* 1548–1554.

Koehler, K. R., Mikosz, A. M., Molosh, A. I., Patel, D., et al. (2013). Generation of inner ear sensory epithelia from pluripotent stem cells in 3D culture. *Nature, 500,* 217–221.

Koh, K., Joiner, W. J., Wu, M. N., Yue, Z., et al. (2008). Identification of SLEEPLESS, a sleep-promoting factor. *Science, 321,* 372–376.

Kohl, M. M., Shipton, O. A., Deacon, R. M., Rawlins, J. N., et al. (2011). Hemisphere-specific optogenetic stimulation reveals left-right asymmetry of hippocampal plasticity. *Nature Neuroscience, 14,* 1413–1415. doi:10.1038/nn.2915. (Erratum in 2011 *Nature Neuroscience, 14,* 1617.)

Kojima, M., Hosoda, H., Date, Y., Nakazato, M., et al. (1999). Ghrelin is a growth-hormone-releasing acylated peptide from stomach. *Nature, 402,* 656–660.

Kokrashvili, Z., Mosinger, B., and Margolskee, R. F. (2009). T1r3 and alpha-gustducin in gut regulate secretion of glucagon-like peptide-1. *Annals of the New York Academy of Sciences, 1170,* 91–94.

Kondo, Y., Sachs, B. D., and Sakuma, Y. (1997). Importance of the medial amygdala in rat penile erection evoked by remote stimuli from estrous females. *Behavioural Brain Research, 88,* 153–160.

Kondoh, K., Lu, Z., Ye, X., Olson, D. P., et al. (2016). A specific area of olfactory cortex involved in stress hormone responses to predator odours. *Nature, 532*(7597), 103–106.

Konishi, M. (1985). Birdsong: From behavior to neuron. *Annual Review of Neuroscience, 8,* 125–170.

Konopka, R. J., and Benzer, S. (1971). Clock mutants of *Drosophila melanogaster. Proceedings of the National Academy of Sciences, USA, 68,* 2112–2116.

Koob, G. F. (1995). Animal models of drug addiction. In F. E. Bloom and D. J. Kupfer (Eds.), *Psychopharmacology: The fourth generation of progress* (pp. 759–772). New York, NY: Raven Press.

Kopell, B. H., Machado, A. G., and Rezai, A. R. (2005). Not your father's lobotomy: Psychiatric surgery revisited. *Clinical Neurosurgery, 52,* 315–330.

Kordower, J. H., Chu, Y., Hauser, R. A., Freeman, T. B., et al. (2008). UK body–like pathology in long-term embryonic nigral transplants in Parkinson's disease. *Nature Medicine, 14,* 504–506.

Korman, M., Doyon, J., Doljansky, J., Carrier, J., et al. (2007). Daytime sleep condenses the time course of motor memory consolidation. *Nature Neuroscience, 10,* 1206–1213.

Korol, D. L., and Pisani, S. L. (2015). Estrogens and cognition: Friends or foes?: An evaluation of the opposing effects of estrogens on learning and memory. *Hormones and Behavior, 74,* 105–115.

Koubeissi, M. Z., Bartolomei, F., Beltagy, A., and Picard, F. (2014). Electrical stimulation of a small brain area reversibly disrupts consciousness. *Epilepsy & Behavior, 37,* 32–35.

Kovelman, J. A., and Scheibel, A. B. (1984). A neurohistological correlate of schizophrenia. *Biological Psychiatry, 19*, 1601.

Krashes, M. J., Lowell, B. B., and Garfield, A. S. (2016). Melanocortin-4 receptor-regulated energy homeostasis. *Nature Neuroscience, 19*(2), 206–219.

Krause, J., Lalueza-Fox, C., Orlando, L., Enard, W., et al. (2007). The derived *FOXP2* variant of modern humans was shared with Neandertals. *Current Biology, 17*, 1908–1912.

Krauss, R. M. (1998). Why do we gesture when we speak? *Current Directions in Psychological Science, 7*(2), 54–60.

Krebs, J. R., Sherry, D. F., Healy, S. D., Perry, V. H., et al. (1989). Hippocampal specialization of food-storing birds. *Proceedings of the National Academy of Sciences, USA, 86*, 1388–1392.

Kreitman, N. (1976). The coal gas story: United Kingdom suicide rates, 1960–71. *British Journal of Preventive & Social Medicine, 30*(2), 86–93.

Kril, J., Halliday, G., Svoboda, M., and Cartwright, H. (1997). The cerebral cortex is damaged in chronic alcoholics. *Neuroscience, 79*, 983–998.

Kringelbach, M. L. (2005). The human orbitofrontal cortex: Linking reward to hedonic experience. *Nature Reviews Neuroscience, 6*, 691–702.

Kringelbach, M. L., Jenkinson, N., Owen, S. L. F., and Aziz, T. Z. (2007). Translational principles of deep brain stimulation. *Nature Reviews Neuroscience, 8*, 623–634.

Kripke, D. F., Garfinkel, L., Wingard, D. L., Klauber, M. R., et al. (2002). Mortality associated with sleep duration and insomnia. *Archives of General Psychiatry, 59*, 131–136.

Krystal, A., Krishnan, K. R., Raitiere, M., Poland, R., et al. (1990). Differential diagnosis and pathophysiology of Cushing's syndrome and primary affective disorder. *Journal of Neuropsychiatry and Clinical Neurosciences, 2*, 34–43.

Kuhl, B. A., Dudukovic, N. M., Kahn, I., and Wagner, A. D. (2007). Decreased demands on cognitive control reveal the neural processing benefits of forgetting. *Nature Neuroscience, 10*, 908–914.

Kulkarni, A., and Colburn, H. S. (1998). Role of spectral detail in sound-source localization. *Nature, 396*, 747–749.

Kuperberg, G. R. (2007). Neural mechanisms of language comprehension: Challenges to syntax. *Brain Research, 1146*, 23–49.

Kupfer, D. J., Frank, E., and Phillips, M. L. (2012). Major depressive disorder: New clinical, neurobiological, and treatment perspectives. *Lancet, 379*(9820), 1045–1055.

Kupfer, D. J., Reynolds, C. F., Ulrich, R. F., Shaw, D. H., et al. (1982). EEG sleep, depression, and aging. *Neurobiology of Aging, 3*, 351–360.

Kutas, M., and Federmeier, K. D. (2011). Thirty years and counting: Finding meaning in the N400 component of the event-related brain potential (ERP). *Annual Review of Psychology, 62*, 621–647.

Kutas, M., and Hillyard, S. A. (1980). Reading senseless sentences: Brain potentials reflect semantic incongruity. *Science, 207*, 203–205.

Kutas, M., and Hillyard, S. A. (1984). Event-related potentials in cognitive science. In M. S. Gazzaniga (Ed.), *Handbook of cognitive neuroscience* (pp. 387–409). New York, NY: Plenum Press.

Kwakkel, G., Veerbeek, J. M., van Wegen, E. E., and Wolf, S. L. (2015). Constraint-induced movement therapy after stroke. *Lancet Neurology, 14*, 224–234. doi:10.1016/S1474-4422(14)70160-7

Kyzar, E. J., Nichols, C. D., Gainetdinov, R. R., Nichols, D. E., et al. (2017). Psychedelic drugs in biomedicine. *Trends in Pharmacological Sciences, 38*(11), 992–1005.

L

LaBar, K. S., Gatenby, J. C., Gore, J. C., LeDoux, J. E., et al. (1998). Human amygdala activation during conditioned fear acquisition and extinction: A mixed-trial fMRI study. *Neuron, 20*, 937–945.

LaFerla, F. M., Green, K. N., and Oddo, S. (2007). Intracellular amyloid-β in Alzheimer's disease. *Nature Reviews Neuroscience, 8*, 499–508.

Lagrèze, W. A., and Schaeffel, F. (2017). Preventing myopia. *Deutsches Arzteblatt International, 114*(35–36), 575–580.

Lai, C. S. L., Fisher, S. E., Hurst, J. A., Vargha-Khadem, F., et al. (2001). A forkhead-domain gene is mutated in a severe speech and language disorder. *Nature, 413*, 519–523.

Landau, B., and Levy, R. M. (1993). Neuromodulation techniques for medically refractory chronic pain. *Annual Review of Medicine, 44*, 279–287.

Langleben, D. D., Schroeder, L., Maldjian, J. A., Gur, R. C., et al. (2002). Brain activity during simulated deception: An event-related functional magnetic resonance study. *NeuroImage, 15*, 727–732.

Larroche, J.-C. (1977). *Developmental pathology of the neonate.* Amsterdam, Netherlands: Excerpta Medica.

Larsson, J., Gulyas, B., and Roland, P. E. (1996). Cortical representation of self-paced finger movement. *NeuroReport, 7*, 463–468.

Larsson, M., and Willander, J. (2009). Autobiographical odor memory. *Annals of the New York Academy of Sciences, 1170*, 318–323.

Lau, H. C., Rogers, R. D., Haggard, P., and Passingham, R. E. (2004). Attention to intention. *Science, 303*, 1208–1210.

Laverty, P. H., Leskovar, A., Breur, G. J., Coates, J. R., et al. (2004). A preliminary study of intravenous surfactants in paraplegic dogs: Polymer therapy in canine clinical SCI. *Journal of Neurotrauma, 21*, 1767–1777.

Lavie, N. (1995). Perceptual load as a necessary condition for selective attention. *Journal of Experimental Psychology: Human Perception and Performance, 21*, 451–468.

Lavie, N., Hirst, A., de Fockert, J. W., and Viding, E. (2004). Load theory of selective attention and cognitive control. *Journal of Experimental Psychology: General, 133*, 339–354.

Lavie, N., Lin, Z., Zokaei, N., and Thoma, V. (2009). The role of perceptual load in object recognition. *Journal of Experimental Psychology: Human Perception and Performance, 35*, 1346–1358.

Lavie, P. (1996). *The enchanted world of sleep* (A. Berris, Trans.). New Haven, CT: Yale University Press.

Lavond, D. G., Kim, J. J., and Thompson, R. F. (1993). Mammalian brain substrates of aversive classical conditioning. *Annual Review of Psychology, 44*, 317–342.

Le Grange, D. (2005). The Maudsley family-based treatment for adolescent anorexia nervosa. *World Psychiatry, 4*, 142–146.

Leask, S. J., and Beaton, A. A. (2007). Handedness in Great Britain. *Laterality, 12*, 559–572.

LeDoux, J. E. (1994). Emotion, memory and the brain. *Scientific American, 270*(6), 50–57.

LeDoux, J. E. (1996). *The emotional brain: The mysterious underpinnings of emotional life.* London, UK: Simon & Schuster.

Lee, E. E., Della Selva, M. P., Liu, A., and Himelhoch, S. (2015). Ketamine as a novel treatment for major depressive disorder and bipolar depression: A systematic review and quantitative meta-analysis. *General Hospital Psychiatry, 37*(2), 178–184.

Lee, H., Kim, D. W., Remedios, R., Anthony, T. E., et al. (2014). Scalable control of mounting and attack by Esr1+ neurons in the ventromedial hypothalamus. *Nature, 509*, 627–632.

Leinders-Zufall, T., Lane, A. P., Puche, A. C., Ma, W., et al. (2000). Ultrasensitive pheromone detection by mammalian vomeronasal neurons. *Nature, 405*, 792–796.

Lepage, J. F., and Theoret, H. (2006). EEG evidence for the presence of an action observation-execution matching system in children. *European Journal of Neuroscience, 23*, 2505–2510.

Lereya, S. T., Copeland, W. E., Costello, E. J., and Wolke, D. (2015). Adult mental health consequences of peer bullying and maltreatment in childhood: Two cohorts in two countries. *Lancet Psychiatry, 2,* 524–531. doi:http://dx.doi.org/10.1016/S2215-0366(15)00165-0

Lescroart, M. D., Stansbury, D. E., and Gallant, J. L. (2015). Fourier power, subjective distance, and object categories all provide plausible models of BOLD responses in scene-selective visual areas. *Frontiers in Computational Neuroscience, 9,* 135.

Lesku, J. A., Roth, T. C., II, Rattenborg, N. C., Amlaner, . J., et al. (2009). History and future of comparative analyses in sleep research. *Neuroscience and Biobehavioral Reviews, 33,* 1024–1036.

Lesné, S., Koh, M. T., Kotilinek, L., Kayed, R., et al. (2006). A specific amyloid-β protein assembly in the brain impairs memory. *Nature, 440,* 352–357.

Leuner, B., Glasper, E. R., and Gould, E. (2010). Sexual experience promotes adult neurogenesis in the hippocampus despite an initial elevation in stress hormones. *PLOS ONE, 5,* e11597.

Leung, C. T., Coulombe, P. A., and Reed, R. R. (2007). Contribution of olfactory neural stem cells to tissue maintenance and regeneration. *Nature Neuroscience, 10,* 720–726.

LeVay, S. (1991). A difference in hypothalamic structure between heterosexual and homosexual men. *Science, 253,* 1034–1037.

Levine, J. D., Gordon, N. C., and Fields, H. L. (1978). The mechanism of placebo analgesia. *Lancet, 2,* 654–657.

Levine, S., Haltmeyer, G. C., and Karas, G. G. (1967). Physiological and behavioral effects of infantile stimulation. *Physiology & Behavior, 2,* 55–59.

Lew, S. M. (2014). Hemispherectomy in the treatment of seizures: A review. *Translational Pediatrics, 3*(3), 208–217.

Lewis, D. O. (1990). Neuropsychiatric and experiential correlates of violent juvenile delinquency. *Neuropsychology Review, 1,* 125–136.

Lewy, A. J., Bauer, V. K., Cutler, N. L., Sack, R. L., et al. (1998). Morning vs evening light treatment of patients with winter depression. *Archives of General Psychiatry, 55,* 890–896.

Lewy, A. J., Rough, J. N., Songer, J. B., Mishra, N., et al. (2007). The phase shift hypothesis for the circadian component of winter depression. *Dialogues in Clinical Neuroscience, 9,* 291–300.

Li, B., Piriz, J., Mirrione, M., Chung, C., et al. (2011). Synaptic potentiation onto habenula neurons in the learned helplessness model of depression. *Nature, 470,* 535–539.

Li, J. Y., Englund, E., Holton, J. L., Soulet, D., et al. (2008). Lewy bodies in grafted neurons in subjects with Parkinson's disease suggest host-to-graft disease propagation. *Nature Medicine, 14,* 501–503.

Li, W., Ma, L., Yang, G., and Gan, W. B. (2017). REM sleep selectively prunes and maintains new synapses in development and learning. *Nature Neuroscience, 20*(3), 427–437.

Li, X., Glaser, D., Li, W., Johnson, W. E., et al. (2009). Analyses of sweet receptor gene (*Tas1r2*) and preference for sweet stimuli in species of Carnivora. *Journal of Heredity, 100*(Suppl. 1), S90–S100.

Liberles, S. D. (2009). Trace amine-associated receptors are olfactory receptors in vertebrates. *Annals of the New York Academy of Science, 1170,* 168–172.

Liberles, S. D., and Buck, L. B. (2006). A second class of chemosensory receptors in the olfactory epithelium. *Nature, 442,* 645–650.

Libet, B. (1985). Unconscious cerebral initiative and the role of conscious will in voluntary action. *Behavioral and Brain Sciences, 8,* 529–566.

Lichstein, K. L. (2017). Insomnia identity. *Behaviour Research and Therapy, 97,* 230–241.

Licht, P., Frank, L. G., Pavgi, S., Yalcinkaya, T. M., et al. (1992). Hormonal correlates of "masculinization" in female spotted hyenas (*Crocuta crocuta*). 2. Maternal and fetal steroids. *Journal of Reproduction and Fertility, 95,* 463–474.

Lichtenstein, P., Yip, B. H., Björk, C., Pawitan, Y., et al. (2009). Common genetic determinants of schizophrenia and bipolar disorder in Swedish families: A population-based study. *Lancet, 373,* 234–239.

Lichtman, J. W., and Purves, D. (1980). The elimination of redundant preganglionic innervation to hamster sympathetic ganglion cells in early post-natal life. *Journal of Physiology (London), 301,* 213–228.

Liddelow, S. A., Guttenplan, K. A., Clarke, L. E., Bennett, F. C., et al. (2017). Neurotoxic reactive astrocytes are induced by activated microglia. *Nature, 541*(7638), 481–487.

Lieberman, P. (1985). On the evolution of human syntactic ability: Its pre-adaptive bases—motor control and speech. *Journal of Human Evolution, 14,* 657–668.

Liégeois, F., Baldeweg, T., Connelly, A., Gadian, D. G., et al. (2003). Language fMRI abnormalities associated with *FOXP2* gene mutation. *Nature Neuroscience, 6,* 1230–1237.

Liepert, J., Bauder, H., Wolfgang, H. R., Miltner, W. H., et al. (2000). Treatment-induced cortical reorganization after stroke in humans. *Stroke, 31,* 1210–1216.

Lim, M. M., and Young, L. J. (2006). Neuropeptidergic regulation of affiliative behavior and social bonding in animals. *Hormones and Behavior, 50,* 506–557.

Lim, M. M., Wang, Z., Olazabal, D. E., Ren, X., et al. (2004). Enhanced partner preference in a promiscuous species by

manipulating the expression of a single gene. *Nature, 429,* 754–757.

Lin, L., Faraco, J., Li, R., Kadotani, H., et al. (1999). The sleep disorder canine narcolepsy is caused by a mutation in the hypocretin (orexin) receptor 2 gene. *Cell, 98,* 365–376.

Linde, K., Allais, G., Brinkhaus, B., Manheimer, E., et al. (2009). Acupuncture for tension-type headache. *Cochrane Database of Systematic Reviews, 1,* CD007587.

Lindemann, B. (1995). Sweet and salty: Transduction in taste. *News in Physiological Sciences, 10,* 166–170.

Lindvall, O., Sawle, G., Widner, H., Rothwell, J. C., et al. (1994). Evidence for long-term survival and function of dopaminergic grafts in progressive Parkinson's disease. *Annals of Neurology, 35,* 172–180.

Lisk, R. D. (1962). Diencephalic placement of estradiol and sexual receptivity in the female rat. *American Journal of Physiology, 203,* 493–496.

Lisman, J., Schulman, H., and Cline, H. (2002). The molecular basis of CAMKII function in synaptic and behavioural memory. *Nature Reviews Neuroscience, 3,* 175–190.

Liu, D., Diorio, J., Tannenbaum, B., Caldji, C., et al. (1997). Maternal care, hippocampal glucocorticoid receptors, and hypothalamic-pituitary-adrenal responses to stress. *Science, 277,* 1659–1662.

Liu, J., Lillo, C., Jonsson, P. A., Vande Velde, C., et al. (2004). Toxicity of familial ALS-linked SOD1 mutants from selective recruitment to spinal mitochondria. *Neuron, 42,* 5–17.

Liu, Y., Gao, J. H., Liotti, M., Pu, Y., et al. (1999). Temporal dissociation of parallel processing in the human subcortical outputs. *Nature, 400,* 364–367.

Liu, Y., Gao, J.-H., Liu, H.-L., and Fox, P. T. (2000). The temporal response of the brain after eating revealed by functional MRI. *Nature, 405,* 1058–1062.

Livingstone, M. S. (2000). Is it warm? Is it real? Or just low spatial frequency? *Science, 290,* 1299.

Llewellyn, S., and Hobson, J. A. (2015). Not only … but also: REM sleep creates and NREM Stage 2 instantiates landmark junctions in cortical memory networks. *Neurobiology of Learning and Memory, 122,* 69–87.

Lloyd, J. A. (1971). Weights of testes, thymi, and accessory reproductive glands in relation to rank in paired and grouped house mice (*Mus musculus*). *Proceedings of the Society for Experimental Biology and Medicine, 137,* 19–22.

Lo, E. H., Dalkara, T., and Moskowitz, M. A. (2003). Mechanisms, challenges and opportunities in stroke. *Nature Reviews Neuroscience, 4,* 399–415.

Lo, J. C., Lee, S. M., Lee, X. K., Sasmita, K, et al. (2018). Sustained benefits of delaying school start time on adolescent sleep and well-being. *Sleep, 41*(6). doi:10.1093/sleep/zsy052

Lockhart, M., and Moore, J. W. (1975). Classical differential and operant conditioning in rabbits (*Oryctolagus cuniculus*) with septal lesions. *Journal of Comparative and Physiological Psychology, 88,* 147–154.

Loconto, J., Papes, F., Chang, E., Stowers, L., et al. (2003). Functional expression of murine V2R pheromone receptors involves selective association with the M10 and M1 families of MHC class Ib molecules. *Cell, 112,* 607–618.

Loeb, G. E. (1990). Cochlear prosthetics. *Annual Review of Neuroscience, 13,* 357–371.

Loewenstein, W. R. (1971). Mechano-electric transduction in the Pacinian corpuscle. Initiation of sensory impulses in mechanoreception. In *Handbook of sensory physiology: Vol. 1. Principles of receptor physiology* (pp. 269–290). Berlin: Springer.

Loftus, E. F. (2003). Make-believe memories. *American Psychologist, 58,* 867–873.

Logan, C. G., and Grafton, S. T. (1995). Functional anatomy of human eyeblink conditioning determined with regional cerebral glucose metabolism and positron emission tomography. *Proceedings of the National Academy of Sciences, USA, 92,* 7500–7504.

Long, M. A., Jutras, M. J., Connors, B. W., and Burwell, R. D. (2005). Electrical synapses coordinate activity in the suprachiasmatic nucleus. *Nature Neuroscience, 8,* 61–66.

Lotto, R. B. and Purves, D. (2000). An empirical explanation of color contrast. *Proceedings of the National Academy of Sciences, USA, 97,* 12834–12839.

Loui, P., Alsop, D., and Schlaug, G. (2009). Tone deafness: A new disconnection syndrome? *Journal of Neuroscience, 29,* 10215–10220.

Lübke, K. T., and Pause, B. M. (2015). Always follow your nose: The functional significance of social chemosignals in human reproduction and survival. *Hormones and Behavior, 68,* 134–144.

Luck, S. J. (2005). *An introduction to the event-related potential technique.* Cambridge, MA: MIT Press.

Luck, S. J., and Hillyard, S. A. (1994). Electrophysiological correlates of feature analysis during visual search. *Psychophysiology, 31,* 291–308.

Lucking, C. B., Durr, A., Bonifati, V., Vaughan, J., et al. (2000). Association between early-onset Parkinson's disease and mutations in the *parkin* gene. *New England Journal of Medicine, 342,* 1560–1567.

Lundberg, U. (1976). Urban commuting: crowdedness and catecholamine excretion. *Journal of Human Stress, 2,* 26–32.

Luria, A. R. (1987). *The mind of a mnemonist.* Cambridge, MA: Harvard University Press.

Lush, I. E. (1989). The genetics of tasting in mice. VI. Saccharin, acesulfame, dulcin and sucrose. *Genetical Research, 53,* 95–99.

Ly, M., Motzkin, J. C., Philippi, C. L., Kirk, G. R., et al. (2012). Cortical thinning in psychopathy. *The American Journal of Psychiatry, 169,* 743–749. DOI: 10.1176/appi.ajp.2012.11111627

Lyamin, O., Pryaslova, J., Lance, V., and Siegel, J. (2005). Continuous activity in cetaceans after birth: The exceptional wakefulness of newborn whales and dolphins has no ill-effect on their development. *Nature, 435,* 1177.

Lynch, G., Larson, J., Staubli, U., and Granger, R. (1991). Variants of synaptic potentiation and different types of memory operations in hippocampus and related structures. In L. R. Squire, N. M. Weinberger, G. Lynch, and J. L. McGaugh (Eds.), *Memory: Organization and locus of change* (pp. 330–363). New York, NY: Oxford University Press.

M

Macdonald, K., Germine, L., Anderson, A., Christodoulou, J., et al. (2017). Dispelling the myth: Training in education or neuroscience decreases but does not eliminate beliefs in neuromyths. *Frontiers in Psychology, 8,* 1314.

MacLean, P. D. (1949). Psychosomatic disease and the "visceral brain": Recent developments bearing on the Papez theory of emotion. *Psychosomatic Medicine, 11,* 338–353.

MacLeod, C. M. (1991). Half a century of research on the Stroop effect: An integrative review. *Psychological Bulletin, 109,* 163–203.

Macmillan, M. (2000). *An odd kind of fame: Stories of Phineas Gage.* Cambridge, MA: MIT Press.

MacNeilage, P. F., Rogers, L. J., and Vallortigara, G. (2009). Origins of the left & right brain. *Scientific American, 301*(1), 60–67.

Maes, M., Bosmans, E., Suy, E., Vandervorst, C., et al. (1991). Depression-related disturbances in mitogen-induced lymphocyte responses and interleukin-1 beta and soluble interleukin-2 receptor production. *Acta Psychiatrica Scandinavica, 84,* 379–386.

Maggioncalda, A. N., and Sapolsky, R. M. (2002). Disturbing behaviors of the orangutan. *Scientific American, 286*(6), 60–65.

Magnusson, A., and Stefansson, J. G. (1993). Prevalence of seasonal affective disorder in Iceland. *Archives of General Psychiatry, 50,* 941–946.

Mahowald, M. W., and Schenck, C. H. (2005). Insights from studying human sleep disorders. *Nature, 437,* 1279–1285.

Maia, T. V., and Conceição, V. A. (2018, March 9). Dopaminergic disturbances in Tourette syndrome: An integrative account. *Biological Psychiatry,* pii: S0006-3223(18)31300-3. [Epub ahead of print]

Mair, W. G. P., Warrington, E. K., and Wieskrantz, L. (1979). Memory disorder in Korsakoff's psychosis. *Brain, 102,* 749–783.

Mak, G. K., Enwere, E. K., Gregg, C., Pakarainen, T., et al. (2007). Male pheromone-stimulated neurogenesis in the adult female brain: Possible role in mating behavior. *Nature Neuroscience, 10,* 1003–1011.

Makino, H., Hwang, E. J., Hedrick, N. G., and Komiyama, T. (2016). Circuit mechanisms of sensorimotor learning. *Neuron, 92*(4), 705–721.

Malenka, R. C., and Bear, M. F. (2004). LTP and LTD: An embarrassment of riches. *Neuron, 44,* 5–21.

Mancuso, K., Hauswirth, W. W., Li, Q., Connor, T. B., et al. (2009). Gene therapy for red-green colour blindness in adult primates. *Nature, 461,* 784–788.

Mani, S. K., Fienberg, A. A., O'Callaghan, J. P., Snyder, G. L., et al. (2000). Requirement for DARPP-32 in progesterone-facilitated sexual receptivity in female rats and mice. *Science, 287,* 1053–1056.

Manoli, D. S., and Tollkuhn, J. (2018). Gene regulatory mechanisms underlying sex differences in brain development and psychiatric disease. *Annals of the New York Academy of Sciences, 1420*(1), 26–45.

Manova, M. G., and Kostadinova, I. I. (2000). Some aspects of the immunotherapy of multiple sclerosis. *Folia Medica, 42*(1), 5–9.

Mantini, D., Gerits, A., Nelissen, K., Durand, J. B., et al. (2011). Default mode of brain function in monkeys. *Journal of Neuroscience, 31,* 12954–12962.

Mantyh, P. W., Rogers, S. D., Honore, P., Allen, B. J., et al. (1997). Inhibition of hyperalgesia by ablation of lamina I spinal neurons expressing the substance P receptor. *Science, 278,* 275–279.

Mao, J. B., and Evinger, C. (2001). Long-term potentiation of the human blink reflex. *Journal of Neuroscience, 21,* RC151.

Marconi, A., Di Forti, M., Lewis, C. M., Murray, R. M., et al. (2016). Meta-analysis of the association between the level of cannabis use and risk of psychosis. *Schizophrenia Bulletin, 42*(5), 1262–1269.

Marcus, G. F., Vijayan, S., Bandi Rao, S., and Vishton, P. M. (1999). Rule learning by seven-month-old infants. *Science, 283,* 77–80.

Marek, G. J., Behl, B., Bespalov, A. Y., Gross, G., et al. (2010). Glutamatergic (*N*-methyl-D-aspartate receptor) hypofrontality in schizophrenia: Too little juice or a miswired brain? *Molecular Pharmacology, 77*(3), 317–326.

Maren, S., and Quirk, G. J. (2004). Neuronal signalling of fear memory. *Nature, 5*, 844–852.

Mariani, J., and Changeaux, J.-P. (1981). Ontogenesis of olivocerebellar relationships. I. Studies by intracellular recordings of the multiple innervation of Purkinje cells by climbing fibers in the developing rat cerebellum. *Journal of Neuroscience, 1*, 696–702.

Mark, V. H., and Ervin, F. R. (1970). *Violence and the brain*. New York, NY: Harper & Row.

Marler, P. (1970). Birdsong and speech development: Could there be parallels? *American Scientist, 58*, 669–673.

Marler, P. (1991). Song-learning behavior: The interface with neuroethology. *Trends in Neurosciences, 14*, 199–206.

Marler, P., and Peters, S. (1982). Developmental overproduction and selective attrition: New processes in the epigenesis of birdsong. *Developmental Psychobiology, 15*, 369–378.

Marler, P., and Sherman, V. (1983). Song structure without auditory feedback: Emendations of the auditory template hypothesis. *Journal of Neuroscience, 3*, 517–531.

Marshall, L., Helgadóttir, H., Mölle, M., and Born, J. (2006). Boosting slow oscillations during sleep potentiates memory. *Nature, 444*, 610–613.

Marsicano, G., Wotjak, C. T., Azad, S. C., Bisogno, T., et al. (2002). The endogenous cannabinoid system controls extinction of aversive memories. *Nature, 418*, 530–532.

Martin, C. K., Heilbronn, L., de Jonge, L., Delany, J. P., et al. (2007). Effect of calorie restriction on resting metabolic rate and spontaneous physical activity. *Obesity (Silver Spring), 15*, 2964–2973.

Martuza, R. L., Chiocca, E. A., Jenike, M. A., Giriunas, I. E., et al. (1990). Stereotactic radiofrequency thermal cingulotomy for obsessive compulsive disorder. *Journal of Neuropsychiatry and Clinical Neurosciences, 2*, 331–336.

Marucha, P. T., Kiecolt-Glaser, J. K., and Favagehi, M. (1998). Mucosal wound healing is impaired by examination stress. *Psychosomatic Medicine, 60*, 362–365.

Maruyama, Y., Pereira, E., Margolskee, R. F., Chaudhari, N., et al. (2006). Umami responses in mouse taste cells indicate more than one receptor. *Journal of Neuroscience, 26*, 2227–2234.

Marzullo, T. C. (2017). The missing manuscript of Dr. Jose Delgado's radio controlled bulls. *Journal of Undergraduate Neuroscience Education, 15*(2), R29–R35.

Maskos, U., Molles, B. E., Pons, S., Besson, M., et al. (2005). Nicotine reinforcement and cognition restored by targeted expression of nicotinic receptors. *Nature, 436*, 103–107.

Masters, W. H., and Johnson, V. E. (1966). *Human sexual response*. Boston, MA: Little, Brown.

Masters, W. H., and Johnson, V. E. (1970). *Human sexual inadequacy*. Boston, MA: Little, Brown.

Masters, W. H., Johnson, V. E., and Kolodny, R. C. (1994). *Heterosexuality*. New York, NY: HarperCollins.

Mastrianni, J. A., Nixon, R., Layzer, R., Telling, G. C., et al. (1999). Prion protein conformation in a patient with sporadic fatal insomnia. *New England Journal of Medicine, 340*, 1630–1638.

Mateo, J. M., and Johnston, R. E. (2000). Kin recognition and the "armpit effect": Evidence of self-referent phenotype matching. *Proceedings of the Royal Society of London. Series B: Biological Sciences, 267*, 695–700.

Matsumoto, K., Suzuki, W., and Tanaka, K. (2003). Neuronal correlates of goal-based motor selection in the prefrontal cortex. *Science, 301*, 229–232.

Mattes, R. D. (2011). Accumulating evidence supports a taste component for free fatty acids in humans. *Physiology & Behavior, 104*(4), 624–631.

Matthews, K. A. (2005). Psychological perspectives on the development of coronary heart disease. *American Psychologist, 60*(8), 783–796.

May, L., Gervain, J., Carreiras, M., and Werker, J. F. (2018). The specificity of the neural response to speech at birth. *Developmental Science, 21*(3), e12564.

May, P. A., and Gossage, J. P. (2011). Maternal risk factors for fetal alcohol spectrum disorders: Not as simple as it might seem. *Alcohol Research & Health, 34*(1), 15–26.

Mayberg, H. S., Lozano, A. M., Voon, V., McNeely, H. E., et al. (2005). Deep brain stimulation for treatment-resistant depression. *Neuron, 45*, 651–660.

Mazur, A., and Booth, A. (1998). Testosterone and dominance in men. *Behavioral and Brain Sciences, 21*, 353–363.

McAllister, A. K., Katz, L. C., and Lo, D. C. (1997). Opposing roles for endogenous BDNF and NT-3 in regulating cortical dendritic growth. *Neuron, 18*, 767–778.

McAlpine, D., Jiang, D., and Palmer, A. R. (2001). A neural code for low-frequency sound localization in mammals. *Nature Neuroscience, 4*, 396–401.

McBurney, D. H., Smith, D. V., and Shick, T. R. (1972). Gustatory cross adaptation: Sourness and bitterness. *Perception & Psychophysics, 11*, 2228–2232.

McCarthy, R. A., and Warrington, E. K. (1990). *Cognitive neuropsychology: A clinical introduction*. San Diego, CA: Academic Press.

McCrae, C. S., Rowe, M. A., Tierney, C. G., Dautovich, N. D., et al. (2005). Sleep complaints, subjective and objective sleep patterns, health, psychological adjustment, and daytime functioning in community-dwelling older adults. *Journals of Gerontology. Series B, Psychological Sciences and Social Sciences, 60*(4), P182–P189.

McDonald, J. J., and Green, J. J. (2008). Isolating event-related potential components associated with voluntary control of visuo-spatial attention. *Brain Research, 1227*, 96–109.

McDonald, J. J., Teder-Sälejärvi, W. A., and Hillyard, S. A. (2000). Involuntary orienting to sound improves visual perception. *Nature, 407*, 906–908.

McDonald, J. J., Teder-Sälejärvi, W. A., and Hillyard, S. A. (2000). Involuntary orienting to sound improves visual perception. *Nature, 407*(6806), 906–908.

McDonald, J. J., Teder-Sälejärvi, W. A., Di Russo, F., and Hillyard, S. A. (2003). Neural substrates of perceptual enhancement by cross-modal spatial attention. *Journal of Cognitive Neuroscience, 15*(1), 10–19.

McDonald, J. J., Teder-Sälejärvi, W. A., Di Russo, F., and Hillyard, S. A. (2005). Neural basis of auditory-induced shifts in visual time-order perception. *Nature Neuroscience, 8*(9), 1197–1202.

McDonald, J. J., Ward, L. M., and Kiehl, K. A. (1999). An event-related brain potential study of inhibition of return. *Perception & Psychophysics, 61*(7), 1411–1423.

McEwen, B. S., and Wingfield, J. C. (2010). What is in a name? Integrating homeostasis, allostasis and stress. *Hormones and Behavior, 57*, 105–111.

McEwen, B. S., Bowles, N. P., Gray, J. D., Hill, M. N., et al. (2015). Mechanisms of stress in the brain. *Nature Neuroscience, 18*(10), 1353–1363.

McFadden, D., and Pasanen, E. (1998). Comparison of the auditory systems of heterosexuals and homosexuals: Click-evoked otoacoustic emissions. *Proceedings of the National Academy of Sciences, USA, 95*, 2709–2713.

McGann, J. P. (2017). Poor human olfaction is a 19th-century myth. *Science, 356*(6338), pii: eaam7263.

McGinty, D. J., and Sterman, M. B. (1968). Sleep suppression after basal forebrain lesions in the cat. *Science, 160*, 1253–1255.

McGowan, P. O., Sasaki, A., D'Alessio, A. C., Dymov, S., et al. (2009). Epigenetic regulation of the glucocorticoid receptor in human brain associates with childhood abuse. *Nature Neuroscience, 12*, 342–348.

McGuigan, F. J., and Lehrer, P. M. (2007). Progressive relaxation: Origins, principles and clinical application. In P. M. Lehrer, R. L. Woolfolk, and W. E. Sime (Eds.), *Principles and practices of stress management* (pp. 57–87). New York, NY: Guilford Press.

McGuire, J. F., Ricketts, E. J., Piacentini, J., Murphy, T. K., et al. (2015). Behavior therapy for tic disorders: An evidenced-based review and new directions for treatment research. *Current Developmental Disorders Reports, 2*(4), 309–317.

McKee, A. C., Cairns, N. J., Dickson, D. W., Folkerth, R. D., et al. (2016). The first NINDS/NIBIB consensus meeting to define neuropathological criteria for the diagnosis of chronic traumatic encephalopathy. *Acta Neuropathologica, 131*(1), 75 86.

McKee, A. C., Cantu, R. C., Nowinski, C. J., Hedley-Whyte, E. T., et al. (2009). Chronic traumatic encephalopathy in athletes: Progressive tauopathy after repetitive head injury. *Journal of Neuropathology and Experimental Neurology, 68*, 709–735.

McKenna, K. (1999). The brain is the master organ in sexual function: Central nervous system control of male and female sexual function. *International Journal of Impotence Research, 11*(Suppl. 1), S48–S55.

McKernan, M. G., and Shinnick-Gallagher, P. (1997). Fear conditioning induces a lasting potentiation of synaptic currents in vitro. *Nature, 390*, 607–611.

McKim, W. A. (1991). *Drugs and behavior: An introduction to behavioral pharmacology* (2nd ed.). Englewood Cliffs, NJ: Prentice Hall.

McLaughlin, S. K., McKinnon, P. J., Spickofsky, N., Danho, W., et al. (1994). Molecular cloning of G proteins and phosphodiesterases from rat taste cells. *Physiology & Behavior, 56*, 1157–1164.

McLellan, T. M., Caldwell, J. A., and Lieberman, H. R. (2016). A review of caffeine's effects on cognitive, physical and occupational performance. *Neuroscience & Biobehavioral Reviews, 71*, 294–312.

McNamara, P., Johnson, P., McLaren, D., Harris, E., et al. (2010). REM and NREM sleep mentation. *International Review of Neurobiology, 92*, 69–86.

Meddis, R. (1975). On the function of sleep. *Animal Behavior, 23*, 676–691.

Meddis, R. (1977). *The sleep instinct*. London, UK: Routledge & Kegan Paul.

Mednick, S. A., Huttunen, M. O., and Machon, R. A. (1994). Prenatal influenza infections and adult schizophrenia. *Schizophrenia Bulletin, 20*, 263–267.

Medori, R., Montagna, P., Tritschler, H. J., LeBlanc, A., et al. (1992). Fatal familial insomnia: A second kindred with mutation of prion protein gene at codon 178. *Neurology, 42*, 669–670.

Mega, M. S., and Cummings, J. L. (1994). Frontal-subcortical circuits and neuropsychiatric disorders. *Journal of Neuropsychiatry and Clinical Neurosciences, 6*, 358–370.

Meguerditchian, A., and Vauclair, J. (2006). Baboons communicate with their right hand. *Behavioural Brain Research, 171*, 170–174.

Mei, L., and Xiong, W.-C. (2008). Neuregulin 1 in neural development, synaptic plasticity and schizophrenia. *Nature Reviews Neuroscience, 9*, 437–452.

Meier, M. H., Caspi, A., Ambler, A., Harrington, H., et al. (2012). Persistent cannabis users show neuropsychological decline from childhood to midlife. *Proceedings of the National Academy of Sciences, USA, 109*, E2657–E2664.

Meisel, R. L., and Luttrell, V. R. (1990). Estradiol increases the dendritic length of ventromedial hypothalamic neurons in female Syrian hamsters. *Brain Research Bulletin, 25*, 165–168.

Meisel, R. L., and Sachs, B. D. (1994). The physiology of male sexual behavior. In E. Knobil and J. D. Neill (Eds.), *The physiology of reproduction* (2nd ed., Vol. 1, pp. 3–105). New York, NY: Raven Press.

Meister, I. G., Boroojerdi, B., Foltys, H., Sparing, R., et al. (2003). Motor cortex hand area and speech: Implications for the development of language. *Neuropsychologia, 41*(4), 401–406.

Mello, C. V., Vicario, D. S., and Clayton, D. F. (1992). Song presentation induces gene expression in the songbird forebrain. *Proceedings of the National Academy of Sciences, USA, 89*, 6818–6822.

Melzack, R. (1984). Neuropsychological basis of pain measurement. *Advances in Pain Research, 6*, 323–341.

Melzack, R. (1990). The tragedy of needless pain. *Scientific American, 262*(2), 27–33.

Melzack, R., and Wall, P. D. (1965). Pain mechanisms: A new history. *Science, 150*, 971–979.

Méndez-Bértolo, C., Moratti, S., Toledano, R., Lopez-Sosa, F., et al. (2016). A fast pathway for fear in human amygdala. *Nature Neuroscience, 19*(8), 1041–1049.

Menninger, W. C. (1948). Facts and statistics of significance for psychiatry. *Bulletin of the Menninger Clinic, 12*, 1–25.

Merchán-Pérez, A., Rodriguez, J. R., Alonso-Nanclares, L., Schertel, A., et al. (2009). Counting synapses using FIB/SEM microscopy: A true revolution for ultrastructural volume reconstruction. *Frontiers in Neuroanatomy, 3*, 18.

Mersch, P. P., Middendorp, H. M., Bouhuys, A. L., Beersma, D. G., et al. (1999). Seasonal affective disorder and latitude: A review of the literature. *Journal of Affective Disorders, 53*, 35–48.

Merzenich, M. M., Schreiner, C., Jenkins, W., and Wang, X. (1993). Neural mechanisms underlying temporal integration, segmentation, and input sequence representation: Some implications for the origin of learning disabilities. *Annals of the New York Academy of Sciences, 682*, 1–22.

Meshberger, F. L. (1990). An interpretation of Michelangelo's *Creation of Adam* based on neuroanatomy. *JAMA, 264*, 1837–1841.

Messias, E., Kirkpatrick, B., Bromet, E., Ross, D., et al. (2004). Summer birth and deficit schizophrenia: A pooled analysis from 6 countries. *Archives of General Psychiatry, 61*, 985–989.

Mesulam, M.-M. (1985). Attention, confusional states and neglect. In M.-M. Mesulam (Ed.), *Principles of behavioral neurology*. Philadelphia, PA: Davis.

Mewton, L., and Andrews, G. (2016). Cognitive behavioral therapy for suicidal behaviors: Improving patient outcomes. *Psychology Research and Behavior Management, 9*, 21–29.

Mez, J., Daneshvar, D. H., Kiernan, P. T., Abdolmohammadi, B., et al. (2017). Clinicopathological evaluation of chronic traumatic encephalopathy in players of American football. *JAMA, 318*(4), 360–370.

Michael, N., and Erfurth, A. (2004). Treatment of bipolar mania with right prefrontal rapid transcranial magnetic stimulation. *Journal of Affective Disorders, 78*, 253–257.

Miczek, K. A., Fish, E. W., De Bold, J. F., and De Almeida, R. M. (2002). Social and neural determinants of aggressive behavior: Pharmacotherapeutic targets at serotonin, dopamine and gamma-aminobutyric acid systems. *Psychopharmacology (Berlin), 163*, 434–458.

Miller, E. K., and Cohen, J. D. (2001). An integrative theory of prefrontal cortex function. *Annual Review of Neuroscience, 24*, 167–202.

Miller, G. F. (2000). *The mating mind: How sexual choice shaped the evolution of human nature*. New York, NY: Doubleday.

Miller, J. M., and Spelman, F. A. (1990). *Cochlear implants: Models of the electrically stimulated ear*. New York, NY: Springer-Verlag.

Miller, N. E., Sampliner, R. I., and Woodrow, P. (1957). Thirst-reducing effects of water by stomach fistula vs. water by mouth measured by both a consummatory and an instrumental response. *Journal of Comparative and Physiological Psychology, 50*(1), 1–5.

Milner, A. D., Perrett, D. I., Johnston, R. S., Benson, P. J., et al. (1991). Perception and action in "visual form agnosia." *Brain, 114*, 405–428.

Milner, B. (1963). Effect of different brain lesions on card sorting. *Archives of Neurology, 9*, 90–100.

Milner, B. (1965). Memory disturbance after bilateral hippocampal lesions. In P. M. Milner and S. E. Glickman (Eds.), *Cognitive processes and the brain; an enduring problem in psychology* (pp. 97–111). Princeton, NJ: Van Nostrand.

Milner, B. (1970). Memory and the medial temporal regions of the brain. In D. H. Pribram and D. E. Broadbent (Eds.), *Biology of memory* (pp. 29–50). New York, NY: Academic Press.

Minzenberg, M. J., Laird, A. R., Thelen, S., Carter, C. S., et al. (2009). Meta-analysis of 41 functional neuroimaging studies of executive function in schizophrenia. *Archives of General Psychiatry, 66,* 811–822.

Mirescu, C., Peters, J. D., and Gould, E. (2004). Early life experience alters response of adult neurogenesis to stress. *Nature Neuroscience, 7,* 841–846.

Mirsky, A. F., and Duncan, C. C. (1986). Etiology and expression of schizophrenia: Neurobiological and psychosocial factors. *Annual Review of Psychology, 37,* 291–321.

Mishkin, M., and Ungerleider, L. (1982). Contribution of striate inputs to the visuospatial functions of parieto-preoccipital cortex in monkeys. *Behavioural Brain Research, 6,* 57–77.

Mishra, J., Zinni, M., Bavelier, D., and Hillyard, S. A. (2011). Neural basis of superior performance of action videogame players in an attention-demanding task. *Journal of Neuroscience, 31,* 992–998.

Mithoefer, M. C., Wagner, M. T., Mithoefer, A. T., Jerome, L., et al. (2013). Durability of improvement in post-traumatic stress disorder symptoms and absence of harmful effects or drug dependency after 3,4 methylenedioxymethamphetamine-assisted psychotherapy: A prospective long-term follow-up study. *Journal of Psychopharmacology, 27,* 28–39.

Miyawaki, Y., Uchida, H., Yamashita, O., Sato, M. A., et al. (2008). Visual image reconstruction from human brain activity using a combination of multiscale local image decoders. *Neuron, 60,* 915–929.

Mogwitz, S., Buse, J., Ehrlich, S., and Roessner, V. (2013). Clinical pharmacology of dopamine-modulating agents in Tourette's syndrome. *International Review of Neurobiology, 112,* 281–349.

Mohammed, A. (2001). Enrichment and the brain. Plasticity in the adult brain: From genes to neurotherapy. 22nd International Summer School of Brain Research, Amsterdam, Netherlands.

Moita, M. A., Rosis, S., Zhou, Y., LeDoux, J. E., et al. (2004). Putting fear in its place: Remapping of hippocampal place cells during fear conditioning. *Journal of Neuroscience, 24,* 7015–7023.

Money, J., and Ehrhardt, A. A. (1972). *Man and woman, boy and girl.* Baltimore, MD: Johns Hopkins University Press.

Monfils, M. H., Plautz, E. J., and Kleim, J. A. (2005). In search of the motor engram: Motor map plasticity as a mechanism for encoding motor experience. *Neuroscientist, 11,* 471–483.

Monks, D. A., and Watson N. V. (2001). N-cadherin expression in motoneurons is directly regulated by androgens: A genetic mosaic analysis in rats. *Brain Research, 895,* 73–79.

Montague, C. T., Farooqi, I. S., Whitehead, J. P., Soos, M. A., et al. (1997). Congenital leptin deficiency is associated with severe early-onset obesity in humans. *Nature, 387,* 903–908.

Montenigro, P. H., Alosco, M. L., Martin, B., Daneshvar, D. H., et al. (2016). Cumulative head impact exposure predicts later-life depression, apathy, executive dysfunction, and cognitive impairment in former high school and college football players. *Journal of Neurotrauma, 34*(2), 328–340. doi:10.1089/neu.2016.4413

Monti, M. M., Vanhaudenhuyse, A., Coleman, M. R., Boly, M., et al. (2010). Willful modulation of brain activity in disorders of consciousness. *New England Journal of Medicine, 362,* 579–589.

Moore, C. L., Dou, H., and Juraska, J. M. (1992). Maternal stimulation affects the number of motor neurons in a sexually dimorphic nucleus of the lumbar spinal cord. *Brain Research, 572,* 52–56.

Moore, G. J., Bebchuk, J. M., Wilds, I. B., Chen, G., et al. (2000). Lithium-induced increase in human brain grey matter. *Lancet, 356,* 241–242.

Moore, R. Y. (2013). The suprachiasmatic nucleus and the circadian timing system. *Progress in Molecular Biology and Translational Science, 119,* 1–28.

Moore, R. Y., and Eichler, V. B. (1972). Loss of circadian adrenal corticosterone rhythm following suprachiasmatic lesions in the rat. *Brain Research, 42,* 201–206.

Moorhead, T. W., McKirdy, J., Sussmann, J. E., Hall, J., et al. (2007). Progressive gray matter loss in patients with bipolar disorder. *Biological Psychiatry, 62,* 894–900.

Moorman, S., Gobes, S. M., Kuijpers, M., Kerkhofs, A., et al. (2012). Human-like brain hemispheric dominance in birdsong learning. *Proceedings of the National Academy of Sciences, USA, 109*(31), 12782–12787.

Moran, J., and Desimone, R. (1985). Selective attention gates visual processing in the extrastriate cortex. *Science, 229,* 782–784.

Morawietz, C., and Moffat, F. (2013). Effects of locomotor training after incomplete spinal cord injury: A systematic review. *Archives of Physical Medicine and Rehabilitation, 94*(11), 2297–2308.

Mori, K., Nagao, H., and Yoshihara, Y. (1999). The olfactory bulb: Coding and processing of odor molecule information. *Science, 286,* 711–715.

Morizane, A., Kikuchi, T., Hayashi, T., Mizuma, H., et al. (2017). MHC matching improves engraftment of iPSC-derived neurons in non-human primates. *Nature Communications, 8*(1), 385.

Morris, B. (2002). Overcoming dyslexia. *Fortune, 145*(10), 1–7.

Morris, R. G., Halliwell, R. F., and Bowery, N. (1989). Synaptic plasticity and learning. II: Do different kinds of plasticity underlie

different kinds of learning? *Neuropsychologia, 27,* 41–59.

Morrison, A. R. (1983). A window on the sleeping brain. *Scientific American, 248*(4), 94–102.

Morrison, A. R., Sanford, L. D., Ball, W. A., Mann, G. L., et al. (1995). Stimulus-elicited behavior in rapid eye movement sleep without atonia. *Behavioral Neuroscience, 109,* 972–979.

Morrison, R. G., and Nottebohm, F. (1993). Role of a telencephalic nucleus in the delayed song learning of socially isolated zebra finches. *Journal of Neurobiology, 24,* 1045–1064.

Moruzzi, G. (1972). The sleep-waking cycle. *Ergebnisse der Physiologie, biologischen Chemie und experimentellen Pharmakologie, 64,* 1–165.

Moruzzi, G., and Magoun, H. W. (1949). Brain stem reticular formation and activation of the EEG. *Clinical Neurophysiology, 1,* 455–473.

Moscovitch, A., Blashko, C. A., Eagles, J. M., Darcourt, G., et al. (2004). A placebo-controlled study of sertraline in the treatment of outpatients with seasonal affective disorder. *Psychopharmacology (Berlin), 171,* 390–397.

Moser, E. I., Moser, M. B., and McNaughton, B. L. (2017). Spatial representation in the hippocampal formation: A history. *Nature Neuroscience, 20*(11), 1448–1464.

Mott, F. W. (1895). Experimental inquiry upon the afferent tracts of the central nervous system of the monkey. *Brain, 18,* 1–20.

Motta, S. C., Guimarães, C. C., Furigo, I. C., Sukikara, M. H., et al. (2013). Ventral premammillary nucleus as a critical sensory relay to the maternal aggression network. *Proceedings of the National Academy of Sciences, USA, 110,* 14438–14443.

Mountcastle, V. B. (1979). An organizing principle for cerebral function: The unit module and the distributed system. In F. O. Schmitt and F. G. Worden (Eds.), *The neurosciences: Fourth study program* (pp. 21–24). Cambridge, MA: MIT Press.

Mountcastle, V. B. (1984). Central nervous mechanisms in mechanoreceptive sensibility. In I. Darian-Smith (Ed.), *Handbook of physiology, Section 1: Vol. 3. Sensory processes* (pp. 789–878). Bethesda, MD: American Physiological Society.

Mounts, J. R. (2000). Attentional capture by abrupt onsets and feature singletons produces inhibitory surrounds. *Perception & Psychophysics, 62,* 1485–1493.

Mueller, H. T., Haroutunian, V., Davis, K. L., and Meador-Woodruff, J. H. (2004). Expression of the ionotropic glutamate receptor subunits and NMDA receptor-associated intracellular proteins in the substantia nigra in schizophrenia. *Brain*

Research. Molecular Brain Research, 121, 60–69.

Muhlert, N., and Lawrence, A. D. (2015). Brain structure correlates of emotion-based rash impulsivity. *NeuroImage, 115,* 138–146.

Mukamal, K. J., Conigrave, K. M., Mittleman, M. A., Camargo, C. A., Jr., et al. (2003). Roles of drinking pattern and type of alcohol consumed in coronary heart disease in men. *New England Journal of Medicine, 348,* 109–118.

Mukhametov, L. M. (1984). Sleep in marine mammals. In A. Borbély and J. L. Valatx (Eds.), *Experimental Brain Research: Suppl. 8. Sleep mechanisms* (pp. 227–238). Berlin, Germany: Springer-Verlag.

Munafo, J., Diedrick, M., and Stoffregen, T. A. (2017). The virtual reality head-mounted display Oculus Rift induces motion sickness and is sexist in its effects. *Experimental Brain Research, 235*(3), 889–901.

Munley, K. M., Rendon, N. M., and Demas, G. E. (2018). Neural androgen synthesis and aggression: Insights from a seasonally breeding rodent. *Frontiers in Endocrinology(Lausanne), 9,* 136.

Münte, T. F., Altenmüller, E., and Jäncke, L. (2002). The musician's brain as a model of neuroplasticity. *Nature Reviews Neuroscience, 3,* 473–478.

Murphy, M. L., Slavich, G. M., Chen, E., and Miller, G. E. (2015). Targeted rejection predicts decreased anti-inflammatory gene expression and increased symptom severity in youth with asthma. *Psychological Science, 26*(2), 111–121.

Muza, R., Lawrence, M., and Drakatos, P. (2016). The reality of sexsomnia. *Current Opinion in Pulmonary Medicine, 22*(6), 576–582.

N

Nader, K., and Hardt, O. (2009). A single standard for memory: The case for reconsolidation. *Nature Reviews Neuroscience, 10,* 224–234.

Naeser, M., and Hayward, R. (1978). Lesion localization in aphasia with cranial computed tomography and the Boston Diagnostic Aphasia Exam. *Neurology, 28,* 545–551.

Naeser, M., Gaddie, A., Palumbo, C., and Stiassny-Eder, D. (1990). Late recovery of auditory comprehension in global aphasia. Improved recovery observed with subcortical temporal isthmus lesion vs. Wernicke's cortical area lesion. *Archives of Neurology, 47,* 425–432.

Naesström, M., Blomstedt, P., and Bodlund, O. (2016). A systematic review of psychiatric indications for deep brain stimulation, with focus on major depressive and obsessive-compulsive disorder. *Nordic Journal of Psychiatry, 70*(7), 483–491.

Nakazato, M., Murakami, N., Date, Y., Kojima, M., et al. (2001). A role for ghrelin in the central regulation of feeding. *Nature, 409,* 194–198.

Naqvi, N. H., Rudrauf, D., Damasio, H., and Bechara, A. (2007). Damage to the insula disrupts addiction to cigarette smoking. *Science, 315,* 531–534.

Naselaris, T., Prenger, R. J., Kay, K. N., Oliver, M., et al. (2009). Bayesian reconstruction of natural images from human brain activity. *Neuron, 63,* 902–915.

Nathans, J. (1987). Molecular biology of visual pigments. *Annual Review of Neuroscience, 10,* 163–194.

Nation, E. F. (1973). William Osler on penis captivus and other urologic topics. *Urology, 2,* 468–470.

National Academy of Sciences. (2003). *The polygraph and lie detection.* Washington, DC: National Academies Press (www.nap.edu/openbook.php?isbn=0309084369).

National Institute of Mental Health. (2017). *Past year prevalence of serious mental illness among U.S. adults (2016).* (Data courtesy of SAMHSA. Last updated November 2017.) Bethesda, MD (www.nimh.nih.gov/health/statistics/prevalence/serious-mental-illness-smi-among-us-adults.shtml).

National Institute on Drug Abuse (NIDA). (2017). National overdose deaths from select prescription and illicit drugs (1999–2016), based on data from CDC/National Center for Health Statistics, CDC Wonder database, 2016. https://www.drugabuse.gov/related-topics/trends-statistics/overdose-death-rates

Nature. (2017). Head injuries in sport must be taken more seriously. *Nature, 548*(7668), 371. doi:10.1038/548371a

Navarro-Lobato, I., and Genzel, L. (2018). The up and down of sleep: From molecules to electrophysiology. *Neurobiology of Learning and Memory,* pii: S1074-7427(18)30067-4.

Neff, W. D., and Casseday, J. H. (1977). Effects of unilateral ablation of auditory cortex on monaural cat's ability to localize sound. *Journal of Neurophysiology, 40,* 44–52.

Neitz, M., Kraft, T.W., and Neitz, J. (1998). Expression of L cone pigment gene subtypes in females. *Vision Research, 38,* 3221–3225.

Nelson, G., Chandrashekar, J., Hoon, M. A., Feng, L., et al. (2002). An amino-acid taste receptor. *Nature, 416,* 199–202.

Nelson, G., Hoon, M. A., Chandrashekar, J., Zhang, Y., et al. (2001). Mammalian sweet taste receptors. *Cell, 106,* 381–390.

Nestler, E. J., and Hyman, S. E. (2010). Animal models of neuropsychiatric disorders. *Nature Neuroscience, 13,* 1161–1169.

Nestor, A., Plaut, D. C., and Behrmann, M. (2016). Feature-based face representations and image reconstruction from behavioral and neural data. *Proceedings of the National Academy of Sciences, USA, 113*(2), 416–421.

Neumeister, A., Bain, E., Nugent, A. C., Carson, R. E., et al. (2004). Reduced serotonin type 1A receptor binding in panic disorder. *Journal of Neuroscience, 24,* 589–591.

Neville, H. J., Bavelier, D., Corina, D., Rauschecker, J., et al. (1998). Cerebral organization for language in deaf and hearing subjects: Biological constraints and effects of experience. *Proceedings of the National Academy of Sciences, USA, 95,* 922–929.

Neville, H. J., Mills, D. L., and Lawson, D. S. (1992). Fractionating language: Different neural subsystems with different sensitive periods. *Cerebral Cortex, 2,* 244–258.

Newsome, W. T., Wurtz, R. H., Dursteler, M. R., and Mikami, A. (1985). Deficits in visual motion processing following ibotenic acid lesions of the middle temporal visual area of the macaque monkey. *Journal of Neuroscience, 5,* 825–840.

Ng, S. F., Lin, R. C., Laybutt, D. R., Barres, R., et al. (2010). Chronic high-fat diet in fathers programs β-cell dysfunction in female rat offspring. *Nature, 467,* 963–966.

Ngandu, T., Lehtisalo, J., Solomon, A., Levälahti, E., et al. (2015). A 2 year multidomain intervention of diet, exercise, cognitive training, and vascular risk monitoring versus control to prevent cognitive decline in at-risk elderly people (FINGER): A randomised controlled trial. *Lancet,* pii: S0140-6736(15)60461-5. doi:10.1016/S0140-6736(15)60461-5

Nguyen, J. D., Bremer, P. T., Hwang, C. S., Vandewater, S. A., et al. (2017). Effective active vaccination against methamphetamine in female rats. *Drug and Alcohol Dependence, 175,* 179–186.

Nichols, M. J., and Newsome, W. T. (1999). The neurobiology of cognition. *Nature, 402,* C35–C38.

Nieto-Sampedro, M., and Cotman, C. W. (1985). Growth factor induction and temporal order in central nervous system repair. In C. W. Cotman (Ed.), *Synaptic plasticity* (pp. 407–457). New York, NY: Guilford Press.

Nietzel, M. T. (2000). Police psychology. In A. E. Kazdin (Ed.), *Encyclopedia of psychology* (Vol. 6, pp. 224–226). Washington, DC: American Psychological Association.

Nishida, M., and Walker, M. P. (2007). Daytime naps, motor memory consolidation and regionally specific sleep spindles. *PLOS ONE, 2,* e341.

Nishimoto, S., and Gallant, J. L. (2011). A three-dimensional spatiotemporal receptive field model explains responses of area MT neurons to naturalistic movies. *Journal of Neuroscience, 31,* 14551–14564.

Nishimoto, S., Vu, A. T., Naselaris, T., Benjamini, Y., et al. (2011). Reconstructing visual experiences from brain activity evoked by natural movies. *Current Biology, 21,* 1641–1646.

Noad, M. J., Cato, D. H., Bryden, M. M., Jenner, M.-N., et al. (2000). Cultural revolution in whale songs. *Nature, 408,* 537–538.

Noguchi, Y., Watanabe, E., and Sakai, K. L. (2003). An event-related optical topography study of cortical activation induced by single-pulse transcranial magnetic stimulation. *NeuroImage, 19,* 156–162.

Nordeen, E. J., Nordeen, K. W., Sengelaub, D. R., and Arnold, A. P. (1985). Androgens prevent normally occurring cell death in a sexually dimorphic spinal nucleus. *Science, 229,* 671–673.

Nottebohm, F. (1980). Brain pathways for vocal learning in birds: A review of the first 10 years. *Progress in Psychobiology and Physiological Psychology, 9,* 85–124.

Nottebohm, F. (1981). A brain for all seasons: Cyclical anatomical changes in song control nuclei of the canary brain. *Science, 214,* 1368–1370.

Numan, M. (2015). Aggressive behavior. In M. Numan (Ed.), *Neurobiology of social behavior* (pp. 63–107). San Diego, CA: Academic Press.

Numan, M., and Numan. M. J. (1991). Preoptic-brainstem connections and maternal behavior in rats. *Behavioral Neuroscience, 105,* 1010–1029.

Nutt, D. J., Lingford-Hughes, A., Erritzoe, D., and Stokes, P. R. (2015). The dopamine theory of addiction: 40 years of highs and lows. *Nature Reviews Neuroscience, 16*(5), 305–312.

Nutt, J. G., Rufener, S. L., Carter, J. H., Anderson, V. C., et al. (2001). Interactions between deep brain stimulation and levodopa in Parkinson's disease. *Neurology, 57,* 1835–1842.

O

O'Connell-Rodwell, C. E. (2007). Keeping an "ear" to the ground: Seismic communication in elephants. *Physiology (Bethesda), 22,* 287–294.

O'Connor, D. B., Archer, J., and Wu, F. C. (2004). Effects of testosterone on mood, aggression, and sexual behavior in young men: A double-blind, placebo-controlled, cross-over study. *Journal of Clinical Endocrinology & Metabolism, 89,* 2837–2845.

O'Craven, K. M., Downing, P. E., and Kanwisher, N. (1999). fMRI evidence for objects as the units of attentional selection. *Nature, 401,* 584–587.

O'Donovan, A., Chao, L. L., Paulson, J., Samuelson, K. W., et al. (2015). Altered inflammatory activity associated with reduced hippocampal volume and more severe posttraumatic stress symptoms in Gulf War veterans. *Psychoneuroendocrinology, 51,* 557–566.

Oades, R. D., and Halliday, G. M. (1987). Ventral tegmental (A10) system:

Neurobiology. 1. Anatomy and connectivity. *Brain Research Reviews, 12,* 117–165.

Oberlander, T. F., Papsdorf, M., Brain, U. M., Misri, S., et al. (2010). Prenatal effects of selective serotonin reuptake inhibitor antidepressants, serotonin transporter promoter genotype (SLC6A4), and maternal mood on child behavior at 3 years of age. *Archives of Pediatrics and Adolescent Medicine, 164,* 444–451.

Ogden, J. (2012). *Health psychology.* New York, NY: Open University Press.

Ojala, K. E., Janssen, L. K., Hashemi, M. M., Timmer, M. H. M., et al. (2018). Dopaminergic drug effects on probability weighting during risky decision making. *eNeuro, 5*(2), pii: ENEURO.0330-18.2018.

Ojemann, G., and Mateer, C. (1979). Human language cortex: Localization of memory, syntax, and sequential motor-phoneme identification systems. *Science, 205,* 1401–1403.

Okano, H., Ogawa, Y., Nakamura, M., Kaneko, S., et al. (2003). Transplantation of neural stem cells into the spinal cord after injury. *Seminars in Cell and Developmental Biology, 14,* 191–198.

O'Keefe, J. H., Bhatti, S. K., Bajwa, A., DiNicolantonio, J. J., et al. (2014). Alcohol and cardiovascular health: The dose makes the poison … or the remedy. *Mayo Clinic Proceedings, 89*(3), 382–393.

O'Keefe, J., and Burgess, N. (2005). Dual phase and rate coding in hippocampal place cells: Theoretical significance and relationship to entorhinal grid cells. *Hippocampus, 15*(7), 853–866.

Olabi, B., Ellison-Wright, I., McIntosh, A. M., Wood, S. J., et al. (2011). Are there progressive brain changes in schizophrenia? A meta-analysis of structural magnetic resonance imaging studies. *Biological Psychiatry, 70*(1), 88–96.

Olanow, C. W., Goetz, C. G., Kordower, J. H., Stoessl, A. J., et al. (2003). A double-blind controlled trial of bilateral fetal nigral transplantation in Parkinson's disease. *Annals of Neurology, 54,* 403–414.

Olds, J., and Milner, P. (1954). Positive reinforcement produced by electrical stimulation of septal area and other regions of rat brain. *Journal of Comparative and Physiological Psychology, 47,* 419–427.

Olender, T., Lancet, D., and Nebert, D. W. (2008). Update on the olfactory receptor (OR) gene superfamily. *Human Genomics, 3*(1), 87–97.

Oler, J. A., Fox, A. S., Shelton, S. E., Rogers, J., et al. (2010). Amygdalar and hippocampal substrates of anxious temperament differ in their heritability. *Nature, 466,* 864–868.

Olfson, M., Marcus, S. C., and Shaffer, D. (2006). Antidepressant drug therapy and suicide in severely depressed children and

adults: A case-control study. *Archives of General Psychiatry, 63,* 865–872.

Olsen, K. L. (1979). Androgen-insensitive rats are defeminised by their testes. *Nature, 279,* 238–239.

Olson, S. (2004). Making sense of Tourette's. *Science, 305,* 1390–1392.

Olsson, A., and Phelps, E. A. (2007). Social learning of fear. *Nature Neuroscience, 10,* 1095–1102.

Oman, C. M. (2012). Are evolutionary hypotheses for motion sickness "just-so" stories? *Journal of Vestibular Research, 22*(2), 117–127.

Opendak, M., and Gould, E. (2015). Adult neurogenesis: A substrate for experience-dependent change. *Trends in Cognitive Science, 19,* 151–161.

Oppenheim, K. (2006, February 3). Life full of danger for little girl who can't feel pain. *CNN* (http://www.cnn.com/2006/HEALTH/conditions/02/03/btsc.oppenheim).

Orlovska, S., Vestergaard, C. H., Bech, B. H., Nordentoft, M., et al. (2017). Association of streptococcal throat infection with mental disorders: Testing key aspects of the PANDAS hypothesis in a nationwide study. *JAMA Psychiatry, 74*(7), 740–746.

O'Shea, J., Revol, P., Cousijn, H., Near, J., et al. (2017). Induced sensorimotor cortex plasticity remediates chronic treatment-resistant visual neglect. *eLife, 6,* pii: e26602.

Osorio, D., and Vorobyev, M. (2008). A review of the evolution of animal colour vision and visual communication signals. *Vision Research, 48,* 2042–2051.

Ossenkoppele, R., Jansen, W. J., Rabinovici, G. D., Knol, D. L., et al. (2015). Prevalence of amyloid PET positivity in dementia syndromes: A meta-analysis. *JAMA, 313,* 1939–1949.

Öst, L. G., Riise, E. N., Wergeland, G. J., Hansen, B., et al. (2016). Cognitive behavioral and pharmacological treatments of OCD in children: A systematic review and meta-analysis. *Journal of Anxiety Disorders, 43,* 58–69.

Osterberg, G. (1935). Topography of the layer of rods and cones in the human retina. *Acta Ophthalmologica Supplement, 13,* 1–102.

Osterhout, L. (1997). On the brain response to syntactic anomalies: Manipulations of word position and word class reveal individual differences. *Brain and Language, 59,* 494–522.

O'Tuathaigh, C. M. P., Moran, P. M., Zhen, X. C., and Waddington, J. L. (2017). Translating advances in the molecular basis of schizophrenia into novel cognitive treatment strategies. *British Journal of Pharmacology, 174*(19), 3173–3190.

Overstreet, D. H. (1993). The Flinders sensitive line rats: A genetic animal model of depression. *Neuroscience and Biobehavioral Reviews, 17,* 51–68.

Ozelius, L. J., Senthil, G., Saunders-Pullman, R., Ohmann, E., et al. (2006). *LRRK2 G2019S* as a cause of Parkinson's disease in Ashkenazi Jews. *New England Journal of Medicine, 354,* 424–425.

P

Pack, A. I. (2003). Should a pharmaceutical be approved for the broad indication of excessive sleepiness? *American Journal of Respiratory and Critical Care Medicine, 167,* 109–111.

Padawer, R. (2016, July 3). Too fast to be female. *New York Times Sunday Magazine* (https://www.nytimes.com/2016/07/03/magazine/the-humiliating-practice-of-sex-testing-female-athletes.html).

Pagel, J. F., and Helfter, P. (2003). Drug induced nightmares—An etiology based review. *Human Psychopharmacology, 18,* 59–67.

Pagel, M., Atkinson, Q. D., Calude, A. S., and Meade, A. (2013). Ultraconserved words point to deep language ancestry across Eurasia. *Proceedings of the National Academy of Sciences, USA, 110*(21), 8471–8476.

Palagini, L., Baglioni, C., Ciapparelli, A., Gemignani, A., et al. (2013). REM sleep dysregulation in depression: State of the art. *Sleep Medicine Reviews, 17*(5), 377–390.

Palaus, M., Marron, E. M., Viejo-Sobera, R., and Redolar-Ripoll, D. (2017). Neural basis of video gaming: A systematic review. *Frontiers in Human Neuroscience, 11,* 248. doi:10.3389/fnhum.2017.00248

Palmer, S. M, Crewther, S. G, Carey, L. M, and the START Project Team. (2015). A meta-analysis of changes in brain activity in clinical depression. *Frontiers in Human Neuroscience, 8,* 1045.

Panksepp, J. (1998). *Affective neuroscience.* New York, NY: Oxford University Press.

Panksepp, J. (2000). Emotions as natural kinds within the mammalian brain. In M. Lewis and J. M. Haviland-Jones (Eds.), *Handbook of emotions* (2nd ed., pp. 137–156). New York, NY: Guilford Press.

Panksepp, J. (2005). Beyond a joke: From animal laughter to human joy? *Science, 308,* 62–63.

Panksepp, J. (2007). Neuroevolutionary sources of laughter and social joy: Modeling primal human laughter in laboratory rats. *Behavioural Brain Research, 182,* 231–244.

Panksepp, J. B., Yue, Z., Drerup, C., and Huber, R. (2003). Amine neurochemistry and aggression in crayfish. *Microscopy Research and Technique, 60,* 360–368.

Panov, A. V., Gutekunst, C.-A., Leavitt, B. R., Hayden, M. R., et al. (2002). Early mitochondrial calcium defects in Huntington's disease are a direct effect of polyglutamines. *Nature Neuroscience, 5,* 731–736.

Pantev, C., Oostenveld, R., Engelien, A., Ross, B., et al. (1998). Increased auditory cortical representation in musicians. *Nature, 392,* 811–814.

Pantle, A., and Sekuler, R. (1968). Size-detecting mechanisms in human vision. *Science, 162,* 1146–1148.

Papez, J. W. (1937). A proposed mechanism of emotion. *Archives of Neurology and Psychiatry, 38,* 725–745.

Papka, M., Ivry, R., and Woodruff-Pak, D. S. (1994). Eyeblink classical conditioning and time production in patients with cerebellar damage. *Society of Neuroscience Abstracts, 20,* 360.

Pare, M., Behets, C., and Cornu, O. (2003). Paucity of presumptive ruffini corpuscles in the index finger pad of humans. *Journal of Comparative Neurology, 456,* 260–266.

Parker, G., Cahill, L., and McGaugh, J. L. (2006). A case of unusual autobiographical remembering. *Neurocase, 12,* 35–49.

Parkes, J. D. (1985). *Sleep and its disorders.* Philadelphia, PA: Saunders.

Parrott, A. C. (2013). Human psychobiology of MDMA or "Ecstasy": An overview of 25 years of empirical research. *Human Psychopharmacology, 28,* 289–307.

Parrott, A. C. (2014). The potential dangers of using MDMA for psychotherapy. *Journal of Psychoactive Drugs, 46*(1), 37–43.

Parton, A., Malhotra, P., and Husain, M. (2004). Hemispatial neglect. *Journal of Neurology, Neurosurgery, and Psychiatry, 75,* 13–21.

Parton, L. E., Ye, C. P., Coppari, R., Enriori, P. J., et al. (2007). Glucose sensing by POMC neurons regulates glucose homeostasis and is impaired in obesity. *Nature, 449,* 228–232.

Pasquinelli, E. (2012). Neuromyths: Why do they exist and persist? *Mind, Brain, and Education, 6*(2), 89–96. doi:10.1111/j.1751-228X.2012.01141.x

Pastalkova, E., Itskov, V., Amarasingham, A., and Buzsáki, G. (2008). Internally generated cell assembly sequences in the rat hippocampus. *Science, 321,* 1322–1327.

Paterson, S. J., Brown, J. H., Gsödl, M. K., Johnson, M. H., et al. (1999). Cognitive modularity and genetic disorders. *Science, 286,* 2355–2358.

Paton, J. J., Belova, M. A., Morrison, S. E., and Salzman, C. D. (2006). The primate amygdala represents the positive and negative value of visual stimuli during learning. *Nature, 439*(7078), 865–870.

Patterson, F., and Linden, E. (1981). *The education of Koko.* New York, NY: Holt, Rinehart, and Winston.

Patterson, P. H. (2007). Maternal effects on schizophrenia risk. *Science, 318,* 576–578.

Pauls, D. L., Abramovitch, A., Rauch, S. L., and Geller, D. A. (2014). Obsessive-compulsive disorder: An integrative genetic and neurobiological perspective. *Nature Reviews Neuroscience, 15*(6), 410–424.

Paus, T., Kalina, M., Patocková, L., Angerová, Y., et al. (1991). Medial vs lateral frontal lobe lesions and differential impairment of central-gaze fixation maintenance in man. *Brain, 114,* 2051–2067.

Paus, T., Keshavan, M., and Giedd, J. N. (2008). Why do many psychiatric disorders emerge during adolescence? *Nature Reviews Neuroscience, 9,* 947–956.

Pedersen, C. B., and Mortensen, P. B. (2001). Evidence of a dose-response relationship between urbanicity during upbringing and schizophrenia risk. *Archives of General Psychiatry, 58,* 1039–1046.

Pediatric Eye Disease Investigator Group. (2005). Randomized trial of treatment of amblyopia in children aged 7 to 17 years. *Archives of Ophthalmology, 13,* 437–447.

Pedreira, C., Mormann, F., Kraskov, A., Cerf, M., et al. (2010). Responses of human medial temporal lobe neurons are modulated by stimulus repetition. *Journal of Neurophysiology, 103,* 97–107.

Peever, J., Luppi, P. H., and Montplaisir, J. (2014). Breakdown in REM sleep circuitry underlies REM sleep behavior disorder. *Trends in Neurosciences, 37,* 279–288.

Pegna, A. J., Khateb, A., Lazeyras, F., and Seghier, M. L. (2005). Discriminating emotional faces without primary visual cortices involves the right amygdala. *Nature Neuroscience, 8,* 24–25.

Peña, J. L., and Konishi, M. (2000). Cellular mechanisms for resolving phase ambiguity in the owl's inferior colliculus. *Proceedings of the National Academy of Sciences, USA, 97,* 11787–11792.

Penadés, R., González-Rodríguez, A., Catalán, R., Segura, B., et al. (2017). Neuroimaging studies of cognitive remediation in schizophrenia: A systematic and critical review. *World Journal of Psychiatry, 7*(1), 34–43.

Penfield, W., and Rasmussen, T. (1950). *The cerebral cortex in man.* New York, NY: Macmillan.

Penfield, W., and Roberts, L. (1959). *Speech and brain-mechanisms.* Princeton, NJ: Princeton University Press.

Peplau, L. A. (2003). Human sexuality: How do men and women differ? *Current Directions in Psychological Science, 12,* 37–40.

Pepper, J., Hariz, M., and Zrinzo, L. (2015). Deep brain stimulation versus anterior capsulotomy for obsessive-compulsive disorder: A review of the literature. *Journal of Neurosurgery, 122,* 1028–1037.

Perani, D., and Abutalebi, J. (2005). The neural basis of first and second language processing. *Current Opinion in Neurobiology, 15,* 202–206.

Perani, D., Farsad, M., Ballarini, T., Lubian, F., et al. (2017). The impact of bilingualism on brain reserve and metabolic connectivity in Alzheimer's dementia. *Proceedings of the National Academy of Sciences, USA, 114*(7), 1690–1695.

Perea, G., Navarrete, M., and Araque, A. (2009). Tripartite synapses: Astrocytes process and control synaptic information. *Trends in Neurosciences, 32,* 421–431.

Perenin, M. T., and Vighetto, A. (1988). Optic ataxia: A specific disruption in visuomotor mechanisms. I. Different aspects of the deficit in reaching for objects. *Brain, 111,* 643–674.

Pernía-Andrade, A. J., Kato, A., Witschi, R., Nyilas, R., et al. (2009). Spinal endocannabinoids and CB1 receptors mediate C-fiber–induced heterosynaptic pain sensitization. *Science, 325,* 760–764.

Peschanski, M., Defer, G., N'Guyen, J. P., Ricolfi, F., et al. (1994). Bilateral motor improvement and alteration of L-dopa effect in two patients with Parkinson's disease following intrastriatal transplantation of foetal ventral mesencephalon. *Brain, 117,* 487–499.

Peter, M. E., Medema, J. P., and Krammer, P. H. (1997). Does the *Caenorhabditis elegans* protein CED-4 contain a region of homology to the mammalian death effector domain? *Cell Death and Differentiation, 4,* 51–134.

Peterhans, E., and von der Heydt, R. (1989). Mechanisms of contour perception in monkey visual cortex. II. Contours bridging gaps. *Journal of Neuroscience, 9,* 1749–1763.

Peters, A., Palay, S. L., and Webster, H. deF. (1991). *The fine structure of the nervous system: Neurons and their supporting cells* (3rd ed.). New York, NY: Oxford University Press.

Peterson, B. S., Warner, V., Bansal, R., Zhu, H., et al. (2009). Cortical thinning in persons at increased familial risk for major depression. *Proceedings of the National Academy of Sciences, USA, 106,* 6273–6278.

Peterson, L. R., and Peterson, M. J. (1959). Short-term retention of individual verbal items. *Journal of Experimental Psychology, 58,* 193–198.

Petit, C., and Richardson, G. P. (2009). Linking genes underlying deafness to hair-bundle development and function. *Nature Neuroscience, 12,* 703–710.

Petitto, L. A., Zatorre, R. J., Gauna, K., Nikelski, E. J., et al. (2000). Speech-like cerebral activity in profoundly deaf people processing signed languages: Implications for the neural basis of human language. *Proceedings of the National Academy of Sciences, USA, 97,* 13961–13966.

Petrides, M., and Milner, B. (1982). Deficits on subject-ordered tasks after frontal- and temporal-lobe lesions in man. *Neuropsychologia, 20,* 249–262.

Petrone, A. B., Simpkins, J. W., and Barr, T. L. (2014). 17β-Estradiol and inflammation: Implications for ischemic stroke. *Aging and Disease, 5,* 340–345.

Petrovic, P., Kalso, E., Petersson, K. M., and Ingvar, M. (2002). Placebo and opioid analgesia imaging—A shared neuronal network. *Science, 295,* 1737–1740.

Pettit, H. O., and Justice, J. B., Jr. (1991). Effect of dose on cocaine self-administration behavior and dopamine levels in the nucleus accumbens. *Brain Research, 539,* 94–102.

Petty, F., Kramer, G., Wilson, L., and Jordan, S. (1994). In vivo serotonin release and learned helplessness. *Psychiatry Research, 52,* 285–293.

Pfaff, D. W. (1980). *Estrogens and brain function: Neural analysis of a hormone-controlled mammalian reproductive behavior.* New York, NY: Springer-Verlag.

Pfaff, D. W. (1997). Hormones, genes, and behavior. *Proceedings of the National Academy of Sciences, USA, 94,* 14213–14216.

Pfeffer, M., Wicht, H., von Gall, C., and Korf, H. W. (2015). Owls and larks in mice. *Frontiers in Neurology, 6,* 101.

Pfefferbaum, A., Sullivan, E. V., Mathalon, D. H., Shear, P. K., et al. (1995). Longitudinal changes in magnetic resonance imaging brain volumes in abstinent and relapsed alcoholics. *Alcoholism: Clinical and Experimental Research, 19,* 1177–1191.

Pfenning, A. R., Hara, E., Whitney, O., Rivas, M. V., et al. (2014). Convergent transcriptional specializations in the brains of humans and song-learning birds. *Science, 346*(6215), 1256846.

Phillips, M. L., Young, A. W., Scott, S. K., Calder, A. J., et al. (1998). Neural responses to facial and vocal expressions of fear and disgust. *Proceedings of the Royal Society of London. Series B: Biological Sciences, 265,* 1809–1817.

Phoenix, C. H., Goy, R. W., Gerall, A. A., and Young, W. C. (1959). Organizing action of prenatally administered testosterone propionate on the tissues mediating mating behavior in the female guinea pig. *Endocrinology, 65,* 369–382. DOI: https://doi.org/10.1210/endo-65-3-369

Pickens, R., and Thompson, T. (1968). Drug use by U.S. Army enlisted men in Vietnam: A followup on their return home. *Journal of Pharmacology and Experimental Therapeutics, 161,* 122–129.

Picton, T. W., Hillyard, S. A., Krausz, H. I., and Galambos, R. (1974). Human auditory evoked potentials. I. Evaluation of components. *Electroencephalography and Clinical Neurophysiology, 26*(2), 179–190.

Pierce, K., Müller, R.-A., Ambrose, J., Allen, G., et al. (2001). Face processing occurs outside the fusiform "face area": Evidence from functional MRI. *Brain, 124,* 2059–2073.

Pierce, R. C., and Kumaresan, V. (2006). The mesolimbic dopamine system: The final common pathway for the reinforcing effect of drugs of abuse? *Neuroscience and Biobehavioral Reviews, 30,* 215–238.

Pinel, P., Fauchereau, F., Moreno, A., Barbot, A., et al. (2012). Genetic variants of *FOXP2* and *KIAA0319/TTRAP/THEM2* locus are associated with altered brain activation in distinct language-related regions. *Journal of Neuroscience, 32,* 817–825.

Pirastu, N., Kooyman, M., Traglia, M., Robino, A., et al. (2016). A Genome-Wide Association Study in isolated populations reveals new genes associated to common food likings. *Reviews in Endocrine and Metabolic Disorders, 17*(2), 209–219.

Pitts, M. A., Padwal, J., Fennelly, D., Martínez, A., et al. (2014). Gamma band activity and the P3 reflect post-perceptual processes, not visual awareness. *NeuroImage, 101,* 337–350.

Pletnikov, M. V., Ayhan, Y., Nikolskaia, O., Xu, Y., et al. (2008). Inducible expression of mutant human *DISC1* in mice is associated with brain and behavioral abnormalities reminiscent of schizophrenia. *Molecular Psychiatry, 13,* 13–186.

Plihal, W., and Born, J. (1999). Effects of early and late nocturnal sleep on priming and spatial memory. *Psychophysiology, 36,* 571–582.

Ploog, D. W. (1992). Neuroethological perspectives on the human brain: From the expression of emotions to intentional signing and speech. In A. Harrington (Ed.), *So human a brain: Knowledge and values in the neurosciences* (pp. 3–13). Boston, MA: Birkhauser.

Plutchik, R. (1994). *The psychology and biology of emotion.* New York, NY: HarperCollins.

Poldrack, R. A., Baker, C. I., Durnez, J., Gorgolewski, K. J., et al. (2017). Scanning the horizon: Towards transparent and reproducible neuroimaging research. *Nature Reviews Neuroscience, 18*(2),115–126.

Polymeropoulos, M. H., Lavedan, C., Leroy, E., Ide, S. E., et al. (1997). Mutation in the alpha-synuclein gene identified in families with Parkinson's disease. *Science, 276,* 2045–2047.

Ponsford, J. (2005). Rehabilitation interventions after mild head injury. *Current Opinion in Neurology, 18,* 692–697.

Poole, J. H., Tyack, P. L., Stoeger-Horwath, A. S., and Watwood, S. (2005). Animal behaviour: Elephants are capable of vocal learning. *Nature, 434,* 455–456.

Pooresmaeili, A., FitzGerald, T. H., Bach, D. R., Toelch, U., et al. (2014). Cross-modal effects of value on perceptual acuity and stimulus encoding. *Proceedings of the National Academy of Sciences, USA, 111,* 15244–15249.

Pope, H. G., Jr., Kouri, E. M., and Hudson, J. I. (2000). Effects of supraphysiologic doses of testosterone on mood and aggression in normal men: A randomized controlled trial. *Archives of General Psychiatry, 57,* 133–140.

Poremba, A., Malloy, M., Saunders, R. C., Carson, R. E., et al. (2004). Species-specific calls evoke asymmetric activity in the monkey's temporal poles. *Nature, 427,* 448–451.

Porta, M., Brambilla, A., Cavanna, A. E., Servello, D., et al. (2009). Thalamic deep brain stimulation for treatment-refractory Tourette syndrome: Two-year outcome. *Neurology, 73,* 1375–1380.

Posner, M. I. (1980). Orienting of attention. *Quarterly Journal of Experimental Psychology, 32,* 3–25.

Posner, M. I., and Cohen, Y. (1984). Components of visual orienting. In H. Bouma and D. Bowhuis (Eds.), *Attention and performance: Vol 10. Control of language processes* (pp. 531–556). Hillsdale, NJ: Erlbaum.

Posner, M. I., and Raichle, M. E. (1994). *Images of mind.* New York, NY: Scientific American Library.

Poulet, J. F. A., and Petersen, C. C. H. (2008). Internal brain state regulates membrane potential synchrony in barrel cortex of behaving mice. *Nature, 454,* 881–885.

Poulos, A. M., and Thompson, R. F. (2015). Localization and characterization of an essential associative memory trace in the mammalian brain. *Brain Research, 1621,* 252–259.

Powell, S. B. (2010). Models of neurodevelopmental abnormalities in schizophrenia. *Current Topics in Behavioral Neurosciences, 4,* 435–481.

Powley, T. L. (2000). Vagal circuitry mediating cephalic-phase responses to food. *Appetite, 34,* 184–188.

Pratt, L. A., Brody, D. J., and Gu, Q. (2011). *Antidepressant use in persons aged 12 and over: United States, 2005–2008* (NCHS Data Brief, No. 76). Hyattsville, MD: National Center for Health Statistics.

Prehn, K., Jumpertz von Schwartzenberg, R., Mai, K., Zeitz, U., et al. (2017). Caloric restriction in older adults: Differential effects of weight loss and reduced weight on brain structure and function. *Cerebral Cortex, 27*(3), 1765–1778.

Premack, D. (1971). Language in a chimpanzee? *Science, 172,* 808–822.

Prendergast, B. J., Onishi, K. G., and Zucker, I. (2014). Female mice liberated for inclusion in neuroscience and biomedical research. *Neuroscience & Biobehavioral Reviews, 40,* 1–5.

Prentice, R. L. (2014). Postmenopausal hormone therapy and the risks of coronary heart disease, breast cancer, and stroke. *Seminars in Reproductive Medicine, 32,* 419–425.

Price, M. A., and Vandenbergh, J. G. (1992). Analysis of puberty-accelerating pheromones. *Journal of Experimental Zoology, 264,* 42–45.

Prudente, C. N., Stilla, R., Buetefisch, C. M., Singh, S., et al. (2015). Neural substrates for head movements in humans: A functional magnetic resonance imaging study. *Journal of Neuroscience, 35,* 9163–9172.

Pugh, K. R., Mencl, W. E., Shaywitz, B. A., Shaywitz, S. E., et al. (2000). The angular gyrus in developmental dyslexia: Task-specific differences in functional connectivity within posterior cortex. *Psychological Science, 11,* 51–56.

Pulak, L. M., and Jensen, L. (2014). Sleep in the intensive care unit: A review. *Journal of Intensive Care Medicine,* pii: 0885066614538749.

Purves, D., and Lotto, B. (2011). *Why we see what we do redux: A wholly empirical theory of vision.* Sunderland, MA: Oxford University Press/Sinauer.

Purves, D., Augustine, G. J., Fitzpatrick, D., Katz, L., et al. (Eds.). (2001). *Neuroscience* (2nd ed.). Sunderland, MA: Oxford University Press/Sinauer.

Purves, D., Shimpi, A., and Lotto, R. B. (1999). An empirical explanation of the Cornsweet effect. *Journal of Neuroscience 19,* 8543–8551.

Putman, C. T., Xu, X., Gillies, E., MacLean, I. M., et al. (2004). Effects of strength, endurance and combined training on myosin heavy chain content and fibre-type distribution in humans. *European Journal of Applied Physiology, 92,* 376–384.

Q

Qi, Y., Zheng, Y., Li, Z., and Xiong, L. (2017). Progress in genetic studies of Tourette's syndrome. *Brain Sciences, 7*(10), pii: E134.

Quraishi, I. H., Benjamin, C. F., Spencer, D. D., Blumenfeld, H., et al. (2017). Impairment of consciousness induced by bilateral electrical stimulation of the frontal convexity. *Epilepsy & Behavior Case Reports, 8,* 117–122.

R

Racette, A., Bard, C., and Peretz, I. (2006). Making non-fluent aphasics speak: Sing along! *Brain, 129,* 2571–2584.

Racine, E., Bar-Ilan, O., and Illes, J. (2005). fMRI in the public eye. *Nature Reviews Neuroscience, 6,* 159–164.

Rafal, R. D. (1994). Neglect. *Current Opinion in Neurobiology, 4,* 231–236.

Rahman, Q. (2005). The neurodevelopment of human sexual orientation. *Neuroscience and Biobehavioral Reviews, 29,* 1057–1066.

Raichle, M. E. (2015). The brain's default mode network. *Annual Review of Neuroscience, 38,* 433–447.

Rainville, P., Duncan, G. H., Price, D. D., Carrier, B., et al. (1997). Pain affect encoded in human anterior cingulate but not somatosensory cortex. *Science, 277,* 968–971.

Raisman, G. (1978). What hope for repair of the brain? *Annals of Neurology, 3,* 101–106.

Raisman, G., and Field, P. M. (1971). Sexual dimorphism in the preoptic area of the rat. *Science, 173,* 731–733.

Raisman, G., and Li, Y. (2007). Repair of neural pathways by olfactory ensheathing cells. *Nature Reviews Neuroscience, 8,* 312–319.

Rakic, P. (1979). Genetic and epigenetic determinants of local neuronal circuits in the mammalian central nervous system. In F. O. Schmitt and F. G. Worden (Eds.), *The neurosciences: Fourth study program* (pp. 21–24). Cambridge, MA: MIT Press.

Ralph, M. R., and Menaker, M. (1988). A mutation of the circadian system in golden hamsters. *Science, 241,* 1225–1227.

Ralph, M. R., Foster, R. G., Davis, F. C., and Menaker, M. (1990). Transplanted suprachiasmatic nucleus determines circadian period. *Science, 247,* 975–978.

Ramachandran, V. S., and Hubbard, E. M. (2001). Psychophysical investigations into the neural basis of synthaesthesia. *Proceedings of the Royal Society of London. Series B: Biological Sciences, 268,* 979–983.

Ramachandran, V. S., and Rogers-Ramachandran, D. (2000). Phantom limbs and neural plasticity. *Archives of Neurology, 57,* 317–320.

Rampon, C., Tang, Y. P., Goodhouse, J., Shimizu, E., et al. (2000). Enrichment induces structural changes and recovery from nonspatial memory deficits in CA1 *NMDAR1*-knockout mice. *Nature Neuroscience, 3,* 238–244.

Rand, M. N., and Breedlove, S. M. (1987). Ontogeny of functional innervation of bulbocavernosus muscles in male and female rats. *Brain Research, 430,* 150–152.

Rao, P. D. P., and Finger, T. E. (1984). Asymmetry of the olfactory system in the brain of the winter flounder *Pseudopleuronectes americanus. Journal of Comparative Neurology, 225,* 492–510.

Rapoport, J. L. (1989). The biology of obsessions and compulsions. *Scientific American, 260*(6), 82–89.

Rasmussen, L. E., and Greenwood, D. R. (2003). Frontalin: A chemical message of musth in Asian elephants (*Elephas maximus*). *Chemical Senses, 28,* 433–446.

Rasmussen, L. E., Riddle, H. S., and Krishnamurthy, V. (2002). Chemical communication: Mellifluous matures to malodorous in musth. *Nature, 415,* 975–976.

Rathelot, J. A., and Strick, P. L. (2006). Muscle representation in the macaque motor cortex: An anatomical perspective.

Proceedings of the National Academy of Sciences, USA, 103, 8257–8262.

Rattenborg, N. C. (2006). Do birds sleep in flight? *Naturwissenschaften, 93,* 413–425.

Rauch, S. L., Shin, L. M., and Wright, C. I. (2003). Neuroimaging studies of amygdala function in anxiety disorders. *Annals of the New York Academy of Sciences, 985,* 389–410.

Recanzone, G. H., Schreiner, D. E., and Merzenich, M. M. (1993). Plasticity in the frequency representation of primary auditory cortex following discrimination training in adult owl monkeys. *Journal of Neuroscience, 13,* 87–103.

Rechtschaffen, A., and Bergmann, B. M. (1995). Sleep deprivation in the rat by the disk-over-water method. *Behavioural Brain Research, 69,* 55–63.

Rechtschaffen, A., and Kales, A. (1968). *A manual of standardized terminology, techniques and scoring system for sleep stages of human subjects.* Bethesda, MD: U.S. National Institute of Neurological Diseases and Blindness, Neurological Information Network.

Redican, W. K. (1982). An evolutionary perspective on human facial displays. In P. Ekman (Ed.), *Emotion in the human face* (2nd ed., pp. 212–280). Cambridge, UK: Cambridge University Press.

Rehkamper, G., Haase, E., and Frahm, H. D. (1988). Allometric comparison of brain weight and brain structure volumes in different breeds of the domestic pigeon, *Columba livia* f. d. (fantails, homing pigeons, strassers). *Brain, Behavior and Evolution, 31,* 141–149.

Reiner, W. G., and Gearhart, J. P. (2004). Discordant sexual identity in some genetic males with cloacal exstrophy assigned to female sex at birth. *New England Journal of Medicine, 350,* 333–341.

Reisberg, D., and Heuer, F. (1995). Emotion's multiple effects on memory. In J. L. McGaugh, N. M. Weinberger, and G. Lynch (Eds.), *Brain and memory: Modulation and mediation of neuroplasticity* (pp. 84–92). New York, NY: Oxford University Press.

Rempel-Clower, N. L., Zola, S. M., Squire, L. R., and Amaral, D. G. (1996). Three cases of enduring memory impairment after bilateral damage limited to the hippocampal formation. *Journal of Neuroscience, 16,* 5233–5255.

Renner, M. J., and Rosenzweig, M. R. (1987). *Enriched and impoverished environments: Effects on brain and behavior.* New York, NY: Springer-Verlag.

Reppert, S. M., and Weaver, D. R. (2002). Coordination of circadian timing in mammals. *Nature, 418,* 935–941.

Revel, F. G., Masson-Pévet, M., Pévet, P., Mikkelsen, J. D., et al. (2009). Melatonin controls seasonal breeding by a network of hypothalamic targets. *Neuroendocrinology, 90,* 1–14.

Rezaie, L., Fobian, A. D., McCall, W. V., and Khazaie, H. (2018). Paradoxical insomnia and subjective-objective sleep discrepancy: A review. *Sleep Medicine Reviews, 40,* 196–202. doi:10.1016/j.smrv.2018.01.002

Richman, D. P., and Agius, M. A. (2003). Treatment of autoimmune myasthenia gravis. *Neurology, 61,* 1652–1661.

Richter, C. (1967). Sleep and activity: Their relation to the 24-hour clock. *Proceedings of the Association for Research in Nervous and Mental Diseases, 45,* 8–27.

Risch, N., Herrell, R., Lehner, T., Liang, K. Y., et al. (2009). Interaction between the serotonin transporter gene (5-HT-TLPR), stressful life events, and risk of depression: A meta-analysis. *JAMA, 301,* 2462–2471.

Rizzolatti, G., and Craighero, L. (2004). The mirror-neuron system. *Annual Review of Neuroscience, 27,* 169–192.

Robertson, D. J., Noyes, E., Dowsett, A. J., Jenkins, R., et al. (2016). Face recognition by metropolitan police super-recognisers. *PLOS ONE, 11*(2), e0150036.

Robins, L. N., and Regier, D. A. (1991). *Psychiatric disorders in America: The epidemiologic catchment area study.* New York, NY: Free Press.

Robinson, D. L., and Petersen, S. E. (1992). The pulvinar and visual salience. *Trends in Neuroscience, 15,* 127–132.

Robinson, R. (2009). Intractable depression responds to deep brain stimulation. *Neurology Today, 9,* 7–10.

Rocca, W. A., Hofman, A., Brayne, C., Breteler, M. M., et al. (1991). The prevalence of vascular dementia in Europe: Facts and fragments from 1980–1990 studies. *Annals of Neurology, 30,* 817–824.

Roenneberg, T., Allebrandt, K. V., Merrow, M., and Vetter, C. (2012). Social jetlag and obesity. *Current Biology, 22,* 939–943.

Roenneberg, T., Kuehnle, T., Pramstaller, P. P., Ricken, J., et al. (2004). A marker for the end of adolescence. *Current Biology, 14,* R1038–R1039.

Roffwarg, H. P., Muzio, J. N., and Dement, W. C. (1966). Ontogenetic development of the human sleep-dream cycle. *Science, 152,* 604–619.

Rogan, M. T., Staubli, U. V., and LeDoux, J. E. (1997). Fear conditioning induces associative long-term potentiation in the amygdala. *Nature, 390,* 604–607.

Rogawski, M. A., and Löscher, W. (2004). The neurobiology of antiepileptic drugs. *Nature Reviews Neuroscience, 5,* 553–564.

Roland, P. E. (1993). *Brain activation.* New York, NY: Wiley-Liss.

Rose, K. A., Morgan, I. G., Smith, W., Burlutsky, G., et al. (2008). Myopia, lifestyle, and schooling in students of Chinese ethnicity in Singapore and Sydney. *Archives of Ophthalmology, 126,* 527–530.

Roseboom, T. J., Painter, R. C., van Abeelen, A. F., Veenendaal, M. V., et al. (2011). Hungry in the womb: What are the consequences? Lessons from the Dutch famine. *Maturitas, 70,* 141–145.

Rosell, D. R., and Siever, L. J. (2015). The neurobiology of aggression and violence. *CNS Spectrums, 20*(3), 254–279.

Roselli, C. E., and Stormshak, F. (2009). The neurobiology of sexual partner preferences in rams. *Hormones and Behavior, 55,* 611–620.

Roselli, C. E., Larkin, K., Resko, J. A., Stellflug, J. N., et al. (2004). The volume of a sexually dimorphic nucleus in the ovine medial preoptic area/anterior hypothalamus varies with sexual partner preference. *Endocrinology, 145,* 475–477.

Rosenbaum, R. S., Köhler, S., Schacter, D. L., Moscovitch, M., et al. (2005). The case of K.C.: Contributions of a memory-impaired person to memory theory. *Neuropsychologia, 43,* 989–1021.

Rosenberg, M. D., Finn, E. S., Scheinost, D., Constable, R. T., et al. (2017). Characterizing attention with predictive network models. *Trends in Cognitive Sciences, 21*(4), 290–302.

Rosenberg, M. D., Finn, E. S., Scheinost, D., Papademetris, X., et al. (2016). A neuromarker of sustained attention from whole-brain functional connectivity. *Nature Neuroscience, 19*(1), 165–171.

Rosenkranz, M. A., Jackson, D. C., Dalton, K. M., Dolski, I., et al. (2003). Affective style and in vivo immune response: Neurobehavioral mechanisms. *Proceedings of the National Academy of Sciences, USA, 100,* 11148–11152.

Rosenzweig, M. R. (1946). Discrimination of auditory intensities in the cat. *American Journal of Psychology, 59,* 127–136.

Rosenzweig, M. R., Bennett, E. L., and Diamond, M. C. (1972). Brain changes in response to experience. *Scientific American, 226,* 22–29.

Rosenzweig, M. R., Krech, D., and Bennett, E. L. (1961). Heredity, environment, brain biochemistry, and learning. In *Current trends in psychological theory* (pp. 87–110). Pittsburgh, PA: University of Pittsburgh Press.

Roses, A. D. (1995). On the metabolism of apolipoprotein E and the Alzheimer diseases. *Experimental Neurology, 132,* 149–156.

Rossi, D. J., Oshima, T., and Attwell, D. (2000). Glutamate release in severe brain ischaemia is mainly by reversed uptake. *Nature, 403,* 316–321.

Rothschild, A. J. (1992). Disinhibition, amnestic reactions, and other adverse reactions secondary to triazolam: A review of the literature. *Journal of Clinical Psychiatry*, *53*, 69–79.

Rouw, R., and Scholter, H. S. (2007). Increased structural connectivity in grapheme-color synesthesia. *Nature Neuroscience*, *10*, 792–797.

Roy, A. (1992). Hypothalamic-pituitary-adrenal axis function and suicidal behavior in depression. *Biological Psychiatry*, *32*, 812–816.

Rozanski, A. (2014). Behavioral cardiology: Current advances and future directions. *Journal of the American College of Cardiology*, *64*(1), 100–110.

Rumbaugh, D. M. (1977). *Language learning by a chimpanzee: The LANA project.* New York, NY: Academic Press.

Rupnick, M. A., Panigrahy, D., Zhang, C. Y., Dallabrida, S. M., et al. (2002). Adipose tissue mass can be regulated through the vasculature. *Proceedings of the National Academy of Sciences, USA*, *99*, 10730–10735.

Rupprecht, R., Rammes, G., Eser, D., Baghai, T. C., et al. (2009). Translocator protein (18 kD) as target for anxiolytics without benzodiazepine-like side effects. *Science*, *325*, 490–493.

Rusak, B., and Zucker, I. (1979). Neural regulation of circadian rhythms. *Physiological Reviews*, *59*, 449–526.

Russell, J. A. (1994). Is there universal recognition of emotion from facial expressions? A review of the cross-cultural studies. *Psychological Bulletin*, *115*, 102–141.

Russell, R., Duchaine, B., and Nakayama, K. (2009). Super-recognizers: People with extraordinary face recognition ability. *Psychonomic Bulletin & Review*, *16*(2), 252–257.

Russo, E. B., Jiang, H. E., Li, X., Sutton, A., et al. (2008). Phytochemical and genetic analyses of ancient cannabis from Central Asia. *Journal of Experimental Botany*, *59*(15), 4171–4182.

S

Saalmann, Y. B., Pinsk, M. A., Wang, L., Li, X., et al. (2012). The pulvinar regulates information transmission between cortical areas based on attention demands. *Science*, *337*(6095), 753–756.

Sack, R. L., Blood, M. L., and Lewy, A. J. (1992). Melatonin rhythms in night shift workers. *Sleep*, *15*, 434–441.

Sack, R. L., Brandes, R. W., Kendall, A. R., and Lewy, A. J. (2000). Entrainment of free-running circadian rhythms by melatonin in blind people. *New England Journal of Medicine*, *343*, 1070–1077.

Sack, R. L., Lewy, A. J., Blood, M. L., Keith, L. D., et al. (1992). Circadian rhythm abnormalities in totally blind people: Incidence and clinical significance. *Journal of Clinical Endocrinology and Metabolism*, *75*, 127–134.

Saha, K. B., Bo, L., Zhao, S., Xia, J., et al. (2016). Chlorpromazine versus atypical antipsychotic drugs for schizophrenia. *Cochrane Database of Systematic Reviews*, *4*, CD010631.

Sahay, A., and Hen, R. (2007). Adult hippocampal neurogenesis in depression. *Nature Neuroscience*, *10*, 1110–1114.

Sakreida, K., Lange, I., Willmes, K., Heim, S., et al. (2018). High-resolution language mapping of Broca's region with transcranial magnetic stimulation. *Brain Structure and Function*, *223*(3), 1297–1312.

Sakurai, T., Amemiya, A., Ishii, M., Matsuzaki, I., et al. (1998). Orexins and orexin receptors: A family of hypothalamic neuropeptides and G protein-coupled receptors that regulate feeding behavior. *Cell*, *92*, 573–585.

Salazar, H., Llorente, I., Jara-Oseguera, A., García-Villegas, R., et al. (2008). A single N-terminal cysteine in TRPV1 determines activation by pungent compounds from onion and garlic. *Nature Neuroscience*, *11*, 255–260.

Salimpoor, V. N., Zald, D. H., Zatorre, R. J., Dagher, A., et al. (2015). Predictions and the brain: How musical sounds become rewarding. *Trends in Cognitive Sciences*, *19*(2), 86–91.

Samad, T. A., Moore, K. A., Sapirstein, A., Billet, S., et al. (2001). Interleukin-1β-mediated induction of Cox-2 in the CNS contributes to inflammatory pain hypersensitivity. *Nature*, *410*, 471–475.

Samaha, F. F., Iqbal, N., Seshadri, P., Chicano, K. L., et al. (2003). A low-carbohydrate as compared with a low-fat diet in severe obesity. *New England Journal of Medicine*, *348*, 2074–2081.

Samson, S., and Zatorre, R. J. (1991). Recognition memory for text and melody of songs after unilateral temporal lobe lesion: Evidence for dual encoding. *Journal of Experimental Psychology. Learning, Memory, and Cognition*, *17*, 793–804.

Samson, S., and Zatorre, R. J. (1994). Contribution of the right temporal lobe to musical timbre discrimination. *Neuropsychologia*, *32*, 231–240.

Sandberg, K., Umans, J. G.; Georgetown Consensus Conference Work Group. (2015). Recommendations concerning the new U.S. National Institutes of Health initiative to balance the sex of cells and animals in preclinical research. *FASEB Journal*, *29*(5), 1646–1652.

Sanders, A. R., Beecham, G. W., Guo, S., Dawood, K., et al. (2017). Genome-wide association study of male sexual orientation. *Scientific Reports*, *7*(1), 16950.

Sanderson, D. J., Good, M. A., Seeburg, P. H., Sprengel, R., et al. (2008). The role of the GluR-A (GluR1) AMPA receptor subunit in learning and memory. *Progress in Brain Research*, *169*, 159–178.

Saper, C. B., Fuller, P. M., Pedersen, N. P., Lu, J., et al. (2010). Sleep state switching. *Neuron*, *68*, 1023–1042.

Sapir, A., Soroker, N., Berger, A., and Henik, A. (1999). Inhibition of return in spatial attention: Direct evidence for collicular generation. *Nature Neuroscience*, *2*, 1053–1054.

Sapolsky, R. M. (1992). Neuroendocrinology of the stress-response. In J. B. Becker, S. M. Breedlove, and D. Crews (Eds.), *Behavioral endocrinology* (pp. 287–324). Cambridge, MA: MIT Press.

Sapolsky, R. M. (2004). *Why zebras don't get ulcers* (3rd ed.). New York, NY: Holt.

Satinoff, E., and Rutstein, J. (1970). Behavioral thermoregulation in rats with anterior hypothalamic lesions. *Journal of Comparative and Physiological Psychology*, *71*, 77–82.

Satinoff, E., and Shan, S. Y. (1971). Loss of behavioral thermoregulation after lateral hypothalamic lesions in rats. *Journal of Comparative and Physiological Psychology*, *77*, 302–312.

Sato, J. R., Salum, G. A., Gadelha, A., Crossley, N., et al. (2015). Default mode network maturation and psychopathology in children and adolescents. *Journal of Child Psychology and Psychiatry, 57*, 55-64. doi:10.1111/jcpp.12444

Saul, S. (2006, March 8). Some sleeping pill users range far beyond bed. *The New York Times*.

Saxe, M. D., Battaglia, F., Wang, J. W., Malleret, G., et al. (2006). Ablation of hippocampal neurogenesis impairs contextual fear conditioning and synaptic plasticity in the dentate gyrus. *Proceedings of the National Academy of Sciences, USA, 103*, 17501–17506.

Saxena, S., Brody, A. L., Ho, M. L., Alborzian, S., et al. (2001). Cerebral metabolism in major depression and obsessive-compulsive disorder occurring separately and concurrently. *Biological Psychiatry*, *50*, 159–170.

Scalaidhe, S. P. O., Wilson, F. A. W., and Goldman-Rakic, P. S. (1997). Areal segregation of face-processing neurons in prefrontal cortex. *Science*, *278*, 1135–1138.

SCENIHR (Scientific Committee on Emerging and Newly Identified Health Risks). (2008, September 23). *Potential health risks of exposure to noise from personal music players and mobile phones including a music playing function*. Brussels, Belgium: European Commission, Directorate General for Health & Consumers Protection (http://ec.europa.eu/health/ph_risk/committees/04_scenihr/docs/scenihr_o_018.pdf).

Schachter, S. (1975). Cognition and peripheralist-centralist controversies in motivation and emotion. In M. S. Gazzaniga and C. Blakemore (Eds.), *Handbook of psychobiology* (pp. 529–564). New York, NY: Academic Press.

Schachter, S., and Singer, J. (1962). Cognitive, social, and physiological determinants of emotional state. *Psychological Review, 69*, 379–399.

Schacter, D. L., Wig, G. S., and Stevens, W. D. (2007). Reductions in cortical activity during priming. *Current Opinion in Neurology, 17*(2), 17–16.

Scharff, C., Kirn, J. R., Grossman, M., Macklis, J. D., et al. (2000). Targeted neuronal death affects neuronal replacement and vocal behavior in adult songbirds. *Neuron, 25*, 481–492.

Scheibel, A. B., and Conrad, A. S. (1993). Hippocampal dysgenesis in mutant mouse and schizophrenic man: Is there a relationship? *Schizophrenia Bulletin, 19*, 21–33.

Schein, S. J., and Desimone, R. (1990). Spectral properties of V4 neurons in the macaque. *Journal of Neuroscience, 10*, 3369–3389.

Schenck, C. H., and Mahowald, M. W. (2002). REM sleep behavior disorder: Clinical, developmental, and neuroscience perspectives 16 years after its formal identification in sleep. *Sleep, 25*, 120–138.

Schieber, M. H, and Hibbard, L. S. (1993). How somatotopic is the motor cortex hand area? *Science, 261*, 489–492.

Schiffman, S. S., Simon, S. A., Gill, J. M., and Beeker, T. G. (1986). Bretylium tosylate enhances salt taste. *Physiology & Behavior, 36*, 1129–1137.

Schildkraut, J. J., and Kety, S. S. (1967). Biogenic amines and emotion. *Science, 156*, 21–30.

Schindler, E. A., Gottschalk, C. H., Weil, M. J., Shapiro, R. E., et al. (2015). Indoleamine hallucinogens in cluster headache: Results of the Clusterbusters Medication Use Survey. *Journal of Psychoactive Drugs, 47*(5), 372–381.

Schlaug, G., Jancke, L., Huang, Y., and Steinmetz, H. (1995). In vivo evidence of structural brain asymmetry in musicians. *Science, 267*, 699–701.

Schnapf, J. L., and Baylor, D. A. (1987). How photoreceptor cells respond to light. *Scientific American, 256*(4), 40–47.

Schneider, K. (1959). *Clinical psychopathology.* New York, NY: Grune & Stratton.

Schneider, P., Scherg, M., Dosch, H. G., Specht, H. J., et al. (2002). Morphology of Heschl's gyrus reflects enhanced activation in the auditory cortex of musicians. *Nature Neuroscience, 5*, 688–694.

Schneps, M. H., Brockmole, J. R., Sonnert, G., and Pomplun, M. (2012). History of reading struggles linked to enhanced learning in low spatial frequency scenes. *PLOS ONE, 7*, e35724.

Schoenbaum, G., Roesch, M. R., Stalnaker, T. A., and Takahashi, Y. K. (2009). A new perspective on the role of the orbitofrontal cortex in adaptive behaviour. *Nature Reviews Neuroscience, 10*, 885–892.

Schramm, E., Schneider, D., Zobel, I., van Calker, D., et al. (2008). Efficacy of Interpersonal Psychotherapy plus pharmacotherapy in chronically depressed inpatients. *Journal of Affective Disorders, 109*(1–2), 65–73.

Schulz, K. M., and Sisk, C. L. (2016). The organizing actions of adolescent gonadal steroid hormones on brain and behavioral development. *Neuroscience & Biobehavioral Reviews, 70*, 148–158.

Schumann, C. M., and Amaral, D. G. (2006). Stereological analysis of amygdala neuron number in autism. *Journal of Neuroscience, 26*, 7674–7679.

Schummers, J., Yu, H., and Sur, M. (2008). Tuned responses of astrocytes and their influence on hemodynamic signals in the visual cortex. *Science, 320*, 1638–1643.

Schuster, C. R. (1970). Psychological approaches to opiate dependence and self-administration by laboratory animals. *Federation Proceedings, 29*, 1–5.

Schwartz, S., and Correll, C. U. (2014). Efficacy and safety of atomoxetine in children and adolescents with attention-deficit/hyperactivity disorder: Results from a comprehensive meta-analysis and metaregression. *Journal of the American Academy of Child and Adolescent Psychiatry, 53*, 174–187.

Schwartzkroin, P. A., and Wester, K. (1975). Long-lasting facilitation of a synaptic potential following tetanization in the in vitro hippocampal slice. *Brain Research, 89*, 107–119.

Sclafani, A., Springer, D., and Kluge, L. (1976). Effects of quinine adulterated diets on the food intake and body weight of obese and non-obese hypothalamic hyperphagic rats. *Physiology & Behavior, 16*, 631–640.

Scott, D. J., Stohler, C. S., Egnatuk, C. M., Wang, H., et al. (2008). Placebo and nocebo effects are defined by opposite opioid and dopaminergic responses. *Archives of General Psychiatry, 65*, 220–231.

Scott, S. K., and Wise, R. J. (2004). The functional neuroanatomy of prelexical processing in speech perception. *Cognition, 92*(1–2), 13–45.

Scoville, W. B., and Milner, B. (1957). Loss of recent memory after bilateral hippocampal lesions. *Journal of Neurology, Neurosurgery and Psychiatry, 20*, 11–21.

Seavey, C., Katz, P., and Zalk, S. R. (1975). Baby X: The effects of gender labels on adult responses to infants. *Sex Roles, 2*, 103–109.

Seeman, P. (1990). Atypical neuroleptics: Role of multiple receptors, endogenous dopamine, and receptor linkage. *Acta Psychiatrica Scandinavica. Supplementum, 358*, 14–20.

Seeman, P., and Tallerico, T. (1998). Antipsychotic drugs which elicit little or no parkinsonism bind more loosely than dopamine to brain D2 receptors, yet occupy high levels of these receptors. *Molecular Psychiatry, 3*, 123–134.

Seiden, R. H. (1978). Where are they now? A follow-up study of suicide attempters from the Golden Gate Bridge. *Suicide and Life Threatening Behavior, 8*, 203–216.

Selkoe, D. J., and Hardy, J. (2016). The amyloid hypothesis of Alzheimer's disease at 25 years. *EMBO Molecular Medicine, 8*(6), 595–608.

Selye, H. (1956). *The stress of life.* New York, NY: McGraw-Hill.

Semendeferi, K., Lu, A., Schenker, N., and Damasio, H. (2002). Humans and great apes share a large frontal cortex. *Nature Neuroscience, 5*, 272–276.

Senju, A., Southgate, V., White, S., and Frith, W. (2009). Mindblind eyes: An absence of spontaneous theory of mind in Asperger syndrome. *Science, 325*, 883–885.

Sessa, B. (2017). MDMA and PTSD treatment: "PTSD: From novel pathophysiology to innovative therapeutics." *Neuroscience Letters, 649*, 176–180.

Seuss, Dr. (1987). *The tough coughs as he ploughs the dough: Early writings and cartoons by Dr. Seuss.* New York, NY: Morrow.

Sexton, C. E., Mackay, C. E., and Ebmeier, K. P. (2013). A systematic review and meta-analysis of magnetic resonance imaging studies in late-life depression. *American Journal of Geriatric Psychiatry, 21*, 184–195.

Seyfarth, R. M., and Cheney, D. L. (2003). Meaning and emotion in animal vocalizations. *Annals of the New York Academy of Sciences, 1000*, 32–55.

Shackman, A. J., Fox, A. S., Oler, J. A., Shelton, S. E., et al. (2013). Neural mechanisms underlying heterogeneity in the presentation of anxious temperament. *Proceedings of the National Academy of Sciences, USA, 110*, 6145–6150.

Shah, D. B., Pesiridou, A., Baltuch, G. H., Malone, D. A., et al. (2008). Functional neurosurgery in the treatment of severe obsessive compulsive disorder and major depression: Overview of disease circuits and therapeutic targeting for the clinician. *Psychiatry (Edgmont), 5*(9), 24–33.

Shallice, T., and Burgess, P. W. (1991). Deficits in strategy application following frontal lobe damage in man. *Brain, 114*, 727–741.

Shammi, P., and Stuss, D. T. (1999). Humour appreciation: A role of the right frontal lobe. *Brain, 122*, 657–666.

Shapiro, R. M. (1993). Regional neuropathology in schizophrenia: Where are we? Where are we going? *Schizophrenia Research, 10*, 187–239.

Shaw, P. J., Tononi, G., Greenspan, R. J., and Robinson, D. F. (2002). Stress response genes protect against lethal effects of sleep deprivation in *Drosophila. Nature, 417,* 287–291.

Shaw, P., Eckstrand, K., Sharp, W., Blumenthal, J., et al. (2007). Attention-deficit/hyperactivity disorder is characterized by a delay in cortical maturation. *Proceedings of the National Academy of Sciences, USA, 104,* 19649–19654.

Shaw, P., Greenstein, D., Lerch, J., Clasen, L., et al. (2006). Intellectual ability and cortical development in children and adolescents. *Nature, 440,* 676–679.

Shaywitz, S. E., Shaywitz, B. A, Fulbright, R. K., Skudlarski, P., et al. (2003). Neural systems for compensation and persistence: Young adult outcome of childhood reading disability. *Biological Psychiatry, 54*(1), 25–33.

Shaywitz, S. E., Shaywitz, B. A., Pugh, K. R., Fulbright, R. K., et al. (1998). Functional disruption in the organization of the brain for reading in dyslexia. *Proceedings of the National Academy of Sciences, USA, 95,* 2636–2641.

Sheikh-Bahaei, N., Sajjadi, S. A., Manavaki, R., McLean, M., et al. (2018). Positron emission tomography-guided magnetic resonance spectroscopy in Alzheimer disease. *Annals of Neurology, 83*(4), 771–778.

Shein-Idelson, M., Ondracek, J. M., Liaw, H. P., Reiter, S., et al. (2016). Slow waves, sharp waves, ripples, and REM in sleeping dragons. *Science, 352*(6285), 590–595.

Sherrington, C. S. (1897). *A textbook of physiology. Part III. The central nervous system* (7th ed.), M. Foster (Ed.). London, UK: Macmillan.

Sherrington, C. S. (1898). Experiments in examination of the peripheral distribution of the fibres of the posterior roots of some spinal nerves. *Philosophical Transactions, 190,* 45–186.

Sherry, D. F. (1992). Memory, the hippocampus, and natural selection: Studies of food-storing birds. In L. R. Squire and N. Butters (Eds.), *Neuropsychology of memory* (2nd ed., pp. 521–532). New York, NY: Guilford Press.

Sherry, D. F., and Vaccarino, A. L. (1989). Hippocampus and memory for food caches in black-capped chickadees. *Behavioral Neuroscience, 103,* 308–318.

Sherry, D. F., Vaccarino, A. L., Buckenham, K., and Herz, R. S. (1989). The hippocampal complex of food-storing birds. *Brain, Behavior and Evolution, 34,* 308–317.

Sherwin, B. B. (1998). Use of combined estrogen-androgen preparations in the postmenopause: Evidence from clinical studies. *International Journal of Fertility and Women's Medicine, 43*(2), 98–103.

Sherwin, B. B. (2002). Randomized clinical trials of combined estrogen-androgen

preparations: Effects on sexual functioning. *Fertility and Sterility, 77*(Suppl. 4), 49–54.

Sherwin, B. B. (2009). Estrogen therapy: Is time of initiation critical for neuroprotection? *Nature Reviews Endocrinology, 5,* 620–627.

Sheth, S. A., Mian, M. K., Patel, S. R., Asaad, W. F., et al. (2012). Human dorsal anterior cingulate cortex neurons mediate ongoing behavioural adaptation. *Nature, 488*(7410), 218–221.

Shic, F., and Scassellati, B. (2007). A behavioral analysis of computational models of visual attention. *International Journal of Computer Vision, 73*(2), 159–177.

Shih, R. A., Belmonte, P. L., and Zandi, P. P. (2004). A review of the evidence from family, twin and adoption studies for a genetic contribution to adult psychiatric disorders. *International Review of Psychiatry, 16,* 260–283.

Shimura, H., Schlossmacher, M. G., Hattori, N., Frosch, M. P., et al. (2001). Ubiquitination of a new form of α-synuclein by parkin from human brain: Implications for Parkinson's disease. *Science, 293,* 263–269.

Shipton, O. A., El-Gaby, M., Apergis-Schoute, J., Deisseroth, K., et al. (2014). Left-right dissociation of hippocampal memory processes in mice. *Proceedings of the National Academy of Sciences, USA, 111,* 15238–15243.

Shu, W., Cho, J. Y., Jiang, Y., Zhang, M., et al. (2005). Altered ultrasonic vocalization in mice with a disruption in the *Foxp2* gene. *Proceedings of the National Academy of Sciences, USA, 102,* 9643–9648.

Siegel, J. M. (1994). Brainstem mechanisms generating REM sleep. In M. H. Kryger, T. Roth, and W. C. Dement (Eds.), *Principles and practice of sleep medicine* (2nd ed., pp. 125–144). Philadelphia, PA: Saunders.

Siegel, J. M. (2005). Clues to the function of mammalian sleep. *Nature, 437,* 1264–1271.

Siegel, J. M., Manger, P. R., Nienhuis, R., Fahringer, H. M., et al. (1999). Sleep in the platypus. *Neuroscience, 91,* 391–400.

Siegel, J. M., Nienhuis, R., Gulyani, S., Ouyang, S., et al. (1999). Neuronal degeneration in canine narcolepsy. *Journal of Neuroscience, 19,* 248–257.

Sierakowiak, A., Monnot, C., Aski, S. N., Uppman, M., et al. (2015). Default mode network, motor network, dorsal and ventral basal ganglia networks in the rat brain: Comparison to human networks using resting state-fMRI. *PLOS ONE, 10,* e0120345.

Sikich, L, Frazier, J. A., McClellan, J., Findling, R. L., et al. (2008). Double-blind comparison of first- and second-generation antipsychotics in early-onset schizophrenia and schizo-affective disorder: Findings from the treatment of early-onset schizophrenia spectrum disorders

(TEOSS) study. *American Journal of Psychiatry, 165,* 1420–1431.

Silva, D. A., and Satz, P. (1979). Pathological left-handedness. Evaluation of a model. *Brain and Language, 7,* 8–16.

Simons, D. J., and Chabris, C. F. (1999). Gorillas in our midst: Sustained inattentional blindness for dynamic events. *Perception, 28,* 1059–1074.

Simons, D. J., and Jensen, M. S. (2009). The effects of individual differences and task difficulty on inattentional blindness. *Psychonomic Bulletin & Review, 16,* 398–403.

Simons, D. J., and Schlosser, M. D. (2017). Inattentional blindness for a gun during a simulated police vehicle stop. *Cognitive Research: Principles and Implications, 2*(1), 37.

Singer, O., Marr, R. A., Rockenstein, E., Crews, L., et al. (2005). Targeting BACE1 with siRNAs ameliorates Alzheimer disease neuropathology in a transgenic model. *Nature Neuroscience, 8,* 1343–1349.

Singer, P. (1975). *Animal liberation: A new ethics for our treatment of animals.* New York, NY: New York Review.

Singer, T., Seymour, B., O'Doherty, J., Kaube, H., et al. (2004). Empathy for pain involves the affective but not sensory components of pain. *Science, 303,* 1157–1162.

Sinopoli, V. M., Burton, C. L., Kronenberg, S., and Arnold, P. D. (2017). A review of the role of serotonin system genes in obsessive-compulsive disorder. *Neuroscience & Biobehavioral Reviews, 80,* 372–381.

Slee, S. J., and Young, E. D. (2014). Alignment of sound localization cues in the nucleus of the brachium of the inferior colliculus. *Journal of Neurophysiology, 111,* 2624–2633.

Smale, L. (1988). Influence of male gonadal hormones and familiarity on pregnancy interruption in prairie voles. *Biology of Reproduction, 39,* 28–31.

Smale, L., Holekamp, K. E., and White, P. A. (1999). Siblicide revisited in the spotted hyaena: Does it conform to obligate or facultative models? *Animal Behaviour, 58,* 545–551.

Smith, C. (1995). Sleep states and memory processes. *Behavioural Brain Research, 69,* 137–145.

Smith, M. A., Brandt, J., and Shadmehr, R. (2000). Motor disorder in Huntington's disease begins as a dysfunction in error feedback control. *Nature, 403,* 544–549.

Smith, S. (1997, September 2). Dreaming awake part 1: Living with narcolepsy. Minnesota Public Radio News (http://news.minnesota.publicradio.org/features/199709/02_smiths_narcolepsy/narco_1.shtml).

Smoller, J. W., and Finn, C. T. (2003). Family, twin, and adoption studies of bipolar disorder. *American Journal of Medical Genetics.*

Part C, Seminars in Medical Genetics, 123, 48–58.

Smyth, K. A., Pritsch, T., Cook, T. B., McClendon, M. J., et al. (2004). Worker functions and traits associated with occupations and the development of AD. *Neurology, 63,* 498–503.

Snyder, J. S., Soumier, A., Brewer, M., Pickel, J., et al. (2011). Adult hippocampal neurogenesis buffers stress responses and depressive behaviour. *Nature, 476,* 458–461.

Snyder, P. J., Bhasin, S., Cunningham, G. R., Matsumoto, A. M., et al. (2018). Lessons from the Testosterone Trials. *Endocrine Reviews.* doi:10.1210/er.2017-00234

Solomon, A. (2001). *The noonday demon: An atlas of depression.* New York, NY: Scribner.

Soltis, J., King, L. E., Douglas-Hamilton, I., Vollrath, F., et al. (2014). African elephant alarm calls distinguish between threats from humans and bees. *PLOS ONE, 9,* e89403.

Somerville, M. J., Mervis, C. B., Young, E. J., Seo, E. J., et al. (2005). Severe expressive-language delay related to duplication of the *Williams-Beuren* locus. *New England Journal of Medicine, 353,* 1694–1701.

Soon, C. S., Brass, M., Heinze, H. J., and Haynes, J. D. (2008). Unconscious determinants of free decisions in the human brain. *Nature Neuroscience, 11,* 543–545.

Sorensen, P. W., and Goetz, F. W. (1993). Pheromonal and reproductive function of F prostaglandins and their metabolites in teleost fish. *Journal of Lipid Mediators, 6,* 385–393.

Sowell, E. R., Kan, E., Yoshii, J., Thompson, P. M., et al. (2008). Thinning of sensorimotor cortices in children with Tourette syndrome. *Nature Neuroscience, 11,* 637–639.

Spalding, K. L., Bergmann, O., Alkass, K., Bernard, S., et al. (2013). Dynamics of hippocampal neurogenesis in adult humans. *Cell, 153*(6), 1219–1227.

Spampinato, D., and Celnik, P. (2018). Deconstructing skill learning and its physiological mechanisms. *Cortex, 104,* 90–102.

Spiegler, B. J., and Mishkin, M. (1981). Evidence for the sequential participation of inferior temporal cortex and amygdala in the acquisition of stimulus-reward associations. *Behavioural Brain Research, 3,* 303–317.

Spiegler, B. J., and Yeni-Komshian, G. H. (1983). Incidence of left-handed writing in a college population with reference to family patterns of hand preference. *Neuropsychologia, 21,* 651–659.

Spitzer, R. L. (2012). Spitzer reassesses his 2003 study of reparative therapy of homosexuality. *Archives of Sexual Behavior, 41,* 757.

Sprague, T. C., Saproo, S., and Serences, J. T. (2015). Visual attention mitigates information loss in small- and large-scale neural codes. *Trends in Cognitive Sciences, 19*(4), 215–226.

Squire, L. R., Amaral, D. G., Zola-Morgan, S., and Kritchevsky, M. P. G. (1989). Description of brain injury in the amnesic patient N.A. based on magnetic resonance imaging. *Experimental Neurology, 105,* 23–35.

Squire, L. R., and Moore, R. Y. (1979). Dorsal thalamic lesion in a noted case of chronic memory dysfunction. *Annals of Neurology, 6,* 503–506.

Squire, L. R., and Zola-Morgan, S. (1991). The medial temporal lobe memor system. *Science, 253,* 1380–1386.

Standing, L. G. (1973). Learning 10,000 pictures. *Quarterly Journal of Experimental Psychology, 25,* 207–222.

Stanovich, K. E. (2009). *What intelligence tests miss: The psychology of rational thought.* New Haven, CT: Yale University Press.

Stansley, B. J., and Conn, P. J. (2018). The therapeutic potential of metabotropic glutamate receptor modulation for schizophrenia. *Current Opinion in Pharmacology, 38,* 31–36.

Stanton, S. J., Beehner, J. C., Saini, E. K., Kuhn, C. M., et al. (2009). Dominance, politics, and physiology: Voters' testosterone changes on the night of the 2008 United States presidential election. *PLOS ONE, 4,* e7543.

Staubli, U. V. (1995). Parallel properties of long-term potentiation and memory. In J. L. McGaugh, N. M. Weinberger, and G. Lynch (Eds.), *Brain and memory: Modulation and mediation of neuroplasticity* (pp. 303–318). New York, NY: Oxford University Press.

Stauffer, V. L., Millen, B. A., Andersen, S., Kinon, B. J., et al. (2013). Pomaglumetad methionil: No significant difference as an adjunctive treatment for patients with prominent negative symptoms of schizophrenia compared to placebo. *Schizophrenia Research, 150,* 434–441.

Stein, B. E., and Stanford, T. R. (2008). Multisensory integration: Current issues from the perspective of the single neuron. *Nature Reviews Neuroscience, 9,* 255–266.

Stein, M., and Miller, A. H. (1993). Stress, the hypothalamic-pituitary-adrenal axis, and immune function. *Advances in Experimental Medicine and Biology, 335,* 1–5.

Stein, M., Miller, A. H., and Trestman, R. L. (1991). Depression, the immune system, and health and illness. Findings in search of meaning. *Archives of General Psychiatry, 48,* 171–177.

Stephan, F. K., and Zucker, I. (1972). Circadian rhythms in drinking behavior and locomotor activity of rats are eliminated by hypothalamic lesions. *Proceedings of the National Academy of Sciences, USA, 69,* 1583–1586.

Sterling, P., and Eyer, J. (1988). Allostasis: A new paradigm to explain arousal pathology. In S. Fisher and J. T. Reason (Eds.), *Handbook of life stress, cognition, and health* (pp. 629–649). Chicester, NY: Wiley.

Stern, K., and McClintock, M. (1998). Regulation of ovulation by human pheromones. *Nature, 392,* 177–179.

Stoeckel, C., Gough, P. M., Watkins, K. E., and Devlin, J. T. (2009). Supramarginal gyrus involvement in visual word recognition. *Cortex, 45,* 1091–1096.

Stranahan, A. M., Khalil, D., and Gould, E. (2006). Social isolation delays the positive effects of running on adult neurogenesis. *Nature Neuroscience, 9,* 526–533.

Substance Abuse and Mental Health Services Administration. (2013). *Results from the 2012 National Survey on Drug Use and Health: Mental health findings* (NSDUH Series H-47, HHS Publication No. [SMA] 13-4805). Rockville, MD: Substance Abuse and Mental Health Services Administration.

Substance Abuse and Mental Health Services Administration (SAMHSA). (2017). *Key substance use and mental health indicators in the United States: Results from the 2016 National Survey on Drug Use and Health* (NSDUH Series H-52, HHS Publication No. [SMA] 17-5044). Rockville, MD: Center for Behavioral Health Statistics and Quality, Substance Abuse and Mental Health Services Administration.

Substance Abuse and Mental Health Services Administration. (2017). *Results from the 2016 National Survey on Drug Use and Health: Key substance use and mental health indicators in the United States* (NSDUH Series H-52, HHS Publication No. [SMA] 17-5044). Rockville, MD: Substance Abuse and Mental Health Services Administration.

Suez, J., and Elinav, E. (2017). The path towards microbiome-based metabolite treatment. *Nature Microbiology, 2,* 17075.

Suk, I., and Tamargo, R. J. (2010). Concealed neuroanatomy in Michelangelo's *Separation of Light from Darkness* in the Sistine Chapel. *Neurosurgery, 66*(5), 851–861.

Sumnall, H. R., and Cole, J. C. (2005). Self-reported depressive symptomatology in community samples of polysubstance misusers who report Ecstasy use: A meta-analysis. *Journal of Psychopharmacology, 19,* 84–92.

Sun, T., Patoine, C., Abu-Khalil, A., Visvader, J., et al. (2005). Early asymmetry of gene transcription in embryonic human left and right cerebral cortex. *Science, 308,* 1794–1798.

Sunn, N., Egli, M., Burazin, T. C. D., Burns, P., et al. (2002). Circulating relaxin acts on subfornical organ neurons to stimulate water drinking in the rat. *Proceedings of the National Academy of Sciences, USA, 99,* 1701–1706.

Sunstein, C. R., and Nussbaum, M. C. (Eds.). (2004). *Animal rights: Current debates and new directions.* Oxford, UK: Oxford University Press.

Sutcliffe, J. G., and de Lecea, L. (2002). The hypocretins: Setting the arousal threshold. *Nature Reviews Neuroscience, 3,* 339–349.

Suzuki, S., Brown, C. M., and Wise, P. M. (2009). Neuroprotective effects of estrogens following ischemic stroke. *Frontiers in Neuroendocrinology, 30,* 201–211.

Svare, B. B. (2013). *Hormones and aggressive behavior.* New York, NY: Plenum.

Svenningsson, P., Chergui, K., Rachleff, I., Flajolet, M., et al. (2006). Alterations in 5-HT1B receptor function by p11 in depression-like states. *Science, 311,* 77–80.

Swedo, S. E., Rapoport, J. L., Leonard, H., Lenane, M., et al. (1989). Obsessive-compulsive disorder in children and adolescents: Clinical phenomenology of 70 consecutive cases. *Archives of General Psychiatry, 46,* 335–341.

Sylvia, K. E., and Demas, G. E. (2018). A gut feeling: Microbiome-brain-immune interactions modulate social and affective behaviors. *Hormones and Behavior, 99,* 41–49.

Szarfman, A., Doraiswamy, P. M., Tonning, J. M., and Levine, J. G. (2006). Association between pathologic gambling and parkinsonian therapy as detected in the Food and Drug Administration Adverse Event database. *Archives of Neurology, 62,* 299–300.

Szente, M., Gajda, Z., Said Ali, K., and Hermesz, E. (2002). Involvement of electrical coupling in the in vivo ictal epileptiform activity induced by 4-aminopyridine in the neocortex. *Neuroscience, 115,* 1067–1078.

T

Taglialatela, J. P., Cantalupo, C., and Hopkins, W. D. (2006). Gesture handedness predicts asymmetry in the chimpanzee inferior frontal gyrus. *NeuroReport, 17,* 923–927.

Takahashi, J. (2018). Stem cells and regenerative medicine for neural repair. *Current Opinion in Biotechnology, 52,* 102–108.

Takahashi, J. S. (1995). Molecular neurobiology and genetics of circadian rhythms in mammals. *Annual Review of Neuroscience, 18,* 531–554.

Takahashi, T., Svoboda, K., and Malinow, R. (2003). Experience strengthening transmission by driving AMPA receptors into synapses. *Science, 299,* 1585–1588.

Takizawa, R., Maughan, B., and Arseneault, L. (2014). Adult health outcomes of childhood bullying victimization: Evidence from a five-decade longitudinal British birth cohort. *American Journal of Psychiatry, 171,* 777–784.

Tam, J., Duda, D. G., Perentes, J. Y., Quadri, R. S., et al. (2009). Blockade of VEGFR2 and not VEGFR1 can limit diet-induced fat tissue expansion: Role of local versus bone marrow-derived endothelial cells. *PLOS ONE, 4,* e4974.

Tanaka, K. (1993). Neuronal mechanisms of object recognition. *Science, 262,* 685–688.

Tanaka, S., Hanako, I., Kazumi, K., Ryo, K., et al. (2013). Larger right posterior parietal volume in action video game experts: A behavioral and voxel-based morphometry (VBM) study. *PLOS ONE, 8,* e66998.

Tanda, G., Munzar, P., and Goldberg, S. R. (2000). Self-administration behavior is maintained by the psychoactive ingredient of marijuana in squirrel monkeys. *Nature Neuroscience, 3,* 1073–1074.

Tang, N. M., Dong, H. W., Wang, X. M., Tsui, Z. C., et al. (1997). Cholecystokinin antisense RNA increases the analgesic effect induced by electroacupuncture or low dose morphine: Conversion of low responder rats into high responders. *Pain, 71,* 71–80.

Tang, Y. P., Shimizu, E., Dube, G. R., Rampon, C., et al. (1999). Genetic enhancement of learning and memory in mice. *Nature, 401,* 63–69.

Tang, Y. P., Wang, H., Feng, R., Kyin, M., et al. (2001). Differential effects of enrichment on learning and memory function in *NR2B* transgenic mice. *Neuropharmacology, 41,* 779–790.

Tanigawa, H., Lu, H. D., and Roe, A. W. (2010). Functional organization for color and orientation in macaque V4. *Nature Neuroscience, 13,* 1542–1548.

Tanji, J. (2001). Sequential organization of multiple movements: Involvement of cortical motor areas. *Annual Review of Neuroscience, 24,* 631–651.

Taub, E. (1976). Movement in nonhuman primates deprived of somatosensory feedback. *Exercise and Sport Sciences Reviews, 4,* 335–374.

Taub, E., Uswatte, G., and Elbert, T. (2002). New treatments in neurorehabilitation founded on basic research. *Nature Reviews Neuroscience, 3,* 228–235.

Teipel, S., Grothe, M. J., Zhou, J., Sepulcre, J., et al. (2016). Measuring cortical connectivity in Alzheimer's disease as a brain neural network pathology: Toward clinical applications. *Journal of the International Neuropsychological Society, 22*(2), 138–163.

Temple, E., Deutsch, G. K., Poldrack, R. A., Miller, S. L., et al. (2003). Neural deficits in children with dyslexia ameliorated by behavioral remediation: Evidence from functional MRI. *Proceedings of the National Academy of Sciences, USA, 100,* 2860–2865.

Templeton, C. N., Greene, E., and Davis, K. (2005). Allometry of alarm calls: Black-capped chickadees encode information about predator size. *Science, 308,* 1934–1937.

Terkel, J., and Rosenblatt, J. S. (1972). Humoral factors underlying maternal behavior at parturition: Cross transfusion between freely moving rats. *Journal of Comparative and Physiological Psychology, 80,* 365–371.

Terpstra, N. J., Bolhuis, J. J., Riebel, K., van der Burg, J. M., et al. (2006). Localized brain activation specific to auditory memory in a female songbird. *Journal of Comparative Neurology, 494,* 784–791.

Terrace, H. S. (1979). *Nim.* New York, NY: Knopf.

Tetel, M. J., de Vries, G. J., Melcangi, R. C., Panzica, G., et al. (2018). Steroids, stress and the gut microbiome-brain axis. *Journal of Neuroendocrinology, 30*(2), e12548.

Thannickal, T. C., Moore, R. Y., Nienhuis, R., Ramanathan, L., et al. (2000). Reduced number of hypocretin neurons in human narcolepsy. *Neuron, 27,* 469–474.

Theunissen, F. E., and Elie, J. E. (2014). Neural processing of natural sounds. *Nature Reviews Neuroscience, 15*(6), 355–366.

Thomas, K., and Gunnell, D. (2010). Suicide in England and Wales 1861–2007: A time-trends analysis. *International Journal of Epidemiology, 39*(6), 1464–1475.

Thomas, R. K. (1994). Pavlov's dogs "dripped saliva at the sound of a bell." *Psycoloquy, 5*(80), Article 4.

Thompson, P. M., Vidal, C., Giedd, J. N., Gochman, P., et al. (2001). Mapping adolescent brain change reveals dynamic wave of accelerated gray matter loss in very early-onset schizophrenia. *Proceedings of the National Academy of Sciences, USA, 98,* 11650–11655.

Thompson, R. F. (1990). Neural mechanisms of classical conditioning in mammals. *Philosophical Transactions of the Royal Society of London. Series B: Biological Sciences, 329,* 161–170.

Thompson, R. F., and Krupa, D. J. (1994). Organization of memory traces in the mammalian brain. *Annual Review of Neuroscience, 17,* 519–549.

Thompson, R. F., and Steinmetz, J. E. (2009). The role of the cerebellum in classical conditioning of discrete behavioral responses. *Neuroscience, 162,* 732–755.

Thompson, T., and Schuster, C. R. (1964). Morphine self-administration, food reinforced and avoidance behaviour in rhesus monkeys. *Psychopharmacologia, 5,* 87–94.

Thornhill, R., and Palmer, C. T. (2000). *A natural history of rape.* Cambridge, MA: MIT Press.

Thornton, A. E., Cox, D. N., Whitfield, K., and Fouladi, R. T. (2008). Cumulative concussion exposure in rugby players: Neurocognitive and symptomatic outcomes.

Journal of Clinical and Experimental Neuropsychology, 30, 398–409.

Thornton-Jones, Z. D., Kennett, G. A., Benwell, K. R., Revell, D. F., et al. (2006). The cannabinoid CB1 receptor inverse agonist, rimonabant, modifies body weight and adiponectin function in diet-induced obese rats as a consequence of reduced food intake. *Pharmacology, Biochemistry, and Behavior, 84*, 353–359.

Thorpe, S. J., and Fabre-Thorpe, M. (2001). Seeking categories in the brain. *Science, 291*, 260–263.

Timmann, D., Drepper, J., Frings, M., Maschke, M., et al. (2010). The human cerebellum contributes to motor, emotional and cognitive associative learning. A review. *Cortex, 46*, 845–857.

Todorov, A., Said, C. P., Engell, A. D., and Oosterhof, N. N. (2008). Understanding evaluation of faces on social dimensions. *Trends in Cognitive Science, 12*, 455–460.

Tolman, E. C. (1949). There is more than one kind of learning. *Psychological Review, 56*, 144–155.

Tolman, E. C., and Honzik, C. H. (1930). Introduction and removal of reward, and maze performance in rats. *University of California Publications in Psychology, 4*, 257–275.

Tom, S. M., Fox, C. R., Trepel, C., and Poldrack, R. A. (2007). The neural basis of loss aversion in decision-making under risk. *Science, 315*, 515–518.

Tomoda, T., Hikida, T., and Sakurai, T. (2017). Role of *DISC1* in neuronal trafficking and its implication in neuropsychiatric manifestation and neurotherapeutics. *Neurotherapeutics, 14*(3), 623–629.

Tootell, R. B. H., Hadjikhani, N. K., Vanduffel, W., Liu, A. K., et al. (1998). Functional analysis of primary visual cortex (V1) in humans. *Proceedings of the National Academy of Sciences, USA, 95*, 811–817.

Tootell, R. B., Silverman, M. S., Hamilton, S. L., De Valois, R. L., et al. (1988). Functional anatomy of macaque striate cortex. III. Color. *Journal of Neuroscience, 8*, 1569–1593.

Tootell, R. B., Silverman, M. S., Switkes, E., and De Valois, R. L. (1982). Deoxyglucose analysis of retinotopic organization in primate striate cortex. *Science, 218*, 902–904.

Tootell, R. B., Tsao, D., and Vanduffel, W. (2003). Neuroimaging weighs in: Humans meet macaques in "primate" visual cortex. *Journal of Neuroscience, 23*, 3981–3989.

Tordoff, M., Rawson, N., and Friedman, M. (1991). 2,5-Anhydro-D-mannitol acts in liver to initiate feeding. *American Journal of Physiology, 261*, R283–R288.

Torrey, E. F., Bowler, A. E., Taylor, E. H., and Gottesman, I. I. (1994). *Schizophrenia and manic depressive disorder*. New York, NY: Basic Books.

Trasande, L., Blustein, J., Liu, M., Corwin, E., et al. (2013). Infant antibiotic exposures and early-life body mass. *International Journal of Obesity (London), 37*(1), 16–23.

Treesukosol, Y., Lyall, V., Heck, G. L., Desimone, J. A., et al. (2007). A psychophysical and electrophysiological analysis of salt taste in *Trpv1* null mice. *American Journal of Physiology, Regulatory, Integrative, and Comparative Physiology, 292*, R1799–R1809.

Treffert, D. A., and Christensen, D. D. (2005). Inside the mind of a savant. *Scientific American, 293*(6), 108–113.

Treisman, A. M. (1996). The binding problem. *Current Opinion in Neurobiology, 6*, 171–178.

Treisman, A. M., and Gelade, G. (1980). A feature-integration theory of attention. *Cognitive Psychology, 12*, 97–136.

Treisman, M. (1977). Motion sickness—Evolutionary hypotheses. *Science, 197*, 493–495.

Tremlett, H., Bauer, K. C., Appel-Cresswell, S., Finlay, B. B., et al. (2017). The gut microbiome in human neurological disease: A review. *Annals of Neurology, 81*(3), 369–382.

Trimble, M. R. (1991). Interictal psychoses of epilepsy. *Advances in Neurology, 55*, 143–152.

Tronick, R., and Reck, C. (2009). Infants of depressed mothers. *Harvard Review of Psychiatry, 17*, 147–156.

Tsai, L., and Barnea, G. (2014). A critical period defined by axon-targeting mechanisms in the murine olfactory bulb. *Science, 344*(6180), 197–200.

Tsuchiya, N., and Adolphs, R. (2007). Emotion and consciousness. *Trends in Cognitive Sciences, 11*, 158–167.

Tuller, D. (2002, January 8). A quiet revolution for those prone to nodding off. *The New York Times* (http://query.nytimes.com/gst/fullpage.html?sec=health&res=980DE5DD1439F93BA35752C0A9649C8B63).

Tully, T. (2003). Reply: The myth of a myth. *Current Biology, 13*(11), r426.

Tulving, E. (1972). Episodic and semantic memory. In E. Tulving and W. Donaldson (Eds.), *Organization of memory* (pp. 381–403). New York, NY: Academic Press.

Tulving, E. (1989). Memory: Performance, knowledge, and experience. *European Journal of Cognitive Psychology, 1*, 3–26.

Tulving, E. (2002). Episodic memory: From mind to brain. *Annual Review of Psychology, 53*, 1–25.

Tulving, E., Hayman, C. A., and Macdonald, C. A. (1991). Long-lasting perceptual priming and semantic learning in amnesia: A case experiment. *Journal of Experimental Psychology: Learning, Memory, and Cognition, 17*, 595–617.

Turgeon, J. L., McDonnell, D. P, Martin, K. A, and Wise, P. M. (2004). Hormone therapy: Physiological complexity belies therapeutic simplicity. *Science, 304*, 1269–1273.

Turner, E. H., Matthews, A. M., Linardatos, E., Tell, R. A., et al. (2008). Selective publication of antidepressant trials and its influence on apparent efficacy. *New England Journal of Medicine, 358*, 252–260.

Tyack, P. L. (2003). Dolphins communicate about individual-specific social relationships. In F. de Waal and P. L. Tyack (Eds.), *Animal social complexity: Intelligence, culture, and individualized societies* (pp. 342–361). Cambridge, MA: Harvard University Press.

U

Umilta, M. A., Kohler, E., Galiese, V., Fogassi, L., et al. (2001). I know what you are doing: A neurophysiological study. *Neuron, 31*, 155–165.

Ungerleider, L. G., Courtney, S. M., and Haxby, J. V. (1998). A neural system for human visual working memory. *Proceedings of the National Academy of Sciences, USA, 95*, 883–890.

Ursin, H., Baade, E., and Levine, S. (1978). *Psychobiology of stress: A study of coping men*. New York, NY: Academic Press.

V

van Anders, S. M., and Watson, N. V. (2006). Social neuroendocrinology: Effects of social contexts and behaviors on sex steroids in humans. *Human Nature, 17*, 212–237.

Van Dongen, H. P., Maislin, G., Mullington, J. M., and Dinges, D. F. (2003). The cumulative cost of additional wakefulness: Dose-response effects on neurobehavioral functions and sleep physiology from chronic sleep restriction and total sleep deprivation. *Sleep, 26*, 117–126.

Van Essen, D. C., and Drury, H. A. (1997). Structural and functional analyses of human cerebral cortex using a surface-based atlas. *Journal of Neuroscience, 17*, 7079–7102.

Van Gaal, L. F., Rissanen, A. M., Scheen, A. J., Ziegler, O., et al. (2005). Effects of the cannabinoid-1 receptor blocker rimonabant on weight reduction and cardiovascular risk factors in overweight patients: 1-year experience from the RIO-Europe study. *Lancet, 365*, 1389–1397.

Van Horn, J. D., Irimia, A., Torgerson, C. M., Chambers, M. C., et al. (2012). Mapping connectivity damage in the case of Phineas Gage. *PLOS ONE, 7*, e37454.

Van Os, J., and Kapur, S. (2009). Schizophrenia. *Lancet, 374*, 635–645.

Van Os, J., Kenis, G., and Rutten, B. P. (2010). The environment and schizophrenia. *Nature, 468*, 203–212.

Van Tol, M. J., van der Wee, N. J., van den Heuvel, O. A., Nielen, M. M., et al. (2010).

Regional brain volume in depression and anxiety disorders. *Archives of General Psychiatry, 67,* 1002–1011.

Van Zoeren, J. G., and Stricker, E. M. (1977). Effects of preoptic, lateral hypothalamic, or dopamine-depleting lesions on behavioral thermoregulation in rats exposed to the cold. *Journal of Comparative and Physiological Psychology, 91,* 989–999.

Vance, C. G., Dailey, D. L., Rakel, B. A., and Sluka, K. A. (2014). Using TENS for pain control: The state of the evidence. *Pain Management, 4,* 197–209.

Vance, C., Rogelj, B., Hortobágyi, T., De Vos, K. J., et al. (2009). Mutations in FUS, an RNA processing protein, cause familial amyotrophic lateral sclerosis type 6. *Science, 323,* 1208–1211.

Vandermosten, M., Boets, B., Poelmans, H., Sunaert, S., et al. (2012). A tractography study in dyslexia: Neuroanatomic correlates of orthographic, phonological and speech processing. *Brain, 135*(Pt. 3), 935–948.

Vandermosten, M., Boets, B., Wouters, J., and Ghesquière P. (2012). A qualitative and quantitative review of diffusion tensor imaging studies in reading and dyslexia. *Neuroscience and Biobehavioral Reviews, 36,* 1532–1552.

Vann, S. D., and Aggleton, J. P. (2004). The mammillary bodies: Two memory systems in one? *Nature Reviews Neuroscience, 5,* 35–44.

Vargha-Khadem, F., Gadian, D. G., Copp, A., and Mishkin, M. (2005). FOXP2 and the neuroanatomy of speech and language. *Nature Reviews Neuroscience, 6,* 131–138.

Vargas, C. D., Aballéa, A., Rodrigues, E. C., Reilly, K. T., et al. (2009). Re-emergence of hand-muscle representations in human motor cortex after hand allograft. *Proceedings of the National Academy of Sciences, USA, 106,* 7197–7202.

Vasey, P. L. (1995). Homosexual behaviour in primates: A review of evidence and theory. *International Journal of Primatology, 16,* 173–204.

Vassar, R., Ngai, J., and Axel, R. (1993). Spatial segregation of odorant receptor expression in the mammalian olfactory epithelium. *Cell, 74,* 309–318.

Vaughan, W., and Greene, S. L. (1984). Pigeon visual memory capacity. *Journal of Experimental Psychology: Animal Behavior Processes, 10,* 256–271.

Veraa, R. P., and Grafstein, B. (1981). Cellular mechanisms for recovery from nervous system injury: A conference report. *Experimental Neurology, 71,* 6–75.

Vernes, S. C., Oliver, P. L., Spiteri, E., Lockstone, H. E., et al. (2011). Foxp2 regulates gene networks implicated in neurite outgrowth in the developing brain. *PLOS Genetics, 7,* e1002145.

Villalobos, M. E., Mizuno, A., Dahl, B. C., Kemmotsu, N., et al. (2005). Reduced functional connectivity between V1 and inferior frontal cortex associated with visuomotor performance in autism. *NeuroImage, 25,* 916–925.

Vincus, A. A., Ringwalt, C., Harris, M. S., and Shamblen, S. R. (2010). A short-term, quasi-experimental evaluation of D.A.R.E.'s revised elementary school curriculum. *Journal of Drug Education, 40,* 37–49.

Visser, S. N., Danielson, M. L., Bitsko, R. H., Holbrook, J. R., et al. (2014). Trends in the parent-report of health care provider–diagnosed and medicated attention-deficit/hyperactivity disorder: United States, 2003–2011. *Journal of the American Academy of Child and Adolescent Psychiatry, 53*(1), 34–46.e2.

Vita, A., Dieci, M., Silenzi, C., Tenconi, F., et al. (2000). Cerebral ventricular enlargement as a generalized feature of schizophrenia: A distribution analysis on 502 subjects. *Schizophrenia Research, 44,* 25–34.

Vitaterna, M. H., King, D. P., Chang, A. M., Kornhauser, J. M., et al. (1994). Mutagenesis and mapping of a mouse gene, Clock, essential for cicadian behavior. *Science, 29,* 719–725.

Vogt, B. A. (2005). Pain and emotion interactions in subregions of the cingulate gyrus. *Nature Reviews Neuroscience, 6,* 533–544.

Volkow, N. D., and Wise, R.A. (2005). How can drug addiction help us understand obesity? *Nature Neuroscience, 8,* 555–560.

Volkow, N. D., Wang, G. J., Kollins, S. H., Wigal, T. L., et al. (2009). Evaluating dopamine reward pathway in ADHD: Clinical implications. *JAMA, 302,* 1084–1091.

Volkow, N. D., Wise, R. A., and Baler, R. (2017). The dopamine motive system: Implications for drug and food addiction. *Nature Reviews Neuroscience, 18*(12), 741–752.

Volkow, N., Benveniste, H., and McLellan, A. T. (2018). Use and misuse of opioids in chronic pain. *Annual Review of Medicine, 69,* 451–465. doi:10.1146/annurev-med-011817-044739

Voytek, B., Kayser, A. S., Badre, D., Fegen, D., et al. (2015). Oscillatory dynamics coordinating human frontal networks in support of goal maintenance. *Nature Neuroscience, 18*(9), 1318–1324.

Vriens, J, and Voets, T. (2018). Sensing the heat with *TRPM3. Pflügers Archiv, 470*(5):799–807.

Vrieze, A., Van Nood, E., Holleman, F., Salojärvi, J., et al. (2012). Transfer of intestinal microbiota from lean donors increases insulin sensitivity in individuals with metabolic syndrome. *Gastroenterology, 143*(4), 913–916.e7.

Vythilingam, M., Anderson, E. R., Goddard, A., Woods, S. W., et al. (2000). Temporal lobe volume in panic disorder—A quantitative magnetic resonance imaging study. *Psychiatry Research, 99,* 75–82.

W

Wada, J. A., and Rasmussen, T. (1960). Intracarotid injection of sodium amytal for the lateralization of cerebral speech dominance: Experimental and clinical observations. *Journal of Neurosurgery, 17,* 266–282.

Wada, J. A., Clarke, R., and Hamm, A. (1975). Cerebral hemispheric asymmetry in humans. Cortical speech zones in 100 adults and 100 infant brains. *Archives of Neurology, 32,* 239–246.

Waddell, J., and Shors, T. J. (2008). Neurogenesis, learning and associative strength. *European Journal of Neuroscience, 27,* 3020–3028.

Wagenmakers, E.-J., Beek, T., Dijkhoff, L., Gronau, Q. F., et al. (2016). Registered Replication Report: Strack, Martin, & Stepper (1988). *Perspectives on Psychological Science, 11,* 917–928.

Wager, T. D., Scott, D. J., and Zubieta, J. K. (2007). Placebo effects on human μ-opioid activity during pain. *Proceedings of the National Academy of Sciences, USA, 104, 11056*–11061.

Wagner, G. C., Beuving, L. J., and Hutchinson, R. R. (1980). The effects of gonadal hormone manipulations on aggressive target-biting in mice. *Aggressive Behavior, 6,* 1–7.

Wahlstrom, K., Dretzke, B., Gordon, M., Peterson, K., et al. (2014). *Examining the impact of later school start times on the health and academic performance of high school students: A multi-site study.* Center for Applied Research and Educational Improvement. St. Paul, MN: University of Minnesota (https://conservancy.umn.edu/bitstream/handle/11299/162769/Impact%20of%20Later%20Start%20Time%20Final%20Report.pdf?sequence=1.pdf).

Waldrop, M. M. (2012). Brain in a box. *Nature 482*(7386), 456–458.

Walker, M. (2017). *Why we sleep: Unlocking the power of sleep and dreams.* New York, NY: Scribner.

Wallis, J. D. (2007). Orbitofrontal cortex and its contribution to decision-making. *Annual Review of Neuroscience, 30,* 31–56.

Walters, R. J., Hadley, S. H., Morris, K. D. W., and Amin, J. (2000). Benzodiazepines act on GABAA receptors via two distinct and separable mechanisms. *Nature Neuroscience, 3,* 1273–1280.

Walther, S., Goya-Maldonado, R., Stippich, C., Weisbrod, M., et al. (2010). A supramodal network for response inhibition. *NeuroReport, 21,* 191–195.

Wang, H., Yu, M., Ochani, M., Amella, C. A., et al. (2003). Nicotinic acetylcholine receptor α7 subunit is an essential regulator of inflammation. *Nature, 421,* 384–388.

Wang, Y. K., Zhu, W. W., Wu, M. H., Wu, Y. H., et al. (2018). Human clinical-grade parthenogenetic ESC-derived dopaminergic neurons recover locomotive defects of nonhuman primate models of Parkinson's disease. *Stem Cell Reports, 11*(1), 171–182. doi:10.1016/j.stemcr.2018.05.010

Warwick, R., and Williams, P. L. (1973). *Gray's Anatomy,* 35th ed. London: Longmans.

Watkins, K. E., Vargha-Khadem, F., Ashburner, J., Passingham, E., et al. (2002). MRI analysis of an inherited speech and language disorder: Structural brain abnormalities. *Brain, 125,* 465–478.

Watson, N. V. (2001). Sex differences in throwing: Monkeys having a fling. *Trends in Cognitive Sciences, 5,* 98–99.

Watson, N. V., Freeman, L. M., and Breedlove, S. M. (2001). Neuronal size in the spinal nucleus of the bulbocavernosus: Direct modulation by androgen in rats with mosaic androgen insensitivity. *Journal of Neuroscience, 21,* 1062–1066.

Webb, W. B. (1992). *Sleep, the gentle tyrant* (2nd ed.). Bolton, MA: Anker.

Wei, F., Wang, G. D., Kerchner, G. A., Kim, S. J., et al. (2001). Genetic enhancement of inflammatory pain by forebrain *NR2B* overexpression. *Nature Neuroscience, 4,* 164–169.

Weinberger, D. R., Aloia, M. S., Goldberg, T. E., and Berman, K. F. (1994). The frontal lobes and schizophrenia. *Journal of Neuropsychiatry and Clinical Neurosciences, 6,* 419–427.

Weinberger, L. E., Sreenivasan, S., Garrick, T., and Osran, H. (2005). The impact of surgical castration on sexual recidivism risk among sexually violent predatory offenders. *Journal of the American Academy of Psychiatry and the Law, 33*(1), 16–36.

Weinberger, N. M. (1998). Physiological memory in primary auditory cortex: Characteristics and mechanisms. *Neurobiology of Learning and Memory, 70,* 226–251.

Weiner, K. S., and Zilles, K. (2016). The anatomical and functional specialization of the fusiform gyrus. *Neuropsychologia, 83,* 48–62.

Weiner, R. D. (1994). Treatment optimization with ECT. *Psychopharmacology Bulletin, 30,* 313–320.

Weiss, L. A., Arking, D. E., and The Gene Discovery Project of Johns Hopkins & the Autism Consortium. (2009). A genome-wide linkage and association scan reveals novel loci for autism. *Nature, 461,* 802–808.

Weitzman, E. D. (1981). Sleep and its disorders. *Annual Review of Neurosciences, 4,* 381–417.

Weitzman, E. D., Czeisler, C. A., Zimmerman, J. C., and Moore-Ede, M. C. (1981). Biological rhythms in man: Relationship of sleep-wake, cortisol, growth hormone, and temperature during temporal isolation. In J. B. Martin, S. Reichlin, and K. L. Bick (Eds.), *Neurosecretion and brain peptides* (pp. 475–499). New York, NY: Raven Press.

Wesensten, N. J., Belenky, G., Kautz, M. A., Thorne, D. R., et al. (2002). Maintaining alertness and performance during sleep deprivation: Modafinil versus caffeine. *Psychopharmacology (Berlin), 159,* 238–247.

West, G. L., Drisdelle, B. L., Konishi, K., Jackson, J., et al. (2015). Habitual action video game playing is associated with caudate nucleus-dependent navigational strategies. *Proceedings of the Royal Society of London. Series B: Biological Sciences, 282*(1808), 20142952.

West, S. L., and O'Neal, K. K. (2004). Project D.A.R.E. outcome effectiveness revisited. *American Journal of Public Health, 94,* 1027–1029.

Westerberg, C. E., Mander, B. A., Florczak, S. M., Weintraub, S., et al. (2012). Concurrent impairments in sleep and memory in amnestic mild cognitive impairment. *Journal of the International Neuropsychological Society, 18,* 490–500.

Wever, R. A. (1979). Influence of physical workload on freerunning circadian rhythms of man. *Pflügers Archiv European Journal of Physiology, 381,* 119–126.

Wexler, N. S., Rose, E. A., and Housman, D. E. (1991). Molecular approaches to hereditary diseases of the nervous system: Huntington's disease as a paradigm. *Annual Review of Neuroscience, 14,* 503–529.

White, N. M., and Milner, P. M. (1992). The psychobiology of reinforcers. *Annual Review of Psychology, 43,* 443–471.

Whitfield-Gabrieli, S., and Ford, J. M. (2012). Default mode network activity and connectivity in psychopathology. *Annual Review of Clinical Psychology, 8,* 49–76.

Whitlock, J. R., Heynen, A. J., Shuler, M. G., and Bear, M. F. (2006). Learning induces long-term potentiation in the hippocampus. *Science, 313,* 1093–1097.

Widge, A. S., Malone, D. A., Jr., and Dougherty, D. D. (2018). Closing the loop on deep brain stimulation for treatment-resistant depression. *Frontiers in Neuroscience, 12,* 175.

Wiesel, T. N., and Hubel, D. H. (1965). Extent of recovery from the effects of visual deprivation in kittens. *Journal of Neurophysiology, 28,* 1060–1072.

Wilens, T. E., Prince, J. B., Spencer, T. J., and Biederman, J. (2006). Stimulants and sudden death: What is a physician to do? *Pediatrics, 118,* 1215–1219.

Will, B., Galani, R., Kelche, C., and Rosenzweig, M. R. (2004). Recovery from brain injury in animals: Relative efficacy of environmental enrichment, physical exercise or formal training (1990–2002). *Progress in Neurobiology, 72,* 167–182.

Williams, J. H., Waiter, G. D., Gilchrist, A., Perrett, D. I., et al. (2006). Neural mechanisms of imitation and "mirror neuron" functioning in autistic spectrum disorder. *Neuropsychologia, 44,* 610–621.

Williams, N. R., and Schatzberg, A. F. (2016). NMDA antagonist treatment of depression. *Current Opinion in Neurology, 36,* 112–117.

Williams, N. R., and Schatzberg, A. F. (2016). NMDA antagonist treatment of depression. *Current Opinion in Neurology, 36,* 112–117.

Williams, T. J., Pepitone, M. E., Christensen, S. E., Cooke, B. M., et al. (2000). Finger-length ratios and sexual orientation. *Nature, 404,* 455–456.

Willis, S. L., Tennstedt, S. L., Marsiske, M., Ball, K., et al. (2006). Long-term effects of cognitive training on everyday functional outcomes in older adults. *JAMA, 296,* 2805–2814.

Wilson, M. L., Boesch, C., Fruth, B., Furuichi, T., et al. (2014). Lethal aggression in *Pan* is better explained by adaptive strategies than human impacts. *Nature, 513*(7518), 414–417.

Wingfield, J. C., Ball, G. F., Dufty, A. M., Hegner, R. E., et al. (1987). Testosterone and aggression in birds. *American Scientist, 75,* 602–608.

Winkowski, D. E., and Knudsen, E. I. (2006). Top-down gain control of the auditory space map by gaze control circuitry in the barn owl. *Nature, 439,* 336–339.

Winslow, J. T., and Insel, T. R. (2002). The social deficits of the oxytocin knockout mouse. *Neuropeptides, 36,* 221–229.

Winocur, G., Wojtowicz, J. M., Sekeres, M., Snyder, J. S., et al. (2006). Inhibition of neurogenesis interferes with hippocampus-dependent memory function. *Hippocampus, 16,* 296–304.

Wisdom, A. J., Cao, Y., Itoh, N., Spence, R. D., et al. (2013). Estrogen receptor-β ligand treatment after disease onset is neuroprotective in the multiple sclerosis model. *Journal of Neuroscience Research, 91,* 901–908.

Witte, A. V., Fobker, M., Gellner, R., Knecht, S., et al. (2009). Caloric restriction improves memory in elderly humans. *Proceedings of the National Academy of Sciences, USA, 106*(4), 1255–1260.

Wolf, M. E. (2016). Synaptic mechanisms underlying persistent cocaine craving. *Nature Reviews Neuroscience, 17*(6), 351–365.

Wolf, S. S., Jones, D. W., Knable, M. B., Gorey, J. G., et al. (1996). Tourette syndrome: Prediction of phenotypic variation in monozygotic twins by caudate nucleus D2 receptor binding. *Science, 273,* 1225–1227.

Wolfe, J. M. (1994). Guided search 2.0: A revised model of visual search. *Psychonomic Bulletin & Review, 1,* 202–238.

Wolfe, J. M., Horowitz, T. S., and Kenner, N. M. (2005). Cognitive psychology: Rare items often missed in visual searches. *Nature, 435,* 439–440.

Wolk, D. A., Price, J. C., Saxton, J. A., Snitz, B. E., et al. (2009). Amyloid imaging in mild cognitive impairment subtypes. *Annals of Neurology, 65,* 557–568.

Wollan, M. (2015, April 10). How to beat a polygraph test. *New York Times Magazine,* p. MM25 (www.nytimes.com/2015/04/12/magazine/how-to-beat-a-polygraph-test.html).

Womelsdorf, T., Anton-Erxleben, K., and Treue, S. (2008). Receptive field shift and shrinkage in macaque middle temporal area through attentional gain modulation. *Journal of Neuroscience, 28,* 8934–8944.

Wood, J. M., Bootzin, R. R., Kihlstrom, J. F., and Schacter, D. L. (1992). Implicit and explicit memory for verbal information presented during sleep. *Psychological Science, 3,* 236–239.

Wood, N., and Cowan, N. (1995). The cocktail party phenomenon revisited: How frequent are attention shifts to one's name in an irrelevant auditory channel? *Journal of Experimental Psychology. Learning, Memory, and Cognition, 21,* 255–260.

Woolf, C. J., and Salter, M. W. (2000). Neuronal plasticity: Increasing the gain in pain. *Science, 288,* 1765–1769.

World Health Organization. (2001). *The world health report.* Geneva, Switzerland: World Health Organization.

Wrangham, R. W. (2018). Two types of aggression in human evolution. *Proceedings of the National Academy of Sciences, USA, 115*(2), 245–253.

Wren, A. M., Seal, L. J., Cohen, M. A., Brynes, A. E., et al. (2001). Ghrelin enhances appetite and increases food intake in humans. *Journal of Clinical Endocrinology and Metabolism, 86,* 5992–5995.

Wren, A. M., Small, C. J., Ward, H. L., Murphy, K. G., et al. (2000). The novel hypothalamic peptide ghrelin stimulates food intake and growth hormone secretion. *Endocrinology, 141,* 4325–4328.

Wright, R. D., and Ward, L. M. (2008). *Orienting of attention.* New York, NY: Oxford University Press.

Wuethrich, B. (2000). Learning the world's languages—before they vanish. *Science, 288,* 1156–1159.

Wurtz, R. H., Goldberg, M. E., and Robinson, D. L. (1982). Brain mechanisms of visual attention. *Scientific American, 246*(6), 124–135.

X

Xerri, C., Stern, J. M., and Merzenich, M. M. (1994). Alterations of the cortical representation of the rat ventrum induced by nursing behavior. *Journal of Neuroscience, 14,* 1710–1721.

Xie, L., Kang, H., Xu, Q., Chen, M. J., et al. (2013). Sleep drives metabolite clearance from the adult brain. *Science, 342,* 373–377.

Y

Yaffe, K., Lui, L. Y., Zmuda, J., and Cauley, J. (2002). Sex hormones and cognitive function in older men. *Journal of the American Geriatrics Society, 50,* 707–712.

Yamazaki, S., Numano, R., Abe, M., Hida, A., et al. (2000). Resetting central and peripheral circadian oscillators in transgenic rats. *Science, 288,* 682–685.

Yang, S. H., Cheng, P. H., Banta, H., Piotrowska-Nitsche, K., et al. (2008). Towards a transgenic model of Huntington's disease in a non-human primate. *Nature, 453,* 921–924.

Yang, T. T., Gallen, C. C., Ramachandran, V. S., Cobb, S., et al. (1994). Noninvasive detection of cerebral plasticity in adult human somatosensory cortex. *NeuroReport, 5,* 701–704.

Yang, Y., and Raine, A. (2009). Prefrontal structural and functional brain imaging findings in antisocial, violent, and psychopathic individuals: A meta-analysis. *Psychiatry Research, 174*(2), 81–88.

Yang, Y., Raine, A., Joshi, A. A., Joshi, S., et al. (2012). Frontal information flow and connectivity in psychopathy. *British Journal of Psychiatry, 201*(5), 408–409.

Ycaza Herrera, A., and Mather, M. (2015). Actions and interactions of estradiol and glucocorticoids in cognition and the brain: Implications for aging women. *Neuroscience & Biobehavioral Reviews, 55,* 36–52.

Yehuda, R. (2002). Post-traumatic stress disorder. *New England Journal of Medicine, 346,* 108–114.

Yin, J. C., Del Vecchio, M., Zhou, H., and Tully, T. (1995). CREB as a memory modulator: Induced expression of a dCREB2 activator isoform enhances long-term memory in *Drosophila. Cell, 81,* 107–115.

Yin, J., Barr, A. M., Ramos-Miguel, A., and Procyshyn, R. M. (2017). Antipsychotic induced dopamine supersensitivity psychosis: A comprehensive review. *Current Neuropharmacology, 15*(1), 174–183.

Young, A. B. (1993). Role of excitotoxins in heredito-degenerative neurologic diseases. *Research Publications—Association for Research in Nervous and Mental Disease, 71,* 175–189.

Young, K. D., Erickson, K., Nugent, A. C., Fromm, S. J., et al. (2012). Functional anatomy of autobiographical memory recall deficits in depression. *Psychological Medicine, 42,* 345–357.

Yu, Y. J., Atwal, J. K., Zhang, Y., Tong, R. K., et al. (2015). Therapeutic bispecific antibodies cross the blood-brain barrier in nonhuman primates. *Science Translational Medicine, 6,* 261ra154.

Yuan, M., Cross, S. J., Loughlin, S. E., and Leslie, F. M. (2015). Nicotine and the adolescent brain. *Journal of Physiology, 593*(16), 3397–3412.

Z

Zaidel, E. (1976). Auditory vocabulary of the right hemisphere following brain bisection or hemidecortication. *Cortex, 12,* 191–211.

Zalocusky, K. A., Ramakrishnan, C., Lerner, T. N., Davidson, T. J., et al. (2016). Nucleus accumbens D2R cells signal prior outcomes and control risky decision-making. *Nature, 531*(7596), 642–646.

Zatorre, R. J., Evans, A. C., and Meyer, E. (1994). Neural mechanisms underlying melodic perception and memory for pitch. *Journal of Neuroscience, 14,* 1908–1919.

Zawilska, J. B. (2014). Mephedrone and other cathinones. *Current Opinion in Psychiatry, 27*(4), 256–262.

Zeki, S., Watson, J. D., Lueck, C. J., Friston, K. J., et al. (1991). A direct demonstration of functional specialization in human visual cortex. *Journal of Neuroscience, 11,* 641–649.

Zeman, A. (2002). *Consciousness: A user's guide.* New Haven, CT: Yale University Press.

Zendel, B. R., and Alain, C. (2009). Concurrent sound segregation is enhanced in musicians. *Journal of Cognitive Neuroscience, 21,* 1488–1498.

Zendel, B. R., Lagrois, M. É., Robitaille, N., and Peretz, I. (2015). Attending to pitch information inhibits processing of pitch information: The curious case of amusia. *Journal of Neuroscience, 35,* 3815–3824.

Zhang, C. L., Zou, Y., He, W., Gage, F. H., et al. (2008). A role for adult TLX-positive neural stem cells in learning and behaviour. *Nature, 451,* 1004–1007.

Zhang, T. Y., and Meaney, M. J. (2010). Epigenetics and the environmental regulation of the genome and its function. *Annual Review of Psychology, 61,* C1–C3.

Zhang, Y., Proenca, R., Maffei, M., Barone, M., et al. (1994). Positional cloning of the mouse *obese* gene and its human homologue. *Nature, 372,* 425–432.

Zhao, G. Q., Zhang, Y., Hoon, M. A., Chandrashekar, J., et al. (2003). The receptors for mammalian sweet and umami taste. *Cell, 115,* 255–266.

Zheng, J., Shen, W., He, D. Z., Long, K. B., et al. (2000). Prestin is the motor protein of cochlear outer hair cells. *Nature, 405,* 149–155.

Zhong, Z., Deane, R., Ali, Z., Parisi, M., et al. (2008). ALS-causing *SOD1* mutants generate vascular changes prior to motor neuron degeneration. *Nature Neuroscience, 11*, 420–422.

Zihl, J., von Cramon, D., and Mai, N. (1983). Selective disturbance of movement vision after bilateral brain damage. *Brain, 106*, 313–340.

Zimmer, C. (2004). *The soul made flesh: The discovery of the brain—and how it changed the world*. New York, NY: Basic Books.

Zimmerman, C. A., Leib, D. E., and Knight, Z. A. (2017). Neural circuits underlying thirst and fluid homeostasis. *Nature Reviews Neuroscience, 18*(8), 459–469.

Zimmerman, C. A., Lin, Y. C., Leib, D. E., Guo, L., et al. (2016). Thirst neurons anticipate the homeostatic consequences of eating and drinking. *Nature, 537*(7622), 680–684.

Zola-Morgan, S., and Squire, L. R. (1986). Memory impairment in monkeys following lesions of the hippocampus. *Behavioral Neuroscience, 100*, 155–160.

Zola-Morgan, S., Squire, L. R., and Ramus, S. J. (1994). Severity of memory impairment in monkeys as a function of locus and extent of damage within the medial temporal lobe memory system. *Hippocampus, 4*, 483–495.

Zorumski, C. F., Izumi, Y., and Mennerick, S. (2016). Ketamine: NMDA receptors and beyond. *Journal of Neuroscience, 36*(44), 11158–11164.

Zucker, I. (1976). Light, behavior, and biologic rhythms. *Hospital Practice, 11*, 83–91.

Zucker, L. M., and Zucker, T. F. (1961). "Fatty," a mutation in the rat. *Journal of Heredity, 52*, 275–278.

Author Index

A

Abbott, S. M., 314
Abe, N., 322
Aben, B., 389
Abramowtiz, J. S., 373
Abutalebi, J., 467
Ackermann, S., 307
Adams, D. L., 42
Ader, R., 341
Adler, E., 174
Adolphs, R., 332, 439
Aflalo, T. N., 145
Agarwal, N., 135
Aggleton, J. P., 384
Ahn, S., 280
Ajslev, T. A., 285
Alain, C., 421
Al-Barazanji, I. A., 278
Albers, G. W., 47
Aldrich, M. A., 312
Almer, G., 304
Almutairi, N., 210
Altemus, M., 365
Altman, N., 465
Altschuler, E. L., 481
Alvarez, J. A., 444
American Psychiatric Association, 110, 284, 348
Amici, R., 299
Amso, D., 465
Amunts, K., 145
Anacker, C., 406
Anand, B. K., 276
Ancoli-Israel, S., 302
Andics, A., 474
Andreasen, N., 8, 355
Andrews, G., 365
Anstey, M. L., 336
Apkarian, A. V., 136
Archer, G. S., 411
Archer, J., 334
Argyll-Robertson, D. M. C. L., 349
Arnone, D., 367
Arnsten, A. F., 436
Asberg, M., 363
Aschwanden, C., 319
Aserinsky, E., 297
Ashmore, J. F., 157

Assaf, Y., 465
Auchus, R. J., 253
Audero, E., 315
Augustine, V., 271
Aungst, J. L., 177
Avila, M. T., 351
Axel, R., 176

B

Baars, B. J., 439
Badre, D., 443, 444
Bagemihl, B., 256
Bailey, C. H., 395
Bailey, J. M., 258
Bailey, K., 431
Baillet, S., 51
Bajbouj, M., 365
Baldermann, J. C., 374
Baldwin, M. W., 174
Ban, T. A., 357
Bancaud, J., 330
Barbeau, H., 480
Bark, N., 349
Barkow, J. H., 10
Barnea, G., 177, 178
Barnett, S. A., 236
Barrett, A. M., 436
Barrio, J. R., 479
Bartels, A., 332
Bartolomeo, P., 436
Bartoshuk, L. M., 173
Basaria, S., 248
Basson, R., 242, 243
Bates, E., 466
Batterham, R. L., 278
Bautista, D. M., 131
Baynes, K. C., 278, 282
Beach, F. A., 235
Bear, M. F., 399
Beaton, A. A., 456
Bedrosian, T. A., 316
Bee, M. A., 421
Beeli, G., 129
Beggs, S., 32
Beggs, W. D., 164
Bellugi, U., 466
Bennett, W., 104
Benney, K. S., 422
Benson, P. J., 351

Benzer, S., 295
Berenbaum, S. A., 255
Bergmann, B. M., 304
Berman, K. F., 355
Bermon, S., 248
Bernal, B., 465
Bernhardt, P. C., 233, 335
Bernstein, I. L., 283
Bernstein, I. S., 335
Bernstein, L. E., 161
Berthold, A., 219
Binder, J. R., 161
Birch, L. L., 281
Birnbaum, R., 351
Bisley, J. W., 434
Bjork, R. A., 307
Blackwell, D. L., 165, 478
Blake, D. T., 129
Blanchard, R., 258
Blaser, M. J., 285
Bleuler, E., 349
Bliss, T. V. P., 398
Bliwise, D. L., 302
Bloom, S. R., 278
Blum, I. D., 296
Blumberger, S. E., 365
Blumstein, S. E., 465
Boddhula, S. K., 132
Boets, B., 477
Bogaert, A. F., 258
Bogenschutz, M. P., 109
Bogin, B., 404
Boldrini, M., 406
Bolhuis, J. J., 475
Bonaz, B., 284
Bonnel, A. M., 421
Boolell, M., 239
Boot, W. R., 431
Booth, A., 335
Borgstein, J., 481
Born, J., 307
Borota, D., 98
Boshuisen, K., 482
Boström, P., 282
Bourke, C. H., 366
Bourque, C. W., 267
Bourque, J., 103
Bouwknecht, J. A., 336
Bower, B., 364

Bowman, M. L., 135
Boyce, R., 307
Boyle, P. C., 277
Braaten, R. F., 422
Brady, T. F., 391
Brainard, D. H., 206
Brandlistuen, R. E., 366
Brasser, S. M., 174
Bray, G. A., 273, 274
Breedlove, S. M., 253, 254, 407
Breier, A., 108
Breitner, J. C., 414
Bremer, F., 308
Bremner, J. D., 371
Brennan, S. C., 171
Brigande, J. V., 168
Briggs, F., 432
Broadbent, D. A., 422
Brobeck, J. R., 276
Broberg, D. J., 283
Brouwer, H., 470
Brown, A. S., 353
Brown, C., 313
Brown, E. C., 465
Brown, J., 389
Brown, R. E., 8
Brown, S. P., 439
Brownlee, S., 112, 134
Bruel-Jungerman, E., 406
Brunetti, M., 435
Bryant, P., 304
Buccino, G., 146, 481
Buchsbaum, M. S., 355
Buchsbaum, B. R., 465
Buchsbaum, M. S., 433
Buck, L., 176
Buck, L. B., 179
Buckner, R. L., 386
Bucy, P. C., 329
Burgdorf, J., 325, 475
Burgess, H. J., 294
Burgess, N., 387
Burgess, P. W., 444
Bushdid, C., 175
Bushman, J. D., 173
Buss, D., 10
Butler, A. C., 365
Byne, W., 257
Byrne, R. W., 474

C

Cade, J. F., 368
Cahill, L., 244, 389, 390
Calvert, G. A., 161
Calvin, W. H., 466, 467
Cameron, J. L., 341
Campbell, F. W., 200
Campbell, J. J., 444
Cannon, T. D., 355
Cannon, W. B., 321
Cantalupo, C., 456
Cantor, J. M., 258
Cao, M., 436
Cao, Y. Q., 133
Caramazza, A., 146
Cardno, A. G., 350
Carey, B., 361
Carhart-Harris, R. L., 108, 109
Carlson, P. J., 108
Carmichael, M. S., 227
Carré, J. M., 334
Carreiras, M., 469
Carretié, L., 426
Carroll, J., 206
Carter, C. S., 227
Cartwright, R. D., 300
Casarosa, S., 479
Casseday, J. H., 164
Castro, J. B., 175
Caterina, M. J., 131
CDC (Centers for Disease Control and Prevention), 106, 361, 365, 479
Celeghin, A., 330
Celnik, P., 386
Centerwall, B. S., 385
Chabris, C. F., 421, 422
Chamberlain, S. R., 373
Champagne, F., 254
Chan, M.Y., 394
Chandrashekar, J., 172, 173, 174
Chang, B. S., 477
Changeux, J.-P., 409, 430
Chapman, C. D., 280
Charney, D. S., 371
Charpentier, P., 357
Chaudhari, N., 174
Chelikani, P. K., 278
Chemelli, R. M., 312
Chen, M., 395
Cheney, D. L., 474
Cherdieu, M., 307
Cherry, E. C., 421
Cheyne, J. A., 313
Cho, I., 285
Choquet, D., 96
Christensen, D. D., 391
Chung, W. S., 32

Chung, Y., 355
Ciccocioppo, R., 112
Clapham, J. C., 274
Clarke, E., 474
Clarke, M. C., 353
Classen, J., 145
Clemente, C. D., 308
Cogan, G. B., 466
Coghill, R. C., 133
Cohen, J. D., 443
Cohen, S., 113, 306, 341
Cohen, Y., 425
Colburn, H. S., 164
Cole, J., 119
Cole, J. C., 108
Cole, K. J., 98
Colman, R. J., 274
Colom, R. 8
Conceição, V. A., 374
Conel, J. L., 409
Conn, P. J., 360
Cooke, B. M., 240
Cooke, J. R., 302
Corballis, M. C., 456, 473
Corbetta, M., 434, 435
Coricelli, G., 446
Corkin, S., 380, 401
Correll, C. U., 100, 357, 437
Coryell, W., 369
Costa, A., 467
Costanzo, R. M., 177
Counotte, D. S., 104
Cowan, N., 421, 422
Cox, J. H., 374
Cox, J. J., 131
Cox, L. M., 285
Cox, S. S., 342
Craighero, L., 146
Crews, F. T., 107
Crick, F. C., 439
Criqui, M. H., 385
Crivelli, C., 327
Crockford, C., 474
Crossley, N. A., 359
Crow, T. J., 349
Cruce, J. A. F., 278
Cummings, D. E., 282
Cummings, J. L., 444
Curcio, C. A., 190
Curran, H.V., 104
Curtis, V., 325
Curtiss, S., 472
Cussotto, S., 284

D

Dabbs, J. M., 334, 335
Dabbs, J. M., Jr., 335
Dabholkar, A. S., 409
Dale, R. C., 373

Dallenbach, K., 307
Damasio, A. R., 333
Damasio, H., 445
Damassa, D. A., 237
Dantz, B., 311
Darwin, C., 324
Davalos, D., 32
Davey-Smith, G., 243
David, L. A., 284
Davidson, J. M., 243
Davis, J. I., 328
Davis, M. C., 100
Davis, N., 132
De Boeck, P., 13
De Felipe, C., 133
de Gelder, B., 194, 330
De Groot, C. M., 374
de Groot, J. H., 179
de Heer, W. A., 466
de Kloet, E. R., 270
de Kluiver, H., 351
de Lecea, L., 312
de Quervain, D., 338
DeValois, K. K., 200, 208, 209
DeValois, R. L., 200, 208, 209
De Win, M. M., 109
Dearborn, G. V. N., 130
Dehaene, S., 430
Dehaene-Lambertz, G., 470
del Campo, N., 437
Delgado, J. M. R., 55
Demas, G. E., 285
Dement, W. C., 307
Den Heijer, A. E., 437
Dennis, S. G., 130
Denton, D., 271
Depaepe, V., 407
DeRubeis, R. J., 365
Desimone, R., 210, 432
Devane, W. A., 103
Devlin, J. T., 468
DeVoogd, T. J., 475
Dewan, A., 179
Dewsbury, D. A., 235
Dhabhar, F. S., 341
Di Marzo, V., 280
Diamond, M. C., 393, 394
Diana, M., 113
Dietz, P. M., 365
Dittmann, R. W., 256
Do, M. T. H., 294
Dohanich, G., 232
Dohrenwend, B. P., 371
Dolan, R. J., 333
Dolder, C. R., 315
Domjan, M., 17
Donaldson, Z. R., 227
Dorsaint-Pierre, R., 455

Dreger, A., 248
Drevets, W. C., 362
Drew, T., 421
Dronkers, N. F., 461, 466
Druckman, D., 307
Du, L., 363
Duchaine, B., 460
Duchamp-Viret, P., 177
Duffy, J. D., 444
Dulac, C.., 178
Dulak, J., 406
Dully, H., 347
Duncan, C. C., 353

E

Eapen, V., 374
Earnest, D. L., 292
Ebbinghaus, H., 4
Edwards, R. R., 306
Ehrhardt, A. A., 249
Eichler, V. B., 292
Eklund, A., 49
Ekman, P., 326
Elbert, T., 129
Elhilali, M., 422
Elie, J. E., 164
Elinav, E., 285
Ellenbogen, J. M., 307
Ellis, H. D., 330
Emborg, M. E., 479
Emens, J. S., 294
Emery, N. J., 330
Emory, E., 444
Engel, J., Jr., 330
Engelmann, T., 301
English, P. J., 278
Epstein, A. N., 270, 271
Erfurth, A., 369
Ernst, T., 105
Erren, T. C., 306
Ervin, F. R., 336
Everitt, B. J., 238
Everson, C. A., 304
Evinger, C., 397
Eybalin, M., 159
Eyer, J., 266

F

Fabre-Thorpe, M., 425
Falk, D., 472
Falkner, A. L., 336
Faraone, S.V., 367
Farbman, A. I., 176
Farrell, A. K., 339
Fay, R. R., 121
Federmeier, K. D., 470
Feinstein, J. S., 319, 332
Felitti, V. J., 341
Felleman, D. J., 201
Feng, W., 426

Ferguson. J. N., 227
Fernández-Espejo, D., 440
Field, P. M., 251
Fields, R. D., 32
Finch, C. E., 411
Finger, S., 460
Fink, H., 280
Fink, M., 363
Finn, C. T., 367
Fisher, S. E., 473, 475
Fishman, R. B., 254
Fitzsimmons, J. T., 271
Flanagan, J. R., 123
Flegal, K. M., 281
Fleming, A. S., 240, 241
Fleming, C., 347
Florence, S. L., 129
Fluharty, S. J., 270
Foerster, O., 78
Foley, C., 351
Ford, J. M., 430, 439
Foreman, D. L., 164
Forger, N. G., 254, 407
Foster, G. D., 274
Foster, R. G., 296
Fothergill, E., 263, 274
Fournier, J. C., 364
Fraher, J. P., 140
Francis, D. D., 412
Frankenhaeuser, M., 339, 340
Franklin, T. R., 104
Franks, N. P., 308
Franssen, C. L., 240
Freedman, M. S., 294
Freitag, J., 175
Freiwald, W. A., 200
French, C. A., 475
Frey, S. H., 129
Fried, I., 79
Friedman, L., 309
Friedrich, F. J., 435
Friston, K. J., 300
Fritz, J., 164
Fryar, C. D., 281
Fukuda, K., 313
Fulton, B. D., 436
Fung, T. C., 285
Furukawa, E., 437
Fuster, J. M., 444

G
Gabel, L. A., 477
Galaburda, A. M., 477
Gallant, J. L., 202, 442
Gallese, V., 146
Gallopin, T., 308
Gangwisch, J. E., 306
Gannon, P. J., 455
Gardner, B. T., 474

Gardner, R. A., 474
Gardner-Medwin, A. R., 398
Garfield, A. S., 280
Garver, D. L., 354, 367
Gasser, P., 109
Gates, N. J., 415
Gauthier, I., 460
Gazzaniga, M. S., 458
Gearhart, J. P., 256
Geers, A. E., 168
Gelade, G., 427
Gelber, R. P., 415
Gelstein, S., 178
Geniole, S. N., 334
Genzel, L., 307
George, D. T., 337
Georgiadis, J. R., 242
Georgopoulos, A. P., 144
Gerashchenko, D., 312
Gerkin, R. C., 175
Geschwind, N., 455, 464
Gibbons, R. D., 364
Gilbertson, M. W., 371
Gildersleeve, K., 243
Gill, R. E., 301
Gillin, J. C., 366
Giustino, T. F., 390
Glaser, R., 341
Glasser, M. F., 45
Glenn, A. L., 336
Glickman, S. E., 334
Glimcher, P. W., 11, 446
Gogtay, N., 410
Goldberg, M. E., 434
Goldin, P. R., 342
Goldstein, J. M., 255
Golomb, J., 413
Gonçalves, T. C., 135
Goodale, M. A., 183
Gooley, J. J., 316
Gordon, T. P., 335
Gorski, R. A., 251
Gorzalka, B. B., 91
Gossage, J. P., 106
Gosseries, O., 440
Goswami, U., 477
Gottesman, I. I., 350
Gottfried, J. A., 446
Gottlieb, J., 434
Gough, P. M., 468
Gougler, M., 322
Gould, E., 406
Goutman, J. D., 159
Grafton, S. T., 387
Gravett, N., 306
Gray, J. D., 11
Gray, N. S., 336
Graybiel, A. M., 148

Graziano, M., 145
Graziano, M. S., 145
Green, J. J., 433, 435
Greene, S. L., 391
Greenough, W. T., 394, 395
Griessenauer, C. J., 481
Grill-Spector, K., 459
Grimm, S., 365
Grob, C. S., 109
Grootendorst, C., 481
Gross, J. J., 342
Grover, G. J., 282
Grumbach, M. M., 253
Grunt, J. A., 237
Grüter, T., 460
Guarner, F., 284
Guillermo, C. J., 243
Gulevich, G., 305
Gunnell, D., 361

H
Haesler, S., 475
Haggard, P., 446
Hagstrom, S. A., 206
Halford, J. C., 282
Hallett, M., 374
Halliday, G. M., 112
Halperin, A., 103
Halsband, U., 145
Hamburger, V., 407
Hamer, D. H., 258
Hamson, D. K., 239, 252
Hancock, R., 477
Hanlon, C. A., 105
Hardt, O., 391
Hardy, J., 415
Hardyck, C., 457
Hare, R. D., 336
Hargrove, M. F., 335
Harold, D., 477
Hartanto, T. A., 437
Hartmann, E., 315
Hartse, K. M., 301
Hayden, B. Y., 11, 446
Haynes, K. F., 220
Hayward, R., 463
He, D. Z., 159
Heath, R. G., 329
Hebb, D. O., 398
Heffner, H. E., 456
Heffner, R. S., 456
Heidenreich, M., 123
Heilbronner, S. R., 11, 446
Heinrichs, R. W., 349
Helfter, P., 300
Heller, S., 168
Helmholtz, H. von, 204, 420
Hen, R., 363
Henry, J. F., 241

Herbst, C. T., 163
Herculano-Houzel, S., 24, 31, 402
Herek, G. M., 256
Heres, S., 359
Herrmann, C., 429
Hertel, P., 359
Hetherington, A. W., 276
Heuer, F., 389
Hewes, G., 473
Hibbard, L. S., 144
Hickey, C., 431
Hickmott, P. W., 129
Hicks, M. J., 113
Hidaka, B. H., 9
Higley, J. D., 336
Hilker, R., 351
Hillhouse, T. M., 365
Hillyard, S. A., 429, 431, 470
Hirtz, D., 9
Hitt, E., 4
Hobson, J. A., 300
Hodgkin, A. L., 61
Hoeft, F., 477
Hoekzema, E., 241
Hofmann, S. G., 342
Hohmann, A. G., 135
Hohmann, G. W., 324
Hollon, S. D., 369
Honey, G. D., 356
Honzik, C. H., 387
Hopfinger, J., 430, 434
Hopfinger, J. B., 431, 434
Hopkins, W. D., 456
Horton, J. C., 42
Howard-Jones, P. A., 19
Howland, R. H., 368
Hsu, M., 446
Hua, J. T., 232
Huang, A. L., 173, 175
Huang, G., 248
Huang, Z. J., 45
Hubel, D. H., 198, 199, 409
Hudspeth, A. J., 159, 160
Huedo-Medina, T. B., 315
Huettel, S. A., 446
Hughes, I. A., 246
Hughes, J., 102
Hülsheger, U. R., 328
Human Rights Watch, 246
Hurtado, M. D., 282
Hussain, S. J., 98
Huth, A. G., 466
Huttenlocher, P. R., 409
Hyde, K. L., 165
Hyde, T. M., 354
Hyman, S. E., 350, 351, 366

I
Imai, T., 177
Imeri, L., 306
Imperato-McGinley, J., 248
Infurna, F. J., 339
Insel, T. R., 227
Insley, S. J., 475
Institute of Medicine, 113, 371
Isles, A. R., 178
Izumikawa, M., 168

J
Jackson, H., 409
Jacobs, G. H., 207
Jacobs, J., 388
Jain, R., 357
James, T. W., 212
James, W., 381, 419
Jamieson, D., 293
Janak, P. H., 330
Jaskiw, G. E., 359
Jasper, H., 79
Jenkins, J., 307
Jensen, M. S., 421
Jentsch, J. D., 360
Jeon, M., 13
Jessen, N. A., 46
Joëls, M., 270
Johansson, R. S., 123
Johnson, L. C., 303
Johnson, M. W., 109
Johnson, V. E., 241, 242
Johnston, R. E., 178
Jones, B. E., 309
Jones, H. J., 103
Jones, P. B., 359
Jones, T. A., 480
Jordan, B. D., 479
Jordan, C. L., 254
Jordt, S.-E., 131
Joseph, J., 351
Joseph, J. S., 426
Julian, T., 335
Justice, J. B., Jr., 112

K
Kaar, G. F., 140
Kable, J. W., 11, 446
Kaiser, D., 299
Kajimura, S., 282
Kales, A., 298, 299, 303
Kales, J., 299, 303
Kandel, E. R., 395
Kandler, K., 164
Kane, J. M., 100
Kang, C., 472
Kanwisher, N., 435
Kapur, S., 367
Karch, S. B., 112

Karlin, A., 73
Karni, A., 307
Karpicke, J. D., 391
Karra, E., 278
Kass, A. E., 284
Katz, B., 61
Katz, D. B., 148
Katzenberg, D., 296
Kaushall, P. I., 384
Kay, K. N., 440, 441
Kaya, E. M., 422
Kaye, W. H., 284
Keane, T. M., 390
Kee, N., 406
Keenan, J. P., 458
Keesey, R. E., 276, 277
Kelly, J. P., 106
Keltner, D., 326
Kempermann, G., 394
Kendler, K. S., 361
Kennedy, D. P., 319
Kennedy, J. L., 351
Kennerknecht, I., 460
Kerns, J. C., 283
Kertesz, A., 480
Kessels, H. W., 400
Kessler, R. C., 9, 348, 367, 372
Kety, S. S., 350, 363
Kheribek, M. A., 371
Kim, D. R., 363
Kim, J. S., 360
Kim, K. H., 472
Kimura, D., 454, 465, 466
Kindt, M., 390
King, A., 176
King, S., 353
Kingsbury, S. J., 367
Kinney, H. C., 315
Kinsey, A. C., 241
Kinsley, C. H., 240
Kirkwood, T. B. L., 411
Kisely, S., 365
Klar, A. J., 457
Klein, M., 395
Klein, R. M., 425
Kleitman, N., 297, 301
Kluger, M. J., 266
Klüver, H., 329
Knecht, S., 459
Knibestol, M., 125
Knight, R., 429
Koch, C., 439
Koch, G., 434
Kodama, T., 310
Koehler, K. R., 168
Kohl, M. M., 456
Kokrashvili, Z., 275
Kondo, Y., 240

Kondoh, K., 178
Konopka, R. J., 295
Koob, G. F., 112
Kopell, B. H., 356
Korman, M., 307
Korol, D. L., 232
Koubeissi, M. Z., 439
Koutstaal, W., 386
Krashes, M. J., 280
Krauss, R. M., 473
Krebs, J. R., 388
Kreitman, N., 361
Kringelbach, M. L., 365, 445
Kripke, D. F., 306, 314
Krupa, D. J., 397
Kuhl, B. A., 391
Kulkarni, A., 164
Kumaresan, V., 329
Kuperberg, G. R., 470
Kupfer, D. J., 361, 366
Kutas, M., 470
Kwakkel, G., 481
Kyzar, E. J., 108

L
LaBar, K. S., 330
Lagrèze, W. A., 213
Lai, C. S. L., 472
Lambert, K. G., 240
Langleben, D. D., 322
Larroche, J.-C., 403
Larsson, J., 145
Larsson, M., 178
Lau, H. C., 443
Lavie, N., 422
Lavie, P., 307
Lavond, D. G., 396
Lawrence, A. D., 11, 446
Le Grange, D., 284
Leask, S. J., 456
LeDoux, J. E., 330, 331
Lee, E. E., 365
Lee, H., 336
Lehrer, P. M., 342
Leinders-Zufall, T., 178
Lepage, J. F., 146
Lereya, S. T., 343
Lescroart, M. D., 442
Lesku, J. A., 301, 306
Leuner, B., 243
Leung, C. T., 177
LeVay, S., 257
Levine, J. D., 135
Levine, S., 340
Levitsky, W., 455
Lew, S. M., 482
Lewis, D. O., 336
Lewis, M. B., 330

Li, B., 367
Li, W., 307
Li, X., 173
Liberles, S. D., 179
Libet, B., 443
Lichstein, K. L., 315
Lichtenstein, P., 367
Lichtman, J. W., 409
Liddelow, S. A., 32
Lieberman, P., 465
Liégeois, F., 472
Liepert, J., 481
Lim, M. M., 227
Lin, L., 312
Linde, K., 135
Linden, E., 474
Lisk, R. D., 238
Lisman, J., 400
Liu, D., 340
Liu, Y., 148, 277, 278
Llewellyn, S., 300
Lloyd, J. A., 335
Lo, J. C., 296
Lockhart, M., 396
Loconto, J., 178
Loeb, G. E., 168
Loewenstein, W. R., 122
Loftus, E. F., 391
Logan, C. G., 387
Lømo, T., 398
Löscher, W., 77
Lotto, R. B., 204
Loui, P., 165
Lübke, K. T., 178
Luck, S. J., 76, 429, 431
Lundberg, U., 340
Luo, L., 45
Luria, A. R., 391
Luthar, S. S., 339
Luttrell, V. R., 238
Ly, M., 336, 337
Lyamin, O., 302
Lynch, G., 401

M
Macdonald, K., 19
MacLean, P. D., 329
Macmillan, M., 445
MacNeilage, P. F., 456
Maggioncalda, A. N., 235
Magoun, H. W., 309
Mahowald, M. W., 313, 314
Maia, T. V., 374
Mair, W. G. P., 384
Makino, H., 386
Malagelada, J. R., 284
Malenka, R. C., 399
Malinow, R., 400
Mancuso, K., 207

Manger, P. R., 301
Mangun, G., 430, 431
Mani, S. K., 238
Manoli, D. S., 11
Mantini, D., 439
Mantyh, P. W., 133
Mao, J. B., 397
Marconi, A., 103
Marcus, G. F., 472
Marek, G. J., 360
Mariani, J., 409
Mark, V. H., 336
Marler, P., 475
Marshall, L., 307
Martin, C. K., 274
Martuza, R. L., 373
Marucha, P. T., 341
Maruyama, Y., 174
Marzullo, T. C., 55
Maskos, U., 104
Masters, W. H., 241, 242
Mastrianni, J. A., 304
Mateo, J. M., 178
Mather, M., 232
Matias, I., 280
Matsumoto, K., 445
Mattes, R. D., 171
Matthews, K. A., 341
May, L., 470
May, P. A., 106
Mazur, A., 335
McBurney, D. H., 174
McCabe, P., 480
McCarthy, R. A., 477
McClintock, M., 178
McCrae, C. C., 303
McDonald, J. J., 129, 426, 430,
    435
McEwen, B. S., 266, 338
McFadden, D., 257
McGann, J. P., 175
McGaugh, J. L., 390
McGinty, D. J., 308
McGowan, P. O., 11, 340, 412
McGuigan, F. J., 342
McGuire, J. F., 374
McKee, A. C., 479
McKenna, K., 239
McKenry, P. C., 335
McKernan, M. G., 401
McKim, W. A., 111
McLaughlin, S. K., 173
McLellan, T. M., 98
McLemore, K. A., 256
McNamara, P., 300
Meany, M. J., 3, 412
Meddis, R., 306, 307
Medori, R., 304

Mega, M. S., 444
Meguerditchian, A., 474
Mei, L., 351
Meier, M. H., 103
Meisel, R. L., 238
Meister, I. G., 467
Melzack, R., 130, 134, 135
Menaker, M., 293
Méndez-Bértolo, C., 330
Menninger, W. C., 100
Merchán-Pérez, A., 394
Meshberger, F. L., 6
Mesulam, M.-M., 436
Mewton, L., 365
Mez, J., 479
Michael, N., 369
Micheyl, C., 421
Miczek, K. A., 91
Miller, E. K., 443
Miller, G. F., 10
Miller, J. M., 168
Miller, N. E., 271
Milner, A. D., 211
Milner, B., 379, 381, 444
Milner, P., 329
Milner, P. M., 8, 329
Minzenberg, M. J., 355
Mirescu, C., 340
Mirsky, A. F., 353
Mishkin, M., 211, 382
Mishra, J., 431
Mithoefer, M. C., 109
Miyawaki, Y., 440, 441, 442
Moffat, F., 480
Mogwitz, S., 374
Mohammed, A., 394
Moita, M. A., 388
Money, J., 249
Monfils, M. H., 145
Monks, D. A., 254
Montague, C. T., 282
Montenigro, P. H., 479
Monti, M. M., 440
Moore, C. L., 254
Moore, G. J., 368
Moore, J. W., 396
Moore, R. Y., 292, 294, 384
Moorhead, T. W., 367
Moorman, S., 475
Moran, J., 432
Morawietz, C., 480
Mori, K., 176, 178
Morizane, A., 479
Morris, B., 477
Morris, R., 334
Morris, R. G., 401
Morrison, A. R., 310
Mortensen, P. B., 352

Moruzzi, G., 306, 309
Moser, A., 387
Mott, F. W., 141
Motta, S. C., 336
Mountcastle, V. B., 43
Mounts, J. R., 432
Mueller, H. T., 360
Muhlert, N., 11, 446
Mukamal, K. J., 106
Mukhametov, L. M., 300, 301
Munafo, J., 171
Munley, K. M., 334
Münte, T. F., 129
Murphy, M. L., 339
Muza, R., 313

N
Nader, K., 391
Naeser, M., 463
Naesström, M., 373
Nakazato, M., 278
Naqvi, N. H., 112
Naselaris, T., 442
Nathans, J., 206
Nation, E. F., 235
National Academy of Sciences,
    322
National Institute of Mental
    Health, 348
Nature, 479
Navarro-Lobato, I., 307
Nee, D. E., 443, 444
Neff, W. D., 164
Neitz, M., 207
Nelson, G., 173, 174
Nelson, M. H., 315
Nestler, E. J., 366
Nestor, A., 442
Neumeister, A., 370
Neville, H. J., 465, 470
Newsome, W. T., 7, 202
NIDA/National Institute on
    Drug Abuse, 102
Ng, S. F., 282
Ngandu, T., 415
Nguyen, J. D., 113
Nichols, M. J., 7
Nienhuis, R., 312
Nietzel, M. T., 322
Nishida, M., 307
Nishimoto, S., 442
Noad, M. J., 475
Noguchi, Y., 51
Nordeen, E. J., 253
Numan, M., 240, 336
Numan, M. J., 240
Nussbaum, M. C., 17
Nutt, D. J., 112

O
Oades, R. D., 112
Oberlander, T. F., 366
O'Connell-Rodwell, C. E., 163
O'Connor, D. B., 334
O'Craven, K. M., 431
O'Donovan, A., 371
Ogden, J., 341
Ojala, K. E., 11, 446
Ojemann, G., 467
Ojemann, G. A., 466
O'Keefe, J., 387
O'Keefe, J. H., 106
Olabi, B., 355
Olds, J., 329
Olender, T., 177
Oler, J. A., 369
Olfson, M., 364
Olsen, K. L., 252
Olson, S., 373
Oman, C. M., 170
O'Neal, K. K., 111
Opendak, M., 406
Opp, M. R., 306
Oppenheim, K., 131
Orlovska, S., 373
O'Shea, J., 436
Osorio, D., 206
Ossenkoppele, R., 415
Osterberg, G., 189
Öst, L. G., 373
Osterhout, L., 470
O'Tuathaigh, C. M. P., 100
Overstreet, D. H., 367
Owen, A. M., 440

P
Pack, A. I., 313
Padawer, R., 248
Pagel, J. F., 300
Pagel, M., 471
Palagini, L., 366
Palaus, M., 431
Palmer, C. T., 234
Palmer, S. M., 362
Panksepp, J., 325, 475
Panksepp, J. B., 336
Pantev, C., 165
Papez, J. W., 329
Papka, M., 387
Pare, M., 123
Parker, G., 391
Parkes, J. D., 314
Parks, T. N., 409
Parrott, A. C., 108, 109
Parton, A., 435
Parton, L. E., 277
Pasanen, E., 257
Pasquinelli, E., 19

Pastalkova, E., 387
Pasternak, O., 465
Paterson, S. J., 472
Paton, J. J., 330
Patterson, F., 474
Patterson, P. H., 353
Pauls, D. L., 373
Paus, T., 410, 434
Pause, B. M., 178
Pedersen, C. B., 352
Pediatric Eye Disease
    Investigator Group, 213
Pedreira, C., 200
Peever, J., 314
Pegna, A. J., 330
Penadés, R., 355
Penfield, W., 39, 78, 79, 466, 467
Peplau, L. A., 242
Pepper, J., 373
Perani, D., 467
Perenin, M. T., 211
Peretz, I., 165
Pernía-Andrade, A. J., 135
Peter, M. E., 407
Peterhans, E., 202
Peters, A., 31
Petersen, C. C. H., 298
Petersen, S. E., 433
Peterson, B. S., 362
Peterson, L. R., 389
Peterson, M. J., 389
Petit, C., 166
Petitto, L. A., 465
Petrides, M., 444
Petrone, A. B., 232
Petrovic, P., 135
Pettit, H. O., 112
Petty, F., 367
Pfaff, D. W., 238, 239
Pfeffer, M., 296
Pfefferbaum, A., 107
Pfenning, A. R., 475
Phillips, A. G., 280
Phoenix, C. H., 249, 250
Pickens, R., 112
Picton, T. W., 76
Pierce, R. C., 329
Pinel, P., 472
Pirastu, N., 171
Pisani, S. L., 232
Pletnikov, M.V., 354
Plihal, W., 307
Ploog, D. W., 474, 475
Plutchik, R., 325
Poldrack, R. A., 49
Ponsford, J., 479
Poole, J. H., 475
Pooresmaeili, A., 426

Pope, H. G., Jr., 232
Popli, A. P., 359
Poremba, A, 456
Porta, M., 374
Porter, J. H., 365
Posner, M. I., 161, 423, 424, 425, 469
Poulet, J. F. A., 298
Poulos, A. M., 396
Powell, S. B., 353
Powley, T. L., 275
Pratt, L. A., 364
Prehn, K., 274
Premack, D., 474
Prendergast, B. J., 244
Prentice, R. L., 232
Prinzmetal, W., 421
Prudente, C. N., 143
Pugh, K. R., 477
Pulak, L. M., 306
Purdy, J. E., 17
Purves, D., 136, 195, 197, 204, 409
Putman, C. T., 139

Q
Qi,Y., 374
Quraishi, I. H., 440

R
Racette, A., 480
Racine, E., 50
Rafal, R. D., 435
Rahman, Q., 257
Raichle, M. E., 12, 161, 438, 469
Raine, A., 336
Raisman, G., 251
Rakic, P., 42
Ralph, M. R., 293
Ramachandran,V. S., 133, 134
Rampon, C., 401
Rand, M. N., 253
Ranson, S. W., 276
Rapoport, J. L., 372
Rasch, B., 307
Rasmussen, T., 39, 459
Rathelot, J. A., 144
Rattenborg, N. C., 301
Rauch, S. L., 369
Rechtschaffen, A., 298, 304
Reck, C., 366
Redican, W. K., 324
Regier, D. A., 365
Reiner, W. G., 256
Reisberg, D., 389
Rempel-Clower, N. L., 383
Renner, M. J., 392
Reppert, S. M., 295
Rezaie, L., 315
Richardson, G. P., 166

Risch, N., 361
Rizzolatti, G., 146
Roberts, A., 293
Roberts, L., 466, 467
Robertson, D. J., 460
Robins, L. N., 365
Robinson, D. L., 433
Robinson, R., 365
Robson, J. G., 200
Rocca, W. A., 414
Roediger, H. L., III, 391
Roenneberg, T., 296
Roffwarg, H. P., 302
Rogan, M. T., 401
Rogawski, M. A., 77
Rogers-Ramachandran, D., 133, 134
Roland, P. E., 51
Rose, K. A., 213
Roseboom, T. J., 341
Rosell, D. R., 336
Roselli, C. E., 257
Rosenbaum, R. S., 385
Rosenberg, M. D., 436
Rosenblatt, J. S., 240, 241
Rosenkranz, M. A., 341
Rosenzweig, M. R., 164, 392, 394
Roses, A. D., 414
Rothschild, A. J., 315
Rumbaugh, D. M., 474
Rupnick, M. A., 282
Rupprecht, R., 370
Rusak, B., 291, 292, 293
Russell, J. A., 326, 327
Russell, R., 460
Russo, E. B., 103
Rutstein, J., 265

S
Saalmann,Y. B., 433
Sachdev, P., 415
Sachs, B. D., 238
Sack, R. L., 294
Saha, K. B., 359
Sahay, A., 363
Saito, M., 282
Sakreida, K., 468
Sakurai, T., 280
Salazar, H., 131
Salimpoor,V. N., 165
Salter, M. W., 133
Samaha, F. F., 274
SAMHSA, 9
Samson, S., 456
Sandberg, K., 244
Sanders, A. R., 258
Sanderson, D. J., 400
Saper, C. B., 312

Sapir, A., 433
Sapolsky, R. M., 235, 342
Satinoff, E., 265
Sato, J. R., 439
Satz, P., 457
Saul, S., 315
Saxe, M. D., 406
Saxena, S., 373
Scalaidhe, S. P. O., 202
Scassellati, B., 422
SCENHIR (Scientific
    Committee on Emerging
    and Newly Identified Health
    Risks), 166
Schachter, S., 323
Schacter, D. L., 386
Schaeffel, F., 213
Schatzberg, A. F., 108, 109
Schein, S. J., 210
Schenck, C. H., 313, 314
Schieber, M. H., 144
Schiffman, S. S., 172
Schildkraut, J. J., 363
Schindler, E. A., 109
Schlaug, G., 455, 456
Schlosser, M. D., 421
Schneider, K., 349
Schneider, P., 165
Schneps, M. H., 477
Schoenbaum, G., 445
Schramm, E., 365
Schrof, J. M., 112, 134
Schulz, K. M., 249
Schummers, J., 32
Schuster, C. R., 111, 112
Schwartz, S., 437
Schwartzkroin, P. A., 398
Sclafani, A., 277
Scott, D. J., 135
Scott, S. K., 468
Scoville, W. B., 379
Seavey, C., 256
Sebastián-Gallés, N., 467
Seeman, P., 358, 359
Seiden, R. H., 361
Selkoe, D. J., 415
Selye, H., 338
Semendeferi, K., 444
Sessa, B., 109
Seuss, Dr., 476
Sexton, C. E., 362
Seyfarth, R. M., 474
Shackman, A. J., 369
Shah, D. B., 373
Shallice, T., 444
Shan, S.Y., 265
Shaw, P., 410
Shaw, P. J., 304
Shaywitz, S. E., 477

Sheikh-Bahaei, N., 415
Shein-Idelson, M., 301
Sherrington, C. S., 141, 392
Sherwin, B. B., 232, 241, 243
Sheth, S. A., 446
Shic, F., 422
Shih, R. A., 369
Shinnick-Gallagher, P., 401
Shipton, O. A., 456
Shors, T. J., 406
Shu, W., 475
Shulman, G. L., 434, 435
Siegel, J. M., 301, 306, 310, 312
Sierakowiak, A., 439
Siever, L. J., 336
Sikich, L., 359
Silva, D. A., 457
Simons, D. J., 421, 422
Singer, J., 323
Singer, O., 415
Singer, P., 17
Singer, T., 133
Sinigaglia, C., 146
Sinopoli, V. M., 373
Sisk, C. L., 249
Slee, S. J., 164
Smith, C., 307
Smith, S., 289
Smoller, J. W., 367
Smylie, C. S., 458
Smyth, K. A., 414
Snyder, J. S., 371
Snyder, P. J., 232
Solomon, A., 361
Soltis, J., 163
Somerville, M. J., 472
Soon, C. S., 443
Sowell, E. R., 374
Spalding, K. L., 406
Spampinato, D., 386
Spelman, F. A., 168
Spiegler, B. J., 382, 456
Spitzer, R. L., 258
Sprague, T. C., 432
Squire, L. R., 383, 384
Stacey, P., 238
Standing, L. G., 391
Stanford, T. R., 129
Stanovich, K. E., 8
Stansley, B. J., 360
Stanton, S. J., 335
Staubli, U. V., 401
Stauffer, V. L., 360
Steen, P. A., 129
Stein, B. E., 129
Steinmetz, J. E., 148, 396
Stephan, F. K., 292
Sterling, P., 266

Sterman, M. B., 308
Stern, K., 178
Stevens-Graham, B., 32
Stoeckel, C., 468
Stormshak, F., 257
Stranahan, A. M., 407
Strick, P. L., 144
Stricker, E. M., 265
Substance Abuse and
    Mental Health Services
    Administration, 111, 348, 361
Suez, J., 285
Suk, I., 6
Sumnall, H. R., 108
Sun, T., 455
Sunn, N., 30
Sunstein, C. R., 17
Sutcliffe, J. G., 312
Suzuki, S., 232
Svare, B. B., 334
Swedo, S. E., 372
Sylvia, K. E., 285

T
Taglialatela, J. P., 474
Takahashi, J., 479
Takahashi, T., 400
Takizawa, R., 343
Tam, J., 282
Tamargo, R. J., 6
Tanaka, S., 431
Tanda, G., 112
Tang, N. M., 135
Tang, Y. P., 401
Tanji, J., 145
Taub, E., 142, 480
Taylor, M. A., 363
Teipel, S., 414
Temple, E., 477
Terkel, J., 240, 241
Terrace, H. S., 474
Tetel, M. J., 285
Thannickal, T. C., 312
Theoret, H., 146
Theunissen, F. E., 164
Thomas, K., 361
Thomas, R. K., 387
Thompson, P. M., 355
Thompson, R. F., 396, 397
Thompson, T., 111, 112
Thornhill, R., 234
Thornton, A. E., 479
Thornton-Jones, Z. D., 282
Thorpe, S. J., 425
Timmann, D., 397
Todorov, A., 325
Tollkuhn, J., 11
Tolman, E. C., 387
Tom, S. M., 446

Tomoda, T., 354
Tootell, R. B., 193, 201
Tootell, R. B. H., 193, 201
Tordoff, M., 280
Torello, A. T., 178
Torrey, E. F., 351, 354
Trasande, L., 285
Treesukosol, Y., 173
Treffert, D. A., 391
Treisman, A. M., 426, 427
Treisman, M., 170
Tremlett, H., 285
Triller, A., 96
Trimble, M. R., 353
Tronick, R., 366
Tsai, L., 178
Tsuchiya, N., 439
Tuller, D., 312
Tully, T., 387
Tulving, E., 385
Turgeon, J. L., 232
Turner, E. H., 363
Tyack, P. L., 475
Tye, K. M., 330

U
Umilta, M. A., 147
Ungerleider, L., 211
Ungerleider, L. G., 202, 211
Ursin, H., 338, 339

V
Valbo, A. B., 125
van Anders, S. M., 335
Van Dongen, H. P., 303
Van Essen, D. C., 201
Van Gaal, L. F., 282
Van Horn, J. D., 445
Van Os, J., 352, 367
Van Tol, M. J., 369
Van Zoeren, J. G., 265
Vance, C. G., 135
Vandermosten, M., 465
Vann, S. D., 384
Vargas, C. D., 457
Vargha-Khadem, F., 473
Vasey, P. L., 256
Vassar, R., 176, 177
Vauclair, J., 474
Vaughan, W., 391
Vernes, S. C., 472
Videnovic, A., 314
Vighetto, A., 211
Villarroel, M. A., 478
Vincus, A. A., 111
Visser, S. N., 437
Vitaterna, M. H., 296
Voets, T., 131
Vogt, B. A., 133
Volkow, N., 135

Volkow, N. D., 112, 280, 282
von der Heydt, R., 202
Vorobyev, M., 206
Voytek, B., 444
Vriens, J., 131
Vrieze, A., 285
Vythilingam, M., 369

W
Wada, J. A., 455, 459
Waddell, J., 406
Wagenmakers, E.-J., 328
Wagner, G. C., 335
Wahlstrom, K., 296
Waldrop, M. M., 12
Walker, M., 315
Walker, M. P., 307
Wall, P. D., 134, 135
Wallis, J. D., 445
Walters, R. J., 101
Walther, S., 435
Wang, Y. K., 406
Ward, L. M., 423
Warrington, E. K., 477
Warwick, R., 33
Watkins, K. E., 468, 473
Watson, N. V., 239, 254, 335,
    456, 465
Weaver, D. R., 295
Webb, W. B., 316
Weinberger, D. R., 351, 354, 356
Weinberger, L. E., 336
Weinberger, N. M., 164
Weiner, K. S., 459
Weiner, R. D., 362
Weitzman, E. D., 294
Wesensten, N. J., 313
West, G. L., 431
West, R., 431
West, S. L., 111
Wester, K., 398
Westerberg, C. E., 302
Wever, R. A., 294
White, N. M., 329
Whitfield-Gabrieli, S., 439
Whitlock, J. R., 401
Widge, A. S., 365
Wiesel, T. N., 198, 199
Will, B., 394
Willander, J., 178
Williams, J. H., 146
Williams, N. R., 108, 109
Williams, P. L., 33
Williams, T. J., 257
Wilson, M. L., 334
Wingfield, J. C., 266, 334
Winocur, G., 406
Winslow, J. T., 227
Wisdom, A. J., 66

Wise, R. J., 280, 282, 468
Witte, A. V., 274
Wojciulik, E., 435
Wolf, M. E., 112
Wolf, S. S., 374
Wolfe, J. M., 422, 426
Wolk, D. A., 415
Wollan, M., 322
Womelsdorf, T., 432
Wood, J. M., 307
Wood, N., 421, 422
Woolf, C. J., 133
World Health Organization, 101
Wrangham, R. W., 335
Wren, A. M., 278

Wright, R. D., 423
Wuethrich, B., 471
Wurtz, R. H., 433

X
Xerri, C., 240
Xie, L., 306
Xiong, W.-C., 351

Y
Yaffe, K., 232
Yamazaki, S., 292
Yang, T. T., 129
Yang, Y., 336
Ycaza Herrera, A., 232
Yehuda, R., 371
Yeni-Komshian, G. H., 456

Yin, J., 357
Young, E. D., 164
Young, K. D., 362
Young, L. J., 227
Young, W. C., 237
Yu, Y. J., 415
Yuan, M., 30, 104

Z
Zaidel, E., 452
Zalocusky, K. A., 446
Zatorre, R. J., 456
Zawilska, J. B., 106
Zeki, S., 210, 332
Zeman, A., 11
Zendel, B. R., 165, 421

Zhang, C. L., 406
Zhang, T. Y., 3, 412
Zhang, Y., 278
Zhao, G. Q., 173
Zheng, J., 159
Zihl, J., 202
Zilles, K., 459
Zimmer, C., 7
Zimmerman, C. A., 269
Zola-Morgan, S., 383
Zorumski, C. F., 108
Zucker, I., 291, 292, 293
Zucker, L. M., 278
Zucker, T. F., 278

Subject Index

Page numbers in *italic* denote entries that are included in a figure or table.

A

A delta (Aδ) fibers, 131, 133
Abducens nerve (cranial nerve VI), 34, 396
Absence attacks, 77
Absolute refractory phase, 61–62, 242
Absorptive phase of insulin release, 275
Abused children, 11, 412
Acamprosate (Campral), 113
Accessory olfactory bulb, 178
Accommodation, 184, 185
Acetaminophen, 135
Acetylcholine (ACh)
  defined, 72, 138
  degradation in the synaptic cleft, 73
  discovery of, 87–88
  functions as a neurotransmitter, 72
  modulation of brain activity, 89–90
  motor neurons and, 139
  parasympathetic system and, 36
  receptors (*see* ACh receptors; Nicotinic ACh receptors)
Acetylcholinesterase (AChE), 73
ACh. *See* Acetylcholine
ACh receptors
  effects of nicotine on, 99
  multiplicity of subtypes in the brain, 90
  poisons that block, 72
  types of, 72–73
  See also Nicotinic ACh receptors
AChE. *See* Acetylcholinesterase
Acid. *See* LSD
Acids, sour taste and, 173
Acquired dyslexia, 476
Acquired prosopagnosia, 459

ACTH. *See* Adrenocorticotropic hormone
Actin, 138, *139*
Action potentials
  all-or-none property, 61
  changes in the postsynaptic membrane potential, 66–68
  compared to a flushing toilet, 65
  conduction velocity, 64–65
  defined, 60–61
  depolarization and the triggering of, 59–61
  electrical characteristics of, *69*
  encoding of sensory stimuli as streams of, 124–125
  firing by postsynaptic neurons, 68–70
  ionic mechanisms underlying, 61–63
  knee-jerk reflex, 55–56, 74, *75*
  neurotransmitter release into the synaptic cleft and, 66, 71–72
  propagation of, 63–65
  refractory period, 65
  in synaptic transmission, 70, *71, 84, 85*
Action video games, 431
Activational effect, 236
Activation-synthesis theory, 300
Acts, 137
Acupuncture, 135, *136*
Adaptation. *See* Sensory adaptation
Addiction. *See* Substance abuse
Adenine, A–1, A–2
Adenosine, 98
Adenosine receptor, 98
ADH. *See* Antidiuretic hormone
ADHD. *See* Attention deficit hyperactivity disorder
Adipose tissue, 273, 278
Adoption studies, of schizophrenia, 350
Adrenal cortex, *218*, 338

Adrenal glands
  congenital adrenal hyperplasia, 246
  endocrine functions, *218*
  stress response, 338, *339*
Adrenal medulla, *218*, 338, 339
Adrenal steroid hormones, 338
Adrenal steroid receptors, 340–341
Adrenaline. *See* Epinephrine
Adrenocorticotropic hormone (ACTH), *221*
Adult neurogenesis, 10, 406–407
Adult-onset diabetes, 275
Affective disorders. *See* Mood disorders
Afferent, 38
Afterpotentials, 61
Age/Aging
  changes in the brain, 414–415
  impact on recovery from brain damage, 480, 481–482
  paternal age and risk of schizophrenia in children, 351
  sleep patterns and, 302–303
Aggression
  androgens and, 334–336
  biopsychology of human violence, 336–337
  brain circuits mediating, 336
  defined, 334
  maternal, 336
Agnosia, 460
Agonists
  agonist drugs, 93, 94, 96
  defined, 72, 93
Agraphia, 460
AgRP, 279
AIS. *See* Androgen insensitivity syndrome
Alarm reaction, 338
Alcohol
  effects as stimulant and depressant, 106–107
  effects on postsynaptic receptors, *99*

Alcohol use disorder
  DSM-5 diagnostic criteria, *110*
  Korsakoff's syndrome, 385
  medical interventions, 113
Alcoholics Anonymous, 113
Aldosterone, 270
"Alertness drug," 312–313
Alexia, 460, 476
Allen Institute, 32
Allomones, 220
Allopregnanolone, 370
All-or-none property, 61, 65
Allostasis, 266
Alpha rhythms, 297
Alprazolam, 89
Altaic language family, *471*
Alternative splicing, A–3
Alzheimer, Alois, 414
Alzheimer's disease, 32, 90, 413, 414–415
Amacrine cells, 185, *186*
Ambien (zolpidem), 315
"Ambien drivers," 315
Amblyopia, 213
American Sign Language (ASL), 465–466, 474–475
Ames, Aldrich, 322
AMH. *See* Anti-müllerian hormone
Amine hormones, 220–222
Amine neurotransmitters
  characteristics of, *86*, 87
  defined, 87
  modulation of brain activity, 89–91
Amino acid neurotransmitters, *86*, 87
Amino acids, 272, A–3
Amnesia
  from damage to the medial diencephalon, 384–385
  from damage to the temporal lobes and hippocampus, 379, 381–382, 383, 385, 401
  defined, 380, 381
  types of, 380–381
Amobarbital, 459
AMPA receptors, *398*, 399–400
Amphetamine psychosis, 358

Amphetamines, *97*, 105–106, 312

Amplitude, of sound, 155

Ampulla, 169, *170*

Amusia, 165

Amygdala
  anxiety disorders and, 369
  changes in activity with depression, 362
  decision making and, *446*
  defined, 43, 330
  emotional enhancement of memory and, 390
  feeding behavior and, 280
  Klüver-Bucy syndrome and, 330
  mediation of emotion and emotion learning, 329, 330–332, 333
  olfactory system and, *176, 178*
  Patient H.M. and memory loss, 381
  post-traumatic stress disorder and, *371*
  substance abuse and, *112*
  vomeronasal system and, 178

Amyloid plaques, *414, 415*

Anafranil. *See* Clomipramine

Analgesia, 134–136

Analgesics, 101–103, 134–135, *136*

Anandamide, 102, 103, 280

Androgen insensitivity syndrome (AIS), 246–247, 249, 255

Androgen receptors, 246–247

Androgens
  aggression and, 334–336
  androgen insensitivity syndrome, 246–247, 249, 255
  congenital adrenal hyperplasia, 246
  defined, 231
  effects of prenatal exposure, 255–258
  human sexual behavior and, 243
  individual differences in mating behavior and, 237
  male sexual behavior and, 238–240, 250–251, 255–258
  masculinization of adult behavior and, 250–251, 255–258
  masculinization of nervous system regions, 251–254
  mechanisms of action, 222

organizational effects on rodent behavior, 250

Angiotensin II (AII), 271, *272*

Anhedonia, 113

Animal Liberation (Singer), 17

Animal models
  in behavioral neuroscience, 15–17
  of depression, 366–367
  of nondeclarative memory, 387–388

Anions, 56

Anomia, 462

Anorexia nervosa, 283–284

Anorexigenic neurons, *279*, 280

ANP. *See* Atrial natriuretic peptide

Antabuse. *See* Disulfiram

Antagonist muscles, 138, *139*

Antagonists
  antagonist drugs, 93, 94, 96
  defined, 72, 93

Anterior, 38

Anterior cingulate cortex
  activation during lying, 322
  changes in activity with depression, 362
  choice system and, 446
  valuation system and, 446

Anterior hypothalamus, 270

Anterior insula, *175*

Anterior pituitary
  defined, 228
  endocrine functions, *218*
  hypothalamic releasing hormones and, 228–230
  regulation of gonadal steroid hormones, *231*
  stress response, 338
  tropic hormones, 228–229

Anterograde amnesia
  from damage to the medial diencephalon, 384
  from damage to the temporal lobes and hippocampus, 381–382, 383, 385
  defined, 381

Anterograde labeling, 30

Anterograde transport, 30

Anterolateral system, 132–133

Antianxiety drugs. *See* Anxiolytics

Antibiotics, impact on gut microbiota, 285

Antibodies, 29, A–6, A–7

Antidepressants
  defined, 100
  effects on transmitter reuptake, *97*

overview and description of, 101, 363–365

Antidiuretic hormone (ADH), 226, 270

Antiepileptic drugs, 77

Anti-inflammatory drugs, *136*

Anti-müllerian hormone (AMH), 244, 245

Anti-obesity drugs, 282

Anti-obesity surgery, 282, *283*

Antipsychotics
  defined, 358
  development of, 356–357
  dopamine hypothesis, 358–359
  effects on transmitter receptors, *99*
  glutamate hypothesis, 359–360
  long-term effects of, 357
  overview and description of, 100
  Tourette's syndrome and, 374
  transmitter system targeted, 93

Anxiety disorders
  defined, 369
  drug treatments, 369–370 (*see also* Anxiolytics)
  exposure to childhood bullying and, *343*
  GABA$_A$ receptors and anxiety relief, 89
  obsessive-compulsive disorder, 372–373
  post-traumatic stress disorder, 370–371
  Tourette's syndrome, 373, 374, 375
  types of, 369

Anxiolytics
  alternatives to benzodiazepines, 370
  benzodiazepines, 89
  mechanisms of action, 369–370
  overview and description of, 101
  transmitter system targeted, 93
  treatment of REM behavior disorder, 314

Apes
  vocal behavior and communication, 474–475
  See also Nonhuman primates

Aphasia
  conduction aphasia, 465
  connectist model of, 464–465

definition and overview of, 460

fluent aphasia, *461, 462, 463*

global aphasia, 462, *463*, 464

nonfluent aphasia, 460–462, *463*

recovery from, 480

Aplysia, 395–396

Apoptosis. *See* Cell death

Appetite control
  effects of social factors on, 280–281
  integration of multiple signals in, 275–276
  other systems in, 280, *281*
  role of hormones in, 278–279, 280
  role of the hypothalamus in, 276–280

Appetite control drugs, 282

Appetite suppression, 278–279, 280

Appetitive behavior, 234, 235

Appetitive learning, 330

Apraxia, 146, 460

Arachnoid, 45

Arcuate fasciculus, 464, 465

Arcuate nucleus, 276–278, 279–280

Area MT, 202

Area V2, 201–202

Area V4, 202, 210

Area V5, 202

Arginine vasopressin (AVP), 226, 270

Aristotle, 5, 219

ASL. *See* American Sign Language

Aspirin, 135

Association areas, 129

Associative learning, 386, 387

Astereognosis, 457

Astrocytes, *31*, 32

Ataxia, 148

Athletes, hyperandrogenism and, 248

Ativan. *See* Lorazepam

Atomexetine (Stratera), 437

Atonia, *310*

Atrial natriuretic peptide (ANP), 271

Attention
  alterations in brain functioning, 428–432
  attention deficit hyperactivity disorder, 374, 436–437
  brain areas that create and direct, 433–437
  brain disorders impairing, 435–436

definition and overview of, 420, *421*
limits on, 420–422
reflexive, 435
stroke and, 419
voluntary, 434–435
ways of deploying, 422–428
William James on, 419
Attention deficit hyperactivity disorder (ADHD), 374, 436–437
Attentional bottleneck, 422
Attentional spotlight, 421–422
Atypical antipsychotics. *See* Second-generation antipsychotics
Auditory canal, 156, *157*
Auditory cortex
in the auditory pathway, *160*
central deafness, 167
complex sound processing, 164–165
connectionist model of aphasia, 464
Auditory N1 effect, 429
Auditory nerves, 159–160
Auditory P300, 429–430
Auditory system
complex sound processing, 164–165
ears and the perception of sound, 154–160
effects of auditory attention on event-related potentials, 429–430
hair cells (*see* Hair cells)
hearing loss, 165–169
pitch discrimination, 162–163
signaling from cochlea to cortex, 160–162
sound localization, 163–164
speech processing and right-ear advantage, 454
tonotopic organization, 161
tuning curves of auditory nerve cells, 160
Aura, 77, 78
Autism spectrum disorder, 437
Autobiographical memory, 385
Autonomic nervous system
bodily responses to emotion and, 320, 321
defined, 33
structure and function, 35–36, *37*
synapse rearrangement, 409
Autoradiography, 29, 222, 223–224
Autoreceptors, 98
Averbia, 462

AVP. *See* Arginine vasopressin
Axo-axonic synapses, 73–74
Axo-dendritic synapses, 73, *74*
Axon collaterals, 25
Axon hillocks
action potentials and, 59
defined, 30, 59
propagation of action potentials away from, 64
summation of local potentials, 67
summation of synaptic inputs, 68–70
Axon terminals
defined, 25
size of, *26*
synapses and, 28, 30
Axonal transport
anterograde and retrograde, 30–31
defined, 30
effects of drugs on, 97–98
Axons
defined, 25
differences with dendrites, *68*
propagation of an action potential, 63–65 (*see also* Action potentials)
size of, *26, 27*
structure and function, 25, 30–31
types of synaptic connections, 73–74
Axo-somatic synapses, 73, *74*
Azolam (Halcion), 315, 370

B
Balance, 169–170
Balint's syndrome, 436, 437
Banting, Frederick, *275*
Bar detectors, 198
Barbiturates, 101, 308, 315
Bard, Philip, 321
Bariatric surgery, 282, *283*
Baroreceptors, *269,* 271, *272*
Bartailed godwit, *301*
Basal, 38
Basal forebrain, 90, 308, *310,* 312
Basal ganglia
adult brain, *41*
defined, 43, 386
extrapyramidal system and, 148–149
mesostriatal pathway and, 91
movement impairments from damage to, 148–149
neuromuscular system and, 138

skill learning and, 386, *388*
Tourette's syndrome and, 374
Basal metabolism, 273–274
Basilar membrane
definition and function of, 156, 157
mechanics of, 158
place coding theory and, 158, 162
sound transduction, 159–160
Bat vocalizations, 162
"Bath salts," 106
Bed-wetting, 313
Behavior
behavioral compensation in homeostasis, 266, *267*
effects of attention on, 420–428
effects of frontal lobe lesions on, 444–446
effects of sleep deprivation on, 303
hormones and, 223–224, 249–251, 255–258 (*see also* Behavioral endocrinology)
movement and, 137
Behavioral endocrinology
gonadal hormones and the sexual differentiation of behavior, 249–251
prenatal exposure to androgens and masculinization of adult behaviors, 255–258
techniques in, 223–224
Behavioral intervention, 14
Behavioral medicine, 341
Behavioral neuroscience
commonplace beliefs about the brain, 19–20
definition and overview of, 4
emerging research areas, 9–12
historical roots and development of, 4–8
key questions in, 18–19
relationship to other fields of science, *5*
research design, 13–20
Békésy, Georg von, 153, 158, 168
Belladonna, 188
Benzodiazepine receptors, 370
Benzodiazepines
alternatives to in the treatment of anxiety, 370
defined, 101
in medical interventions for addiction, 113
as sleeping pills, 315

transmitter system targeted, 93
treatment of anxiety disorders, 89
treatment of REM behavior disorder, 314
Berthold, Arnold, 219, 223–224
Best, Charles, *275*
Beta activity, 297, *298*
Beta-amyloid, 415
Beta-blockers, 389
Beta-endorphin, 91
Between-participants experiments, 14
Biceps, *139*
Biggest Loser, The (television show), 263, 274
Bilateral lesions, effects on attention, 436
Bilateral occipitotemporal cortex, 386
Bilateral temporal cortex, *337*
Binaural processing, *160,* 161
Binding affinity, 94
Binding problem, 426, *427*
Binge eating, 284
Binocular, 192, 193
Bioavailability, of drugs, 94
Biological psychology. *See* Behavioral neuroscience
Biological rhythms
circadian rhythms and the endogenous clock, 290–292
definition and overview, 290
suprachiasmatic nucleus and circadian rhythms, 292–296
Biomedical science, male bias in, 244
Biotransformation, 95
Bipolar cells
concentric receptive fields and lateral inhibition, 195–197
defined, 185
on-center and off-center cells, 194–195
organization in the retina, 185, *186*
Bipolar disorder, 367–369
Bipolar neurons, 27, 28
Birds
attentional spotlight, 422
unilateral sleep, 301
vocalizations, 475
Bitter taste, 171, 174
Black widows, *97*
Blind spot, *189,* 190, *191*
Blindness, 212–213, 294

Blindsight, 194
Blood plasma, 268
Blood pressure
    effects of angiotensin II on, 271
    lie detectors and, 322
Blood supply, brain and, 46
Blood supply, stroke and, 47
Blood-brain barrier, 46, 96
Blotting
    defined, A–4
    Northern blots, A–6, A–7
    Southern blots, A–4, A–7
    Western blots, A–6, A–7
Body temperature
    effects of sleep deprivation on, 304
    thermoregulation, 264, 265, 266, 267
Botox, 98
Bottlenose dolphins, 302
Botulinum toxin, 98
Boxers, 479
Brain
    actions of drugs in, 92–99
    areas activated during consciousness, 438–440
    areas involved in memory and learning, 388
    areas that create and direct attention, 433–437
    blood supply, 46
    cellular structure of, 29–30
    central nervous system, 33
    cerebrospinal fluid, 45–46
    changes associated with schizophrenia, 353–356
    changes in activity with depression, 362
    circuits mediating aggression, 336
    circuits mediating emotions, 328–333
    connectome, 45
    effects of sleep, 306
    electroencephalograms, 75–76
    environmental enrichment and neuroplasticity, 392–394, 395
    functional organization, 42–45
    gonadal hormones and the sexual differentiation of, 249–251
    imaging techniques, 48–51
    labeled lines and, 121
    myelination by oligodendrocytes, 31

neuroactive drugs, 100–113 (see also Neuroactive drugs)
    neurotransmitter receptors and, 73
    neurotransmitter systems, 88–92
    orientations for viewing, 38
    outer surface, 36, 39–40
    protective membranes, 45
    reaction-time circuit, 425
    seizures (see Epilepsy; Seizures)
    size of, 26
    stroke (see Stroke)
    subdivisions, 40–41
Brain and behavior. See Behavioral neuroscience
Brain damage
    amnesia from damage to the medial diencephalon, 384–385
    amnesia from damage to the temporal lobes and hippocampus, 379, 381–382, 383, 385, 401
    effects of frontal lobe lesions on behavior, 444–446
    effects on emotions in monkeys, 329–330
    impact of age on recovery from, 480, 481–482
    recovery of function, 478–480
    rehabilitation and retraining, 480–481
    types of cognition affected by right hemisphere lesions, 457–460
Brain development
    adult neurogenesis, 406–407
    changes with aging, 413–415
    interactions of genes with experience, 410–413
    overview, 402–403, 404
    stages of, 404–406
    synapse formation and rearrangement, 407–410
Brain extraction kit, 5
Brain imaging
    studies of deception, 322
    techniques, 48–51
Brain mapping
    origins of and the homunculus, 78–79
    studies of language areas, 466–468
Brain plate, 403
Brain potentials (brain waves), 75–76
Brain self-stimulation, 328, 329

Brain size, intelligence and, 8
Brain stimulation
    deep brain stimulation, 365, 373, 374
    electrodes and the work of José Delgado, 55, 56
    repetitive transcranial magnetic stimulation, 113, 363, 368–369
    self-stimulation, 328, 329
    studies of the language areas, 466–468
    transcranial magnetic stimulation, 51, 467–468
Brain waves. See Brain potentials
Brainstem
    arousal from sleep and, 308, 309, 310
    defined, 40
    extrapyramidal system, 143
    eye-blink reflex and, 396–397
    fluid regulation and, 272
    functional organization, 44
    gustatory system, 175
    neuromuscular system and, 138
    post-traumatic stress disorder and, 371
    pyramidal system and, 142
    synapse rearrangement, 409
Branson, Sir Richard, 476
Bremer, Frédéric, 308, 309
Brightness
    defined, 204
    effects of context on the perception of, 196, 197
Broca, Paul, 8, 460–461
Broca's aphasia, 460–462, 463
Broca's area
    Broca's aphasia, 460–462, 463
    conduction aphasia, 465
    connectionist model of aphasia, 464, 465
    defined, 461
    differences between the cerebral hemispheres, 455–456
    fMRI studies of language processing, 468–469
    subregions, 468
Bromodeoxyuridine, 406
Buccal branch of the trigeminal nerve, 327
Buffers, 169
Bufotenine, 107
Bulbocavernosus, 253–254
Bulimia (bulimia nervosa), 284
Bullying, 343
Bungarotoxin, 72, 73

Bungarus multicinctus, 72
Buspirone (Buspar), 370

C
C fibers, 131, 133
Caffeine, 97, 98
CAH. See Congenital adrenal hyperplasia
Calcium channel blockers, 97, 98
Calcium ions
    defined, 71
    distribution inside and outside neurons, 57
    long-term potentiation and, 398, 399, 400
    in sound transduction, 159
    in synaptic transmission, 70, 71, 84, 85
Caloric restriction, 274
Campral. See Acamprosate
Canine narcolepsy, 312
Cannabidiol (CBD), 102, 103
Cannabinoid receptors, 102, 103, 135
Cannabinoids, 103–104, 135, 136
Cannabis (Cannabis sativa), 102, 103–104, 135, 280
Cannon, Walter, 321
Cannon-Bard theory of emotional responses, 321
Capgras delusion, 330
Capillaries, in the brain, 46
Capsaicin, 131
Carbon monoxide, 92
"Carolina Reaper" pepper, 132
Carotid arteries, 46, 47
CART, 279
Castration
    defined, 218
    effects on testosterone and sexual behavior, 236
    experiments illustrating the functions of hormones, 219
CAT scans. See Computerized axial tomography
Cataplexy, 289, 311, 312, 313
Cathinones, 106
Cations, 56
Cats
    sleep and dreaming, 310
    split-brain studies, 452
    visual receptive fields, 198–199
Cauda equina, 33
Caudal, 38
Caudate nucleus, 43, 374
Causality, 14, 15

CBD. *See* Cannabidiol
CBT. *See* Cognitive-behavioral therapy
CCK. *See* Cholecystokinin
Celexa. *See* Citalopram
Cell body (soma), 25
Cell death
 in brain development, 404, *405*, 407
 defined, 407
Cell differentiation
 in brain development, 404, 405
 defined, 405, A–3
Cell membrane
 defined, 56
 ionic basis of the resting potential of neurons, 57–59
 selective permeability, 58
Cell migration, in brain development, 404–405
Cell nucleus, A–2
Cell-cell interactions, in brain development, 405–406
Central canal, *403*
Central deafness, 166, 167
Central gray, *136*
Central injection of drugs, *95*
Central modification of sensory information, 126
Central nervous system (CNS)
 defined, 32, 33
 divisions in the embryo and the adult, *41*
 pathways and levels of sensory processing, 126–129
 structure of the brain, 36, 39–41 (*see also* Brain)
Central sulcus, 39, *77, 78*
Cephalic phase of insulin release, 275
Cerebellum
 defined, 44, 148, 386
 in the embryo and the adult, *41*
 extrapyramidal system and, 148
 eye-blink conditioning and, 387
 eye-blink reflex and, 396–397
 neuromuscular system and, 138
 nondeclarative memory and, 386, 387, *388*
 sensorimotor skill learning and, 386
 structure and function, 44
 synapse rearrangement, 409
Cerebral aqueduct, 46
Cerebral arteries, 46, *47*

Cerebral cortex
 abnormalities associated with dyslexia, 477
 abnormalities associated with schizophrenia, 355–356
 adult brain, *41*
 auditory pathway from the cochlea, 160–162
 changes with depression, 362
 defined, 36
 development, *409*
 emotional processing and, 321
 environmental enrichment and neuroplasticity, 393–394, *395*
 fatal familial insomnia and, 304
 function, 39
 functional organization, 42–43
 mapping of, *77, 78*
 nicotine and, 104
 structure, 36, 39–40
 synapse rearrangement, 409–410
 thickness of, *26*
Cerebral hemispheres, 36
 See also Left cerebral hemisphere; Right cerebral hemisphere
Cerebral lateralization
 defined, 451, 452
 handedness and, 456–457
 hemisphere differences in auditory specializations, 455–456
 hemisphere differences in information processing, 454–455
 left hemisphere language abilities and aphasia, 460–470
 split-brain studies of hemisphere specializations, 452–454
 types of cognition affected by right hemisphere lesions, 457–460
 Wada tests, 458, 459
Cerebral ventricles, 45–46
Cerebrospinal fluid, 45–46, 306
Cervical dermatome, *127*
Cervical spinal segments, 35
c-fos protein, 29
Chacam baboons, *325*
Chemical communication, 220
Chemical neurotransmission, 84–92

Chemical sensory systems
 modalities and sensed stimuli, *120*
 olfaction, 175–179
 taste, 171–175
Chemical synapses, 73–74
 See also Synapses
Chemical transmitters. *See* Neurotransmitters
Children
 abuse victims and epigenetics, 11, 412
 effects of maternal deprivation on adult stress responses, 340–341
 long-term consequences of bullying, 343
 recovery from hemispherectomy, 481–482
Chili peppers, 131, 132
Chimpanzees
 asymmetry in the planum temporale, 455–456
 facial expressions and emotions, 324–325
 inter-male aggression, 334
 vocal behavior and communication, 474–475
 See also Nonhuman primates
Chloride ions, 57, 68
Chlorinated drinking water, 285
Chlorpromazine (Thorazine), 100, 357, *359*
Choice system, 446
Cholecystokinin (CCK), 92, 280
Cholesterol, 232
Cholinergic, 90
Cholinergic neurons, *89, 90*
Cholinergic receptors, 72–73
Chomsky, Noam, 475
Choroid plexus, 46
Chromosomes
 chromosome 7, 206
 definition and description of, A–2
 Y chromosomes, 244
 See also X chromosomes
Chronic alcoholism, 106–107
Chronic pain, 136
Chronic stress, 341–342
Chronic traumatic encephalopathy (CTE), 479
Chukchee-Kamchtkan language family, *471*
Ciliary muscle, 184, 185
CIMT. *See* Constraint-induced movement therapy
Cingulate cortex
 abnormalities in psychopaths, *337*

 activation by emotions, 333
 cingulotomy and obsessive-compulsive disorder, 373
 consciousness and, 439
 decision making and, 446
 deep brain stimulation treatment of depression, 365
 defined, 133
 executive control and, 444
 limbic system and the mediation of emotion, 329
 pain processing, 133
Cingulate gyrus, 43
Cingulotomy, 373
CIP. *See* Congenital insensitivity to pain
Circadian rhythms
 defined, 290
 endogenous clock and, 290–292
 molecular basis, 295–296
 suprachiasmatic nucleus and, 292–295
 value of, 292
Circumvallate papillae, 172, *173*
Circumventricular organs, 270, 271, *272*
Citalopram (Celexa), 101
City living, risk of schizophrenia and, 352
Classic antipsychotics, 93
Classical conditioning, 8, 386, 387, *388*, 396–397
Claustrum, 439
Climbing fibers, 397
Clitoris
 androgen insensitivity syndrome and, 247
 in congenital adrenal hyperplasia, 246
 defined, 242
 differentiation of, 245
 in human sexual behavior, 242
Cloacal exstrophy, 217, 218, 256
Clock protein, 295, 296
Clomipramine (Anafranil), 373
Clones, 411, A–3
Clozapine, 359
CNS. *See* Central nervous system
Coca, 104
Cocaine, *97, 102,* 104–105
Coccygeal spinal segments, 35
Cochlea
 auditory pathway to the brain, 160–162
 defined, 156

effects of loud noise on, 166–167
Georg von Béskéy and the cochlear wave, 158
hearing loss and deafness, 166–167
perception of pitch and, 162
restoring auditory stimulation in deafness, 168
sound transduction, 159–160
structure and function, 156–157
Cochlear implants, 168, 169
Cochlear nuclei, 160–161
Cochrane, Kent (Patient K.C.), 385
Cocktail party effect, 420
Codons, A–2, A–3
Cognitive maps, 387
Cognitive skills, 386
Cognitive theory, of emotions, 323–324
Cognitive-behavioral therapy (CBT), 365, 366, 369, 373
Cognitively impenetrable functions, 440
Colchicine, 97
Collateral sprouting, 478
Collip, James, 275
Co-localization, 90
Color, 204
Color blindness, 206, 207, 210
Color vision
    in animals, 207
    color blindness, 206, 207, 210
    cone photoreceptors and, 204–206
    dimensions of, 204
    spectral opponent cells, 208–209
    visual cortex processing, 209–210
    wavelengths of light and, 203–204
Color-deficient vision, 207, 210
Color-opponent cells, 208–209
Coma, 439, 440
Combat fatigue, 370
Communication
    defined, 451, 452
    functions of facial expressions, 326–327
    nonhuman primates, 474–475
Complex cortical cells, 198, 199
Complex environment. See Enriched condition
Complex partial seizures, 77
Compulsions, 372, 374

Computerized axial tomography (CAT or CT), 48
Concentric receptive fields, 195–197, 198, 199
Conceptual priming, 386
Concordance, 350–351, 361
Concussion, 479
Conditioned response (CR), 387, 396–397
Conditioned stimulus (CS), 387, 396, 397
Conduction aphasia, 465
Conduction deafness, 166, 168
Conduction velocity, 64–65
Conduction zone, 25, 27
Cones
    color vision and, 204–206
    defined, 185
    in the fovea, 189–190
    organization in the retina, 185, 186
    photopic system, 186, 187
    the question of correcting color blindness, 210
    response to light, 186–187, 195
    spectral opponency and, 208–209
Confabulation, 384–385
Congenital adrenal hyperplasia (CAH), 246, 255–256
Congenital insensitivity to pain (CIP), 131
Congenital prosopagnosia, 459–460
Conjunction searches, 426, 427
Connectist model of aphasia, 464–465
Connectome, 45
Consciousness
    brain regions activated during, 438–440
    defined, 438
    easy problem of consciousness, 440, 441, 442
    elements of, 438
    emerging research in, 11–12
    frontal lobes and the executive system, 444
    hard problem of consciousness, 441, 443
    introduction, 437
    neuroeconomics and decision making, 446
Consolidation, in the memory system, 389
Constraint-induced movement therapy (CIMT), 480–481
Constrictor vestibuli, 254
Contralateral, 38, 452

Control group, 14
Convergence, 186
Coolidge effect, 234, 235
Coprolalia, 374
Copulation
    defined, 234
    intromission and ejaculation, 235
    in rats, 236
    testosterone and, 223–224
    See also Male sexual behavior; Reproductive behavior
Copulatory lock, 235
Cornea, 184–185
Coronal plane, 38
Corpora lutea, 230, 231, 232
Corpus callosum
    abnormalities associated with schizophrenia, 355
    defined, 39, 452
    normal function connecting the hemispheres, 453, 455
    split-brain studies and, 452–454
    split-brain surgery and, 452, 454
Correlation, 14–15
Cortical columns, 42–43
Cortical deafness, 166, 167
Cortical stimulation. See Brain stimulation
Corticospinal system, 142–143
Cortisol, 338, 339, 371
Courtship behavior, of ring-doves, 233
Covert attention, 420, 421
COX-1, 135
COX-2, 135
Crack, 104
Cranial nerve I. See Olfactory nerve
Cranial nerve II. See Optic nerve
Cranial nerve III. See Oculomotor nerve
Cranial nerve IV. See Trochlear nerve
Cranial nerve IX. See Glossopharyngeal nerve
Cranial nerve V. See Trigeminal nerve
Cranial nerve VI. See Abducens nerve
Cranial nerve VII. See Facial nerve
Cranial nerve VIII. See Vestibulocochlear nerve
Cranial nerve X. See Vagus nerve

Cranial nerves
    control of facial expressions, 327
    defined and described, 34–35
    gustatory system, 175
    motor nuclei and the eye-blink reflex, 396, 397
    See also individual cranial nerves
Crib death, 315
Cribriform bone, 176
Critical period, 472
Cross-tolerance, 96
Cryptochrome, 295
CT scans. See Computerized axial tomography
CTE. See Chronic traumatic encephalopathy
Cue-induced drug use, 112
Culture, facial expressions and, 326–327
Curare, 72, 73, 99
Cycle protein, 295
Cyclooxygenase enzymes, 135
Cymbalta. See Duloxetine
Cytosine, A–1, A–2

D

Dams, 240
Darwin, Charles, 324
DBS. See Deep brain stimulation
Deaf community, 168
Deaf people, 465–466
Deafness
    overview, 165–167
    restoring auditory stimulation in, 168
Death genes, 407
Decibel (dB), 154, 155, 167
Decision making, 11, 443, 445–446
Declarative memory
    amnesia from damage to the medial diencephalon, 384–385
    brain structures underlying, 383, 385
    defined, 382
    subtypes, 385, 388
Decomposition of movement, 148
Decorticate rage, 329
Deep brain stimulation (DBS), 365, 373, 374
Deep dyslexia, 476
Deep facial muscles, 327
Default mode network, 438–439
Degradation
    defined, 73

effects of drugs on, *97, 98*
Delayed non-matching-to-sample task, 382
Delgado, José, 55, *56, 78–79*
Delta waves, 297 298
Delta-9-tetrahydrocannabinol (THC), 102, 103
Delusions, 349
Dementia, 314, 414
Dementia pugilistica, 479
Dendrites
    definition and description, 25
    dendritic branches, 394, *395*
    dendritic spines, 70
    dendritic trees, 28
    differences with axons, *68*
    input zone of neurons and, *27, 28*
    neuronal integration of synaptic inputs and, 70
    size of, *26*
    synapses and, 28
    types of synaptic connections, 73, 74
Dendro-dendritic synapses, 74
Dentate gyrus, 399, *406*
Deoxyribonucleic acid (DNA)
    cloning and sequencing, A–3
    defined, A–1
    duplication, *A–2*
    Southern blots, A–4, A–7
    storage of genetic information in, A–1
    transcription, A–2
Dependent variable, 13
Depolarization
    defined, 59
    production of an excitatory postsynaptic potential and, 67
    triggering of an action potential, 59–61
Depressants, 101
Depression
    animal models, 366–367
    changes in brain activity, 362
    defined, 361
    exposure to childhood bullying and, *343*
    genetic studies, 361–362
    reuptake of neurotransmitters and, 73
    sex differences, 365–366
    sleep and, 366
    suicide and, 361
    treatments, 362–365 (*see also* Antidepressants)
Depth perception, 192
Dermatomes, 126, *127*

Descartes, René, 7
Desynchronized EEG, 297
Developmental dyslexia, 477
"D.F.," 183, 202, 211–212
DHT. *See* Dihydrotestosterone
Diabetes mellitus, 275
Diabetes-induced blindness, 213
Diacetylmorphine. *See* Heroin
Diagnostic and Statistical Manual of Mental Disorders (DSM-5), 110, 348
Diazepam (Valium), 101, 314, *370*
Dichotic presentation, 421, 454, 455
Dichromatic color vision, 207
Diencephalon, 40, *41, 403*
Dieting, 263, 273–274
Diffusion, 58, 268
Diffusion tensor imaging (DTI), *48, 49, 465*
Digestive phase of insulin release, 275
Dihydrotestosterone (DHT), 244, 245, 247
DISC1 gene, 351, 354
Disease model of substance abuse, 111
Disrupted in schizophrenia 1 (DISC1) gene, 351, 354
Distal, 38
Disulfiram (Antabuse), 113
Diurnal animals, 290
Divide-attention tasks, 421
Dizygotic twins. *See* Fraternal twin studies
DNA. *See* Deoxyribonucleic acid
DNA sequencing, A–4
Dogs
    decorticate rage, 329
    narcolepsy and, 312
    olfactory receptor neurons, 176
    word learning, 474
Dolphins, sleep in, 301, 302
Dominance, 335
Dopamine
    ADHD and, 437
    antidepressants and, 101
    antipsychotics and, 358–359
    defined, 91
    effects of cocaine on reuptake, 105
    learned helplessness and, 367
    modulation of brain activity, 89–90, 91

reuptake in the synaptic cleft, 73
    substance abuse and, 112
Dopamine D$_2$ receptors
    antipsychotics and, 100, 358
    positive reinforcement and, 91
    Tourette's syndrome and, 374
    valuation system and, 446
Dopamine hypothesis, 358–359
Dopamine receptors
    antipsychotics and, *99, 357, 358*
    multiplicity of subtypes in the brain, *90*
    See also Dopamine D$_2$ receptors
Dopamine-mediated reward system
    ADHD and, 437
    brain self-stimulation and the mediation of emotions, 329
    feeding behavior and, 280
    valuation system and, 446
Dopaminergic neurons/circuits
    brain self-stimulation and the mediation of emotions, 329
    modulation of brain activity, 91
    pathways in the brain, *89*
    Tourette's syndrome and, 374
Dorsal, 38
Dorsal cingulate cortex, 446
Dorsal column system, 126, *127*
Dorsal frontoparietal network, 433, 434–435
Dorsal parietal cortex, 211
Dorsal prefrontal cortex, 443
Dorsal root, *127, 403*
Dorsolateral prefrontal cortex, 444, *445, 446*
Dorsomedial thalamus, 384–385
Dose-response curves, of drugs, 94, *95*
Double hand transplants, 457
Down-regulation, 96, 99
Dravidian language family, *471*
Drinking behavior, 271–272
Drosophila melanogaster, 295
Drug pumps, *275*
Drug tolerance, 96
Drugs
    actions in the brain, 92–99
    administration and elimination of, 94–96
    agonistic and antagonistic actions, 93

analgesics, 101–103, 134–135, *136*
    basis of the behavioral effects of, 83
    effects depend on dose, 94, *95*
    effects on postsynaptic processes, 98–99
    effects on presynaptic processes, 97–98
    examples, 93
    interactions with receptor subtypes, 93–94
    meanings of the term, 93
    neuroactive, 100–113 (*see also* Neuroactive drugs)
    tolerance, 96
    See also Antidepressants; Antipsychotics; Anxiolytics
Drugs of abuse, 93
DTI. *See* Diffusion tensor imaging
DTI tractography, 465
Dualism, 7
Dully, Howard, 347, *348, 357*
Duloxetine (Cymbalta), 365
Dura mater, 45
Dutch famine children, 341
Dynamic endorphins, 103
Dynorphins, 91, 103
Dyskinesia, 357
Dyslexia, 476–478
Dysphoria, 111

E
Ear canal, 156, *157*
Eardrum, 156, 157
Early-selection model of attention, 422
Ears
    perception of sound, 154–160
    sound localization, 163–164
Easy problem of consciousness, 440, *441*, 442
Eating disorders, 283–284
Ecological niche, 306
Ecstasy. *See* MDMA
ECT. *See* Electroconvulsive shock therapy
Ectoderm, 402, *403*
Ectopias, *477*
Ectotherms, 264, 266, *267*
Edema, 32
Edge detectors, 198
EEGs. *See* Electroencephalograms
Effective dose, *95*
Efferent, 38
Effexor. *See* Venlafaxine
Efficacy, 94

Eggs. *See* Ova
Egypt, ancient, 4, *5*
Eisenhower, Dwight, *156*
Ejaculation, 234, 235, 239, 242
Ekman, Paul, 326
Elbow muscles, *139*
Electric neurons
  gross potentials, 75–79
  ionic basis of polarization, 56–59
  ionic mechanisms underlying an action potential, 61–63
  propagation of an action potential, 63–65
  spatial and temporal summation of synaptic inputs, 68–70
  synapses and changes in the postsynaptic membrane potential, 66–68
  synaptic transmission, 70–75
  triggering on an action potential, 59–61
Electrical sensory system, *120*
Electrical stimulation
  in pain control, 135, *136*
  studies of the brain's language areas, 466–467 (*see also* Brain stimulation)
Electroconvulsive shock therapy (ECT), 362–363
Electrodes, 55, *56*
Electroencephalograms (EEGs)
  defined and described, 75–76, 297
  of seizure disorders, *77*
  studies of attention, 428–429
  studies of decision making, 443
  studies of sleep, 297, 298, 299
Electromyography (EMG), 137
Electrostatic pressure, 58
Elephant seals, *334*
Elephant vocalizations, 162–163
Embryo
  brain development, 402, *403*
  defined, 402
Embryonic stem cells, 479
EMG. *See* Electromyography
Emotional learning, 330–332
Emotions
  adaptive value, 325
  bodily responses to, 320–322
  brain circuits mediating, 328–333
  cognitive theory of, 323–324
  consciousness and, *438*
  core set of, 324–328

defined, 320
  effects of frontal lobe injury on, 445
  effects on health, 341
  facial expressions, 324–325, 326–328
  memory and, 389, 390
Empathy, *438*
EnChroma, 210
Encoding, in the memory system, 389
Endocannabinoids, 103, 280
Endocrine, 220
Endocrine communication, 220
Endocrine glands
  defined, 218
  functions of, *218*
  secretions of, 225–233
  See also individual glands
Endocrine system
  actions on cellular mechanisms, 221–225
  actions throughout the body, 218–221
  endocrine glands and their functions, *218*
  endocrine glands and their secretions, 225–233
  interactions with the nervous system, 232–233
  See also Hormones
Endoderm, *403*
Endogenous attention. *See* Voluntary attention
Endogenous opioids, 102–103, 135, *136*
Endogenous substances, 83, 84
Endorphins, 102–103, 134
Endotherms
  defined, 264
  thermoregulation, 264, 265, 266
Energy conservation, sleep and, 306
Engram, 391
Enkephalins, 102
Enriched condition (IC), 393–394, *395*
Enterotype, 284–285
Entrainment
  defined, 291
  light and, 293–295
Environmental enrichment, neuroplasticity and, 392–394, *395*
Enzymes, A–1
Ependymal layer. *See* Ventricular zone
Epididymis, 245
Epidural injections, 134

Epigenetic regulation, 340–341
Epigenetic transmission, 282
Epigenetics
  brain development and, 412
  defined, 11, 412
  effects of maternal care on adult stress reactivity, 3, 11, 340–341, 412
  effects of maternal care on child brain development, 412
  emerging research in, 11
  paternal age and risk of schizophrenia in children, 351
Epilepsy
  causes and types of seizures, 76–77
  defined, 76
  hemispherectomy in children, 481–482
  neurosurgery and, 77
  Patient H.M., 379
  split-brain surgery and, 452, 454
Epinephrine
  defined, 338
  emotional enhancement of memory and, 389, 390
  stress response and, 338, 339, *340*
Episodic memory, 385, *388*
EPSP. *See* Excitatory postsynaptic potential
Equilibrium potential, defined, 58–59
ER-fMRI. *See* Event-related functional MRI
ERPs. *See* Event-related potentials
Essential amino acids, 272
Estradiol, *221, 232*
Estrogens
  definition and functions of, 232
  mechanisms of action, 222
  regulation of, *231*
  sexual behavior and, 236, 243
Estrus, 235
Eszopiclone (Lunesta), 315
Ethics, animal research and, 17
Eukaryotes, A–2
Eunuchs, 219
Event-related functional MRI (ER-fMRI), 434, 435
Event-related potentials (ERPs)
  attention and, 429–431
  definition and overview of, 76, 429
  time base for language processing, 470

Evolutionary psychology, 10
Evolutionary theory, 15
Excitatory neurons, 67
Excitatory postsynaptic potential (EPSP)
  defined, 67
  electrical characteristics of, *69*
  production of, 67
  spatial and temporal summation of, 68–70
  in synaptic transmission, 70, *71*
Executive function, 389, 444
Executive system, 444
Exocrine glands, 218
Exocytosis, 85
Exogenous attention. *See* Reflexive attention
Exogenous substances, 83, 84
Expression, A–3
Expression of the Emotions in Man and Animals, The (Darwin), 324
External ears, *154,* 156, *157,* 164
Extracellular compartment, 268
Extracellular fluid
  as a buffer, 269
  defined, 56, 268
  hypovolemic thirst and, 269, 270–271
  osmotic thirst and, 269–270
  salt concentration, 269
Extraocular muscles, 185
Extrapyramidal system
  defined, 143
  description of, 142, 143
  motor functions, 148
  movement impairments from damage to, 148–149
Extrastriate cortex, 192, 193, 201–202
Eye patches, 213
Eye-blink conditioning, 387
Eye-blink reflex, 396–397
Eyes
  sensitivity to light intensity, 188–189
  structure and function, 184–186 (*see also* Retina)

F
F5 neurons, 146–147
Face blindness. *See* Prosopagnosia
Facial expressions
  functions in communication, 326–327
  mediation by facial muscles, cranial nerves, and CNS pathways, 327–328

in nonhuman primates, 324–325

universal expressions, *326*

Facial feedback hypothesis, 328

Facial muscles, 327

Facial nerve (cranial nerve VII)
control of facial expressions, 327

eye-blink reflex, 396

function, *34, 35*

gustatory system, *175*

Fallopian tubes, 245

False memories, 391

Family studies
of schizophrenia, 349–350

of Tourette's syndrome, 374

Fasciculation, 140

Fast-twitch fibers, 139

Fat cells, 278

Fat tissue, 273

Fatal familial insomnia, 304

Fats, *273*

Fear, 319, 325

Fear conditioning, 330, *331, 332,* 371, 390

Fearlessness, 319, 332

Feature searches, 426, *427*

Fecal transplantation, 285

Feedback control, of hormone secretion, 227–228, 230

FEF. *See* Frontal eye field

Fentanyl, 135

Fetal alcohol spectrum disorder, 106

Fetus
brain development, 402, *403, 404*

defined, 402

Fevers, 266

Fiber tracking, 465

Fight-or-flight response, 36, 338

Final common pathway, 140, 142–143

First-generation antipsychotics, 100, 357, 358, 359, 374

Fisher, Carrie, *369*

5-HT. *See* Serotonin

Flashbulb memories, 390

Flavors, 171

Flinders Sensitive Line, 367

Florez, Guillermo F., 464

Fluent aphasia, *461, 462, 463*

Fluid regulation
drinking behavior, 271–272

overview of, *272*

salt concentration of extracellular fluid, 269

types of thirst, 269–271

water movement between body compartments, 267–269

Fluoxetine (Prozac)
a selective serotonin reuptake inhibitor, 101, 239, 363

transmitter system targeted, 93

treatment of anxiety disorders, 370

treatment of obsessive-compulsive disorder, 373

Fluvoxamine (Luvox), 373

fMRI. *See* Functional MRI

Foliate papillae, 172, *173*

Follicles, 230, *231,* 232

Follicle-stimulating hormone (FSH)
definition and functions of, 230

oral contraceptives and, 232

ovulatory cycle and, *231,* 232

regulation of gonadal steroid hormones, *231*

ringdove courtship behavior and, *233*

Food and energy regulation
appetite control and the hypothalamus, 276–281

basal metabolism and dieting, 273–274

eating disorders, 283–284

glucose and, 273, 275

gut microbiota, 284–285

importance and complexity of, 272

obesity and its treatment, 281–283

role of insulin in, 273, 275–276

Football players, 479

Forebrain
activation by emotions, 332–333

defined, 40, 402

development, 402, *403*

divisions in the embryo and the adult, *41*

extrapyramidal system, 143

slow wave sleep and, 308–309, *310*

Fornix, 43, 329

Fourth ventricle, 46

Fovea, *184,* 189–190, 193

FoxP2 gene, 475

FOXP2 gene, 472, 473, 475

Fractional anisotropy, 465

Fraternal birth order effect, 258

Fraternal twin studies, of schizophrenia, 350

Free nerve endings, *122, 123,* 130–131

Free will, 11, 443, 446

Freeman, Walter, 347, *356*

Free-running cycles, 291, 294–295

Frequency
frequencies of mammal vocalizations, 162–163

of sound waves, 155, 162

Frontal eye field (FEF), 434

Frontal lobe
abnormalities associated with schizophrenia, 355–356

abnormalities in psychopaths, *337*

autobiographical memory and, 385

conceptual priming and, 386

decision making and, 443

defined, 39

emotional, motor, and cognitive changes from damage to, 444–446

executive system and, 444

frontal eye field, 434

Korsakoff's syndrome and, 385

pyramidal system and, 142

Frontal operculum, *175*

Frontal plane, 38

Frontoparietal cortex, 385

Frontoparietal network, consciousness and, 439

Fruit flies, genetic basis of circadian rhythms, 295

FSH. *See* Follicle-stimulating hormone

Functional MRI (fMRI)
of the brain's language areas, 468–470

defined and described, *48, 49*

event-related, 434, 435

studies of deception, 322

Functional tolerance, 96

Fundamental, 155

Fungiform papillae, 172, *173*

Fuseli, Henry, *300*

Fusiform gyrus
face processing and, 431

prosopagnosia and, 458–459, 460

G

G protein–coupled receptors (GPCRs), 176

GABA. *See* Gamma-aminobutyric acid

GABA receptors
anxiolytics and, 370

effects of alcohol on, 106

multiplicity of subtypes in the brain, *90*

GABA$_A$ receptors
anxiety relief and, 89

anxiolytics and, 370

benzodiazepines and, 101

sleep and the tuberomammillary nucleus, 308

Gage, Phineas, 445

Galápagos marine iguanas, *267*

Galen, 5–6

Gallant, Jack, 442

Gametes, 236

Gamma-aminobutyric acid (GABA)
anxiety disorders and, 370

benzodiazepines and, 101

defined, 88

inhibition of motor neurons during REM sleep and, 310

modulation of brain activity, 88

sleep and the basal forebrain, 308, *310*

Gamma-hydroxybutyrate (Xyrem), 312

Gandhi, Mahatma, 319

Ganglia, 40

Ganglion cells
concentric receptive fields and lateral inhibition, 195–197

defined, 185

on-center and off-center cells, 194–195

optic tract, 192

organization in the retina, 185, 186

retinohypothalamic pathway, 294

spectral opponent cells and color vision, 208, *209*

Gardner, Randy, 304–305

Gas neurotransmitters, *86, 87,* 92

Gated ion channels, 57

Gel electrophoresis, A–4, *A–5*

Gender, genitals and, 217

Gene expression
defined, 11, A–3

epigenetics and, 11 (*see also* Epigenetics)

regulation by experience in brain development, 3, 411–413

General anesthetics, 308

Generalized anxiety disorder, 369
Genes
 defined, A–1
 DNA and genetic information, A–1
 interactions with experience, 3, 410–413
 Southern blots, A–4, A–7
 See also Molecular biology
Genetic disorders, 411
Genetic sex, *246*
Genetics
 depression and, 361–362
 schizophrenia and, 349–351, 353
 Tourette's syndrome and, 374
Genital tubercle, 244, 245
Genitals, gender and, 217
Genome, A–3
Genotype, 411
George VI (king of England), *472*
GH. *See* Growth hormone
GHB. *See* Gamma-hydroxybutyrate
Ghrelin, 278–279, 280, *282, 283*
Gibbons, 474
Giffords, Gabrielle, *478*
Gill withdrawal response, 395–396
Glial cells (glia)
 definition and description, 24
 myelination and, 31–32
 problems caused by, 32
 sleep and, 306
 types of, 31
Global aphasia, 462, *463*, 464
Globus pallidus, 43
Glomerulus, olfactory, *176, 177*–178
Glossopharyngeal nerve (cranial nerve IX), *34, 35, 175*
Glucagon, 272, 273
Glucagon-like peptide, 282
Glucocorticoid receptors, 412
Glucocorticoids, 412
Glucodetectors, 275
Glucose
 defined, 272
 energy regulation and, 273
 insulin and, 273, 275
Glucose transporters, 275
Glutamate
 defined, 88
 long-term potentiation and, *398, 399, 400*
 modulation of brain activity, 88–89

receptors, 88–89, *90* (*see also* Glutamate receptors)
 in signaling between retinal cells, 194–195
 umami taste and, 174
Glutamate hypothesis, 359–360
Glutamate receptors
 antipsychotics and, 359–360
 description of, 88–89
 multiplicity of subtypes in the brain, *90*
Glycine, 310
Glycogen, 272, 273
Glymphatic system, 46, 306
GnRH. *See* Gonadotropin-releasing hormone
Goal-directed behavior, 443, 445–446
Golgi stains, 29
Golgi tendon organs, 140, 141–142
Gonadal hormones
 organizational effect and sexual differentiation of the brain and behavior, 249–251
 overview, 230–232
 sexual differentiation of the body and, 244–245
 See also Androgens; Estrogens; Testosterone
Gonadal sex, *246*
Gonadotropin-releasing hormone (GnRH)
 action on the anterior pituitary, 230
 defined, 230
 oral contraceptives and, 232
 regulation of gonadal steroid hormones, *231*
 ringdove courtship behavior and, 233
Gonadotropins, 233
Gonads
 actions of tropic hormones on, 230
 endocrine functions, *218*
 gonadal hormones and sexual differentiation of the body, 244–245
 sequence of sexual differentiation and, 245–246
 sex chromosomes and the differentiation of, 244
 steroid hormones produced by, 230–232
Gorillas. *See* Great apes
GPCRs. *See* G protein–coupled receptors
Graded response, 60

Grammar, 451, 452, 470, 472
Grand mal seizures, 77
"Grandmother cells," 200
Gray matter
 abnormalities associated with schizophrenia, 355
 in the brain, 39–40
 defined, 39
 thinning in the cerebral cortex during brain development, 409–410
Great apes
 vocal behavior and communication, 474–475
 See also Nonhuman primates
Grid cells, 388
Gross neuroanatomy, 32, 33
Gross potentials, 75–76
Growth hormone (GH), 230, 302, 306
Guanine, A–1, A–2
Guevedoces, 247–248
Guinea pigs
 gonadal hormones and sexual differentiation of the brain and behavior, 249
 individual differences in mating behavior, 237
Gulf War veterans, 371
Gustatory cortex, *175*
Gustatory system, 171–175
Gut
 endocrine functions, *218*
 microbiota, 284–285
Gut liners, *283*
Gyri (sing. gyrus), 36

H
Habituation, 395–396
Hair cells
 defined, 156, 157
 effects of loud noise on, *167*
 inducing new growth of, 168
 inner hair cells, *157*, 159, 160
 outer hair cells, *157*, 159–160
 sensorineural deafness, 166–167
 in sound transduction, 159–160
Halcion. *See* Azolam
Haldol. *See* Haloperidol
"Halle Berry neurons," 200
Hallucinogens, 107–109
Haloperidol (Haldol)
 effects on dopamine receptors, 99, 100, *359*
 transmitter system targeted, 93
 treatment of schizophrenia, 100

treatment of Tourette's syndrome, 374
Hamburger, Viktor, 407
Hamsters
 circadian rhythms, 291, 293
 infradian rhythms, 291
 tau mutant, 293, 296
Hand transplants, 457
Handedness, 456–457
Hard problem of consciousness, *441*, 443
Harmonic, 155
Hashish, 103
Head movements, 169, *170*
Health psychology, 341
Hearing. *See* Auditory system
Hearing aids, 168
Hearing loss
 overview, 165–167
 restoring auditory stimulation in deafness, 168
Heart
 discovery of acetylcholine and, 87–88
 hypovolemic thirst and, 271
Heart rate, lie detectors and, 322
Hebb, Donald O., 8–9, 398
Hebbian synapses, 398–401, 409
Helena Fourment as Aphrodite (Rubens), *283*
Helmholtz, Hermann von, 204, 205
Hemiparesis, 146, 461
Hemiplegia, 146, 461
Hemispatial neglect, 435–436, 476
Hemispherectomy, 481–482
Hemorrhagic stroke, *47*
Hering, Ewald, 205, 210
Heroin, 101, *102*, 103, 113
Hertz (Hz), 154, 155
Heschl's gyrus, 165, *477*
Heterocyclics, *363*
Hierarchical cognitive control, 444
"High road" of emotional processing, 330, *331*
High-definition television (HDTV), 200
Hindbrain, 40, *41, 402, 403*
Hippocampal formation, 399–401, 413
Hippocampus
 anterograde amnesia from damage to, *380*, 381, 383, 385, 401
 changes with depression, 362

declarative memory and, 383, 385

defined, 43, 381

effects of environmental enrichment on, 394

long-term potentiation in, 399–401

memory consolidation and, 390

place cells, 387–388

post-traumatic stress disorder and, 371

sexual activity and adult neurogenesis, 243

shrinkage during aging, 413

Hippocrates, 5

Histology, 29

Hofmann, Albert, 108

Homeostasis
definition and overview, 264

fluid regulation, 267–272

food and energy regulation, 272–285

negative feedback control, 264–265

obligatory losses and, 267

redundancy and, 264

thermoregulation, 264, 265, 266, 267

Homosexual behavior, 256–258

Homunculus, 78

Horizontal cells, 185, 186

Horizontal plane, 38

Hormones
activational effects, 236

appetite control and, 278–279, 280

chemical communication and, 220

classification by chemical structure, 220–221

defined, 218

examples of major classes, 221

experiments adding to an understanding of, 219

feedback control mechanisms, 227–228, 230

interaction with neural systems, 232–233

mechanisms of action, 221–222

pituitary gland hormones, 225–230

stress response, 338–339, 340

techniques of behavioral endocrinology, 223–224

Hot peppers, 131, 132

Hubel, David, 198–199

Hue, 204, 210

Hummingbirds, 174

Hunger center, 276

Hunger control. See Appetite control

Huntington's disease, 149

Hybridization
defined, A–2

in Southern blots, A–4, A–5

Hydrocephalus, 46

Hydrogen ions, sour taste and, 173

5- Hydroxytryptamine. See Serotonin

Hyperandrogenism, 248

Hyperpolarization
defined, 59

effect on a neuron, 59–60

of photoreceptors, 187

production of an inhibitory postsynaptic potential and, 67–68

Hypertonic solutions, 270

Hypnosis, 136

Hypocretin, 312
See also Orexin

Hypofrontality hypothesis, 355–356

Hypoglossal nerve, 34

Hypoglycemia, 275

Hypothalamic-pituitary portal system, 229, 230, 233

Hypothalamus
appetite control and, 276–280

connection to the pituitary gland, 225, 226

control of body temperature, 265, 266

coordination of sleep, 308, 310, 311, 312, 313

definition and overview of, 43

endocrine feedback loops and, 228

endocrine functions, 218

fluid regulation and, 270, 271, 272

INAH-3 and homosexual behavior, 257

limbic system and the mediation of emotion, 329, 331

neuroendocrine cells and gonadotropin-releasing hormone, 230

neuroendocrine cells and the posterior pituitary, 225, 227

olfactory system and, 176, 178

oral contraceptives and, 232

ovulatory cycle and, 231, 232

production of peptide hormones, 92

regulation of gonadal steroid hormones, 231

releasing hormones and the anterior pituitary, 228–230

ringdove courtship behavior and, 233

stress response and, 338, 339

suprachiasmatic nucleus and circadian rhythms, 292–295

supraoptic and paraventricular nuclei, 226

vomeronasal system and, 178

Hypotonic solutions, 271

Hypovolemic thirst, 269, 270–271, 272

I

ICC. See Immunocytochemistry

Iconic memories, 388, 389

Identical twin studies, of schizophrenia, 350, 351

IDs. See Interaural intensity differences

Iguanas, 266, 267

IHC. See Immunohistochemistry

IHC afferents, 159, 160

IHC efferents, 159

Imipramine, 101

Imitation, 438

Immediate early gene, 29

Immune system
effects of sleep deprivation on, 304

stress and, 341–342

Immunization, 113

Immunocytochemistry (ICC), 224, 225, A–6, A–7

Immunoglobulins. See Antibodies

Immunohistochemistry (IHC), 29

Impoverished condition (IC), 393, 395

In situ hybridization, 29, 224, 225, A–6

INAH-3. See Third interstitial nucleus of the anterior hypothalamus

Inattentional blindness, 421

Incus, 156, 157

Independent variable, 13

Indifferent gonads, 244

Indo-European language family, 471

Infants, sleep patterns, 301–302

Inferior, 38

Inferior colliculi, 44, 160, 161

Inferior temporal lobe, 425

Infradian rhythms, 290

Ingestion, of drugs, 95

Inhalation, of drugs, 95

Inhibition of return, 425

Inhibitory neurons, 67–68

Inhibitory postsynaptic potential (IPSP)
defined, 68

electrical characteristics of, 69

production of, 67–68

spatial and temporal summation of, 68–70

in synaptic transmission, 70, 71

Inner ear
cochlear wave and pitch coding, 158

defined, 156

Georg von Békésy's experiments, 153, 158

sense of balance, 169–170

sound transduction, 159–160

structure and function of the cochlea, 156–157
See also Cochlea

Inner hair cells, 157, 159, 160

Innervate, 30

Input zone, 25, 27, 28

Insomnia, 302, 314–315

Instrumental conditioning, 387

Insula, 112, 333

Insulin
in appetite control, 278, 279

defined, 272

role in food and energy regulation, 273, 275–276

Insulin pumps, 275

Integration zone, 25, 27

Intelligence quotient (IQ), 8, 410

Intensity
interaural intensity differences, 163–164

of sound, 155

Interaural intensity differences (IDs), 163–164

Interaural temporal differences (ITDs), 163–164

Intermale aggression, 334

Interneurons, 27

Intersex condition, 246

Interstitial fluid, 268

Intracellular compartment, 268

Intracellular fluid, 56

Intrafusal muscle fibers, 140, 141

Intraparietal sulcus (IPS), 434, *435*, 443, 446
Intrathecal injections, 134
Intrinsic activity, 94
Intromission, 234, 235
Inuit-Yupik language family, *471*
Invertebrate nervous systems, synaptic plasticity in, 394–396
Ion channels
  defined and described, 57–58
  ionotropic receptors, 85–86
  size of, *26*
  in sound transduction, 159
Ionotropic receptors
  AMPA receptors, 88
  characteristics of, 85–86
  defined, 85
  glutamate receptors, 88, *90*
Ions
  defined, 56
  distribution inside and outside a neuron, *57*
  ionic basis of polarization, 56–59
  ionic mechanisms underlying an action potential, 61–63
IPS. *See* Intraparietal sulcus
Ipsilateral, 38
IPSP. *See* Inhibitory postsynaptic potential
IQ. *See* Intelligence quotient
Iris, *184,* 188
Ischemic stroke, *47*
Isolated brain, 308
Isolated condition. *See* Impoverished condition
Isolated forebrain brain, 308, *309*
Isotonic solutions, 169
ITDs. *See* Interaural temporal differences

J
James, William, 8, 321, 419
James-Lange theory of emotional responses, 321, 324
Johnson, Virginia, 241, 242
Juvenile-onset diabetes, 275

K
K complexes, 297, *298*
Kandel, Eric, 395
Kartvelian language family, *471*
KE family, 472, *473*
Keller, Helen, *156*
Kennedy, Rosemary, *356*
Ketamine (Special K), *108–109,* 360, 365
Ketones, 273

Khat, 105, 106
Kidneys, fluid regulation and, 270, 271, *272*
Killer whales, 302
King's Speech, The (film), *472*
Kinsey, Alfred, 241
Klüver-Bucy syndrome, 330
Knee-jerk reflex, 55–56, 74, *75*
Knightley, Keira, *283*
Knockout organisms, 222, 223
Kokumi, 171
Korsakoff's syndrome, 384–385

L
L cones, *205,* 206, 208, *209,* 210
Labeled lines, 121, 124, 174–175
Labia, 246, 247
Lamellated corpuscle. *See* Pacinian corpuscle
Lange, Carl, 321
Language
  acquisition of, 472
  basic features of, 471–472
  consciousness and, *438*
  defined, 451, 452
  evolution and major families, *471*
  inborn and learned components, 472–475
Language behavior
  aphasia, 460–466 (*see also* Aphasia)
  brain imaging studies, 468–470
  brain mapping studies, 466–468
  cerebral lateralization and, 452–453, 454–455
  introduction, 470
  left hemisphere and, 452, 453, 454, 455, 459 (*see also* Left cerebral hemisphere)
  models of speech mechanisms, 464–466
  prosody, 456
  reading skills, 476–478
  sense of self and, 451
  See also Speech processing; Vocal behavior
"Larks," 296
Lashley, Karl, 8
Lateral, 38
Lateral frontal cortex, 440
Lateral geniculate nucleus (LGN)
  concentric receptive fields of neurons, 195, *198, 199*
  defined, 193
  reaction-time circuit, *425*

spectral opponent cells and color vision, 208
  visual system, 192, 193
Lateral hypothalamus (LH), 276–277, 280
Lateral inhibition, 196, *197*
Lateral intraparietal area (LIP), 434, 446
Lateral tegmental area, 91
Lateral ventricle, 46, 354
Late-selection model of attention, 422
Lazy eye, 213
Leaky ion channels, 57–58
Learned helplessness, 367
Learning
  defined, 380, 381
  nonassociative, 395–396
  sleep and, 307
  spatial learning, 387–388
  summary of brain regions involved in, 388
  types of, 386–387
Leborgne, M., *461*
Left cerebral hemisphere
  aphasia, 460–466 (*see also* Aphasia)
  brain imaging studies, 468–470
  brain mapping studies, 466–468
  language behavior and, 452, 453, 454, 455, 459, 466–470
  models of speech mechanisms, 464–466
  planum temporale and auditory specialization, 455–456
  right-ear advantage, 454
  split-brain studies of hemisphere specializations, 452–454
  See also Cerebral lateralization
Left frontal cortex, 386
Left-ear advantage, 454
Left-handedness, 456–457
Lens, 184, 185
Leonardo da Vinci, 6
Leptin, 278, *279,* 280
Lesbians, 257–258
Lethal dose, *95*
Letter-by-letter reading, 476
Leu-enkephalin, 91
Levels of analysis, 17–18
Leydig cells, 231
LGN. *See* Lateral geniculate nucleus
LH. *See* Lateral hypothalamus; Luteinizing hormone

Licking and grooming behavior, 340
Lie detectors, 322
Ligand-binding sites, 72
Ligands, 72, 93
Light
  entrainment of the circadian clock, 293–295
  resetting of the endogenous clock, 291
  response of photoreceptors to, 186–187, 195
  visual sensitivity to light intensity, 188–189
  wavelengths and color vision, 203–204
  as a zeitgeber, 291
Limbic system
  adult brain, *41*
  defined, 43, 329
  mediation of emotions, 329–330
LIP. *See* Lateral intraparietal area
Lipids, 273
Liraglutide (Saxenda), 282
Lithium, 367, 368
Lithium chloride, 99
Liver, glucodetectors cells, 275
Lobes, 36
Lobotomy, 347, *348,* 356, 357, 373
Local potentials, 60, 67
Localization of function, 7–8
Locus coeruleus, 91, 309–310, 312
Loewi, Otto, 83, 87–88
Long-term habituation, 395, *396*
Long-term memory
  defined, 389
  kinds of, 382, *388* (*see also* Declarative memory; Nondeclarative memory)
  memory consolidation and, 390
  Patient H.M. and, 381
  reconsolidation, 391
  storage capacity, 390–391
  synaptic changes and, 392
Long-term potentiation
  definition and overview of, 398
  mechanisms in, *398,* 399–401
  memory formation and, 401
Lorazepam (Ativan)
  activation of GABA$_A$ receptors, 89, 101
  a benzodiazepine, 89, 101, 370
  dose-response curve, *95*

transmitter system targeted, 93

Lordosis
  defined, 236
  effects of in utero exposure to testosterone on, 249, 250
  regulation by neural circuitry, 238, *239*

Loudness
  defined, 155
  interaural intensity differences, 163–164
  sensorineural deafness and, 166–167

"Low road" of emotional processing, 330, *331*

Loxapine (Loxitane), 100

Loxitane. *See* Loxapine

LSD (lysergic acid diethylamide)
  definition and effects of, 108
  effect on serotonin receptors, 99
  possible clinical applications, *108–109*

Lumbar dermatome, *127*

Lumbar spinal segments, 35

Lunesta (eszopiclone), 315

Luteinizing hormone (LH)
  definition and functions of, 230
  oral contraceptives and, 232
  regulation of gonadal steroid hormones, *231*
  ringdove courtship behavior and, *233*

Luvox. *See* Fluvoxamine

Lysergic acid diethylamide. *See* LSD

M

M cones, *205*, 206, *207*, 208, *209*, 210

Macaques, *201*

Magentoenecephalography (MEG), 51

"Magic" mushrooms, 107, *108–109*

Magnesium ions, long-term potentiation and, *398*, 399, 400

Magnetic resonance imaging (MRI), *48*, 49

Magnetic sensory system, *120*

Male sexual behavior
  androgens and, 238–240, 250–251, 255–258
  medial preoptic area and, 224, 238–239, 240

testosterone and, 223–224, 233, 236, 237, 243
  See also Copulation; Reproductive behavior

Malleus, 156, *157*

Mammillary bodies, 384–385

Mandibular branch of the trigeminal nerve, *327*

Mania, 367

Manic depression, 367

MAO. *See* Monoamine oxidase

MAO inhibitors. *See* Monoamine oxidase inhibitors

Marijuana. *See* Cannabis

Marine mammals, sleep in, *300*, 301, 302

Masculinization
  androgens and masculinization of adult behavior, 250–251, 255–258
  androgens and masculinization of nervous system regions, 251–254
  gonadal hormones and the organizational effect, 249–251

Master gland, 225

Master, William, 241, 242

Masturbation, 242, 243

Maternal aggression, 336

Maternal behavior
  epigenetic effects on adult stress reactivity, 3, 11, 340–341, 412
  epigenetic effects on child brain development, 412
  regulation of by sex-related hormones, 240–241

Mating behavior. *See* Copulation; Male sexual behavior; Reproductive behavior

Maudsley therapy, 284

McGill Pain Questionnaire, 130

MDMA (3,4-methylenedioxymethamphetamine), 108–109

Meadow vole (*Microtus pennsylvanicus*), 227, *228*

Meaney, Michael, 340, 412

Mechanical receptors, 126

Mechanical sensory system, *120*

Meddis, Ray, 307

Medial, 38

Medial amygdala
  defined, 240, 336
  male arousal in rodents and, *239*, 240
  mediation of aggression in mice, 336

Medial diencephalon, 384–385

Medial forebrain bundle, 329

Medial frontal cortex, 439, *445*

Medial geniculate nuclei, *160*, 161

Medial preoptic area (mPOA)
  defined, 238
  male reproductive behavior and, 224, 238–239, 240

Medial temporal area (area MT), 202

Medial temporal lobes
  declarative memory and, 383
  memory consolidation and, 390
  memory loss from damage to, 382–381, 383, 401

Median eminence, 229, 230

Medulla
  defined, 44
  in the embryo and the adult, *41*
  pyramidal tract, 142–143
  in somatosensory processing, *127*

MEG. *See* Magentoenecephalography

Meissner's corpuscles, 122–123

Melanopsin, 316

Melatonin, 294

Memory
  Alzheimer's disease and, 414–415
  amnesia and damage to the medial diencephalon, 384–385 (*see also* Amnesia)
  defined, 380, 381
  emotion and, 389, 390
  episodic and semantic memory, 385, *388*
  false memories, 391
  impairment with aging, 413
  kinds of, 382 (*see also* Declarative memory; Nondeclarative memory)
  long-term potentiation and, 398–401
  neural mechanisms of, 392–402
  Patient H.M., 379, 380–382, 383, 384, 401
  Patient K.C., 385
  Patient N.A., 384
  post-traumatic stress disorder and, 371
  processes of the memory system, 388–391
  sleep and, 302, 307
  summary of brain regions involved in, 388

Memory trace, 391

Meninges, 45

Meningioma, 45, 49

Meningitis, 45

Menopause, 243

"Meow meow," 106

Mephedrone, 106

Meprobamate (Miltown), 370

Merkels discs, 122–123

Mescaline, 107, 108

Mesoderm, *403*

Mesolimbocortical pathway
  description of, 91
  music perception and, 165
  substance abuse and, 112, 113

Mesostriatal pathway, 91

Messenger RNA
  defined, A–2
  DNA sequencing and, A–4
  formation of, A–2, *A–3*
  formation of proteins and, A–2
  Northern blots, A–6
  in situ hybridization, A–6

Meta-analyses, 364

Metabolic tolerance, 96

Metabotropic glutamate receptors (mGluRs), 89, 360

Metabotropic receptors, *85*, 86, *90*

Metacognition, *438*

Met-enkephalin, 91

Methadone, 113

Methamphetamine ("meth"), *102*, 105–106

Methylation, 11, 412

3,4-Methylenedioxymethamphetamine. *See* MDMA

Methylphenidate (Ritalin), 437

mGluRs. *See* Metabotropic glutamate receptors

Mice
  aggression, *335*, 336
  effects of maternal care on pup brain development, 412
  obese gene, 278
  olfactory receptor neurons, 176
  trace amine–associated receptors, 178–179
  See also Rodents

Michelangelo, 6

Microbiome, 284–285

Microelectrodes, 56–57

Microglial cells, *31*, 32

Micropolygyria, *477*

Microtus ochrogaster (prairie vole), 227, *228*

Microtus pennsylvanicus (meadow vole), 227, *228*
Microvilli, 172, *173*
Midbrain
    defined, 40, 402
    development, 402, *403*
    in the embryo and the adult, *41*
    functional organization, 43–44
    mesolimbocortical pathway and, 91
    mesostriatal pathway and, 91
    in somatosensory processing, *127*
Middle canal, 156, *157*
Middle ear, 156, *157*
Mild traumatic brain injury (mTBI), 479
Milk letdown reflex, 226, *227*, 240
Millivolts, 57
Miltown. *See* Meprobamate
Mindfulness-based stress reduction, 342
Minimally consciousness states, 440
Mirror neurons, 146–147
Mirror recognition, *438*
Mirror-reversed text, 381, *382*
Mirror-tracing task, 381
Mitosis, 404
Mitral cells, *176*
Modafinil (Provigil), 312–313
Molaison, Henry (Patient H.M.), 379, 380–382, 383, 384, 401
Molecular biology
    genes and proteins, A–1
    methods in, A–3
Molly. *See* MDMA
Monaural presentation, 454
Monkeys
    color vision, 207, 208–209
    default mode network and consciousness, 439
    effects of brain lesions on emotions, 329–330
    effects of cocaine on the brain, *105*
    effects of orbitofrontal lesions on behavior, 445
    visual brain areas, *201*
Monoamine hypothesis of depression, 363
Monoamine neurotransmitters, *86*
Monoamine oxidase (MAO), 100, 363

Monoamine oxidase (MAO) inhibitors, *97*, 101, 363
Monoamine transmitters, 105
Monopolar neurons. *See* Unipolar neurons
Monosodium glutamate (MSG), 174
Monozygotic twins. *See* Identical twin studies
Mood disorders
    antidepressants and, 101 (*see also* Antidepressants)
    bipolar disorder, 367–369
    depression, 361–367
Moral model of substance abuse, 111
Morphemes, 470, 471
Morphine, 101, 188
Morris water maze test, 401
Moser, May-Britt and Edvard, 388
Motion, visual perception of, 202
Motion sickness, 170–171
Motivation, 264
Motoneurons. *See* Motor neurons
Motor cortex
    abnormalities in Tourette's syndrome, 374
    connectionist model of aphasia, 464
    control of facial expressions and, 327
    motor functions, 144–146
    sensorimotor skill learning and, 386, *388*
    strokes and, 146
Motor end plates, *139*
Motor homunculus, *143*, 144
Motor nerves, 33
Motor neurons (motoneurons)
    defined, 27, 138
    inhibition during REM sleep, 310
    innervation of muscles, *139*
    motor units, 139–140
    muscle contraction and, 139
    reaction-time circuit, 425
    synapse rearrangement, 408–409
Motor perseveration, 444
Motor plans (motor programs), 137
Motor theory of language, 465–466, 468, 473
Motor tics, *374*
Motor units, 139–140
Movement
    behavior and, 137

    defined, 137
    effects of damage to the extrapyramidal systems on, 148–149
    effects of frontal lobe injury on, 444
    effects of stroke on, 146
    functions of the motor cortex, 144–146
    importance of proprioceptors in control of, 141–142
    subcortical systems involved in, 148
    tracking in others with mirror neurons, 146–147
    See also Neuromuscular system
mPOA. *See* Medial preoptic area
MRI. *See* Magnetic resonance imaging
MSG (monosodium glutamate), 174
mTBI. *See* Mild traumatic brain injury
Müllerian ducts, 244, 245
Multiple sclerosis, 65, 66
Multipolar neurons, 27, 28
Muscarine, 107
Muscarinic ACh receptors, *90*
Muscle contraction, 139
Muscle fibers, 139–140, 141
Muscle spindles, 140–141, 142
Muscles
    antagonists and synergists, 138
    monitoring of length, 140, 141
    monitoring of tension, 140, 141–142
    neuromuscular system and, 137
Musical perception, 165, 456
My Lobotomy (Dully and Fleming), 347
Myelin
    brain development and, 410
    defined, 31, 65
    glial cells and, 31–32
    motor neurons, 140
    multiple sclerosis and, 65, 66
    propagation of an action potential and, *64*, 65
Myopia, 185, 213
Myosin, 138, *139*

N
N1 wave, 429, 430
N2 wave, 431
N400 responses, 470

Naloxone (Narcan), 103, 113, 135
Narcan. *See* Naloxone
Narcolepsy, 289, *310*, 311–313
Nasal hemiretina, 192
Nature-nurture controversy, 3
NE. *See* Norepinephrine
Neandertals, 473
Nearsightedness, 185, 213
Negative feedback
    control of homeostasis, 264–265
    defined, 228, 264
    regulation of hormone secretion, 228, 230
Negative symptoms, 349, *350*
Neologisms, 462
Neonatal, 249
Neonatal period, 249
Neonatal sex reassignment, 217, 256
Nerve fibers. *See* Axons
Nerves, defined, 33, 40
Nervous system
    androgens and sexual dimorphism, 251–254
    cellular components, 24–32
    effects of social influences on the sexual differentiation of, 254–255
    functional organization, 42–46
    interaction with the endocrine system, 232–233
    large scale structure, 32–41
Neural crest, *403*
Neural groove, 402, *403*
Neural plasticity. *See* Neuroplasticity
Neural plate, *403*
Neural tube, 40, 402, *403*
Neuroactive drugs
    antidepressants, 101 (*see also* Antidepressants)
    antipsychotics, 100 (*see also* Antipsychotics)
    anxiolytics, 101 (*see also* Anxiolytics)
    cannabinoids, 103–104
    hallucinogens, 107–109
    opiates, 101–103
    problems of substance abuse and addiction, 109–113
    stimulants, 104–106
    See also Drugs
Neurodmodulators, 98
Neuroeconomics, 11, 446
Neuroendocrine cells
    definition and function of, 225

hormone release from the pituitary gland and, 225–226, 229–230
hypothalamic and gonado-tropin-releasing hormone, 230
Neurofibrillary tangles, *414*, 415
Neurogenesis
adult neurogenesis, 10, 406–407
in brain development, 404, *405*
Neuroleptics, 100
Neuromuscular junctions, 138, 139
Neuromuscular system
extrapyramidal systems, 148–149
functions of the motor cortex, 144–146
mirror neurons, 146–147
muscles, muscle contraction, and motor units, 138–140
organization, 137–138
proprioceptors, 140–142
spinal cord pathways, 142–143
Neuron doctrine, 24
Neurons
axon hillocks, 31
cell death in brain development, 404, *405*, 407
collateral sprouting, 478
cortical, 42–43
definition and description of, 15, 24
dendritic trees, 28
effects of attention on the activity of, 431–432
glial cells and, 31
interactions with the endocrine cells, 233
invertebrate nervous systems, 394–396
mechanistic approach to research and, 15
neurogenesis, 10, 404, *405*, 406–407
principle divisions and types of, 24–25, 27–28
size of, *26*
structure and function of axons, 30–31 (*see also* Axons)
synapses (*see* Synapses)
thickness of membranes, *26*
visualizing in the brain, 29–30
Neuropathic pain, 133, *134*
Neuropeptide Y (NPY), 92

Neurophysiology
classic pattern of neural function, 55–56
defined, 55, 56
electric neurons, 56–70
Neuroplasticity
defined, 10, 30, 392
emerging research in, 10
environmental enrichment and, 392–394, *395*
long-term potentiation, 398–401
neuropathic pain, 133
Neuroscience, 4
Neurosurgery
brain mapping and, *77*, 78
hemispherectomy, 481–482
lobotomy, 347, *348*, 356, 357, 373
for seizures, 77
split-brain surgery, 452, 454
Neurotensin, 92
Neurotransmitter receptors
in the brain, 73
characteristics of, 86
definition and function of, 30, 72, 85
degradation and reuptake of, 73
diversity of receptor subtypes, 86
effects of drugs on, 99
ionotropic and metabotropic, 85–86
ligand-binding sites, 72
properties of, 72–73
in synaptic transmission, 70, *71, 84*, 85
types of, 72–73, *86*, 87
Neurotransmitters
in the brain, 88–92
co-localization, 90
defined, 30, 66, 85
discovery of acetylcholine, 87–88
effects of drugs on, 97–98
effects on the postsynaptic membrane potential, 66–68
as endogenous substances, 83
excitatory or inhibitory effects of, 68
graded release by photoreceptors, 185, *186*, 187
knee-jerk reflex and, 56
properties of receptors, 72–73
release into the synaptic cleft, 66, 71–72

of the sympathetic and parasympathetic systems, 36
in synaptic transmission, *28*, 30, 70, *71, 84*, 85
Neurotrophic factors, *107, 108*, 410
Niche adaptation, 306
Nicotine, 72, *99*, 104
Nicotine patches, 113
Nicotinic ACh receptors
characteristics of, 72–73
effects of curare on, 99
functions of, *90*
nicotine and, 104
"Night owls," 296
Night terrors, 300
Nightmare, The (Fuseli), *300*
Nightmares, 300
Nissl stains, 29
Nitric oxide, 92
NMDA receptors
defined, 399
effects of phencyclidine on, 360
functions of, *90*
glutamate and, 88
long-term potentiation and, *398*, 399, 400, 401
Nociceptors, 130–131
See also Free nerve endings
Nocturnal animals, 290
Nodes of Ranvier, 31, *64*, 65
Nonassociative learning, 395–396
Nondeclarative memory
animal research, 387–388
defined, 382
types of, 386–387, *388*
Nonfluent aphasia, 460–462, *463*
Nonhuman primates
asymmetry in the planum temporale, 455–456
color vision, 207, 208–209
facial expressions and emotions, 324–325
fetal brain development, *404*
handedness, 456
vocal behavior and communication, 474–475
Nonprimary motor cortex, 138, 145
Nonprimary sensory cortex, 128, 129
Non-REM sleep, 297, *299*, 300
Nonsleepers, 307
Noradrenaline. *See* Norepinephrine
Noradrenergic neurons, *89*, 91

Norepinephrine (NE)
ADHD and, 437
antidepressants and, 101
defined, 91, 338
effects of cocaine on reuptake, 105
emotional enhancement of memory and, 390
modulation of brain activity, 89–90, 91
reuptake in the synaptic cleft, 73
stress response, 338, 339, *340*
sympathetic system and, 36
Norepinephrine receptors, *90*
Normal flora, 284
Northern blots, A–6, A–7
Nose, 175–178
NPY. *See* Neuropeptide Y
NPY neurons, 279, 280
Nucleotides
defined, A–1
in DNA, A–1
DNA sequencing and, A–4
in RNA, A–2
Nucleus (central nervous system), 40
Nucleus accumbens
brain self-stimulation and the mediation of emotions, 329
defined, 112, 329
substance abuse and, 112
valuation system and, 446
Nucleus of the solitary tract, *175, 279*, 280
Nutrients, 272

O

obese gene, 278
Obesity
dieting and basal metabolism, 263, 274
epigenetic transmission, 282
gut microbiota and, 285
as a public health epidemic, 263, 281–282
treatments, 282–283, 285
Object recognition task, 382
Obsessions, 372
Obsessive-compulsive disorder (OCD), 372–373, 374
Occipital chiasm, *189*, 190
Occipital cortex, 190, 191, *201*, 430
Occipital lobe, 39
Occipitotemporal cortex, 386
OCD. *See* Obsessive-compulsive disorder
Oculomotor apraxia, 436

Oculomotor nerve (cranial nerve III), 34
Odorants, 176, 177
Odors, 175
Off-axis sounds, 163
Off-center bipolar cells, 194, 195
Off-center ganglion cells, 195
Off-center/on-surround receptive field, 195, *196, 198*
OHC afferents, 159
OHC efferents, 159–160
O'Keefe, John, 388
Old World monkeys, color vision, 207
Olfaction
    defined, 175
    description of, 175–178
    effects of pregnancy on, 240–241
Olfactory bulb, 43, *176,* 177–178
Olfactory cilia, *176*
Olfactory epithelium
    definition and description of, 175–177
    trace amine–associated receptors, 178–179
Olfactory mucosa, *176*
Olfactory nerve (cranial nerve I), 34
Olfactory receptor neurons, 175–177
Olfactory system, 175–178
Olfactotopic map, 178
Oligodendrocytes, 31
On-center bipolar cells, 194–195
On-center ganglion cells, 194–195
On-center/off-surround receptive field, 195, *196, 198*
Ongoing phase disparity, 163
Onset disparity, 163
Ontogeny, 15
Onuf's nucleus, 254
Operant conditioning, 387
Opiate antagonists, 103
Opiates
    addiction, 112
    medical interventions for addiction, 113
    overview and description of, 101–103
    in pain control, 134–135, *136*
Opioid peptide, 91
Opioid peptide neurotransmitters, *86*
Opioid receptors, 102, 103
Opium, 101, 315

Opium poppy, 101
Opponent-process hypothesis, 205
Opsins, *187,* 205
Optic ataxia, 211–212, 436
Optic chiasm, 191, *192*
Optic disc, *184, 189,* 190, *191*
Optic nerve (cranial nerve II), 34, *184,* 185, 191
Optic radiations, 192, 193
Optic tract, 192
Optogenetics, 336
Oral contraceptives, 232
Orangutans. *See* Great apes
Orbitofrontal cortex
    decision making and, *446*
    effects of lesions on behavior, 445
    olfactory system and, *176, 178*
Orexigenic neurons, 279–280
Orexin, 280, *310,* 312, 313
Organ of Corti
    effects of loud noise on, *167*
    sound transduction, 159–160
    structure and function, 156–157
Organum vasculosum of the lamina terminalis (OVLT), 270, *272*
Orgasm, 241, 242
Orlistat (Xenical), 282
Osmosensory neurons, *269,* 270, *272*
Osmosis, 268
Osmotic pressure, 268
Osmotic thirst, 269–270, *272*
Ossicles, 156, 157, 168
Otolithic membrane, 169
Ototoxic, 166
Outer hair cells, *157,* 159–160
Output zone, defined, 25, *27*
Ova (eggs)
    defined, 236
    fusion with sperm, 236
    release in the ovulatory cycle, *231,* 232
Oval window, 156, *157*
Ovaries
    actions of tropic hormones on, 230
    defined, 232
    endocrine functions, *218*
    sex chromosomes and the differentiation of, 244
    steroid hormones and, *231,* 232
Overt attention, 420
Oviducts, 245

OVLT. *See* Organum vasculosum of the lamina terminalis
Ovulation, 236
Ovulatory cycle, *231, 232*
Oxycodone (OxyContin), 101, 135
OxyContin. *See* Oxycodone
Oxytocin, 92, 226–227

P
P1 wave, 429, 430
P3 effect, 429–430
P3 wave, 429–430
P600 response, 470
Pacinian corpuscles, 122, *123,* 126
Pain
    chronic, 136
    control of, 134–136
    defined, 130
    neuropathic, 133, *134*
    significance and dimensions of, 130
Pain pathway
    anterolateral system, 132–133
    effects of eating super-hot chili peppers, 132
    nociceptors, 130–131
    overview, 126, 128
Painkillers. *See* Opiates
Pair-bonds, 227, *228*
Pancreas, *218,* 273, 278
Panic disorder, 369
Papez, James, 329
Papillae, 172, *173*
Parabiotic, 240, *241*
Para-chlorophenylalanine, *97*
Paradoxical sleep, 297, 299
    See also Rapid-eye-movement sleep
Parahippocampal place area, 431
Paralysis, curare and, 99
Paralytic dementia, 349
Paraphasia, 460, 462
Parasympathetic nervous system
    bodily responses to emotion and, 320, 321
    defined, 36, 320
    neurotransmitter of, 36
    stress response and, 338, *339*
    structure and function, 36, 37
Paraventricular nuclei
    in appetite control, *279,* 280
    fluid regulation and, *272*
    neuroendocrine function, 226, *227*
"Parentese," 472

OVLT. *See* Organum vasculosum of the lamina terminalis
Paresis, 146
Parietal lobe
    abnormalities associated with dyslexia, 477
    Alzheimer's disease and, 414
    autobiographical memory and, 385
    bilateral lesions and Balint's syndrome, 436
    brain mapping and, *77, 78*
    defined, 39
    effects of right hemisphere lesions on spatial cognition, 457–458
    networks generating and directing attention, 433–435
Parietal temporal cortex, 362
Parieto-occipital cortex, 385
Parkinson's disease
    basal ganglia and, 148
    defined, 148
    REM behavior disorder and, 314
    substantia nigra and, 44
Paroxetine (Paxil), 370
Partial agonists, 93
Paternal age, risk of schizophrenia in children and, 351
Patient H.M. (Henry Molaison), 379, 380–382, 383, 384, 401
Patient K.C. (Kent Cochrane), 385
Patient N.A., 384
Pattern coding, 174, 175
Pavlov, Ivan, 8, 387
Pavlovian conditioning, 386
Paxil. *See* Paroxetine
PCP. *See* Phencyclidine
PCR. *See* Polymerase chain reaction
Peek, Kim, 391
Penfield, Wilder, 77, 78
Penis
    cloacal exstrophy and, 217, 218
    defined, 242
    differentiation of, 245
    human sexual behavior and, 242
    5-alpha-reductase deficiency and, 248
Peptide hormones, 220, 221–222
Peptide neurotransmitters, *86,* 87, 91–92
Peptide receptors, *90*
Peptides, A–2, A–3
Perceptual priming, 386
Perceptual skills, 386
Periaqueductal gray

defined, 44, 238
lordosis circuit and, 238, *239*
opioid receptors and, 102
in pain control, 134
pain perception and, 133, 134
Period, of cycles, 291
Period protein, 295, 296
Peripheral injection, of drugs, *95*
Peripheral nervous system, 33–36
Peripheral spatial cuing, 424–425
Perseverate, 444
Personal agency, 443, 446
Personal memory, 385
PET. *See* Positron emission tomography
Petit mal seizures, 77
Phallus
    in congenital adrenal hyperplasia, 246
    defined, 242
    in human sexual behavior, 242
    5-alpha-reductase deficiency and, 247, 248
Phantom limb pain, 133, *134*
Pharmacokinetics, 95
Phase shifts, 291
Phasic receptors, 125
Phencyclidine (PCP), 359–360
Phenobarbital, *95, 101*
Phenotype, 411
Phenotypic sex, *246*
Phenylalanine, 411
Phenylketonuria (PKU), 411
Pheromones
    chemical communication and, 220
    male arousal in rodents and, 239–240
    vomeronasal system and, 178–179
Phillips, Tina Geula, 451, 462, 464
Phobic disorders, 369
Phonemes, 470, 471
Photic sensory system, *120*
Photopic system, 186, *187, 188*
Photopigments, color vision and, 205, 206, 207
Photoreceptor adaptation, 188–189
Photoreceptors
    adaptation, 188–189
    defined, 185
    graded release of neurotransmitters, 185, *186,* 187

organization in the retina, 185, 186
receptive fields, 194–195
response to light, 186–187, 195
scotopic and photopic systems, 186, *187*
types of, 185
Phrenology, 7, 8
Physical dependence model of substance abuse, 111, 112
Physiological psychology. *See* Behavioral neuroscience
Physiological saline solutions, 169
Pia mater, 45
Pigeons, 391
Pigmented epithelium, *186*
Pineal gland, *218,* 293–294
Pinnae, *154, 156, 157,* 164
Pitch (head motion), 169, *170*
Pitch (sound)
    defined, 155
    perception of, 162–163, 165
Pitch coding, 158
Pittsburgh Blue dye, 415
Pituitary gland
    anterior pituitary hormones and actions, 228–230 (*see also* Anterior pituitary)
    defined, 225
    endocrine functions, *218*
    feedback control mechanisms, 227–228
    ovulatory cycle and, *231,* 232
    posterior pituitary hormones and actions, 226–227, *228*
    production of peptide hormones, 92
    ringdove courtship behavior and, 233
    stress response and, 338, *339*
Pituitary stalk, 225, *226*
PKU. *See* Phenylketonuria
Place cells, 387–388
Place coding theory, 162
Placebo effect, 135
Placebos, 135, *136*
"Plant food," 106
Planum temporale, 455–456, *477*
Plegia, 146
POA. *See* Preoptic area
"Poison hypothesis" of motion sickness, 170
Poisons, actions on neurotransmitter receptors, 72
Polarization, ionic basis of, 56–59
Polygraphs, 322

Polymerase chain reaction (PCR), A–4
Polymodal neurons, 129
POMC neurons, 279, 280
Pons (pontine system)
    defined, 44
    in the embryo and the adult, *41*
    REM sleep and, 308, 309–311
Pontine center, 313
Positive reinforcement, mesolimbocortical pathway and, 91
Positive reward model of substance abuse, 111–112
Positive symptoms, 349, *350*
Positron emission tomography (PET), 48, 49, 51
Posner, Michael, 423–424
Postcentral gyrus
    brain mapping and, 77, 78
    defined, 39
    somatic sensation and, 457
Postcopulatory behaviors, 235
Posterior, 38
Posterior parietal cortex, 414
Posterior pituitary, *218,* 226–227, *228*
Posterior temporal cortex, 362
Postmenopausal treatment, 232, 243
Postpartum depression, 365–366
Postsynaptic, 28, 67
Postsynaptic cell, 67
Postsynaptic membrane, *28, 30,* 70, *71*
Postsynaptic neurons
    effects of drugs on, 98–99
    long-term potentiation, 398–400
    spatial and temporal summation of synaptic inputs, 68–70
    in synaptic transmission, 28, 30, 70, *71*
Postsynaptic potential
    changes in caused by neurotransmitter release into the synapse, 66–68
    defined, 67
    excitatory or inhibitory, 67–68 (*see also* Excitatory postsynaptic potential; Inhibitory postsynaptic potential)
    spatial and temporal summation of, 68–70

Post-traumatic stress disorder (PTSD)
    definition and description of, 370–371
    emotional enhancement of memory and, 390
    fear conditioning and, 330, 332
Potassium ions
    defined, 58
    distribution inside and outside a neuron, 57
    ionic basis of the resting potential of neurons, 58–59
    in sound transduction, 159
Potency, *95*
Pragmatics, 472
Prairie vole (*Microtus ochrogaster*), 227, *228*
Precentral gyrus
    brain mapping and, 77, 78
    connections from the arcuate fasciculus, 465
    defined, 39, 144
    primary motor cortex, 143, 144
Predators, visual field, 191
Prefrontal cortex
    activation by emotions, 333
    activation during lying, *322*
    consciousness and, 439
    decision making and, 446
    defined, 444
    development, 410
    effects of chronic pain, 136
    emotional, motor, and cognitive effects of lesions, 444–446
    executive system and, 444
    reaction-time circuit, 425
    visual region, 202
Pregnancy, effects on odor discrimination, 240–241
Premotor cortex
    defined, 145
    mirror neurons, 146–147
    motor functions, 145
    reaction-time circuit, 425
Preoptic area (POA)
    control of body temperature in rats, 265
    fluid regulation and, 270, 271, *272*
    homosexual behavior and, 257
    sexual dimorphism in rats, 251–253
Prepyriform cortex, *176, 178*
Presynaptic, 28, 67, 85
Presynaptic cell, 67

Presynaptic membrane
  defined, 30
  in synaptic transmission, *28,
    30, 84,* 85
Presynaptic neurons
  effects of drugs on, 97–98
  long-term potentiation and,
    398, 400
  neurotransmitter release into
    the synaptic cleft, 71–72
  in synaptic transmission, 28,
    30, 70, *71*
Prey animals, visual field, 191
Primary auditory cortex (A1)
  connectionist model of
    aphasia, 464
  defined, 161
  planum temporale and au-
    ditory specialization of the
    hemispheres, 455–456
  responses to sound, 161
Primary motor cortex
  body map and motor ho-
    munculus, *143,* 144
  motor representations in,
    144–145
  neuromuscular system and,
    138
  nonfluent aphasia and, 461
  pyramidal tract and, 143
  reaction-time circuit, 425
Primary olfactory cortex, *176,
  178*
Primary sensory cortex, 128
Primary somatosensory cortex
  abnormalities in Tourette's
    syndrome, 374
  defined, 129
  organization and represen-
    tation of the body surface,
    128–129
  in somatosensory processing,
    127, 128
Primary visual cortex (V1)
  color perception and,
    209–210
  connection to the temporo-
    parietal junction, 435
  defined, 193
  effects of attention on recep-
    tive fields of neurons, 432
  extrastriate regions and, *201*
  mesostriatal pathway, 91
  reaction-time circuit, 425
  receptive fields of neurons,
    198–199
  synapse rearrangement, 409
  topographic projection of
    visual space, 193
  visual processing, 192–193

what and *where* processing
    streams, 211–212
Primates. *See* Nonhuman pri-
  mates
Primers, A–4
Priming, 386, *388*
Principles of Psychology (James),
  8
Proactive aggression, 335
Probes, A–4
Procedural memory. *See* Non-
  declarative memory
Proceptive, 234, 235
Progesterone, *231,* 236
Progestins, 232
Project D.A.R.E., 111
Propranolol, 389, 390
Proprioception, 119, 140–142
Prosody, 456, 472
Prosopagnosia, 458–460
Proteins
  defined, A–1
  formation of, A–2
  Western blots, A–6, A–7
Protons, sour taste and, 173
Provigil. *See* Modafinil
Proximal, 38
Prozac. *See* Fluoxetine
Psilocybe, 108
Psilocybin, 107, *108–109*
Psychiatric disorders
  anxiety disorders, 369–375
  biological perspective, 349
  incidence, *9*
  mood disorders, 361–369
  neuroactive drugs and,
    100–103
  prevalence, 348–349
  schizophrenia, 349–360 (*see
    also* Schizophrenia)
Psychoactive drugs, 93
  See also Neuroactive drugs
Psychogenic pain control, *136*
Psychoneuroimmunology, 341
Psychopaths, 336, *337*
Psychopharmacology, 100–113
  See also Neuroactive drugs
Psychosomatic medicine, 341
Psychotomimetics, 359–360
PTSD. *See* Post-traumatic stress
  disorder
Puberty
  guevedoces and 5-alpha-re-
    ductase deficiency, 247–
    248, 249, 256
  as a sensitive period, 249–
    250
  shift in the circadian rhythm
    of sleep, 296

Pulvinar, 433
Punch-drunk syndrome, 479
Pupil, *184,* 188
Pure tone, 155
Putamen, 43
Pyramidal cells, 42
Pyramidal system (pyramidal
  tract), 142–143, 144
PYY$_{3-36}$, 278–279, 280, 282

Q
Qat, 105, 106
Qualia, 443
Quaternary amine neurotrans-
  mitters, *86*

R
Ramón y Cajal, Santiago, 24
Range fractionation, 188
Raphe nuclei, 91
Rapid-cycling bipolar disorder,
  367
Rapid-eye-movement (REM)
  sleep
  defined, 297
  depression and, 366
  description of, 298–299
  in different species, 301
  dreaming and, 300
  in infants, 302
  learning and, 307
  narcolepsy and, 311–312
  the pons and, 308, 309–311
  properties of, *299*
  in sleep recovery, 305
Rats
  adult neurogenesis, 407
  animal model of depression
    and, 367
  appetite control and the hy-
    pothalamus, 276–277
  cannabinoid receptors in the
    brain, *103*
  default mode network and
    consciousness, 439
  effects of sleep deprivation
    on, 304
  effects of social experience
    on sexual differentiation of
    the nervous system, 254
  environmental enrichment
    and neuroplasticity, 392–
    394, *395*
  epigenetic effects of maternal
    care, 3, 11
  Flinders Sensitive Line, 367
  hippocampal place cells,
    387–388
  hypothalamus and control of
    body temperature, 265

individual differences in
    mating behavior, 237
  lordosis, 236, 238, *239*
  olfactory system, *177*
  opioid receptors in the brain,
    102
  reproductive behavior, 236
  sexual dimorphism the spi-
    nal nucleus of the bulbo-
    cavernosus, 253–254
  sexually dimorphic nucleus
    of the POA, 251–253
  stress immunization, 339–
    340
  See also Rodents
Reaction-time responses, 425
Reactive aggression, 335
Reading skills, 476–478
Receptive fields
  concentric, 195–197
  defined, 125, 194
  effects of attention on, 432
  in extrastriate areas, 201–202
  of the lateral geniculate nu-
    clei, 195
  of the photopic and scotopic
    systems, *187*
  of retinal cells, 194–197
  of the somatosensory sys-
    tem, *124,* 125
  of the visual cortex, 198–199
Receptor agonists, 93, 99
Receptor antagonists, 93, 99
Receptor cells
  adaptation to unchanging
    stimuli, 125–126
  defined, 120
  function of, 120
  labeled lines and, 121
  sensory transduction,
    122–123
Receptor subtypes, 86, *90*
Receptor supersensitivity, 357
Reconsolidation, of long-term
  memories, 391
Recovered memories, 391
Recovery of function, 478–480
Red nucleus, 143
5-alpha-Reductase
  defined, 244
  guevedoces and deficiency in,
    247–248, 249, 256
  sexual differentiation of the
    body and, 245
Reductionism, 17
Redundancy, homeostasis and,
  264
Reflexes
  defined, 137

effects of spinal injuries on, 143

eye-blink reflex, 396–397

knee-jerk reflex, 55–56, 74, *75*

milk letdown reflex, 226, *227*, 240

spinal circuits in, 142

Reflexive attention, 424–426, 435

Refraction, 184–185

Refractory period

absolute refractory phase, 61–62

action potential compared to a flushing toilet, 65

defined, 61

relative refractory phase, 62

Refractory phase, 234, 235, 242

Relative refractory phase, 62

Relaxation training, 342

Releasing hormones, 228–230

REM behavior disorder, 313–314

REM sleep. *See* Rapid-eye-movement sleep

Repetition priming, 386

Repetitive transcranial magnetic stimulation (rTMS), 113, 363, 368–369

Reproductive behavior

fusion of gametes and, 236

human sexual behavior, 241–243

individual differences in, 237

in rats, 236

regulation by neural circuitry, 238–241

stages of, 234–235

steroid hormones and, 230–232, 236, 243

See also Copulation; Male sexual behavior

Research design

animal research, 15–17

challenges in behavioral neuroscience, 13

levels of analysis, 17–18

theoretical orientations, 15

types of study designs, 13–15

Reserpine, *97*

Respiratory rate, lie detectors and, 322

Rest-and-digest response, 36

Resting potential, 56–59

Reticular formation (reticular activating system)

arousal from sleep and, 309, *310*

connections to the hypothalamic sleep center, 312

defined, 44, 309

extrapyramidal system, 143

Retina

defined, 184

lateral inhibition between receptor cells, 196, *197*

neural connections to the brain, 191–192

optic disc and the blind spot, *189*, 190, *191*

photoreceptors (*see* Photoreceptors)

receptive fields of bipolar and ganglion cells, 194–197

scotopic and photopic systems, 186, *187, 188*

structure and function, 185–186

visual acuity and the fovea, 189–190

visual field and, 193

Retinohypothalamic pathway, 294

Retinotopic mapping, 193

Retrieval, in the memory system, 389

Retrograde amnesia, 380–381

Retrograde labeling, 30

Retrograde transmitters, 92, 400

Retrograde transport, 31

Reuptake

defined, 73, 85

effects of amphetamine on, 105

effects of cocaine on, 105

effects of drugs on, *97, 98*

in synaptic transmission, *84,* 85

Reuptake inhibitors, *97, 98*

Reward system. *See* Dopamine-mediated reward system

Rhodopsin, 187

Ribonucleic acid (RNA)

defined, A–2

Northern blots, A–6, A–7

Ribosomes, A–2

Right cerebral hemisphere

linguistic ability and, 452–453

perception of music and prosody, 456

planum temporale and auditory specialization, 456

spatial cognition and, 453–454, 455, 457–458

split-brain studies of hemisphere specializations, 452–454

types of cognition affected by damage to, 457–460

See also Cerebral lateralization; Right-hemisphere lesions

Right tempoparietal network, 433, *434,* 435

Right-ear advantage, 454

Right-handedness, 456–457

Right-hemisphere lesions

hemispatial neglect, 435–436

types of cognition affected by, 457–460

Ringdove courtship behavior, 233

Risperidone, *359*

Ritalin. *See* Methylphenidate

Rodents

adult neurogenesis, 406–407

circadian rhythms, 290–291

effects of maternal care on pup brain development, 412

gonadal hormones and sexual differentiation of the brain and behavior, 249, 250, 251

individual differences in mating behavior, 237

lordosis, 236, 238, *239*

oxytocin and social behavior, *227, 228*

regulation of maternal behavior by sex-related hormones, 240

reproductive behavior, 236

See also Mice; Rats

Rods

defined, 185

organization in the retina, 185, 186

response to light, 186–187, 195

scotopic system, 186, *187*

variation in density across the retina, *189,* 190

Roll (head motion), 169, *170*

Rostral, 38

Round window, *157*

Roux-en-Y bypass surgery, *283*

rTMS. *See* Repetitive transcranial magnetic stimulation

Rubens, Peter Paul, *283*

Ruffini corpuscles, *122,* 123

S

S cones, *205,* 206, 208, *209*

Saccule, 169, *170*

Sacral dermatome, *127*

Sacral spinal segments, 35

SAD. *See* Seasonal affective disorder

Sagittal plane, 38

Salt (sodium chloride)

concentration in extracellular fluid, 269

hypertonic solutions, 270

hypotonic solutions, 271

osmotic thirst and, 269–270

Saltatory conduction, *64,* 65, 66

Salty taste, 171, 172–173

Salvia divinorum, 108

Satiety center, 276

Satiety hormones, 278–279, 280

Saturation, 204

Savants, 391

Saxenda (liraglutide), 282

Scala media, 156, *157*

Scala tympani, 156, 157

Scala vestibuli, 156, 157

Scalp whorl, *457*

Schacter, Stanley, 323–324

Schizophrenia

abnormal P3 responses, 430

antipsychotics and, 100, 356–360

changes in brain structure and function, 353–356

defined, 349

emerging research in, 9

genetic studies, 349–351, 353

integrative model of, 353

lobotomy and, 347, *348,* 356, 357

mesolimbocortical pathway and, 91

prevalence, *348,* 349

stress and, 352, 353

symptoms, 349, *350*

Schwann cells, 31

SCN9A gene, 131

Scotomas, 193–194, 480

Scotopic system, 186, *187, 188*

Scrotum, 245

Sea slugs, 395–396

Seasonal affective disorder (SAD), 366

Seawater, salt concentration, 270

Second messengers

defined, 222

effects of drugs on, 99

mechanisms of hormone action and, 222

metabotropic receptors and, *85,* 86, 89

Secondary sensory cortex. *See* Nonprimary sensory cortex

Second-generation antipsychotics, 100, 357, 359, 374

Seizures
 causes and types of, 76–77
 defined, 23
 hemispherectomy in children, 481–482
 split-brain surgery and, 452, 454
 from tumors, 23, 49

Selective permeability, 58

Selective serotonin reuptake inhibitors (SSRIs)
 debate on the efficacy of, 364
 defined, 101, 363
 risks of prenatal exposure to, 366
 side effects, 239
 treatment of depression, 363
 treatment of obsessive-compulsive disorder, 373

Selectively permeable membranes, 268

Selye, Hans, 337–338

Semantic memory, 385, *388*

Semen, 234, 235

Semenya, Mokgadi Caster, 248

Semicircular canals, 169, *170*

Seminal vesicles, 245

Semipermeable membranes, 268

Senile dementia, 302

Sense of balance, 169–170

Sense of self, language and, 451

Sensitive period, 249–250, 472

Sensorimotor skills, 386

Sensorineural deafness, 166–167, 168

Sensory adaptation, 125–126

Sensory buffers, 388, *389*

Sensory conflict theory, 170–171

Sensory cortical maps, 124–125, 128–129

Sensory homunculus, 128–129

Sensory nerves, 33

Sensory neurons
 defined, 27
 encoding of stimuli as streams of action potentials, 124–125
 labeled lines and, 121
 receptive fields, *124*, 125

Sensory organs, diversity in, 120–121

Sensory processing
 adaptation of receptor cells to unchanging stimuli, 125–126

changes in sensory brain regions with experience and over time, 129
 encoding of stimuli as streams of action potentials, 124–125
 labeled lines and, 121
 pathways and levels of in the central nervous system, 126–129
 sensory organs and the detection of stimuli, 120–121
 sensory transduction, 122–123
 suppression of systems, 126

Sensory systems, classification of, *120*

Sensory transduction, 122–123

Serotonergic neurons, 89, *91*

Serotonin (5-HT)
 aggression and, 336
 antidepressants and, 101
 depression and, 363
 inhibition of synthesis by drugs, *97*
 learned helplessness and, 367
 modulation of brain activity, 89–90, *91*
 obsessive-compulsive disorder and, 373
 reuptake in the synaptic cleft, 73

Serotonin receptors
 5-HT$_{1A}$ receptors, 370
 5-HT$_{2A}$ receptors, 99, 108, 359
 buspirone and, 370
 clozapine and, 359
 LSD and, 99, 108
 multiplicity of subtypes in the brain, *90*

Serotonin-norepinephrine reuptake inhibitors (SNRIs), *363*, 365

Sertoli cells, 231

Set point, 264

Set zone, 265

Sex, issues in defining, 248–249

Sex chromosomes
 differentiation of the gonads, 244
 sequence of sexual differentiation and, 245–246
 Turner's syndrome, 245
 See also X chromosomes

Sex drive, 242

Sex offenders, 336

Sex reassignment, neonatal, 217, 256

"Sexsomnia," 313

Sexual attraction, 234–235

Sexual behavior
 human, 241–243
 See also Copulation; Male sexual behavior; Reproductive behavior

Sexual differentiation
 androgen insensitivity syndrome, 246–247, 249, 255
 androgens and sexual dimorphism in the nervous system, 251–254
 congenital adrenal hyperplasia, 246, 255–256
 defined, 244
 defining sex and, 248–249
 effects of social influences on nervous system differentiation, 254–255
 gonadal hormones and sexual differentiation of the body, 244–245
 gonadal hormones and the organizational effect, 249–251
 guevedoces and 5-alpha-reductase deficiency, 247–248, 256
 male bias in biomedical science and, 244
 prenatal exposure to androgens and masculinization of adult human behaviors, 255–258
 sequence of, 245–246
 sex chromosomes and differentiation of the gonads, 244
 Turner's syndrome, 245

Sexual dimorphism, 251–254

Sexual orientation, factors shaping, 256–258

Sexual therapy, 242

Sexually dimorphic nucleus of the POA (SDN-POA), 251–253

Sexually receptive, 235

Shadowing, 420–421

Sham rage, 329

Sharpness of vision, 189–190

Sheep, homosexual behavior and, 256–257

Shell shock, 370

Shepherds (*silbadores*), 469–470

Sherrington, Charles, 392

Short-term habituation, 395, *396*

Short-term memory
 defined, 389

memory consolidation and, 390
 Patient H.M. and, 381
 working memory and, 389

Siberian hamsters, *290*

SIDS. *See* Sudden infant death syndrome

Silbadores (shepherds), 469–470

Silbo Gomero, 469–470

Sildenafil, 239

Simple cortical cells, 198, *199*

Simple partial seizures, 77

Simultagnosia, 436, 437

Simultaneous extinction, 435, 436

Singer, Peter, 17

Siphon, 395, *396*

Sistine Chapel, 6

Skeletal muscles
 electromyography, 137
 innervation, *139*
 proprioceptors, 140–141
 structure, contraction, and motor units, 138–140

Skill learning, 386, *388*

Skin conductance, lie detectors and, 322

Skin receptors, 122–123

Skinner, B. F., 387

Skinner box, 387

Sleep
 biological functions of, 305–307
 changes across the life span, 301–303
 depression and, 366
 in different species, 301
 neural systems underlying, 308–311, 312, *313*
 nonsleepers, 307
 puberty and a shift in the circadian rhythm of, 296
 sleep disorders, 311–315
 sleep hygiene, 315–316
 stages of, 297–300
 See also Sleep deprivation

Sleep apnea, 315

Sleep deprivation
 effects of, 303–304, 306
 sleep recovery and, 304–305

Sleep disorders, 311–315

"Sleep drunkenness," 315

Sleep enuresis, 313

Sleep hygiene, 315–316

Sleep paralysis, 313

Sleep recovery, 304–305

Sleep spindles, 297, *298*

Sleep state misperception, 315

Sleep walking, 313

Sleeping pills, 315
Sleep-maintenance insomnia, 315
Sleep-onset insomnia, 315
Slow wave sleep (SWS)
    definition and description of, 297–298
    in different species, 301
    dreaming and, 300
    in the elderly, 302
    forebrain and, 308–309, 310
    memory consolidation and, 307
    sleep dysfunctions, 313
    in sleep recovery, 304–305
Slow-twitch fibers, 139
S.M. (patient lacking fear), 319, 332
SMA. See Supplementary motor area
Smell
    olfactory system, 175–178
    vomeronasal system, 178–179
Smooth muscle, 138–139
Snoring, 315
SNRIs. See Serotonin-norepinephrine reuptake inhibitors
Social behavior, posterior pituitary hormones and, 226–227, 228
Social experience
    impact on feeding patterns, 280–281
    impact on sexual differentiation of the nervous system, 254–255
Social neuroscience, 10
Sodium channel blockers, 98
Sodium chloride. See Salt
Sodium ion channels, 172
Sodium ions
    aldosterone and the conservation of, 270
    defined, 58
    distribution inside and outside a neuron, 57
    excitatory postsynaptic potential and, 67
    generation of an action potential and, 61, 62
    propagation of an action potential and, 64
    salty taste and, 172–173
Sodium-potassium pump, 58, 59
Solutes, 268
Solvents, 268
Soma. See Cell body
Somatic intervention, 13–14

Somatic nervous system, 33, 34–35
Somatosensory system
    encoding of stimuli as streams of action potentials, 124
    pathways of and levels processing in the central nervous system, 126–129
    receptive fields, 124, 125
Somnambulism, 313
Songbirds, 475
Sound
    basic properties of, 155
    ears and the perception of, 154–160
Sound localization, 163–164
Sound shadows, 163, 164
"Soups," 83, 87, 88
Sour taste, 171, 173
Southern, Edward, A–6
Southern blots, A–4, A–7
"Sparks," 83, 87, 88
Spatial cognition
    defined, 451, 452
    right cerebral hemisphere and, 453–454, 455, 457–458
Spatial learning, 387–388
Spatial resolution, 428
Spatial summation, 68, 69
Spatial-frequency analysis, 199–200
Special K. See Ketamine
Spectral filtering, 164
Spectral opponent cells, 208–209
Speech processing
    auditory cortex and complex sound processing, 164
    models of, 464–466
    right-ear advantage, 454
    See also Language behavior
Speechless (documentary film), 464
Sperm, 236, 351
Sperry, Roger, 452
Spike, 61
    See also Action potential
Spinal block, 134, 136
Spinal cord
    anterolateral system and pain perception, 132–133
    central nervous system, 33
    development, 402, 403
    lordosis circuit and, 238, 239
    mediation of genital reflexes, 239
    motor neurons, 140

myelination by oligodendrocytes, 31
    neuromuscular system and, 138, 142–143
    in pain control, 134
    sexual dimorphism in mammals, 253–254
    in somatosensory processing, 126, 127
    structure, 35
Spinal cord injuries
    effects of, 143
    rehabilitation and retraining, 480–481
Spinal cord reflexes
    effects of spinal injuries on, 143
    knee-jerk reflex, 55–56, 74, 75
    stretch reflex, 142
    See also Reflexes
Spinal nerves
    anterolateral system and pain perception, 132–133
    in appetite control, 279
    defined, 35
    dermatomes, 126, 127
Spinal nucleus of the bulbocavernosus (SNB), 253–254
Spinothalamic system, 132–133
Split-brain individuals, 452–454
Spotted hyenas, 246
SRY gene, 244
SSRIs. See Selective serotonin reuptake inhibitors
Stage 1 sleep, 297, 298
Stage 2 sleep, 297, 298
Stage 3 sleep, 297–298
    See also Slow wave sleep
Stains, 29
Standard condition (IC), 393, 395
Stapedius, 156, 157
Stapes, 156, 157
Stem cells, 406
Stereocilia, 157, 159, 167
Steroid hormones
    chemical structure, 221
    defined, 221
    examples of, 221
    interactions among, 232
    mechanisms of action, 222
    regulation of, 231
    reproductive behavior and, 230–232, 236, 243
    See also Androgens; Estrogens
Stimulants, 104–106, 437
Stimuli
    adaptation of receptor cells to unchanging stimuli, 125–126

defined, 120
    detection by receptor cells, 120
    encoding as streams of action potentials, 124–125
    receptor cells and sensory transduction, 122–123
    suppression of sensory activity and, 126
Stomach, secretion of ghrelin, 278
Strain Black6 mice, 412
Stratera. See Atomexetine
Stress
    chronic stress, 341–342
    defined, 339
    effects on health, 341–342
    epigenetic effects of maternal care and, 3, 11, 340–341, 412
    individual differences in the stress response, 339–341
    pain control and, 135, 136
    risk of schizophrenia and, 352, 353
    stages of the stress response, 338–339, 340
    studies of, 337–338
Stress immunization, 339–340
Stretch reflex, 142
Striate cortex. See Primary visual cortex
Stroke
    attention and, 419
    definition and description of, 47
    effects from injury to the motor cortex, 146
    effects on V5 and motion perception, 202
    Wada test simulation, 459
    See also Brain damage
Stuttering, 472, 473
Subcortical systems, attention and, 433
Subfornical organ, 271, 272
Substance abuse
    as a global social problem, 109–111
    medical interventions, 113
    models of, 111–112
    neural pathway implicated in, 112
Substance P, 92, 133
Substance use disorder, 110
Substantia nigra
    defined, 44, 91, 148
    extrapyramidal system and, 148
    mesostriatal pathway and, 91

Parkinson's disease and, 148
Subthalamic nucleus, 148
Subtractive analysis, 50
Sudden infant death syndrome (SIDS), 315
Suicidality
  depression and, 361
  epigenetic effects of maternal care and, 11, 340–341, 412
  exposure to childhood bullying and, 343
  warning signs, 362
Sulci (sing. sulcus), 36
Suparoptic nucleus, 270, 272
Superficial facial muscles, 327
Super-hot chili peppers, 132
Superior, 38
Superior colliculus, 44, 192, 433
Superior olivary nuclei, 160, 161
Superior temporal cortex, 465
Supersensitivity psychosis, 357
Supplementary motor area (SMA), 145, 461
Suprachiasmatic nucleus, 292–295
Supraoptic nuclei, 226
Surface dyslexia, 476
Surgery. See Anti-obesity surgery; Neurosurgery
Sustained-attention tasks, 422, 423, 431
Sweet taste, 171, 173
SWS. See Slow wave sleep
Sylvian fissure, 39
Symbolic cuing, 423–424
Sympathetic ganglia, 36, 37
Sympathetic nervous system
  defined, 36, 320
  neurotransmitter of, 36
  stress response, 338, 339
  structure and function, 36, 37
Synapse rearrangement, 404, 405, 408–410
Synapses
  in brain development, 404, 405, 407–410
  chemical communication and, 220
  definition and description of, 24, 85, 220
  neurotransmitter release and changes in the postsynaptic membrane potential, 66–68
  structure and function, 28, 30
  synaptogenesis, 404, 405
  See also Synaptic cleft; Synaptic plasticity; Synaptic transmission

Synaptic boutons. See Axon terminals
Synaptic cleft
  defined, 30, 71
  degradation and reuptake of transmitters, 73
  release of neurotransmitters into, 66, 71–72
  size of, 26
  in synaptic transmission, 28, 30, 84, 85
Synaptic delay, 71
Synaptic plasticity
  eye-blink reflex, 396–397
  invertebrate nervous systems, 394–396
  long-term potentiation, 398–401
  types of changes associated with memory storage, 392, 393
Synaptic remodeling. See Synapse rearrangement
Synaptic transmission
  action potentials and neurotransmitter release, 71–72
  degradation and reuptake of transmitters, 73
  effects of drugs on, 97, 98, 100, 101
  neurotransmitter release and changes in the postsynaptic membrane potential, 66–68
  overview of, 28, 30, 70–71, 84, 85
  properties and types of neurotransmitter receptors, 72–73, 85–86 (see also Neurotransmitters)
  spatial and temporal summation of synaptic inputs, 68–70
  types of chemical synapses, 73–74
Synaptic transmitters. See Neurotransmitters
Synaptic vesicles
  defined, 30, 71
  neurotransmitter release into the synaptic cleft, 71–72
  in synaptic transmission, 28, 30, 70, 71, 84, 85
Synaptogenesis, 404, 405
Synergist muscles, 138, 139
Synesthesia, 129
Syntax, 472
Synthetic opiates, 101–102
Syphilis, 349

T
T1R taste receptors, 173, 174
T2R taste receptors, 173, 174
TAARs (trace amine–associated receptors), 178–179
Tachistoscope test, 454–455
Tactile corpuscles, 122–123
Tardive dyskinesia, 357
Task shifting, 444
Tastants, 172, 173
Taste, 171–175
Taste buds, 172, 173, 174
Taste pores, 172, 173
Taste receptors, 172–175
tau hamster mutant, 293, 296
Tau protein, 479
Tauopathy, 479
TBI. See Traumatic brain injury
Tectorial membrane, 157, 159
Tectum, 44
Tegmentum, 44
Telencephalon, 40, 41, 403
Temporal branch of the trigeminal nerve, 327
Temporal coding theory, 162
Temporal hemiretina, 192
Temporal lobe
  abnormalities associated with dyslexia, 477
  abnormalities in anxiety disorders, 369
  Alzheimer's disease and, 414
  declarative memory and, 383
  defined, 39
  dysfunctions and violence, 336
  effects of right hemisphere lesions on spatial cognition, 457
  mediation of emotion, 329–330
  memory loss from damage to, 379, 381–382, 383, 385, 401
  visual regions, 201
Temporal resolution, 428
Temporal summation, 69
Temporoparietal cortex, 470
Temporoparietal junction (TPJ), 435
TENS. See Transcutaneous electrical nerve stimulation
Tensor tympani, 156, 157
Testes
  actions of tropic hormones on, 230
  definition and function of, 231
  effects of castration, 218, 219, 236

endocrine functions, 218
  ringdove courtship behavior and, 233
  sex chromosomes and the differentiation of, 244
  sexual differentiation of the body and, 245
  steroid hormones released by, 231–232
  testosterone and copulatory behavior, 223–224
Testosterone
  aggression and, 334–336
  bodily indicators of prenatal exposure, 257
  conversion to dihydrotestosterone, 247
  defined, 231, 334
  functions, 231–232
  individual differences in mating behavior and, 237
  male sexual behavior and, 223–224, 233, 236, 237, 243
  masculinization of nervous system regions, 251–254
  organizational effects on rodent behavior, 249, 250
  prenatal exposure and the masculinization of adult human behaviors, 255–258
  regulation of, 231
  sexual differentiation of the body and, 245
  stress response and, 338, 339
Testosterone patches, 243
Tetanus, 398, 399–400, 401
Tetrachromats, 207
Tetraiodothyronine, 221
Tetrodotoxin, 97, 98
Thalamus
  defined, 43, 128
  fatal familial insomnia and, 304
  functions, 43
  gustatory system and, 175
  lateral geniculate nucleus (see Lateral geniculate nucleus)
  limbic system and the mediation of emotion, 329, 330, 331
  neuromuscular system and, 138
  olfactory system and, 176, 178
  pain pathway and, 133
  in sensory processing, 128
  in somatosensory processing, 127

THC. *See* Delta-9-tetrahydro-cannabinol
Theory of mind, *438*
Therapeutic index, *95*
Thermal sensory system, *120*
Thermoregulation, 264, 265, 266, *267*
Thiamine, 385
Thioridazine, *359*
Third interstitial nucleus of the anterior hypothalamus (INAH-3), 257
Third ventricles, 46
Third-generation antipsychotics, 100
Thirst
    hypovolemic, 269, 270–271
    osmotic, 269–270
Thompson, Polly, *156*
Thoracic dermatome, *127*
Thorazine. *See* Chlorpromazine
Threshold, 60, 65, 122
Throacic spinal segments, 35
Thunderclap headaches, 132
Thymine, A–1, A–2
Thyroid, *218*
Thyroxine, *221*
TIA. *See* Transient ischemic attack
Timbre, 155
Tinnitus, 166, 167
TMS. *See* Transcranial magnetic stimulation
Tobacco, 104
Tone-deafness, 165
Tongue, 172, *173*, *175*
Tonic receptors, 125
Tonic-clonic seizures, 77
Tonotopic organization, 161
Tool use, *438*
Topographic projection, 193
Tourette's syndrome, 373, 374, 375
Tower of Hanoi problem, 386
Toxic dose, *95*
TPJ. *See* Temporoparietal junction
Trace amine–associated receptors (TAARs), 178–179
Tract tracing, 29–30
Tracts, 40
Transcranial magnetic stimulation (TMS), 51, 467–468
Transcript, A–2
Transcription, A–2, *A–3*
Transcutaneous electrical nerve stimulation (TENS), 135, *136*
Transduction
    defined, 155, 184

by the inner ear, 155
    of sound into electrical signals by hair cells, 159–160
    visual, 184
Transgenic, A–4
Transient ischemic attack (TIA), 47
Transient receptor potential (TRP) ion channels
    type M3, 131
    vanilloid type 1, 131, 172–173
Translation, A–2
Transmitters. *See* Neurotransmitters
Transporters
    defined, 73, 85
    in synaptic transmission, *84*, 85
Transverse plane, 38
Traumatic brain injury (TBI), 478, 479
    See also Brain damage
Triceps, *139*
Trichromatic color vision, 207
Trichromatic hypotheses, 204, 205
Tricyclics, 101, 363
Trigeminal nerve (cranial nerve V)
    branches of, *327*
    control of facial expressions, 327
    eye-blink reflex, 396, *397*
    function, *34*, 35
Trochlear nerve (cranial nerve IV), 34
Trophic factors. *See* Neurotrophic factors
Tropic hormones, 228–229
TRP ion channels. *See* Transient receptor potential ion channels
Tryptophan hydroxylase, *97*
Tuberomammillary nucleus, 308, *310*, 312
Turbinates, *176*
Twin studies, of schizophrenia, 350–351
Tylenol, 135
Tympanic canal, 156, 157
Tympanic membrane, 156, 157
Type 1 diabetes, 275
Type 2 diabetes, 275
Typical antipsychotics. *See* First-generation antipsychotics

U
Ultradian rhythms, 290
Umami taste, 171, 174

Unconditioned response (UR), 387
Unconditioned stimulus (US), 387, 396, 397
Unilateral sleep, 301
Unipolar neurons (monopolar neurons), 27
Units of measure, *26*
Unmyelinated axons, *64*, 65
Up-regulation, 96, 99
Uracil, A–2
Uralic language family, *471*
Urea, 368
Uterus, 245
Utricle, 169, *170*

V
V1. *See* Primary visual cortex
V1R and V2R receptor proteins, 178
Vaccines, in medical interventions for addiction, 113
Vagina
    defined, 234
    differentiation, 245
    human sexual behavior and, 242
    intromission and, 235
Vagus nerve (cranial nerve X)
    in appetite control, *279*
    discovery of acetylcholine and, 87–88
    function, *34*, 35
    gustatory system and, *175*
    stimulation in treatment of depression, 365
Valium. *See* Diazepam
Valuation system, 446
Vanilloid receptor 1, 131
Vas deferens, 245
Vasoactive intestinal peptide (VIP), 92
Vasopressin
    defined, 226
    functions of, 92, 226, 227, *228*
    hypovolemic thirst and, 271
    osmotic thirst and, 270, *272*
    treatment of sleep enuresis, 313
Vegetative state, *439*, 440
Venlafaxine (Effexor), 101, 365
Ventral, 38
Ventral frontal cortex, 435
Ventral palladium, *228*
Ventral tegmental area (VTA)
    defined, 91
    mesolimbocortical pathway, 91
    nicotine and, 104
    substance abuse and, 112

Ventricular system
    abnormalities associated with schizophrenia, 354–355
    abnormalities in bipolar disorder, 367
    defined, 45–46
Ventricular zone, 404, *405*
Ventromedial hypothalamus (VMH)
    appetite control and, 276–277
    defined, 238, 336
    lordosis circuit and, 238, *239*
    mediation of aggression in mice, 336
Ventromedial prefrontal cortex, 446
Verapamil, *97*
Verbal tics, *374*
Vertebral arteries, 46
Vertex spikes, 297, *298*
Vesalius, Andreas, *33*
Vestibular canal, 156, 157
Vestibular nuclei, 169
Vestibular system
    definition and description of, 169–170
    motion sickness, 170–171
Vestibulocochlear nerve (cranial nerve VIII)
    auditory connections to the inner ear, *157*, 159–160
    auditory pathway from the cochlea to the cortex, 160
    connection to the vestibular nuclei, 169
    defined, 159
    function, 34
VFC. *See* Ventral frontal cortex
Viagra, 239
Video games, 431
Vietnam War veterans, 371
Violence
    biopsychology of, 336–337
    See also Aggression
VIP. *See* Vasoactive intestinal peptide
Vision
    case of "D.F.," 183, 202, 211–212
    color vision, 203–211
    introduction, 183–184
    visual analysis, 194–202
    visual system, 184–194
    what and *where* processing streams, 211–212

Vision impairments
amblyopia, 213
case of "D.F.," 183, 202, 211–212
color blindness, 206, 207, 210
myopia, 185, 213
optic ataxia, 211–212
visual neuroscience and the alleviation of, 212–213
Visual acuity, *187*, 189–190
Visual analysis
cortical receptive fields, 198–199
effects of context on the perception of brightness, 196, *197*
hierarchical model and spatial-frequency analysis, 199–200
perception of motion, 202
receptive fields in extrastriate areas, 201–202
retinal receptive fields and lateral inhibition, 194–197
Visual attention
brain areas creating and directing, 433–437
effects on event-related potentials, 430–431
effects on the activity of neuron, 431–432
See also Attention
Visual cortex. *See* Primary visual cortex
Visual fields
defined, 193
of predators and prey, 191
scotoma, 193–194, 480
Visual P1 effect, 430
Visual searches, 426–428
Visual system
hemispheric differences in the perception of linguistic stimuli, 454–455

mapping of the visual field, 193–194
neural connections from the retina to the brain, 191–193
optic disc and the blind spot, 190, *191*
overview, 184–185
response of photoreceptors to light, 186–187
sensitivity to light intensity, 188–189
structure and function of the retina, 185–186
visual acuity, 189–190
visual searches, 426–428
VMH. *See* Ventromedial hypothalamus
VNO. *See* Vomeronasal organ
Vocal behavior
features of human language, 471–472
frequencies used by mammals, 162–163
inborn and learned components of language, 472–475
of nonhuman primates, 473–475
vocal communication by animal species, 475
See also Language behavior
Voles, 227, *228*
Voltage-gated calcium channels, 70, *71*, *84*, *85*
Voltage-gated sodium channels
defined, 61
excitatory postsynaptic potential and, 67
generation of an action potential and, 61, 62–63
propagation of an action potential and, 63, 64, 65

Voluntary attention, 423–424, 426, 434–435
Vomeronasal organ (VNO), 178, 179, 239–240
Vomeronasal receptor proteins, 178
Vomeronasal system, 178–179, 239–240
Voxels, 442
VTA. *See* Ventral tegmental area

W
Wada tests, 458, 459
War neurosis, 370
Water
movement between body compartments, 267–268
See also Fluid regulation
Waterman, Ian, 119, 140
Wavelengths, of light, 203–204
Weight loss, basal metabolism and, 273–274
Wernicke, Carl, 462
Wernicke-Geschwind model, 464–465
Wernicke's aphasia, *461*, 462, *463*
Wernicke's area
conduction aphasia, 465
connectionist model of aphasia, 464, 465
defined, 462
planum temporale and, 455
processing of word meaning, 470
Wernicke's aphasia, *461*, 462, *463*
Western blots, A–6, A–7
What visual processing stream, 211–212
Where visual processing stream, 211–212
Whistled surrogate languages, 469–470

White matter, 40, 465
Wiesel, Torsten, 198–199
Williams syndrome, 472, *473*
Willis, Thomas, 7
Wisconsin Card Sorting Task, 355–356
Withdrawal symptoms, 111, 113
Within-participants experiments, 14
Wolffian ducts, 244, 245, 247
Women, depression and, 365–366
Word blindness, 462
Word deafness, 166, 167, 462
Word meaning, 470
Words, 471–472
Working memory, 389
Wound healing, effects of stress on, 341

X
X chromosomes
color vision and, 206, 207
differentiation of the gonads and, 244
Turner's syndrome, 245
Xq28 region and sexual orientation, 258
Xanax, 89, 370
Xenical (orlistat), 282
Xyrem (gamma-hydroxybutyrate), 312

Y
Y chromosomes, 244
Yaw, 169, *170*

Z
Zeitgeber, 291
Zolpidem (Ambien), 315
Zygomatic branch of the trigeminal nerve, *327*
Zygote, 236